T0344789

Microbial Transmission

Microbial Transmission

Editors

Fernando Baquero

Emilio Bouza

J.A. Gutiérrez-Fuentes

Teresa M. Coque

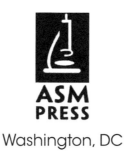

ASM
PRESS

Washington, DC

Library of Congress Cataloging-in-Publication Data

Names: Baquero, F. (Fernando), editor. | Bouza, Emilio, editor. | Gutierrez Fuentes, Jose Antonio, editor. | Coque, Teresa M., editor.
Title: Microbial transmission / editors: Fernando Baquero, Emilio Bouza, Jose Antonio Gutierrez and Teresa M. Coque.
Description: Washington, DC : ASM Press, [2019] | Includes index.
Identifiers: LCCN 2018051708 (print) | LCCN 2018054163 (ebook) | ISBN 9781555819743 (ebook) | ISBN 9781555819736 (print : alk. paper)
Subjects: LCSH: Communicable diseases--Transmission. | Infection. | Pathogenic bacteria.
Classification: LCC RB153 (ebook) | LCC RB153 .M53 2019 (print) | DDC 616.9/0471--dc23
LC record available at https://lccn.loc.gov/2018051708

Address editorial correspondence to
ASM Press, 1752 N St., N.W.,
Washington, DC 20036-2904, USA

Send orders to ASM Press, P.O. Box 605, Herndon, VA 20172, USA
Phone: 800-546-2416; 703-661-1593
Fax: 703-661-1501
E-mail: books@asmusa.org
Online: http://www.asmscience.org

Contents

Contributors

Nacho Aguilo
University of Zaragoza
Department of Microbiology
CIBER in Respiratory Diseases (CIBERES)
Zaragoza, Spain

Dan I. Andersson
Uppsala University
Medical Biochemistry and Microbiology
Uppsala, Sweden

Patricia Antunes
Faculdade de Ciências de Nutrição e Alimentação
Universidade do Porto, Portugal

Eric Bapteste
Sorbonne Universités, UPMC Univ Paris 06, CNRS
Evolution Paris Seine - Institut de Biologie Paris Seine (EPS - IBPS)
Paris, France

Fernando Baquero
Institute Ramon y Cajal for Health Research (IRYCIS)
University Ramon y Cajal Hospital
Department of Microbiology
CIBER in Epidemiology and Public Health (CIBERESP)
Madrid, Spain

Cédric Bicep
Newcastle University
Institute for Cell and Molecular Biosciences
Faculty of Medical Sciences
Newcastle, United Kingdom

Frederick M. Cohan
Wesleyan University
Biology
Middletown, Connecticut

Eduardo Corel
Sorbonne Universités, UPMC Univ Paris 06, CNRS
Evolution Paris Seine - Institut de Biologie Paris Seine (EPS - IBPS)
Paris, France

Francisco Cortés
University of Salamanca
Department of Classical and Indoeuropean Philology
Salamanca, Spain

Fernando de la Cruz
Universidad de Cantabria
Instituto de Biomedicina y Biotecnologia de Cantabria
Santander, Spain

Rosa del Campo
Institute Ramon y Cajal for Health Research (IRYCIS)
University Ramon y Cajal Hospital
Department of Microbiology
Madrid, Spain

Teresa M. Coque
Institute Ramon y Cajal for Health Research (IRYCIS)
University Ramon y Cajal Hospital
Department of Microbiology
CIBER in Epidemiology and Public Health (CIBERESP)
Madrid, Spain

Rafael Delgado
Hospital Universitario 12 de Octubre (i+12)
Microbiology Department
Madrid, Spain

Médéric Diard
ETH Zurich
Institute of Microbiology
Zurich, Switzerland
University of Basel, Biozentrum
Basel, Switzerland

Darío García de Viedma
Gregorío Marañón University Hospital
Clinical Microbiology and Infectious
Diseases Department
Gregorio Marañón Health Research Institute
(IiSGM)
Madrid, Spain

Francisco García-del Portillo
Centro Nacional Biotecnologia-CSIC
Laboratory of Intracellular Bacterial Pathogens
Madrid, Spain

María Getino
University of Surrey
Department of Microbial and Cellular Sciences
Guildford
Surrey, United Kingdom

Jesus Gonzalo-Asensio
University of Zaragoza
Microbiology Department
CIBER in Respiratory Diseases (CIBERES)
Zaragoza, Spain

Wolf-Dietrich Hardt
ETH Zurich
Institute of Microbiology
Zurich, Switzerland

Diarmaid Hughes
Uppsala University
Medical Biochemistry and Microbiology
Uppsala, Sweden

Maureen Laroche
Institut Hospitalo-Universitaire
Méditerranée Infection
Marseille, Bouches du Rhône, France

Amparo LaTorre
Institute of Integrative Systems Biology
University of Valencia
Valencia, Spain
Foundation for the Promotion of Sanitary and Biomedical Research of
Valencian Community (FISABIO)
Valencia, Spain
CIBER in Epidemiology and Public Health (CIBERESP) Madrid, Spain

Pablo Llop
Foundation for the Promotion of Sanitary and Biomedical Research of
Valencian Community (FISABIO)
Valencia, Spain

Philippe Lopez
Universités, UPMC Univ Paris 06, CNRS,
Evolution Paris Seine - Institut de Biologie Paris Seine (EPS - IBPS),
Paris, France

R. Craig MacLean
Oxford University
Department of Zoology
Oxford, United Kingdom

Dessislava Marinova
University of Zaragoza
Microbiology Department
CIBER in Respiratory Diseases (CIBERES)
Zaragoza, Spain

Carlos Martin
University of Zaragoza
Department of Microbiology
CIBER in Respiratory Diseases (CIBERES)
Zaragoza, Spain

Jose Luis Martinez
Centro Nacional de Biotecnología (CNB)-CSIC
Departamento de Biotecnologia Microbiana
Madrid, Spain

Laura Martínez-García
Institute Ramon y Cajal for Health Research (IRYCIS)
University Ramon y Cajal Hospital
Department of Microbiology
Madrid, Spain

Andres Moya
Institute of Integrative Systems Biology
University of Valencia
Valencia, Spain
Foundation for the Promotion of Sanitary and Biomedical Research of
Valencian Community (FISABIO)
Valencia, Spain
CIBER in Epidemiology and Public Health (CIBERESP) Madrid, Spain

Fernando Navarro
Cabrerizos
Salamanca, Spain

Carla Novais
Faculdade de Farmácia. Universidade do Porto
Departamento de Ciências Biológicas
Porto, Portugal

Philippe Parola
Institut Hospitalo-Universitaire *Méditerranée Infection*
Marseille, France

Luísa Peixe
Faculdade de Farmácia
Universidade do Porto
Departamento de Ciências Biológicas
Porto, Portugal

Laura Pérez Lago
Gregorio Marañón University Hospital
Department of Clinical Microbiology and Infectious Diseases
Gregorio Marañón Health Research Institute (IiSGM)
Madrid, Spain

Johann D. D. Pitout
University of Calgary
Pathology and Lab Medicine
Alberta, Canada

M. Graciela Pucciarelli
Universidad Autónoma de Madrid
Departamento de Biología Molecular
Madrid, Spain

Didier Raoult
Institut Hospitalo-Universitaire *Méditerranée Infection*
Marseille, France

Alvaro San Millan
Institute Ramon y Cajal for Health Research
University Ramon y Cajal Hospital
Department of Microbiology
Madrid, Spain

Ana María Sánchez-Díaz
Institute Ramon y Cajal for Health Research (IRYCIS)
University Ramon y Cajal Hospital
Department of Microbiology
Madrid, Spain

Fernando Simón
Ministry of Health, Consumers and Social Welfare
Center for Health Alerts and Emergencies Coordination
CIBER in Epidemiology and Public Health (CIBERESP)
Madrid, Spain

Chloé Vigliotti
Universite Pierre et Marie Curie
IBPS
Paris, France
ICAN, 47-83 boulevard de l'hôpital,
Paris, France

Joaquín Villalba
University of Extremadura
Department of Sciences of Antiquity
Cáceres, Spain

Mark Woolhouse
University of Edinburgh
Usher Institute of Population
Health Sciences and Informatics
Edinburgh, United Kingdom

Preface: Transmission and Interaction

This edited volume from ASM Press is inspired by and partly based on the 26th International Scientific Symposium "Transmission," organized by the Life and Matter Sciences Division of the Ramón Areces Foundation (http://www.fundacionareces.es/fundacionareces/cargarAplicacionAgendaEventos.do?verPrograma=1&idTipoEvento=1&identificador=1754&nivelAgenda=2) jointly with the Spanish Research Council (CSIC) Foundation and the Institute for Knowledge and Development, currently the GADEA for Science Foundation (http://gadeaciencia.org), in Madrid, May 7–8, 2015. For this book, we selected the most significant contributions to the symposium, and this work was complemented by articles authored by other invited contributors.

The word *transmission* has been extensively used in the life sciences since the 18th century, with different usages that paralleled the growing complexity of the scientific disciplines. The main objective of *Microbial Transmission* is to emphasize the generality of transmission processes acting in all domains of nature, enabling different events on disparate scales, from evolution in the chemical world or among living organisms to the direct and/or indirect spread and distribution of pathogenic microbes in humans and animals. In essence, the processes of transmission provide the possibility of crossing spaces: micro-spaces inside a cell, meso-spaces between organisms, macro-spaces on a global scale. The elements crossing these spaces range from molecules to genes, mobile genetic elements, viruses, bacterial clones, and microbial communities as well as their vectors and hosts. Crossing spaces allows interactions with new environments and, more importantly, interactions of the transmitted elements with other elements encountered in other locations. Interaction is the basic condition for evolution.

The book begins in Section 1 with a comprehensive analysis of the origins, history, and meanings of the word *transmission* that reveals two major connotations of this term, *space* and *genetic legacy*, inherent in all the uses of the word in medical, veterinary, and environmental microbiology. Evolution progresses in the time dimension (survival of the fittest implies time) but is not understandable without interactions between living beings, which implies transmission. The other dimension of evolution is space: space is obtained and occupied because of transmission events. This is the cornerstone of the primary hypothesis proposed by Lourens Baas Becking in 1934 to explain microbial distribution patterns. His microbial tenet, "Everything is everywhere, but the environment selects," contributed to explaining the universal spatial distribution of microorganisms, suggested by Martinus Beijerinck in 1913, as a result of interactions and dispersion over time. In transmission, both dimensions, space and time, are intertwined, as the elements in nature are transmitted and evolve in space and time; without changes in space or changes in time, these elements will be doomed to niche extinction or evolutionary stasis.

The abstract concept of *transmission*, when considered apart from the elements that are transmitted or the pathways involved in the transmission, certainly carries a powerful heuristic value and is considered in the second section of this book ("Basic Processes of Transmission"). Here the analysis of the general causes of transmission provides a background for understanding the universality of the process and for establishing the possibilities of transmission control in cases where it negatively affects both individual and global health. This section also includes a few key cases related to transmission of genetic material between bacterial organisms (plasmids) or transmission of microbial pathogens from cell to cell or from host to host (e.g., *Salmonella*).

As mentioned above, the space in which transmission occurs is an environment that certainly influences the process. Therefore, we considered the "ecology" of transmission in the third section of the book ("Scenarios of Transmission"). Here cases in point are presented, from the micro- and meso-spaces—considering the ecology of chromosome gene transfer between bacterial cells—to the role of food as a driver of transmission of microbes and insects as vectors facilitating microbial spread. Water is also a main transmission pathway, but in recognition of the extensive reviews published recently about this topic, it is not included in this book.

Section 4 is devoted to the prevention and detection of microbial transmission events in a clinical setting ("Patient-to-Patient Transmission"). This section focuses our topic on the field of infectious diseases and clinical microbiology, where the word *transmission* has extensively been used in one of its most fundamental meanings in medical sciences. Although the term *transmissible (infectious) diseases* has long been accepted, the expression *diseases caused by transmissible (infectious) agents* would better reflect the specific interaction of the microbial etiological agent with a particular host required to trigger the disease. The "Semmelweis gap," consisting of specifically approaching infectious disease from the perspective of either the physician (the syndrome) or the microbiology-based epidemiologist (the etiological agent), limits the understanding of the microbe-host interactions and, thus, the development of key effective measures to combat infectious diseases.

Another chapter analyzes the biology of microbial hand transmission, a landmark topic in infectious diseases first addressed by Ignaz Semmelweis in 1847, who suggested handwashing as a key preventive measure to limit interhost transmission of diseases (specifically, puerperal fever, which caused a high mortality rate at that time). The success of Semmelweis's findings toward control of this disease led epidemiologists to consider irrelevant the question of what in fact was prevented from being transmitted—that is, the microbe. Semmelweis's hypothesis was only widely accepted after Louis Pasteur discovered the origin of many other transmissible diseases and demonstrated the possibility of interrupting transmission of such infections by vaccines, which is another topic of this fourth section. Also described in this section are methods to trace transmission, facilitating "transmission surveillance," and the relation between pathogenicity and host-to-host transmission in the light of the experience in Ebola epidemics.

The fifth and final section of the book ("Experimental and Theoretical Modes of Transmission") analyzes the possibilities of experimental transmission models, the methods for quantifying transmission, the use of network analysis in transmission studies, and the application of these models to understand transmission as a key feature of the evolution of bacterial diversity.

In the fight against infectious diseases, we are moving from disrupting the structure of biological organisms (as with many antibiotics or biocides) to controlling the biological processes that are essential for the replication and propagation of these agents. The foremost of these processes is transmission. Analysis of the events involved in transmission processes, as well as comprehension of current microbial distribution patterns that result from multiple transmission events through time, should facilitate the design of accurate interventions to reduce the spread of pathogenic or potentially dangerous microorganisms in humans, animals, and the Earth's microbiosphere. With the use of such interventions, the scope of interactions—and consequently the evolution of colonization, pathogenicity, and antimicrobial resistance—will be limited. This is why transmission is becoming one of the key topics in medical and microbiological research and constitutes a cornerstone in the development of precision public health.

Fernando Baquero and Teresa M. Coque

About the Editors

Fernando Baquero
Dr. Baquero graduated in Medicine at the Complutensis University in Madrid, and received his PhD in Medical Microbiology (1973) from the Autonomous University of Madrid. He was Director of the Department of Microbiology in the Ramón y Cajal University Hospital (1977-2008) and Scientific Director of the Ramón y Cajal Health Research Institute (IRYCIS) (2008-2015). He was Senior Scientist in Evolutionary Biology at the Center for Astrobiology. From 2008 to the present, he is Research Professor in Microbial Evolution and Director of the Division of Microbial Biology and Evolution of Microorganisms. He has received several international honors and awards, including the Excellence Awards of the American ASM-ICAAC, Award of Excellence of European Society for Clinical Microbiology and Infectious Diseases, Garrod Medal of the British Society for Antimicrobial Chemotherapy, Descartes Award of the EU Commission for International Collaborative Research, Medal and Honorary ISC Membership of the International Society for Chemotherapy, Excellence Award of the Spanish Society of Microbiology, Lilly Foundation Award to Distinguished Scientific Carrier, FENIN Award to Technological Innovation in Health, Lwoff Award and Medal of the European Federation of Microbiological Societies (2015), ESCMID Fellow (2017), and Arima Award for Applied Microbiology of the International Union of Microbiological Societies (2017). His major research interests focus on the biochemistry, genetics, population biology, epidemiology, ecology, evolutionary biology, and modelization of antibiotic resistance and virulence. The resulting publications (490 referenced in PubMed) results in an H-index of 100 (Google Scholar), with more than 35,000 citations. As side-interests, he has also published in the fields of philosophy of science, particularly in epistemology of complex biological systems.

Emilio Bouza
Dr. Bouza is Professor in the Department of Medicine, Universidad Complutense, Madrid, and Research Consultant in the Department of Infectious Diseases and Clinical Microbiology at the Hospital Gregorio Maranon in Madrid. Dr. Bouza obtained his degree and performed his residency training in Internal Medicine in Madrid. He is also a certified specialist in Clinical Microbiology and did his Fellowship in Infectious Diseases at the Center for the Health Sciences (UCLA Los Angeles, California). He founded in 1977, within the Department of Microbiology of Ramón y Cajal Hospital in Madrid, one of the first multidisciplinary Infectious Diseases Units in Europe. From 1984 to 2017 he was the founder and chief of the Division of Clinical Microbiology and Infectious Diseases of

Hospital Gregorio where he directs an Observership of Clinical Microbiology and Infectious Diseases. He was President of the Spanish Society for Infectious Diseases and Clinical Microbiology (SEIMC) and Secretary General of the European Society of Clinical Microbiology and Infectious Diseases (ESCMID). He directed three major medical journals: *Revista Clínica Española, Enfermedades Infecciosas y Microbiología Clínica* (EIMC) and *Clinical Microbiology and Infection* (CMI). Member of the Board of the Ramón Areces Foundation and is an ESCMID Fellow, he obtained the ESCMID Award to "one life devoted to Infectious Diseases" in 2012. He has more than 800 indexed publications in different research areas, including bacteremia and endocarditis, catheter-related infections, ventilator-associated pneumonia, and infections caused by *Staphylococcus, Clostridium difficile,* and *Candida,* with an H-index over 70. He is particularly interested in infections in Intensive Care Unit patients in the immunocompromised host and particularly in patients with solid-organ transplants.

J.A. Gutiérrez-Fuentes

Dr. Gutiérrez-Fuentes earned his Doctor and Bachelor of Medicine from the Universidad Complutense de Madrid. He is an Academic of the Royal Academy of Doctors of Spain, and Founding trustee and Director of the Foundation GADEA for Science. Dr. Gutiérrez-Fuentes was a Founder, and former Director of the Lilly foundation for Biomedical Research, Former Director General of the Carlos III National Institute of Health of Spain, President of the DRECE Institute of Biomedical studies, President and founder of the National Center Foundation for Oncology Research (CNIO), and Cardiovascular Research (CNIC) of the Carlos III Institute (CNIO). He is the author of numerous communications and scientific books. In addition, he is the Director of the Project Diet and Risk of Cardiovascular Disease in Spain (DRECE), involving the Ministries of Health, Agriculture, and the National Institute for Health in Spain.

Teresa M. Coque

Teresa M. Coque is Senior Research Scientist at the Microbiology Department of the Ramón y Cajal University Hospital within the Division of Microbial Biology and Infections at the Ramón y Cajal Institute for BioHealth Research (IRYCIS, www.irycis.es) in Madrid (Spain), leading a research group focused on Population Biology of Human Bacterial Pathogens and their mobile genetic elements. Her special interests and expertise include molecular epidemiology, evolutionary biology, and microbial ecology, with the emphasis on the genetic basis for transmission of antibiotic resistance and the adaptation of commensal and pathogenic bacteria to different hosts. Advanced genomics and metagenomics to be applied to the diagnosis of antibiotic-resistant bacterial pathogens and as predictive markers of infection under the personalized medicine perspective are a priority in the group in the last years. Dr. Coque has published more than 150 articles in refereed journals and 10 book chapters, co-edited special issues on antibiotic resistance, and regularly participates in international events in the field of antibiotic resistance and plasmid biology. She is member of the Scientific Board Committee of the Joint Programming Initiative on Antimicrobial Resistance (JPIAMR, http://www.jpiamr.eu/ 2015-19), Study Groups of the European Society for Clinical Microbiology and Infectious Diseases (ESCMID), and the Scientific Board of Gadea for Science Foundation (http://gadeaciencia.org). She is a leading investigator of research grants funded by national agencies since 1999 and has participated in 8 EU projects (6FPEU, 7FPEU, H2020, ERA-Net). The group is also involved in Spanish Networks (CIBER-ESP, http://www.ciberesp.es/, www.ingemics.es) working on different aspects of antibiotic resistance (epidemiology, public health biology of mobile genetic elements, and system biology). She has directed 10 doctoral theses and coordinates research projects of students associated funded by European programs (Leonardo da Vinci, Erasmus, FEMS, H2020) and universities from Europe and South America. Her Twitter handle is @TMcoque.

INTRODUCTION

Origin, History, and Meanings of the Word *Transmission*

1

JOAQUÍN VILLALBA,[1] FERNANDO A. NAVARRO,[2] and FRANCISCO CORTÉS[3]

The origin of the words *transmit* and *transmission* and their derivatives can be traced to the Latin *transmittere*, in turn formed by prefixing the preposition *trans* ("across or beyond") to the verb *mittere* ("to let go or to send"). The >400 cases we have documented in Latin literature through the 4th century C.E. attest to its use throughout Roman history. The earliest records date back to Archaic Latin (3rd to 2nd centuries B.C.E.) and more specifically to Plautus's comedies, a fragment by tragic poet Pacuvius, and some of Lucilius's satires. In light of such frequent use of the verb, the sparing instances found of the respective nouns, *transmissio* and *transmissus*, is intriguing. The former was found in barely a couple of cases in Cicero's prose, while the latter was used only once each by Pacuvius, Caesar, and Aulus Gellius.

Transmittere, moreover, has not only existed since the dawn of Latin literature, but has also been "transmitted" to the Romance languages[a] and from there to English. It remains in common usage today, both in everyday language and especially in scientific and technological jargon.

[1]Department of Sciences of Antiquity, University of Extremadura, Spain; [2]Cosnautas, Cabrerizos (Salamanca), Spain; [3]Department of Classical Philology and Indoeuropean Studies, University of Salamanca, Spain.
[a]Spanish *transmitir*, French *transmettre*, Portuguese *transmitir*, Italian *trasmettere*, Romanian *transmite*, Catalonian *transmetre*, Corsican *trasmèttala*.

Microbial Transmission in Biological Processes
Edited by Fernando Baquero, Emilio Bouza, J.A. Gutiérrez-Fuentes, and Teresa M. Coque
© 2018 American Society for Microbiology, Washington, DC
doi:10.1128/microbiolspec.MTBP-0004-2016

ORIGIN AND MEANING OF *MITTERE*

The uncertain etymology of *mittere* has induced scholars to propose a number of hypotheses around the true Indo-European origin of the verb, two of which are set out below.

Some linguists contend that its Indo-European root is **smeit-* or **smit*, meaning "to throw," which would have lost the initial *s* as it evolved into Latin. Further to that proposal, the same root would be found in some Germanic verbs with a similar meaning: the Dutch *smitjen* or German *schmeissen*. Identical origin would be attributed to the English verb *to smite*, whose specific meaning ("to strike") would be the immediate outcome of throwing something at someone.[b]

Be that as it may, the conversion from the original sense of **smeit-* into "to let go" or "to release" would appear to be reasonable. That meaning is also found in the Avestan *āmiϑnāiti* and in some compound forms of *mittere*, such as *manumittere* and *manumissio* (English, *to manumit, manumission*), whose definition, "to free a slave," derives from the literal "to let go of someone's hand."

For others, in contrast, *mittere* would stem from another Indo-European root, **mit(h)-*, "to leave," found in German verbs such as *meiden* ("to leave aside," "to avoid") or *vermissen* ("to miss"). That original meaning could feasibly have evolved into "to lose" (see *amittere* or *omittere* below) and from there into "to let go" and ultimately into "to send," which is the first dictionary definition of *mittere* and the one that has persisted in modern languages.

That meaning lasted in the form of any number of terms deriving from the past participle *missus*, which were taken up into English directly or through French: words such as *mission, missionary*, or *missile* (which in Latin referred to any hurled weapon and today is applied to self-propelled projectiles) or *missive*, from the expression *littera missiva* ("letters sent"), eventually converted into a noun, as in the French *(lettre) missive* or the Spanish *(carta) misiva*. The notion of "sending" is also present in the English *message*, a derivative of the Medieval Latin *missaticum*, introduced through French in the 14th century. This "French connection" was common to other words such as *voyage* (French *voyage*, Latin *viaticum*) or *savage* (French *sauvage*, Latin *silvaticum*). Lastly, *mass* (French *messe*, Spanish *misa*) stems from the noun taken from the feminine participle *missa*, pronounced at the end of the Eucharist: *Ite, missa est*. Whilst its origin is certain, the interpretation of the phrase is less so, for it may mean either "Go, (the prayer) has been sent" or "Go, it is the dismissal."[c] Either way, the term was first used to mean "Eucharistic celebration" in the 4th century C.E. by St. Ambrose in his letters. *Christmas*, in turn, a derivative of *mass*, means "celebration of the birth of Christ."

The Middle Ages witnessed a significant variation: the original meaning of *mittere*, "to send," was attributed to other verbs such as *inviare* (literally, "to set on its way") or *mandare*, in which the meaning "to command" was clearly replaced by the notion "to send." Both verbs were successfully introduced into most Latin languages: Spanish *enviar, mandar*; French *envoyer, mander*; and Italian *inviare, mandare*.

Even so, *mittere* did not disappear altogether, although its use changed to mean "to send something to the table," "to set on the table," or simply "to put." This latter meaning has survived in the French *mettre*, "to put," and derivatives such as *mettable* ("wearable"), *metteur* ("director"), or *mise en scène* ("put on

---

[b] Oxford English Dictionary (OED) online (1), under "smite": "The development of the various senses is not quite clear, but that of throwing is perh. the original one."

[c] The latter would allude to the Catechumenal farewell (*missa cathecumenorum*), initially pronounced after the sermon, although the meaning was ultimately extended to the celebration of the entire mass, as noted by Ernout-Meillet and Blaise in the entries in their respective dictionaries (2, 3).

stage"). The Spanish verb *meter* ("to put into"), in turn, gives rise to *remeter* ("to tuck in"), *arremeter* ("to attack"), or the expressive adjective *meterete* ("busybodying").

The meaning "to set on the table" was present in early Latin in *missorium* ("dish") and *missus* ("course"). It is the root of the French *mets* ("dish"), introduced into English as *mess*, which changed from the original sense of "army officers' dining hall" to a "chaotic mix of things." *Mets* also gave rise to *entremets*, courses served between the main dish and dessert. That in Spanish became *entremés*, which is applied both in the culinary context and to a type of skit very popular in 16th- and 17th-century Spain, performed between acts in a longer play (*interlude* in English).

ORIGIN AND MEANING OF *TRANS-*

The root proposed by linguists, **ter-* ("to go through, to cross"), and its variation **tra-*, would give rise to the Latin *intrare* ("to enter"). Further to that theory, *intrare* would derive from *trare*, whose present participle *trans* would ultimately become a preposition.[d] Its significance in any event is clear: "through," "across," "beyond." Hence the Latin *traducere* ("to lead or convey across") and other more abstract conceits denoting progression, such as *transformare* ("to change in shape"), or duration, *transcurrere* ("to elapse").

The root **ter-* is present in other Indo-European languages in prepositions equivalent to *trans*, such as the German *durch* or the English *through*. It also appears in *avatar* (Sanskrit *avatarah*, "descent," from *avá*, "off, down" + *tarah*, "crossover"), a term applied to the terrestrial incarnation of deities. Hence

the modern meaning of transformation into another being. In its transferal into the Romance languages, *trans* gave rise to the French *très* (the origin of whose meaning, "very," lies in "from one place to another," which in turn yields the more abstract conceit "throughout, completely," and hence "more intense") and the Spanish *tras* (from the notion "beyond").

In English, the presence of *trans* is not confined to the words introduced in the past from Latin or French; it is also found in words formed directly in English, such as *transatlantic*, *transnational*, *transpersonal*, or *transship*. And it is still being used today in electronics (*transducer*, *transponder*, *transceiver*) and science. In chemistry, for instance, *trans-* is the opposite of *cis-* ("on this side"), describing the arrangement of atoms in a molecular structure, as in *cis-trans* isomerism. It is widespread in medicine and biology: *transaminase*, *transcranial*, *transcriptase*, *transcriptome*, *transcytosis*, *transdermal*, *transection*, *transfection*, *transferase*, *transferrin*, *transfusion*, *transgenesis*, *transgenic*, *translocation*, *transmembrane*, *transpiration*, *transplantation*, *transposition*, *transposon*, and so on. And in recent years it has found its way into the terminology denoting sexual identity with terms such as *transgender*, *transsexual*, *transvestism*, *transman*, *transwoman*, and *transphobia*.

DERIVATIVES OF THE VERB *MITTERE*

Languages draw from a number of morphological mechanisms to create new from existing words with which they are etymologically and semantically related. That resource contributes decisively to the enhancement of language, for the creation of vocabulary entails the inclusion of nuances in word meanings and therefore greater precision in the verbal depiction of reality.

In traditional grammar, the three morphological processes for creating new words were composition, derivation, and parasynthesis, to

---

[d]This is not uncommon. Other instances of participles converted into prepositions include English *during* (Spanish *durante*) and Latin *versus*. Other authors, including Ernout-Meillet (2), reject this theory, contending that *intrare* derives from *intra*.

which a fourth, acronymy,[e] might be added. Structural semantics (4), in turn, also defines three processes, modification, development, and composition.[f] Our interest here focuses on the first of the three. More specifically, it hinges on the modification of verbs, the process of creating new verbs by adding prefixes or suffixes that alter the meaning of the base word, as in *transmittere* from *mittere*. In Latin, the mechanism normally involved in verbal modification consisted in adding a preverb to a verb. In English, the mechanism often involves the generation of *phrasal verbs*, i.e., associating an existing verb with another word or phrase. The two procedures are analogous, as the following examples show:

ire, "to go"/*exire*, "to go out"
rumpere, "to break"/*perrumpere*, "to break through"

Before addressing the modifications of *mittere*, we should say that preverbs and prepositions have a single underlying meaning from which more or less interrelated notions derive. According to linguists such as Pottier, prepositions can express space, time, or notion (5). Hence, in connection with the Latin *ante* and its equivalent *before*:

Space. "in front of": *ante aedes*, "before the house"
Time. "preceding in time": *ante meridiem*, "before midday"
Notional. "in preference to": *ante omnia*, "before anything else"

Mittere stands as indisputable proof of how productive verbal modification was in Latin. In this study, we documented 23 preverbal modifications that add some nuance to the meaning of *mittere*, most of which have been carried over into modern languages. In English, all these derivatives were introduced as learned words directly from Latin or via other languages, French in particular. Some of the most prominent are listed below.

Admittere. The original meaning of the modifier *ad-* ("toward") would yield the notion "to allow entry" (as in English *admittance*). A derivative of that initial idea would be "to accept," present in most modern languages, English among them (as in *admit*, *admission*, *admissible*, and *inadmissible*).

Committere. Attached to this preverb ("with"), *mittere* became "to join, to put together" (found in the English noun *commissure*). This notion would ield "to engage" (observed in Latin in *committere proelium*, "to engage in battle"), which ultimately became associated with "to begin, to carry out" (Spanish *acometer*, "to undertake"). More specifically, it became associated with something reprehensible: *to commit* a crime, suicide, or in Spanish *decomiso*, "confiscation," drawn from the Latin phrase *de commisso crimine*, "to confiscate goods related to the commission of a crime." A third meaning, "to trust, entrust," is present in *commitment*, which evolved from the delivery of something to the state for custody to today's more figurative notion, "engagement." The words *committee* and *commission* ("group of people in charge of something") also convey that idea, as do *commissary* (once "officer in charge of food supply," now "officers' dining hall"), *commis* ("junior chef"), and *committal* (both "imprisonment" and "burial"). In Spanish, the conceit is inherent in the words *comisario* ("police superin-

---

[e] Composition consists in forming a word by joining two or more, such as in *heartache*. In derivation words are formed by adding prefixes or suffixes to existing words, as in *unmyelinated*. Parasynthesis would be the simultaneous deployment of composition and derivation, as in *nearsightedness*. Acronomy is the creation of words from the initial letter or letters of each of the parts or major parts of a compound term, as in *dopa* (di-OH-phenylalanine).

[f] In modification the derived and original words are the same part of speech (e.g., the creation of *to react* from *to act*). Development entails a change in part of speech (e.g., the adjective *microbial* from the noun *microbe*). Lastly, composition is the joining of two lexemes, as in *earwax*.

tendent"), *cometido* ("task"), and *fideicomiso* ("trusteeship").

Demittere. The preverb *de-* ("downwards") vests the word with the meaning "to send down, to drop." It has persisted, but only barely. In Spanish, *demisión* ("despondency") refers to a person's mood; in English, to *demit* and *demission*, to relinquishment of a position or job.

Dimittere. With the modifier *dis-* ("in different directions"), the verb means "to send apart." English took *dismiss* from the French *demettre*, giving it essentially two meanings: "to withdraw" and "to remove." Oddly, the latter is the opposite of the Spanish *dimitir*, meaning "to resign," which is not at all the same as being fired. The literal sense of the Latin verb persists in English in the adjective *dismissive* as well as in *demise*, a euphemism for death borrowed from French and originally meaning the conveyance of goods, which normally occurs after the death of their owner.

Emittere. With the addition of the prefix *ex-* ("out of," "from within"), the meaning is clearly "to send out, to let go" (Latin *emissarium*, hence *emissary*). The same idea is conveyed by *emit* and *emission*, used in English in the context of global warming ("emit GHGs," "emissions trading") and in other modern languages in telecommunications (Spanish *emisora*, for "broadcasting station").

Immittere. *In-* ("into," "in") affords the verb an obvious meaning: "to send into a place, to introduce." In English, while to *immit* and *immission* are now archaic, *immitance* is used in electronics as a synonym of impedance. In Spanish, *inmisión* refers to the pollution concentrated in a given time and place.

Intermittere. When the verb is prefixed by *inter-* ("among," "between"), its meaning is "to suspend temporarily, to pause for a moment," which persists in the English *intermit* and *intermission*. The words *intermittence* and *intermittent* are also associated with discontinuity, such as in rain or, in medicine, the temporary easing of symptoms. *Inter-* also conveys the idea of "being in the midst," "mediating in something." Hence *intermise* in English; *entremise* in French, for "intercession"; and in Spanish, to refer to someone who interferes in others' affairs, *entremetimiento* ("meddlesomeness"), *entremeter* ("to meddle"), and *entremetido* ("meddler").

Intromittere. The meaning here is similar to *immittere*. In English, *intromit* and *intromission* are applied in medicine to mean the penetration of one body part by another (such as the vagina by the penis). The usage differs widely in colloquial Spanish, where *intromisión* is "interference" and *entrometido* a synonym of *entremetido* (derived from *intermittere*).

Omittere. With the preverb *ob-* ("toward, over, against, in the way of"), the meaning is clearly "to lay aside" and thus "to refrain from doing something, willingly or otherwise," "to neglect," "to disregard." The word is widely used in the Romance languages (Spanish *omitir*, French *omettre*), from where it was introduced into English in the 14th century (*to omit*, *omission*). Shakespeare coined the term *omittance*, authoring the proverb "Omittance is no quittance."

Permittere. The preverb *per-* ("through") modifies *mittere* to mean "to let pass or go through," and hence "to allow, to give consent." The words to *permit*, *permission*, *permissible*, and *permissive* were introduced into English from French in the 15th century. The verb is extensively used in Latin languages (French *permettre*, Italian *permettere*, Spanish *permitir*).

Praemittere. The definition of *prae-* ("before") explains the meaning of *praemittere*, "to send forward or before." It persists in *premise* (French *premisse*, Spanish *premisa*), a term used in logic to signify the two propositions of a syllogism from which a conclusion is drawn. In archaic legal language, premises meant the property conveyed by bequest or deed, from which present usage, introduced in the 18th century ("land, appurtenances, and structures"), stems.

Praetermittere. *Praeter-*, "beyond," is a modifier meaning "to let pass." In English, to *pretermit* and *pretermission* convey the idea "to disregard intentionally," which in certain contexts may be synonymous with *to omit.* In rhetoric, *pretermission* is another word for *preterition* or *paraleipsis*, the intention to omit something.

Promittere. With *pro-* ("forward, forth, before") as a prefix, the verb assumes the meaning "to let go forward, to say beforehand," "to foretell," which even in Latin conveyed the idea of "promise" as "guaranteeing in advance that something would/would not occur." This is the notion that prevails in modern languages: Spanish *prometer* and French *promettre*, lent to English as *promise*, from the past participle *promesse* (Latin *promissum*). It is found in phrases such as *promised land*, alluding to God's announcement of Canaan to the people of Israel, and *promissory note* ("IOU"), common in business language.

Promittere, in turn, yields *compromittere* (literally "mutual consent to arbitration"), applied to the intention of litigants to honor a judge's decision. In English, *compromise* ("to adjust or settle by partial mutual relinquishment of principles, position, or claims") comes from the French *compromis*, in turn a derivative of the Latin participle *compromissum.* In Spanish, for instance, that initial legal sense has since acquired today's moral connotations: *compromiso* ("commitment") and *comprometido* ("committed"). *To compromise* also means "to put at risk"; hence in medicine the participle *compromising* is used to refer to any harmful element that may affect another body part.

Remittere. With the addition of *re-* ("back to the original place, again"), the original meaning is "to let go/to send back," i.e., to reposition something in its original place (French *remise*, "garage") or "to release from burden or guilt" and therefore "to forgive" in legal or religious domains (English *remissible*). "To weaken" or "to lose energy" is a related meaning, which when applied to adverse developments is equivalent in a way to returning something to its natural state. Hence *to remit*, said of a storm that abates or a disease whose intensity declines (as in *remittent*), but also *remiss*, "negligent in the performance of one's work," and *unremitting*, "relentless." The notion "to send" conveyed by *mittere* also persists in the context of money or goods (*to remit*, *remittance*, Spanish *remesa*), correspondence (Spanish *remitente*, "sender"; *remite*, "return address"), and the referral to authority for consideration (*to remit*).

Submittere. This verb, like its equivalent in English, *to submit*, bears two main meanings, deriving from the two senses of the preverb *sub-* ("under" and "forth, up"). The first would be "to place under the control of another" and therefore "to yield, lower, let down" (as in *submission, submittee, submittal, submittance*, and *submissive*). The second is "to send forth from below, to produce," meaning "to send or commit for consideration, study, or decision," found as well in *resubmit* and *submissible.*

TRANS + MITTERE = TRANSMITTERE

And that brings us to *transmittere*. The many meanings listed in dictionaries can be grouped under two main headings.

1. *"To send across, to transfer."* Given its spatial dimension, its use to refer to food digestion is striking (Celsus: *"alvus nihil reddit, ac ne spiritum quidem transmittit"* ["the bowels cannot evacuate and do not even permit the escape of flatulence"]). Notionally, it serves to transfer intangibles, such as vices (Justin: *"Asia cum opibus suis vitia Romam transmisit"* ["Asia brought Rome its vices along with its wealth"]). And it also bears the meaning "to hand over, to entrust" as a synonym of *committere* (Tacitus: *"munia imperii transmittere"* ["to transfer the functions of government"]), whereby it entered the realm of law and hereditary conveyance (Plinius the Younger: *"Hereditas transmittenda filiae fratris"* ["inheritance passed on to his brother's daughter"]).

2. *"To cross over."* It was used in the spatial sense, as in *"flumen ponte transmitti"* ("The river is crossed by a bridge"), but also to express time (Seneca: *"vitam per obscurum transmittere"* ["to spend life in obscurity"]). Lastly, the verb was used figuratively to mean "to pass." Referring to turncoats, Velleius Paterculus wrote: *"transmittere ad Caesarem"* ("to go over to Caesar's side"). Silius Italicus, using the word to mean "to pass over, leave disregarded," claimed: *"Haud fas, Bacche, tuos tacitum tramittere honores"* ("Bacchus, I must not ignore your honors"). The verb was also applied to mean "to feel," both in positive ("to enjoy," as in Pliny the Younger: *"secessus uoluptates transmittere"* ["to *enjoy the pleasures of retirement*"]) and negative contexts ("to bear", again in Pliny the Younger: *"ardorem transmittere"* ["to endure the heat of fever"]).

In the transition from Latin to modern languages, only the first meaning of the verb persisted. The second was replaced in English by *to cross*, in French by *traverser*, and in Spanish by *atravesar*. In English, the use of *to transmit* has been verified from the 15th century, whereas *transmission* appeared later. The verb bears two connotations, one spatial, meaning to send something tangible to another place (to transmit a letter, a message), and the other notional, the transfer of ideas or feelings. It also persisted as the transmission of a legacy, and by extension genetic legacy. Today its use is associated primarily with disciplines such as physics, telecommunications, mechanical engineering, and medicine.

TO TRANSMIT AND TRANSMISSION IN NATURAL SCIENCE

According to the *Oxford English Dictionary* (*OED*) (1), the first documented use of the verb *to transmit* in English dates from 1400 to 1450. In *The Wars of Alexander*, written in Middle English, it means "to cause (a thing) to pass," a conceit unrelated to this discussion. Its next documented usage, in 1565, conveys the same meaning, although in the context of transmitting impurities or sins. The second definition given in the *OED*, documented since 1629, refers to inheritance law, which as discussed below is related to the subsequent use of the verb in the context of disease. The meaning acquired by the word in physics or mechanics (third definition in the *OED*, documented since at least 1664) to describe the transfer of sound, light, or heat is closer to medical usage, for it was later applied in physiology and then in pathology. Both the legal and mechanical meanings are found in classical Latin, as noted, and were introduced into modern languages (English, French, Spanish, Italian) via learned channels through Renaissance Latin.

According to the *OED*, the first documented appearance of the noun *transmission* dates to 1611. Used to mean the "action of transmitting," "passage through a medium," it was later applied more specifically to mechanics (first documented in 1704). Oddly, the *OED* makes no mention of the use of these words in biology or pathology, despite the firmly established usage in those contexts in English. The disease-related examples for the entries *transmissible* and *transmissibility* in this very dictionary and for the verb *to transmit* in *Webster's Third International Dictionary of the English Language* (6) stand as proof of such usage. The omission may be partly explained by the fact that these entries are still to be revised further to a note in the *OED*. Interestingly, the subsequent use of the terms associated with the transfer of a disease has a precedent in classical Latin, in which the verb was also used to mean "conveying something in silence,"[g] as is generally the case of diseases passing from an ill to a healthy person.

To explain the progressive and specialized use of the verb *to transmit* and the noun *transmission* in medical contexts, we reviewed the appearance of both in medical treatises from the 15th to the 19th centuries in Latin, English, Spanish, French, and Italian[h] to acquire a historical overview of the matter. Bearing in mind that until the 18th century Latin was the language used in scientific literature intended for an international readership, the specialized terms used by a scientist in one language tended to appear in parallel form in another, usually within a narrow time frame.

In classic, late, and Medieval Latin, neither the verb *transmittere* nor the noun *transmissio* appeared with specialized meanings associated with medicine. No precedents of the modern use of these terms in connection with disease were found until the 16th century.

In the Renaissance, Girolamo Fracastoro introduced the word *syphilis* in medicine in 1530 with his most famous work, the poem

Syphilis sive morbus Gallicus (*Syphilis or the French disease*). He also authored a book in 1546 on contagion entitled *De contagione et contagiosis morbis* (*On Contagion and Contagious Diseases*) (8), in which he distinguished between fevers caused from within and those prompted by external agents such as the air, germs, or vapors, noting that the latter could be "transmitted" from one person to another (*febris in nobis primo pestilens sit et ab uno in alium transmittitur*). In another context, he described the passage of fever from one area of the body to another, affecting different body parts. This notion of the conveyance of disease or its symptoms from one place to another connects with the aforementioned use of the term in mechanics and physics. Fracastoro in fact wrote about *transmissio caloris* ("heat transmission"). This mechanics-related meaning of the Latin verb applied to physiology can also be found in a treatise published in 1628 by William Harvey that revolutionized the understanding of the circulatory system. The English translation of his *De motu cordis et sanguinis* (*On the Motion of the Heart and Blood*) reads:

> although some state that the lungs, arteries, and heart have the same function, they also say that the heart is the factory of spirits and that the arteries contain and transmit them...
> To desire that waste vapors from the heart and air to the heart be transmitted by this same conduit is opposed to Nature which nowhere has made but a single vessel or way for such contrary movements and purposes. (9)

Fracastoro was apparently ahead of his times in the pathological use of the Latin verb *transmittere* and noun *transmissio*, which did not become widespread until the 18th century. French physician Nicolas Chesnau (10), in a treatise written in Latin, used the phrase *qualitatis malignae transmissionem* ("transmission of malignancy") to refer to epilepsy and the mechanics of its flow to the brain.

Another significant text found in a 1725 treatise by a doctor to the Spanish court,

---

[g]The eighth sense in the *Oxford Latin Dictionary* (7).
[h]From GoogleBooks and medical publications listed in archive.org.

Martín Martínez, attempted to explain fever in terms of its transmission from a number of sites within the body (11). An Italian medical text dated in 1746 on the transmission of fever also used the verb *transmettere* (12). Although we searched in English, we were unable to find a single clear example of such usage, a failing we would attribute to documentary shortcomings.

In 1774, we found the following sentence in a book on popular medicine: "What a dreadful inheritance is the gout, the scurvy, or kings-evil, to transmit to our offspring" (13).

The second edition of a treatise by an Irish physician published in 1777 used the word *transmission* to refer to interpersonal conveyance of what causes disease: "These morbific matters which are found capable of producing, occasionally, particular species of diseases, are of two sorts, native and adventitious; the first appear to be formed within the body, the second are communicated from without; either by the transmission of a subtile matter, or by actual contact with a diseased subject" (14).

By the late 18th century the verb and noun began to be used in their modern medical meaning, i.e., under the entry *transmit* in *Webster's* (6), "to give or convey (a disease or infection) to another person or organism."

From then on the use of these terms in pathology became increasingly popular and more abundant. In 1796, a medical journal contended: "the [venereal] disease or its consequences are frequently transmitted to the offspring, and often when the parents have no symptoms indicating its presence."

These examples show that the two senses of the Latin verb converge in the pathological use of these terms. The meanings in both inheritance law, "to convey property or rights," and in physics and mechanics (likewise documented in medicine in texts on physiology such as Harvey's) are now applied to the mechanisms whereby disease is conveyed from the ill to the healthy.

Before *transmission* and *to transmit* in the sense studied here came into general use, the Latin word applied since ancient times to refer to the conveyance of disease from one person to another was *contagio*. Etymologically speaking, the term implies physical contact, for it is a nominal derivative of *contingere* (comprising *tangere*, "to touch," and, to reinforce the notion of contact, the preverb *cum*, "with"). Hence, "to touch," "to be in contact with." From Medieval Latin it made its way into modern languages: *contagion* is documented in French since 1375 (15), *contagio* in Spanish since 1490 (16, 17), *contagion* in English since 1522 (1), and so on. We believe that *transmission* was introduced with its new pathological meaning as a generic term that embraced the conveyance of disease through both inheritance and contagion. *Transmission* and *to transmit* were also useful when it was unclear whether propagation entailed the direct contact between the ill and the healthy intrinsic to the word *contagion*. Both terms, *transmission* and *contagion*, were found in the following text written in 1821: "The plague is by most writers considered as the consequence of pestilential contagion, which is propagated from one person to another by association, or by coming near infected materials … but the laws of its transmission are not more accurately known than the specific nature of the contagion" (18).

In short, we believe that the introduction of the pathological use of *transmission* and *to transmit* was a response to the gradual deepening of the understanding of disease propagation. That led to a need for generic terms applicable to the conveyance of disease, whether through inheritance or through proximity (with or without physical contact) between the healthy and the ill.

Accustomed today to conceits such as airborne transmission, blood-borne transmission, fecal-oral transmission, and vertical transmission, many biomedical professionals tend to restrict the term *transmission* to mean microbial transmission. Like them, many a layperson appears to find it difficult to distinguish between *transmissible* (or in English, also *communicable*), *contagious*, and *infectious*, which are frequently used interchangeably, as if they were synonyms. Actually, however, the three are not strictly equivalent and their subtle differences should be borne in mind when precision of language is a concern. The adjective *infectious* refers to a disease caused by pathogenic microorganisms, be they bacteria, viruses, fungi, or protozoa. Such microorganisms are transmitted from one individual to another via immediate (direct contact) or mediate contagion. In the latter case, the mechanism may consist of hydric contagion, fomites, droplets, used/shared syringes, blood transfusion, organ transplant, or other channels of indirect contagion. All infectious diseases are, then, by definition, contagious and transmissible, but the contrary is not true. Inherent in the adjective *contagious* is the notion of disease transmission via direct or indirect contact between two people, although not necessarily involving the intervention of a pathogenic microorganism. Contagious diseases have been known in medicine, in fact, since the age of Hippocrates, whereas infectious disease as a conceit first appeared in the 19th century. The difference can be seen more clearly when we consider that both laughter and hysterics are contagious, but certainly not infectious. Lastly, the adjective *transmissible* is applicable to any disease that can be conveyed from one individual to another, via contagion (infectious or otherwise) or genetics. Huntington's chorea, for instance, is a genetically transmissible disease, but it is neither contagious nor infectious.

Hereditary transmission, linked to nucleic acids, is crucial today in fields such as clinical genetics, molecular biology, and biotechnology. But it dates back 150 years, when Augustin monk Gregor Mendel published his "Versuche über Pflanzen-Hybriden" (19) (Experiments on plant hybrids) in the *Proceedings of the Natural History Society of Brünn*. Over 8 years of experimentation, Mendel examined upward of 20,000 green and yellow peas and took detailed notes of their *Charaktere*, or phenotypical characteristics.

The mathematical analysis of his results enabled him to deduce the laws whereby certain *Elemente* (today we call them *genes* or *alleles*) determine how characteristics are inherited or transmitted from parents to offspring. Initially his paper went unnoticed, for contemporary scientists were unable to perceive the significance of experiments with hybrid plants and Mendel died before his talents as a naturalist could be acknowledged. It was not until 1900 when three botanists and pioneering geneticists, Hugo de Vries (20, 21) in The Netherlands, Carl Correns (22) in Germany, and Erich von Tschermak (23) in Austria, independently rediscovered Mendel's works and paved the way for the spectacular development of genetics, today the foremost discipline in biological science and the driver of modern biotechnology.

The transmission of pathogenic microorganisms and of genetic material are two fundamentals of biomedical science and can be found in such widely used expressions as *sexually transmitted diseases (STDs)* in connection with the former and the *transmission of plasmid-mediated resistance* with the latter. The use of the term *transmission* in science and technology does not by any means end there, however. The prevalence of the usage of *transmission* in modern science is readily visible in countless specialized terms in all realms of biology and other technical and scientific disciplines: in mechanics and engineering it is applied to energy, electricity, mechanical force, and electromagnetic waves; in botany, to pollen from a flower's stamen to its stigma; and in physiology, to nerve pulses across neuron synapses and of electrical stimuli from auricles to ventricles through the conductive tissue in the heart. In a similar vein, transmission electron microscopy is a type of microscopy in which a beam of electrons is transmitted through an ultrathin specimen. And we call acetylcholine, adrenaline, dopamine, γ-aminobutyric acid (GABA), glycine, histamine, and serotonin *neurotransmitters* because they are the chemical substances involved in neurotransmission, i.e., specific chemical agents that cross a synapse to inhibit or stimulate the postsynaptic nerve cell. Even the notion of cell signaling, a complex system of communication that governs basic cellular activities and coordinates cell actions, can essentially be interpreted as intracellular signal transmission.

From the times of Ancient Rome in the 3rd century B.C.E., the Latin word *transmissio* has been "transmitted" (through Romance languages such as French, Italian, Spanish, and Portuguese) to all the major languages of culture, English among them. And through English, the international language of biomedical science in the 21st century, the term *transmission* is increasingly present today in some of the most dynamic disciplines of modern natural science, including genomics, molecular microbiology, hospital epidemiology, molecular genetics, biotechnology, evolutionary biology, and systems biology. In conjunction with the meanings of *transmission* ushered in by new concepts, the progressive development of every scientific discipline entails a growing degree complexity in the understanding of all the senses of the word. One immediate example can be found in this work, in which the kaleidoscopic reality of transmission processes in the specific realm of microbial biology is addressed from a host of perspectives.

CITATION

Villalba J, Navarro FA, Cortés F. 2017. Origin, history, and meanings of the word *transmission*. Microbiol Spectrum 5(6):MTBP-0004-2016.

REFERENCES

1. **Oxford English Dictionary (OED) online.** 2016. Oxford University Press. http://www.oed.com/. Accessed 28 November 2017.
2. **Ernout A, Meillet A.** 1967. *Dictionnaire étymologique de la langue latine: histoire des mots*, 4th ed. Klincksieck, Paris, France.
3. **Blaise A.** 1954. *Dictionnaire latin-français des auteurs chrétiens*. Brepols, Turnhout, Belgium.
4. **Coseriu E.** 1991. *Principios de semántica estructural*. Gredos, Madrid, Spain.
5. **Pottier B.** 1962. *Systématique des éléments de relation. Étude de morphosyntaxe structurale romane*. Klincksieck, Paris, France.
6. **Gove PB (ed).** 1981. *Webster's Third New International Dictionary of the English Language Unabridged*. G. & C. Merriam Co, Springfield, MA.
7. **Glare PG (ed).** 1982. *Oxford Latin Dictionary*. Oxford University Press, New York, NY.
8. **Fracastoro G.** 1584. *De contagionibus & contagiosis morbis. In Hieronymi Fracastorii Veronensis Opera Omnia*, Venetiis, Apud Iuntas, p 89a.
9. **Harvey W.** 1928. *Exercitatio anatomica de motu cordis et sanguinis in animalibus*. Leake CD, trans, annot, p 12 and 17 of the facsímile and p 10 and 19 of the translation. Charles C Thomas, Springfield, IL.
10. **Chesnau N.** 1719. *Observationum medicarum libri*, p 88. Lugduni Batavorum, Leiden, The Netherlands.
11. **Martínez M.** 1725. *Medicina sceptica*, **II**, p 265. Madrid, Spain.
12. **Moreali G.** 1746. *Delle febbri maligne e contagiose*, p 145. Venice.
13. **Buchan W.** 1774. *Domestic Medicine, or the Family Physician*, p 6. Philadelphia, PA.
14. **MacBride D.** 1777. *A Methodical Introduction to the Theory and Practice of the Art of Medicine*, 2nd ed, p 19, 60. Dublin, Ireland.
15. **Dictionnaires Le Robert.** 2016. *Le Grand Robert de la langue française*. www.lerobert.com/le-grand-robert. Accessed 28 November 2017.
16. **Real Academia Española.** 2016. *Corpus diacrónico del español* (CORDE). http://corpus.rae.es/cordenet.html. Accessed 28 November 2017.
17. **Instituto de Investigación Rafael Lapesa y Real Academia Española.** 2013. *Corpus del Nuevo diccionario histórico* (CDH); version 3.1. http://web.frl.es/CNDHE/view/inicioExterno.view. Accessed 28 November 2017.
18. **Thomas R.** 1821. *In The Modern Practice of Physic... Improved Method of Treating the Diseases of All Climates*, 7th ed, p 279. Longman, London, United Kingdom.
19. **Mendel G.** 1866. Versuche über Pflanzen-Hybriden. *Verh Naturforsch Ver Brunn* **4:**3–47.
20. **De Vries H.** 1900. Sur la loi de disjonction des hybrides. *C R Acad Sci* **130:**845–847.
21. **De Vries H.** 1900. Das Spaltungsgesetz der Bastarde. *Ber Dtsch Bot Ges* **18:**83–90.
22. **Correns C.** 1900. Mendel's Regel über das Verhalten der Nachkommenschaft der Rassenbastarde. *Ber Dtsch Bot Ges* **18:**158–167.
23. **Tschermak E.** 1900. Über künstliche Kreuzung von Pisum sativum. *Zeitschr Landwirtsch Versuchsw Osterr* **3:**465–555.

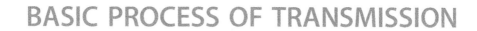

BASIC PROCESS OF TRANSMISSION

Causality in Biological Transmission: Forces and Energies

2

FERNANDO BAQUERO[1]

The immediate mental representation of the concept of transmission for the public health epidemiologist, clinical microbiologist, or infectious diseases specialist concerns its application to the transmission of pathogenic microorganisms or the transmission of infections. Note that the widely used term "transmissible diseases" is certainly most inappropriate. Disease is the result of particular cross talk between microbe and host and is never transmissible as such. The infective process is what the microbe produces inside a particular host, which is well illustrated in the Latin origin of the word "infection," derived from *inficere* (*in* + *facere*): "to put in, to dip into, to do an action inside." Microbes are transmissible, not the infection. In general biology, the most frequent use of "transmission" applies to the transmission of hereditary characters (to the progeny), as in population genetics (1). To our knowledge, a broad conceptual understanding of transmission has not yet been attempted, although Hugh Dingle has approached the need of expanding the transmission-related concept of migration to different hierarchical levels (2). In this review, I intend to present the concept of transmission in a broad perspective, as a basic biological and evolutionary process, focusing particularly on the causes (forces and

[1]Department of Microbiology, Hospital Universitario Ramón y Cajal (IRYCIS) and Centro de Investigacion Biomedica en Red (CIBERESP), Madrid, Spain.
Microbial Transmission in Biological Processes
Edited by Fernando Baquero, Emilio Bouza, J.A. Gutiérrez-Fuentes, and Teresa M. Coque
© 2018 American Society for Microbiology, Washington, DC
doi:10.1128/microbiolspec.MTBP-0018-2016

energies) governing transmission, a hitherto neglected field in biological and epidemiological research. For this purpose, it is appropriate to review what we collectively have in mind when considering the concept of transmission.

THE COGNITIVE REPRESENTATION OF THE CONCEPT OF TRANSMISSION

Thinking about a concept implies a cognitive representation, producing mental particulars with semantic properties (3), allowing the intelligibility of complex, polysemic processes (4). Paraphrasing Wittgenstein, the limits of our knowledge correspond to the limits of our words, our synthetic cognitive representations. In the case of the concept of transmission, we inevitably construct our cognitive representation with a quite diverse array of "transsumptions" involving knowledge and experiences of different origins that are for natural scientists transposed to the domain of biology (5).

The word "transmission" evokes the movement of a particle or a wave from one part of space to another. Particulate transmission occurs in nuclear fission; transmission (transport) of molecules in the cytoplasm or across cell membranes; transmission of pheromones; neurotransmission in synapsis; transmission of phages and plasmids across bacteria; and transmission of genes and gene sequences between genomes, including fertilization of ovules. Transmission is typically host-to-host transmission of microbes by insects or by microdrops in the air, transmission of multiresistant bacteria in hospitals, mother-child transmission of microbiota, or transmission of bacterial communities from farms to environmental water bodies. Also, there is transmission of gametes by pollinator insects, transmission of seeds by fruits, and transmission of fungal spores. In addition, there are bird migrations and globalized human journeys. Nonparticulate transmission occurs in the oscillatory waves produced by

vibration after a stone impacts water, or propagation of a sound, electric light, or radio waves; transmission in the wheels of machines or mechanisms; and fire-to-the-teapot heat transmission. Also, there is cultural transmission of knowledge, cultural values, or even stupid behavior in society. In short, transmission is movement; and life is replication and change, movement.

COMPONENTS OF THE TRANSMISSION PROCESS

Transmission has a site of origin and a termination, a site of end. Reducing our view to biological particulate transmitted entities (ranging from biomolecules to biological ecosystems), and in order to facilitate a general view on transmission, we consider these sites as "patches," in the meaning used in metapopulation biology. A patch is here defined as a part of space that is occupied by the transmitted entity and separated by an unfit space from other patches that might be able to receive this object (6). Note that this concept of transmission between patches diverges from mere "dispersal"—dispersal is not transmission if a receiving patch does not interact with the transmitted object. Therefore, transmission implies a patch of departure, a nonpatched space to cross, and a patch of reception (7, 8).

This view is obviously inspired from information theory (9, 10), with the classic tripartite composition: a sender or transmitter, located in a particular patch of space, which is the source of the transmitted object; the message; and a receiver patch that interacts with the message. I would like to insist on the point that transmission is only completed if the message is received, that is, if the transmitted entity to a certain extent integrates into (modifies) the receiver patch.

This key message can be supported by the etymological analysis of the word "transmission." This analysis is provided in another article in this issue thematically devoted to transmission (11). It shows that it derives from the Latin *transmittere*, in turn formed by prefixing the preposition *trans* ("across" or "beyond") to the verb *mittere* ("to let go" or "to send"). The Latin meaning might suggest that transmission is not only "to throw," "to release," "to let go," but also "to send" (to cause something to go from one place to another). The equivalent term in Greek is *metádosi* (μετάδοση), and in this language the meaning implies more a type of sharing or exchange as a result of transmission, so that when something is transmitted it migrates from one place (patch) to another one.

As stated above, transmission occurs if the message is received, that is, if the transmitted entity to a certain extent integrates into (modifies) the receiver patch. The sense of the word "information" fully corresponds to this condition of reception. This word derives from the Latin verb *informare* ("to inform") in the meaning of "to put form in," "to give form." It implies "to give ordered form," to create a type or order influenced by the reception of a message, an informative coded message composed by an ordered array of meaningful symbols (http://the informationalturn.net/philosophy_information/the-meaning-and-etymology-of-information/#sthash.igXsN5ga.dpuf). The reception of the message might imply a decoding process (a translation from its original form to another form meaningful for the receiver), but there is also the possibility that the message can act as a compact "brick" altering the structure of a passive receiver in a particular way, as I consider next.

BIOLOGICAL ENTITIES AS MESSAGES

In the previous paragraph, I stated that I am considering the transmission of biological entities (from biomolecules to biological ecosystems) as particulate objects of transmission. This implies that the "messages" transmitted between (among) patches are biological entities. This is the basic concept of biosemiotics (12, 13). Biological individuals, at the different levels of the hierarchy, act as messages; that is, their topological features, chemical structure, or chemical periphery (eventually resulting from their activity) act as an encoded informative system, potentially providing signs (information) and signals (instructions) to the receiver entity. In fact, pathogenesis of infectious diseases is based on the reception of these instructions and information by the host cells. Note that to produce a biological effect, the information contained in the transmitted signs and signals should be able to modify the activity of the receiver; the information should be "expressed." However, how permanent this modification is depends on the robustness or the reiteration of the message.

Until recently, the concept of "code" in biology was almost totally restricted to the genetic code, able to ensure ribosomal translation of particular DNA sequences into proteins. However, many other biological processes use the structure of biological entities as codes: it is clearly incorrect to suppose that all biological systems are encoded by DNA alone (14, 15). In the field of microbiology, examples of this are the synthesis by assembly of the different structural components of phages, the synthesis of the multiple parts of the ribosome, the physical construction of the bacterial cell, or, on a larger scale, the building up and the reconstruction of complex microbial ensembles in the animal or vegetal microbiota or the construction of integrated holobionts (16). Note that these building codes correspond to ensembles. Finally, everything is constituted by "pieces" that following particular codes associate in "patterns" (17). The patterns are selectable complexes, so that selection of a complex array of integrated pieces also means selection of the code giving rise to such efficient organization. Is it also important to consider that biological entities (individuals) correspond to different (embedded) hierarchical levels, as genes, mobile genetic elements, viruses, plasmids, chromosomes, cells, cell populations, or integrated multispecies ensembles. The notion of a biological or evolutionary individual applies to the group of biological entities that, at different hierarchical levels, fulfill the criteria of Stephen Jay Gould of (i) reproduction, (ii) inheritance, (iii) variation, and (iv) interaction (18, 19). These entities are in fact selfish individuals, evolving as independent units, that is, units of selection and evolution (20). Note that the notion of independent evolutionary units does not deny the effect of the surrounding units of lower and higher hierarchical levels but stresses the fact that under these "ecological" conditions, the units are able to evolve independently. Most importantly, these biological entities are transmitted and received, either at their hierarchical level (*cis*-acting transmission) or across hierarchical levels (*trans*-acting transmission), as we will see below.

CIS-ACTING AND *TRANS*-ACTING TRANSMISSION

Two main types of hierarchical relation between the emitter and receiver linked by the process of transmission can be distinguished. The terms "*cis*-acting" and "*trans*-acting" modes of transmission are coined on the bases of the Latin prefixes *cis* (in the sense of "on the same level") and *trans* ("across levels") (Fig. 1).

cis-acting transmission occurs when unenclosed patches acting as emitter and receiver entities of the same hierarchical level are linked across the space. For instance, a bacterial strain that is being transmitted (message) in the hospital from a patient (emitter patch) to another host (receiver patch) is linking *cis*-linked patches. It also occurs when bacteria translocate (are transmitted) from one part of the human or animal body (as the intestine) to an internal organ. It is the same case when a conjugative plasmid or a phage is transmitted between bacterial strains. In some cases, the

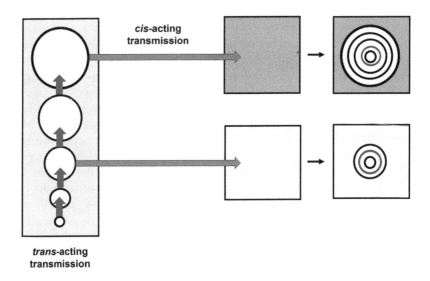

FIGURE 1 *trans*- and *cis*-acting modes of transmission. In *trans*-acting transmission, biological individuals (circles) belonging to different hierarchical levels (different sizes) are transmitted from one individual to another of a different level, giving rise to embedded entities acting as new complex individuals. In *cis*-acting transmission, biological individuals of different complexities are transmitted from a patch to another one, keeping their hierarchical level.

space between emitter and receiver patches can be very small (as in mosaic patches), and we can denominate this situation (a variant of *cis*-acting transmission) *para*-acting transmission—transmission events of mobile genetic elements in bacterial biofilms, in sexually transmitted diseases in humans, or when an almost complete bacterial system (such as the intestinal microbiome) is transmitted from mother to child.

trans-acting transmission occurs between embedded emitter-receiver systems, that is, between biological individuals of different hierarchical level, closely located within an external common limit (such as a cell membrane). The lower-rank entity penetrates (21) into the one of higher rank, the receiver patch, which results in embedded or nested structures. The word "introgression" originates from the Latin *introgredior*, meaning "to go inside." Introgressive events facilitate fusion, merging of biological elements belonging to different lineages and hierarchical levels that now replicate and are transmitted as a single corporate entity (20, 22).

Examples of this are the transmission of genes from a bacterial chromosome into a plasmid or the integration of a virus sequence in the genome of a human cell. *trans*-acting transmission is a major contributor to evolutionary progress, for instance, in the origin of bacterial endosymbionts in aphid insects or in the prokaryotic origin of mitochondria in eukaryotic cells or chloroplasts in green algae and plants.

CAUSALITY OF TRANSMISSION: FORCES AND ENERGIES

The investigation of the causal structure of transmission events is a promising open field of theoretical and experimental research in ecology, epidemiology, and evolutionary biology. In the preceding paragraphs, I stated that transmission requires an accomplished emitter-receiver interaction, so that if the message is not received (decoded,

admitted, or integrated), transmission is not fulfilled, or not proficient, in a sense is aborted. I am proposing that transmission (emigration) is the effect of centrifugal or repelling forces, and reception (immigration) is the effect of centripetal or attractive energies.

Emission requires a power, a directed action, which is the cause of the movement from the emitter patch to the receiver patch. But when the transmitted entity reaches the receiver, the decoding process, admission, and integration of the message (requiring a certain deformation of the receiver itself) *also* requires a power, a directed action. These powers can be described, respectively, as "forces" (to start emission, and the whole dynamics of transmission) and "energies" (to accomplish reception). These designations roughly correspond to the use of these terms in Aristotle's terminology. A force is the cause of a displacement, "whatever is capable of changing the state of a body," according to Euler (23), producing an emission with a possibility of reaching a goal (*potentia*). Energy is from the Greek *energeia*, "active internal working, activity," from *en* ("in") + *ergon* ("work"), in the sense of something that is being accomplished, realized (*actus*), integrated, or received. Energy is, according to Euler, "rather the contrary of force" (23). The "pieces in a puzzle" metaphor (Fig. 2) provides a good image of the energy working at the receptor patch. During the process of puzzle construction, or replacement of one or more pieces, the integration (reception) of an incoming piece, the object of transmission, depends on the matching of its shape (information, a message) with the shape of the empty place resulting from the borders of already installed pieces, as in codon-anticodon recognition. Once the new piece is received, it remains bound to the others by a kind of energy. In fact, if an external perturbation influences the puzzle (as by bending the whole construction), there will be a resistance to destructure the links between pieces,

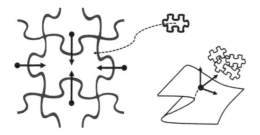

FIGURE 2 A puzzle representation of centripetal energies in the receiver patch. (Left) Reception of the transmitted entity (broken line, small puzzle piece) in the organized puzzle pattern is assured by local energies (centripetal bonding arrows). (Right) The organized puzzle is bent by external influences, arriving at a catastrophic event leading to a local disintegration of the puzzle pieces, liberating the centripetal energies and eventually creating forces (centrifugal arrows) for new transmission events.

so that many will remain bound. In fact, the equilibrium between external shear force (transverse to the plane of the puzzle) and internal normal energy (along the plane) will be broken (Fig. 2) by disbalancing the "bending moment" created by these opposing powers (24, 25). Note that the "linking energy" of puzzle pieces the received depends on the "code versus anticode" shapes of the transmitted object and the receiver structure, in other words, their informative content. A complex shape of a piece, determining a large number of interactions with neighboring pieces, will produce more constraints for its integration, but if it is accomplished, the linking energy is increased, and therefore also resistance to disbalance the bending moment.

Information creates energy. The forces invested in creating the message are converted into energy, capability of changing. This Einsteinian-like conversion has been shown using a Maxwell demon generated particle. This particle can exert work only by receiving information, rather than energy, and the conversion exchange rate occurs as one bit of information being equivalent to 0.28 kT ln 2 J of energy (26). Certainly the

"ordering" energy is invested in the reduction of entropy, triggering evolution (27).

THE CAUSAL QUESTIONS IN TRANSMISSION

An appropriate example, almost a metaphor, suggested by Ernst Mayr, which might help in understanding causality of transmission is the case of human or animal migrations (28). Emigrants are displaced from their patch source (transmitter) by transmission forces. After a process of emigration in a particular ecological landscape with certain risks, they reach the receiver patch (immigration), where local energies, such as conspecific attraction or interspecific facilitation, influence the final establishment (colonization) (8) as well as its later consequences, cross-information, deterritorialization, and hybridity (29).

Of course, it is legitimate to query the causal reasons of transmission (such as migration) events (29). The causal question "Why?" applied to transmission has distinguished precedents, such as Ernst Mayr, using the example of a perching bird, a warbler, starting its migration from New Hampshire (30). He was differentiating functional biology from evolutionary biology. The first answers the question "How?" concerning the operation and interaction of structural elements of biological individuals, from molecules to whole organisms. The second addresses the question "Why?" by analyzing the ultimate and proximate causes of the phenomenon (28, 31).

THE ULTIMATE CAUSE OF TRANSMISSION

The ultimate cause of transmission is replication. In other words, replication is a prerequisite for transmission. Biological individuals are replicators, and they are transmitted because they replicate. Replication is normally understood as propagation (transmission) along the time frame. However, replication has immediate consequences for the occupation of space, as every individual entity requires its own physical and functional (for instance, nutritional) space. Particularly in microbial asexual organisms (where death is elusive), this need for space for the progeny might even compete with the space occupied by the ancestors, giving rise to interesting ancestors-progeny antagonistic dynamics (32). To a certain extent, the gain of space because of replication has inspired the self-replicating computer programs that compete for "space" in the central processing unit, so that time is the fuel needed for their replication (33). Transmission in time and space is in fact the "phenotype" of replication. As I will consider below, the "biology of the space" frequently determines transmission events.

THE PROXIMATE CAUSES OF TRANSMISSION

I will analyze below a number of emission forces and reception energies, providing a kind of "causal frame" of transmission events in biology, which ideally should be applicable to any of the different biological entities of different hierarchical levels, from genes to superior organisms or consortia (34). These causal reasons are certainly without "purposes" but obviously not without effects. Certainly, the confusion between cause and purpose should be avoided, but inevitably a certain "teleological flavor" contaminates any discussion about causes. If this might occur reading the following part of this section, it should be understood as an undesired secondary effect of my heuristic intention to help the understanding of the bases of the transmission process (31). In addition, in the list presented in the following sections there is some redundancy and overlapping in analyzing the causes, because there are

frequently associated causalities, or even causes that might only differ by our way of representing them. Unfortunately, theoretical research on transmission processes in a wide sense has been hampered by the quite different types of studies focused on transmission of pathogenic microorganisms between humans or animals, or involving specific changes in biodiversity in the field of landscape ecology, animal migrations over long distances, or transmission of inheritable characters to the progeny (transmission genetics). As a result, the general meaning of "transmission" as a basic biological process has been underestimated. This "basic biology of transmission" remains a "black box" that has only recently been reopened (7).

PROXIMATE CAUSES OF EMISSION

What are the forces that influence biological entities to decline to remain stable in their original suitable patches and push them to enter into uncertain transmission processes? As stated by Bruce Levin (35), "Why be a vagabond when you can stay at home?" In other words, why does emission take place? Causes (forces) encompass individuals, populations, and the characteristics of the emitter patch. Note that to keep a general message I have not comprehensively illustrated each one of the causal forces that I describe (just an indicative example for each one), but different types of biological scientists will easily recognize known cases in each instance.

Causes Originated by the Size, Quality, and Location of the Emitter Patch

Patch size limitation
At every level of the hierarchy of biological entities, each individual incorporates an associated space, so that the patch is occupied by the entity and its associated space. Patches limited in size force the replicating

local entities to leave the patch to be transmitted (37).

Local demographics: Overpopulated patch
This is related to the above cause; if the patch is overcrowded, independently of its components and size, transmission is favored. Intraspecific population overcrowding and the resulting kin competition is alleviated by dispersal (36). On the other hand, dense populations might have easier access to suboptimal secondary niches, a kind of "mass effect" (37).

Breeding requirements; Progeny crowding
The biological individuals resulting from replication of the patch-installed entity (progeny) might produce a reduction of available space-for-individual; in this case, they will tend to be transmitted (38).

Nutrient shortage; Unfit patch conditions
Patches differ in their ability to renovate nutrients and eliminate toxic end products; differences between open, closed, and enclosed patches are relevant here. Also, patches can be submitted to physical, chemical, and biological (including immunological) fluctuations, eventually cyclic ones, altering the fitness of the installed biological individuals. Reduced fitness leads to stress, and stress is a known trigger of transmission, including gene transmission (recombination) (42). Nutrient shortage increases transmission mechanisms, including motility (39).

Distance between emitter and receiver patches: Mosaics and gradients
The "visibility" of an alternative, better-quality patch close to the original one favors transmission, and that is expected to occur in "wall-to-wall" or mosaic patches; transmission might even be enhanced along highly connected "gradient patches," gradually differing from the neighboring ones in their qualitative composition. Transmission between neighboring patches is greatly influenced by the patch (habitat) "edge effects," where the populations more prone to be transmitted are located (44, 45). Also, shorter distance between patches increases the density of transmitted entities, a prediction of the Allee effect (40).

Causes Originated in Populations' Conflicts within the Emitter Patch

Local negative interactions
Local conflicts, as competition between local populations, parasitism, amensalism, or predation, increase local stress, which can be relaxed by promoting transmission. Competition-colonization trade-off ecological models suggest that inferior competitors will be superior transmitter dispersers (41).

Cooperation for transmission
Transmission of a given biological entity can be enhanced by association with a highly transmissible one (cotransmission, mobilization) (42). This association can occur, for instance, by aggregation in a single transmitted entity; transmission as groups has been termed budding dispersal (43).

Patch deconstruction
Habitat destruction, or patch deconstruction, favors transmission (44, 45). Shortsighted evolution of local populations, oriented to obtain immediate benefits (such as full exploitation of local nutrients), might result in deleterious effects, irretrievably altering the conditions for survival in the patch, as in highly lethal infections (46). This "niche deconstruction" forces transmission as a survival strategy.

Displacement from the patch
Eventually a biological individual arrives into the patch with the possibility of displacing the first indigenous ones. If competitive displacement does not produce the extinction of the former population, their components will be forced to transmit

in order to find unoccupied or tolerant patches. Residual populations at the patch of origin can eventually be restored later by retransmission from these newly colonized patches, a process known as the rescue effect (53).

Causes Related to the Lifestyle of Biological Individuals

Search for optimal or exclusive patches
Transmission is triggered to fulfill the reproductive optimality of the biological individual, which is dependent on the optimal environment. After colonization of suboptimal patches, the search (transmission) for higher reproductive fitness will be maintained until reaching the one in which the population will reach its maximal fitness level.

Search for patches enabling genetic diversification and evolution
An attractive concept is that the search for patches with optimal conditions for genetic diversification and genetic exchange and recombination acts as an emission force. For instance, environmental-triggered hormonal changes can promote migration, as there is an "ecology of fertility" (47). Of course, replication is the major driver for transmission, but search for variability assures long-term broad-spectrum adaptation, as genetic isolation and stagnation reduce evolvability (48).

Vagility: Explorer life plan strategy
Biological individuals can be broadly classified in terms of "life plans" as explorers or exploiters, roughly related to, respectively, the r or K strategies used by ecologists (49). Individuals belonging to the explorer life plan possess traits (for instance, larger, multifunctional genomes in bacteria) to be efficiently transmitted to a wide spectrum of possible environments. Note once more that we would not like to identify biological individuals with organisms *only*. For instance, the basic individuals (replicators) are genes, but even here we can distinguish groups of genes more prone to be transmitted, as the accessory genes in genomes, "exploring" different landscapes to provide advantages to higher-rank individuals (50).

THE PROXIMATE CAUSES OF INTEGRATION AND PERMANENCE IN THE PATCH

Rephrasing the Levin sentence quoted earlier, "Why stay at home when there is a wealth of possibilities outside?" Below I list a number of causes, acting as centripetal local energies, which oppose centrifugal transmission but also act as energies able to integrate incoming biological entities into the receiver patch. Of course, to a certain extent, these energies are orthogonal to the forces triggering transmission, but I present them separately for heuristic reasons.

Causes Originated by the Size, Quality, and Location of the Hosting Patch

Stability and sustainability
Biological individuals tend to remain attached to stable and sustainable patches, thus allowing a constant but controlled rate of reproduction. These patches frequently possess some kind of buffered physicochemical stability and homeostasis, ensuring constant flows of incoming nutrients and regular elimination of wastes. Under conditions of patch stability, transmission propensity is decreased (51).

Shielded environments
Closely related to the previous cause, patches protected from deleterious biological or ecological external influences are "safe" and the installed biological individuals do not face risks of extinction, hence increasing the long-term possibility of stable permanence. Spatial habitat isolation selects against dispersal (52).

Specific and rare hosting patches
Environmental specialization of biological individuals in particular environments might decrease the possibility of successful transmission after migratory events. In these cases, concerted evolution of the biological individual with their host patch is expected to occur, repressing the transmission strategies for survival.

Host patches with predictable fluctuation
As a variant of stable patches sustaining biological entities, unstable patches presenting highly predictable regular variation can be permanently linked to particular biological individuals adapted to these changes, not needing transmission to overcome changes.

Niche construction
The patch containing, over a sufficient period of time, particular biological individuals tends to be modified by these entities to better fit with the needs of the population. This "niche construction" process increases the mutual population-host specificity, assuring stable, long-term maintenance in the patch (53).

Causes Originated in Interactions within the Host Patch

Stable or cooperative interactions with local biological entities
A receiver patch might already contain established biological entities, eventually interconnected by cooperative interactions. The transmission of each one of these entities out of the patch is hampered by the mutual needs of maintaining the interactive network, which can be considered as an individual entity of higher level in the hierarchy (as populations in the microbiota). This network ensures in fact a "complex system homeostasis" (54) where different functions are distributed among members. An incoming, newly transmitted element can be rejected or accepted by the network, if its presence is neutral with respect to the overall functioning of the system, and particularly if there is an empty function that can be covered by the incoming element, it is accepted. Probably the spontaneous "construction" of complex systems such as the intestinal microbiota follows this process (55).

Patch allowing low-cost replication
The transmitted entity might reach a receiving patch where the establishment and maintenance are ensured because of the abundant provision of resources, for instance, if nutrients or basic functions are provided by the host. In the absence of consistent competition, the exploitation of these rich patches tends to fix the transmitted entity and prevents further transmission events. Certainly this is the case for members of normal microbiota (56); also, long-term dominance of cyanobacterial organisms (blue-green algae) occurs in freshwater environments under nutrient-rich eutrophic conditions (57).

Causes Related to Biological Individuals

Exploiter life plan strategy
The exploiter strategy of life is the opposite of the explorer life plan strategy (58). Exploiters are K-strategists (49) evolved to extract all possible energy in the colonized patch. The patch is deeply exploited and the highest carrying capacity is reached, that is, the highest density of individuals that can be supported at the population equilibrium. The exploiter strategy leads to specialization, eventually to genomic reduction, and that is associated with prevention of transmission. At the gene-individual scale, the core genes in genomes are historical exploiters of specific organisms and are rarely transmitted (50), and there are also near-core genes that are kept for sufficient time to be the origin of further clonal speciation.

VEHICLES AS CAUSES OF TRANSMISSION

Transmission occurs between emitter and receiver patches. As stated before, these patches are frequently separated by an unfit space (6) that can only be crossed with the help of "bridge" or "shuttle" vehicles. Note that the vehicle itself is frequently a transitory colonizable patch. In the conventional sense of vehicle, as understood in epidemiology, a vehicle should firstly be considered as a passively "contaminated" inanimate object (typically a fomite). Passive interaction of the transmitted entity with inanimate (or near-inanimate, as skin surfaces) vehicles might be relatively complex, due to a number of factors, such as the ability of the transmitted entity to adhere multiply or being inhibited in contact with the vehicle. Vehicles can also be animated objects, acting as vectors, as in the case of arthropods serving as vehicles of transmission of microorganisms from an animal to a human host (59). As stated before, the transmitted biological entity frequently interacts in some specific way with the vehicle, eventually replicating within it, particularly in the case of vectors. In this case, the vector is an intermediate receiver patch, which is converted to an "emitter" to reach the ultimate receiver patch. This receiver-emitter consecutive duality is an interesting trait of vector vehicles that should be understood in light of the constellation of transmission forces and energies considered in previous sections. Of course, we should acknowledge transmission without vehicles; for instance, if biological particles are released by the emitter patch (acting as reservoir) and dispersed in air or water flows, the success of transmission depends on the ability of the transmitted entity to survive (eventually to multiply) in these environments.

The classic epidemiological notion of vehicle or vector, when referring to biological entities, as stated in the former paragraph, is in fact fully compatible with the concept first coined by Richard Dawkins (60). In his view, genes are replicative entities (replicators). Other biological entities, such as cells, are simply the vehicles ensuring the propagation of the replicators. As stated earlier in this review, above the gene level, other replicators (biological individuals) such as mobile genetic elements, viruses, plasmids, chromosomes, cells, populations of cells, or integrated multispecies ensembles should be considered. These are embedded individuals (the one inside the other in the hierarchy), but they eventually maintain distinct evolutionary trajectories. Interestingly, each individual entity is a vehicle for the lower entity and a transmitted object for the highest entities in the hierarchy.

In this perspective, a vehicle is any discrete individual biological entity that houses replicator biological entities of lower hierarchical levels, an entity that can be regarded as a machine that preserves ("survival machine") and propagates the replicators that ride inside it (60). The term "propagates" emphasizes the term "vehicle" as a tool for transmission. Indeed, the notion of vehicles inside vehicles is a good description of the complexities of transmission processes in biology, in which each one of the internal vehicles influences the global phenotype of the more external vehicle. Transmission of an embedded ensemble of replicators contained in a single vehicle implies transmission of all of them. However, each one of these individual replicators can *also* be transmitted individually. For instance, transmission of a single bacterial population between microbiomes in hospital patients implies transmission of all plasmids and genes it might contain. Plasmids carrying specific genes can, however, be independently transmitted from one bacterial population to another, the new population serving as a new vehicle to expand the genes in other types of hosts or environments. In these new hosting entities, genes from one plasmid can move into another, and this one into a successive series of entities along the hierarchy. This example points out the transmission independence (not opposed to interdependence, considering the hierarchical levels) of biological individuals (61).

TRANSMISSION AND THE CAUSES OF NATURAL SELECTION: *CIS*- AND *TRANS*-EVOLUTION

The subject of causes of natural selection was analyzed a long time ago by Wade and Kalisz (62). Certainly, evolution is *caused* by a "lack of fit" between biological individuals and their environments (63), and in fact the interplay between evolutionary and ecological dynamics of biological populations constitutes the "newest evolutionary synthesis" (64, 65). Transmission is a (the?) key process in evolution, as transmission is involved in both the creation of genetic diversity (recombination and introgression) and the exposure to novel and alternative patches-environments (migration). In fact, transmission is the main evolutionary method to solve the problems of ecologically unfit populations: either by changing the biological individual to survive (be selected) in the nonoptimal patch; or by changing the patch, seeking a better (alternative) one, while maintaining (essentially) the same type of individual. In general, the first strategy, modification of the individual (eventually giving rise to a complex one), can be achieved by events of *cis*-acting transmission, and the second, dispersal, by events of *trans*-acting transmission, so that we can claim two dimensions of evolution: *cis*- and *trans*-evolution. Both dimensions, independently and in combination, are highly relevant as drivers of biological changes. Certainly *cis*-evolution, acting across hierarchical levels, is responsible for most of the major transitions in evolution (66). The concept of major transitions reflects the innovative change in the type of individual, as in the shift from prokaryotic to eukaryotic cellular organization, or from unicellular to cell-differentiated organisms, frequently by introgressive events (67), resulting in a complexification, *ex pluribus unum* dynamics (19). *trans*-evolution acts by moving the individual across more or less distant patches and is more related to the progressive differentiation of evolutionary individuals, being involved in evolutionary processes of structured populations, leading to clonalization or speciation (76–78), in *ex unibus plurum* dynamics (19).

CODA: CAUSES AND EFFECTS

This mostly conceptual review focuses on the general causes (qualities) and not on the effects (quantities) of the transmission processes. In contrast to conceptual works, the studies on transmission numbers and, in general, transmission dynamics are extremely abundant. There are significant reviews addressing this area in the fields of ecology, epidemiology, and infectious diseases (68–74). In a number of cases, these studies are supported by mathematical modeling, certainly requiring a high complexity in order to include *cis*-evolutionary events. This has been recently addressed by the application of membrane computing methods (75), in which different embedded biological "objects" are surrounded by virtual cell-like membrane structures and can be "transmitted" across membranes (patches) according to preestablished rules (76). If the advance of biological sciences is frequently based on comprehensive collections and careful analysis of relevant quantitative data, the contribution of qualitative theoretical studies should synergize these studies, and project them to future research, by increasing the "intelligibility" (mental representation) of complex but universal processes in the biological universe (4, 77).

ACKNOWLEDGMENTS

This work was supported by funding from the Instituto de Salud Carlos III (projects FIS [PI15-00818] and CIBERESP [CB06/02/0053] cofinanced by the European Social Fund and the European Development Regional Fund "A way to achieve Europe").

CITATION

Baquero F. 2018. Causality in Biological Transmission: Forces and Energies. Microbiol Spectrum 6(5):MTBP-0018-2016.

REFERENCES

1. **Pierce BA.** 2009. *Transmission in Population Genetics: A Conceptual Approach*, 4th ed. W.H. Freeman and Co, New York, NY.

2. **Dingle H, Drake VA.** 2007. What is migration? *Bioscience* **57:**113–121.

3. **Margolis E, Laurence S.** 2007. The ontology of concepts—abstract objects or mental representations? *Noûs* **41:**561–593.

4. **Baquero F, Moya A.** 2012. Intelligibility in microbial complex systems: Wittgenstein and the score of life. *Front Cell Infect Microbiol* **2:** 88.

5. **De Libera A.** 2014. Analogy, p 31–33. *In* Cassin B (ed), *Dictionary of Untranslatables: A Philosophical Lexicon*. Princeton University Press, Princeton, NJ.

6. **Hanski I, Semberloff D.** 1997. The metapopulation approach, its history, conceptual domain, and application to conservation, p 5–26. *In* Hanski IA, Gilpin ME (ed), *Metapopulation Biology: Ecology, Genetics, and Evolution*. Academic Press, San Diego, CA.

7. **Antonovics J.** 2017. Transmission dynamics: critical questions and challenges. *Philos Trans R Soc Lond B Biol Sci* **372:**20160087.

8. **Ims RA, Yoccoz NG.** 1997. Studying transfer processes in metapopulations: emigration, migration, and colonization, p 247–264. *In* Hanski IA, Gilpin ME (ed), *Metapopulation Biology: Ecology, Genetics, and Evolution*. Academic Press, San Diego, CA.

9. **Pierce JR.** 1980. *An Introduction to Information Theory: Symbols, Signals, and Noise*. Dover Publications, New York, NY.

10. **Shannon C, Weaver W.** 1949. *The Mathematical Theory of Communication*. Urbana University Press, Urbana, IL.

11. **Villalba J, Navarro FA, Cortés F.** 2017. Origin, history and meanings of the word "transmission." *Microbiol Spec* **5**(6).

12. **Barbieri M.** 2008. Biosemiotics: a new understanding of life. *Naturwissenschaften* **95:**577–599.

13. **Cariani P.** 1998. Towards an evolutionary semiotics: the emergence of new functions in organisms and devices, p 359–377. *In* Van de Vijver G, Salthe S, Delpos M (ed), *Evolutionary Systems*. Kluwer, Dordrecht, The Netherlands.

14. **Noble D.** 2011. Differential and integral views of genetics in computational systems biology. *Interface Focus* **1:**7–15.

15. **Baquero F.** 2014. Genetic hyper-codes and multidimensional Darwinism: replication modes and codes in evolutionary individuals of the bacterial world, p 165–180. *In* Trueba G (ed), *Why does Evolution Matter? The Importance of Understanding Evolution*. Cambridge Scholars Publishing, Newcastle upon Tyne, United Kingdom.

16. **Richardson LA.** 2017. Evolving as a holobiont. *PLoS Biol* **15:**e2002168.

17. **Baquero F.** 2004. From pieces to patterns: evolutionary engineering in bacterial pathogens. *Nat Rev Microbiol* **2:**510–518.

18. **Gould SJ.** 2002. *The Structure of Evolutionary Theory*. Harvard University Press, Cambridge, MA.

19. **Baquero F.** 2011. The 2010 Garrod Lecture: the dimensions of evolution in antibiotic resistance: *ex unibus plurum et ex pluribus unum*. *J Antimicrob Chemother* **66:**1659–1672.

20. **Okasha S.** 2006. *Evolution and the Levels of Selection*. Oxford University Press, Oxford, United Kingdom.

21. **Bapteste E, Lopez P, Bouchard F, Baquero F, McInerney JO, Burian RM.** 2012. Evolutionary analyses of non-genealogical bonds produced by introgressive descent. *Proc Natl Acad Sci U S A* **109:**18266–18272.

22. **Bapteste E.** 2014. The origins of microbial adaptations: how introgressive descent, egalitarian evolutionary transitions and expanded kin selection shape the network of life. *Front Microbiol* **5:**83.

23. **Balibar F.** 2014. Force and energy, p 343–349. *In* Cassin B (ed), *Dictionary of Untranslatables: A Philosophical Lexicon*. Princeton University Press, Princeton, NJ.

24. **Beer FP, Johnston ER, DeWolf JT.** 2004. *Mechanics of Materials*, 3rd edition, p 322–323. McGraw-Hill, New York, NY.

25. **Saunders PT.** 1980. *An Introduction to Catastrophe Theory*, p 41–60. Cambridge University Press, Cambridge, United Kingdom.

26. **Toyabe S, Sagawa T, Ueda M, Muneyuki E, Sano M.** 2010. Experimental demonstration of information-to-energy conversion and validation of the generalized Jarzynski equality. *Nat Phys* **6:**988–992.

27. **Collier JD.** 1986. Entropy in evolution. *Biol Philos* **1:**5–24.

28. **Mayr E.** 1961. Cause and effect in biology. *Science* **134:**1501–1506.

29. **Papastergiadis N.** 2013. *The Turbulence of Migration: Globalization, Deterritorialization*

and Hybridity. John Wiley & Sons, Hoboken, NJ.

30. **Mayr E.** 1965. Cause and effect in biology, p 33–50. *In Cause and Effect.* Free Press, New York.

31. **Brandon RN.** 1998. Biological teleology: questions and explanations, p 79–97. *In* Allen C, Bekoff M, Lauder J (ed), *Nature's Purposes.* MIT Press, Cambridge MA.

32. **Baquero F, Lemonnier M.** 2009. Generational coexistence and ancestor's inhibition in bacterial populations. *FEMS Microbiol Rev* **33:**958–967.

33. **Lenski RE, Ofria C, Collier TC, Adami C.** 1999. Genome complexity, robustness and genetic interactions in digital organisms. *Nature* **400:**661–664.

34. **Daubin V, Ochman H.** 2004. Bacterial genomes as new gene homes: the genealogy of ORFans in *E. coli. Genome Res* **14:**1036–1042.

35. **Levin BR, Bergstrom CT.** 2000. Bacteria are different: observations, interpretations, speculations, and opinions about the mechanisms of adaptive evolution in prokaryotes. *Proc Natl Acad Sci U S A* **97:**6981–6985.

36. **Bach LA, Thomsen R, Pertoldi C, Loeschcke V.** 2006. Kin competition and the evolution of dispersal in an individual-based model. *Ecol Modell* **192:**658–666.

37. **Shmida AV, Wilson MV.** 1985. Biological determinants of species diversity. *J Biogeogr* **12:**1–20.

38. **Dingle H.** 2014. *Migration: The Biology of Life on the Move,* 2nd ed, p 324. Oxford University Press, Oxford, United Kingdom.

39. **Hibbing ME, Fuqua C, Parsek MR, Peterson SB.** 2010. Bacterial competition: surviving and thriving in the microbial jungle. *Nat Rev Microbiol* **8:**15–25.

40. **Taylor CM, Hastings A.** 2005. Allee effects in biological invasions. *Ecol Lett* **8:**895–908.

41. **Harbison CW, Bush SE, Malenke JR, Clayton DH.** 2008. Comparative transmission dynamics of competing parasite species. *Ecology* **89:**3186–3194.

42. **Herre EA, Knowlton N, Mueller UG, Rehner SA.** 1999. The evolution of mutualisms: exploring the paths between conflict and cooperation. *Trends Ecol Evol* **14:**49–53.

43. **Gardner A, West SA.** 2006. Demography, altruism, and the benefits of budding. *J Evol Biol* **19:**1707–1716.

44. **Tilman D, Lehman CL, Yin C.** 1997. Habitat destruction, dispersal, and deterministic extinction in competitive communities. *Am Nat* **149:**407–435.

45. **Warren PH.** 1996. Dispersal and destruction in a multiple habitat system: an experimental approach using protist communities. *Oikos* **77:**317–325.

46. **Levin BR, Bull JJ.** 1994. Short-sighted evolution and the virulence of pathogenic microorganisms. *Trends Microbiol* **2:**76–81.

47. **Low BS, Clarke AL, Lockeridge NA.** 1992. Towards an evolutionary demography. *Popul Dev Rev* **18:**1–31.

48. **Cody ML, Overton JM.** 1996. Short-term evolution of reduced dispersal in island plant populations. *J Ecol* **84:**53–61.

49. **Pianka ER.** 1970. On *r*- and *K*-selection. *Am Nat* **104:**592–597.

50. **Lanza VF, Baquero F, de la Cruz F, Coque TM.** 2017. AcCNET (Accessory Genome Constellation Network): comparative genomics software for accessory genome analysis using bipartite networks. *Bioinformatics* **33:**283–285.

51. **Friedenberg NA.** 2003. Experimental evolution of dispersal in spatiotemporally variable microcosms. *Ecol Lett* **6:**953–959.

52. **Hargreaves AL, Eckert CG.** 2014. Evolution of dispersal and mating systems along geographic gradients: implications for shifting ranges. *Funct Ecol* **2:**5–21.

53. **Odling-Smee FJ, Laland KN, Feldman MW.** 2003. *Niche Construction: The Neglected Process in Evolution.* Monographs in Population Biology no. 37. Princeton University Press, Princeton, NJ.

54. **Levin SA.** 1998. Ecosystems and the biosphere as complex adaptive systems. *Ecosystems* **1:**431–436.

55. **Baquero F, Nombela C.** 2012. The microbiome as a human organ. *Clin Microbiol Infect* **18**(Suppl 4):2–4.

56. **Sonnenburg JL, Xu J, Leip DD, Chen CH, Westover BP, Weatherford J, Buhler JD, Gordon JI, Gordon JI.** 2005. Glycan foraging in vivo by an intestine-adapted bacterial symbiont. *Science* **307:**1955–1959.

57. **Sharma NK, Choudhary KK, Bajpai R, Rai AK.** 2010. Freshwater cyanobacterial blooms: causes, consequences and control, p 73–95. *In* El Nemr A (ed), *Impact, Monitoring and Management Impact of Environmental Pollution.* Nova Science Publishers Inc, Hauppauge, NY.

58. **Andrews JH, Harris RF.** 1986. *r*- and *K*-selection and microbial ecology, p 99–147. *In* Nelson KE (ed), *Advances in Microbial Ecology.* Springer US, New York, NY.

59. **Wilson AJ, Morgan ER, Booth M, Norman R, Perkins SE, Hauffe HC, Mideo N, Antonovics J, McCallum H, Fenton A.** 2017. What is a vector? *Philos Trans R Soc Lond B Biol Sci* **372:**20160085.

60. **Dawkins R.** 1982. Replicators and vehicles, p 45–64. *In* King's College Sociobiology Group (ed), *Current Problems in Sociobiology*. Cambridge University Press, Cambridge, United Kingdom.

61. **Baquero F, Tedim AP, Coque TM.** 2013. Antibiotic resistance shaping multi-level population biology of bacteria. *Front Microbiol* **4:**15.

62. **Wade MJ, Kalisz S.** 1990. The causes of natural selection. *Evolution* **44:**1947–1955.

63. **Bell G.** 1997. *The Basics of Selection*, p 31–33. Chapman and Hall, New York, NY.

64. **Schoener TW.** 2011. The newest synthesis: understanding the interplay of evolutionary and ecological dynamics. *Science* **331:**426–429.

65. **Saccheri I, Hanski I.** 2006. Natural selection and population dynamics. *Trends Ecol Evol* **21:**341–347.

66. **Szathmáry E, Smith JM.** 1995. The major evolutionary transitions. *Nature* **374:**227–232.

67. **Bapteste E, O'Malley MA, Beiko RG, Ereshefsky M, Gogarten JP, Franklin-Hall L, Lapointe FJ, Dupré J, Dagan T, Boucher Y, Martin W.** 2009. Prokaryotic evolution and the tree of life are two different things. *Biol Direct* **4:**34.

68. **Antia R, Levin BR, May RM.** 1994. Within-host population dynamics and the evolution and maintenance of microparasite virulence. *Am Nat* **144:**457–472.

69. **Keesing F, Ostfeld RS.** 2012. Disease ecology, p 217–230. *In* Ingram JC, DeClerck F, Rumbaitis del Rio C (ed), *Integrating Ecology and Poverty Reduction: Ecological Dimensions*. Springer, New York, NY.

70. **Anderson RM, May RM, Joysey K, Mollison D, Conway GR, Cartwell R, Thompson HV, Dixon B.** 1986. The invasion, persistence and spread of infectious diseases within animal and plant communities. *Philos Trans R Soc Lond B Biol Sci* **314:**533–570.

71. **Anderson RM.** 1995. Evolutionary pressures in the spread and persistence of infectious agents in vertebrate populations. *Parasitology* **111**(Suppl):S15–S31.

72. **Anderson RM.** 1982. Transmission dynamics and control of infectious disease agents, p 149–176. *In* Anderson RM, May RM (ed), *Population Biology of Infectious Diseases*. Springer, Berlin, Germany.

73. **Anderson RM, May RM.** 1992. *Infectious Diseases of Humans: Dynamics and Control*, vol 28. Oxford University Press, Oxford, United Kingdom.

74. **Read JM, Keeling MJ.** 2003. Disease evolution on networks: the role of contact structure. *Proc Biol Sci* **270:**699–708.

75. **Zhang G, Pérez-Jiménez MJ, Gheorghe M.** 2017. *Real-Life Applications with Membrane Computing*, p 1–9. Springer, Berlin, Germany.

76. **Campos M, Llorens C, Sempere JM, Futami R, Rodriguez I, Carrasco P, Capilla R, Latorre A, Coque TM, Moya A, Baquero F.** 2015. A membrane computing simulator of trans-hierarchical antibiotic resistance evolution dynamics in nested ecological compartments (ARES). *Biol Direct* **10:**41.

77. **Baquero F.** 2017. Basic sciences fertilizing clinical microbiology and infection management. *Clin Infect Dis* **65**(Suppl 1):S80–S83.

78. **Okasha S.** 2012. Emergence, hierarchy and top-down causation in evolutionary biology. *Interface Focus* **2:**49–54.

79. **Hanski I.** 1998. Metapopulation dynamics. *Nature* **396:**41–49.

80. **Zhong W, Priest NK.** 2011. Stress-induced recombination and the mechanism of evolvability. *Behav Ecol Sociobiol* **65:**493–502.

81. **Fagan WF, Cantrell RC, Cosner C.** 1999. How habitat edges change species interactions. *Am Nat* **153:**165–182.

82. **Levin SA (ed).** 2009. *The Princeton Guide to Ecology*, p 780. Princeton University Press, Princeton, NJ.

83. **Brown JH, Kodric-Brown A.** 1977. Turnover rates in insular biogeography: effect of immigration on extinction. *Ecology* **58:**445–449.

84. **Johnson ML, Gaines MS.** 1990. Evolution of dispersal: theoretical models and empirical tests using birds and mammals. *Annu Rev Ecol Syst* **21:**449–480.

85. **Wright S.** 1943. Isolation by distance. *Genetics* **28:**114–138.

86. **Winker K.** 2000. Migration and speciation. *Nature* **404:**36.

87. **Brown JS, Pavlovic NB.** 1992. Evolution in heterogeneous environments: effects of migration on habitat specialization. *Evol Ecol* **6:**360–382.

Natural and Artificial Strategies to Control the Conjugative Transmission of Plasmids

3

MARÍA GETINO[1,2] and FERNANDO DE LA CRUZ[2]

INTRODUCTION

Antibiotics have saved the lives of countless people suffering from bacterial infections since Alexander Fleming discovered penicillin in 1928 (1). Nevertheless, this success was accompanied by the emergence of antibiotic resistance (AbR). It is thought that AbR arose originally as a self-protection mechanism of producer organisms (2). AbR genes rapidly disseminated through the biosphere as a result of the selection pressure established by human application of antibiotics (3). Resistance mechanisms capable of rendering newly discovered drugs ineffective emerged with astonishing speed, rapidly reaching human pathogens and increasingly invalidating newer antimicrobial therapies (4). Altogether, >20,000 potential resistance genes of nearly 400 types have been predicted from bacterial genome sequences (5). The danger created by the ever-increasing number of pathogens resistant to conventional antibiotics is further increased by a significant drop in the development of new antimicrobial compounds (6). This situation demands solutions to prevent the hundreds of thousands of people dying each year as a result of AbR from becoming millions (7).

[1]School of Biosciences and Medicine, University of Surrey, Guildford, United Kingdom; [2]Instituto de Biomedicina y Biotecnología de Cantabria, Universidad de Cantabria–Consejo Superior de Investigaciones Científicas, Santander, Spain.

Microbial Transmission in Biological Processes
Edited by Fernando Baquero, Emilio Bouza, J.A. Gutiérrez-Fuentes, and Teresa M. Coque
© 2018 American Society for Microbiology, Washington, DC
doi:10.1128/microbiolspec.MTBP-0015-2016

Proposed strategies include more-accurate prescription policies and a controlled use and release of antibiotics in animal husbandry and agriculture, restrictions difficult to implement on a global scale (3).

Alternatives to conventional antibiotics are emerging to treat this global crisis. For example, inhibitors of bacterial virulence are promising alternatives with an advantage over antibiosis in that selection for resistance might not occur because pathogen growth would not be impaired (8). Additional lines of attack under development are vaccines (9), phage therapy (10), predatory bacteria (11), and antiplasmid strategies (12–14), among others. In this context, this review focuses on natural and artificial strategies that could be employed in Gram-negative bacteria to control the transmission of conjugative plasmids, the main propagation devices involved in AbR dissemination.

HORIZONTAL GENE TRANSFER

AbR genes are transferred either vertically when bacteria divide or laterally from one bacterium to another through horizontal gene transfer (HGT), an important source of bacterial variability (15). HGT is mediated by mobile genetic elements (MGEs), that is, DNA devices for the intra- or intercellular movement of DNA (16). Intracellular mobility is produced by transposons, DNA fragments with the ability to move from one genome location to another, including different replicons of the same cell. Intercellular mobility occurs by one of three main processes: transformation, conjugation, or transduction. Transformation involves extracellular DNA uptake, integration, and functional expression. Bacteria must be in a physiological state of competence to acquire exogenous DNA, which could be natural or artificially induced. Most naturally transformable bacteria develop competence in response to

specific environmental conditions, such as altered growth conditions, nutrient access, cell density, or starvation (13). Conjugation requires genetic elements encoding the apparatus needed for their transfer from a donor to a recipient cell through direct contact (16). Transduction is mediated by bacteriophages when they accidentally pack segments of host DNA and inject them into a new host. Transduction may be generalized or specialized, depending on whether any gene may be transferred or only those located near the site of prophage integration (17).

BACTERIAL CONJUGATION

Conjugation is arguably the most common mechanism of HGT (18), and that with the broadest host range (19). Encoded either in autonomously replicating conjugative plasmids or in integrative and conjugative elements (ICEs) inserted in the bacterial chromosome, conjugation systems allow the transfer of large DNA fragments containing diverse adaptive traits (20). Indeed, they are major vehicles for the spread of AbR genes (21, 22).

Either double-stranded DNA (dsDNA) or single-stranded DNA (ssDNA) molecules can be transported from donor to recipient cells. dsDNA conjugation was described in Actinobacteria. The translocation mechanism involves a single protein, a plasmid-encoded septal DNA translocase similar to the segregation ATPase FtsK, unlike the complex machinery needed for "classic" ssDNA conjugation (23). Conjugative systems involved in ssDNA conjugation carry two sets of genetic components: mobility (MOB) for conjugative DNA processing, and mating-pair formation (MPF) for DNA delivery through the membranes of donor and recipient bacteria. The MOB component includes an origin of transfer (*oriT*), a short DNA sequence required in *cis* for plasmid transfer (24); a relaxase to initiate conjugation; and a type IV coupling protein (T4CP) to interconnect DNA processing with DNA transport. MPF genes code for a complex of proteins that build the type IV secretion system (T4SS).

Plasmids can be classified into three mobility categories: conjugative, mobilizable, and nonmobilizable. A conjugative plasmid contains the two sets of components necessary for its own transfer, whereas a mobilizable plasmid lacks MPF genes and uses the T4SS of a coresident self-transmissible element, thus escaping from pilus synthesis burden (20). In general, conjugative plasmids are large (>30 kb) and of low copy number, while mobilizable plasmids are small (<15 kb) and have relatively higher copy number. Plasmids unable to transfer by conjugation or mobilization are called nonmobilizable (20). Nevertheless, nonmobilizable plasmids may be transferred by physical association with a transmissible plasmid (the process is called cointegration, if the resulting plasmid maintains the physical association, or conduction, if the two plasmids resolve in recipient cells) (25).

Conjugative Transfer, the Process

The initial requirement for bacterial conjugation is the expression of MPF genes in donor cells. Four MPF classes are found in conjugative systems from *Proteobacteria*: MPF_T (whose prototype is T-DNA transfer system of *Agrobacterium tumefaciens* pTi plasmid), MPF_F (exemplified by conjugative plasmid F), MPF_I (exemplified by IncI plasmid R64), and MPF_G (related to a broad family of ICEs whose prototype is ICE *Hin1056* of *Haemophilus influenzae*) (20). The MPF_T class encodes the simplest T4SS, consisting of 11 proteins called VirB1 to VirB11 from *A. tumefaciens* T4SS (26). The T4SS complex can be divided in four parts: the pilus, the core channel complex, the inner membrane platform, and the cytoplasmic ATPases that supply the energy for pilus biogenesis and substrate transport

(27). The conjugative pilus is the appendage that extends from the donor cell to reach the recipient cells within its proximity and subsequently retracts it to facilitate cell-to-cell contact (28). Retraction has not been demonstrated for all types of pili (29). Pilus morphology determines the ability of plasmids to transfer in liquid media or on solid surfaces (such as biofilms). Plasmids that determine rigid pili (Inc groups M, N, P, and W) or thick flexible pili (Inc groups C, D, F, H, J, T, V, and X) transfer better on solid media, while plasmids encoding thin flexible pili (Inc groups I, B, and K) transfer equally well in both situations (30, 31). This feature, added to plasmid host range (32), and the contribution of pili to establishing bacterial biofilms (33), are important determinants for plasmid dissemination in the environment (22). Once donor-recipient contact is established, the next step in conjugation is DNA processing (Fig. 1), driven by the MOB proteins. Based on MOB sequences and DNA-processing mechanism, transmissible plasmids are classified into six MOB families: MOB_F, MOB_H, MOB_Q, MOB_C, MOB_P, and MOB_V (34). The key protein for DNA transfer initiation, present in all transmissible plasmids, is the relaxase. Together with specific auxiliary factors, the relaxase assembles a nucleoprotein complex on the *oriT* called the relaxosome. The relaxase is directed to the *nic* site within the *oriT* by auxiliary factors, such as TrwA and the chromosomally encoded integration host factor (IHF) in the case of plasmid R388 (35), where the relaxase cleaves the phosphodiester bond of the DNA strand to be transferred (T-strand) (36). The transesterification reaction results in a covalent link between relaxase and ssDNA (37), followed by DNA replication from the 3' end of the cleaved strand, using the complementary circular strand as a template. A helicase domain, usually present at the C terminus of the relaxase domain (34), unwinds DNA to displace the T-strand (38). Then, the relaxase produces a second cleavage at the *nic*

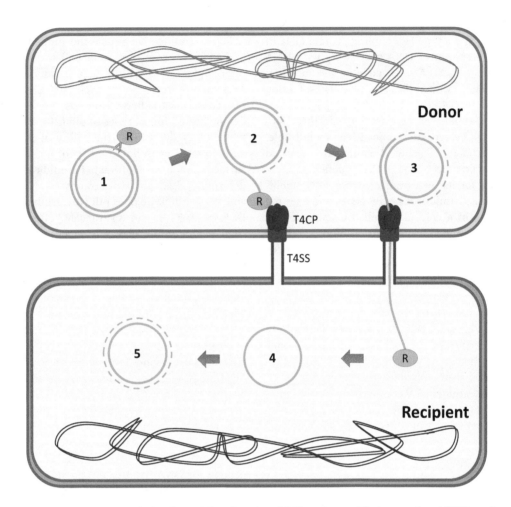

FIGURE 1 DNA processing during bacterial conjugation. (1) The relaxase (R) cleaves plasmid DNA at the *nic* **site and forms a covalent intermediate with the 5′ end of the** *oriT***. (2) The T4SS protein machinery recruits the relaxosome through interaction with the T4CP, while the donor DNA is replicated using the uncleaved DNA strand as a template. (3) The relaxase releases the T-strand by a second cleavage reaction at the** *nic* **site and acts as pilot protein for the ssDNA to be transferred through the T4SS, helped by the T4CP pumping activity. (4) In the recipient cell, the relaxase carries out the reverse nicking reaction to recircularize the T-strand. (5) The transferred ssDNA is replicated to generate a complete copy of the original plasmid.**

site to release the T-strand from the newly formed strand (39).

After the nicking reaction, the T4CP recruits the relaxosome to the T4SS (40) in order to start the DNA transfer process. Then, the nucleoprotein complex is delivered to the inner membrane platform at the base of the T4SS to cross the channel that connects donor with recipient cells (29). According to the shoot-and-pump model (40), once

the relaxase is shot through the channel acting as a pilot protein for the T-strand, T4CP pumps remaining ssDNA using the energy derived from ATP hydrolysis. When a complete copy of plasmid ssDNA reaches the recipient cell, the relaxase recognizes the *nic* site as a termination site and carries out the reverse nicking reaction, resolving the covalent intermediate relaxase-DNA and resulting in recircularization of the T-strand in the recipient cell (41, 42). Finally, a second strand is synthesized by rolling-circle replication to generate a copy of the original conjugative plasmid in the recipient cell, thus turning it into a new donor.

NATURAL STRATEGIES THAT CONTROL CONJUGATION

Several strategies, called eco-evo (based on an ecological and evolutionary perspective), have been explored with the aim of restoring antibiotic susceptibility in the environment (14). Since conjugation is a key mechanism involved in AbR dissemination (18, 22), this review focuses on both natural and artificial strategies to control this process (Fig. 2). Natural strategies can be defined as mechanisms that bacteria already employ in the environment to prevent conjugation (for instance, exclusion systems), while artificial strategies are human-based strategies not used by nature for this purpose (for example, antibodies targeting conjugative relaxases). It is worth noting that environmental factors like temperature, pH, chemical and physical composition, redox status, or moisture, as well as anthropogenic factors (e.g., organic or inorganic pollutants),

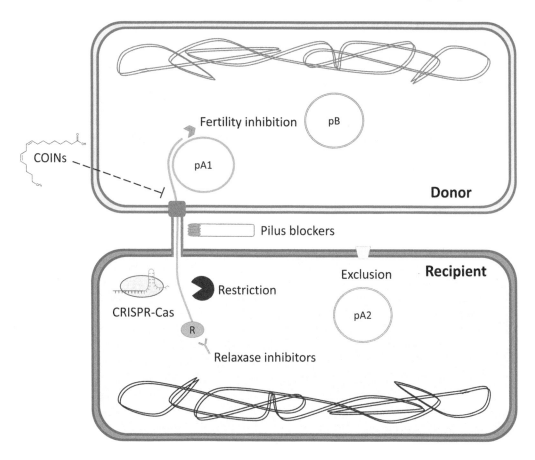

FIGURE 2 **Natural and artificial mechanisms that control the transmission of conjugative plasmids. Natural mechanisms include RM and CRISPR-Cas systems (encoded by the recipient chromosome), exclusion systems (used to prevent the entrance of related plasmids in the same recipient), and fertility inhibition systems (encoded by plasmids in donor bacteria). Artificial mechanisms interfere with key components of the conjugative process, such as the relaxase, the pilus, or conjugation-related ATPases.**

significantly influence conjugation rates (43–45). Besides, the type of environment (human and animal microbiota, rhizosphere, manure, soil, wastewater treatment plants, aquatic environments that receive waste streams, etc.) is also an essential factor determining conjugation dynamics (17, 46). However, these factors are out of this review's scope due to the variability of effects in different conjugative systems and the difficulty of designing a strategy to control conjugation based on environmental factors. The genetic determinants that are the basis of natural strategies can be located in the host chromosome (host strategies) or in the plasmid genome (plasmid strategies). Among host strategies, restriction-modification (RM) and CRISPR-Cas systems are the most common mechanisms to prevent stable acquisition of foreign DNA in bacteria. Conjugative plasmids display mechanisms that regulate their own transfer, block the entry of related plasmids into the same cell, or inhibit conjugative transfer of plasmids present in the same donor bacteria. Regulatory networks for bacterial conjugation comprise a set of complex responses to maximize DNA transport and minimize the burden to cells carrying the conjugative machinery (47). However, plasmid regulatory factors are diverse between different groups of conjugative systems. To give an example, the regulatory proteins encoded by prototype plasmids F, RP4, and R388 bear no homology relationship whatsoever. Another example of this diversity could be the specific antagonistic signaling of the pair cCF10/iCF10 pheromone-inhibitor peptides in the regulation of the conjugative plasmid pCF10 of *Enterococcus faecalis* (48). Therefore, our analysis of plasmid barriers will focus on exclusion and fertility inhibition systems, which are more conserved between different conjugative plasmids.

Host Strategies: Restriction

Restriction was first observed in the 1950s when bacteriophage λ, propagated in *Escherichia coli* B, was found to grow poorly on *E. coli* K-12 (49). RM systems code for a diverse group of enzymes, ubiquitous among prokaryotes, involved in defense against invading genomes, such as phages or plasmids (50). They comprise two opposing enzymatic activities, restriction endonuclease (REase) and methyltransferase (MTase) (51). The REase recognizes and cleaves foreign DNA at a specific site, whereas the MTase confers protection from cleavage to host genome by methylating a defined adenine or cytosine residue within the specificity site. Due to their ability to recognize self from nonself DNA, RM systems are considered a primitive, innate immune system (52). They are classified in four types, based on molecular structure, sequence recognition, cleavage position, and cofactor requirements (53).

RM systems are major players in the coevolutionary interaction between MGEs and their hosts (54). RM systems may have additional roles (51). For example, MGE-encoded RM systems act as toxin-antitoxin stability systems. During cell division, the failure to segregate RM systems efficiently results in postsegregational killing of the progeny lacking the RM-containing plasmids. This is due to the higher stability of the REase (toxin), which attacks the unmodified host genome of the progeny lacking the MTase (antitoxin) (55). Thus, the MGE is stabilized by the RM system and the RM system acquires the ability to be transferred. Although this role contributes to the stability of RM-containing plasmids instead of being a barrier to conjugation, it seems to be a minor role, since only 10% of the plasmids encode RM systems, whereas 69% of the chromosomes do so (54).

While host defense against bacteriophage infection has been extensively described (56), inhibition of bacterial conjugation by RM systems has been reported to a lesser extent. Several reports revealed that inactivation of restriction systems in recipient cells (57–62) or deletion of methylation systems in donor cells (63) increases conjugation frequency, while others showed a reduction in conjugative transfer when the number of restriction sites in the donor plasmid was increased (64–66). Accordingly, the ability of phages and plasmids to escape restriction highlights the importance of RM systems as defense devices against foreign DNA. The mechanisms used in this coevolutionary arms race between bacteria and parasitic DNA molecules to avoid restriction include four different strategies (Table 1). A number of conjugative plasmids encode antirestriction proteins, named Ard (alleviation of restriction of DNA). ArdA and ArdB, encoded by conjugative transposons and plasmids of the IncN, IncI, and IncF groups, are examples of direct inhibitors of REases that mimic DNA after their rapid expression in recipient cells (67, 68). ArdC protein from IncW plasmid pSa protects incoming T-strand by transient occlusion of restriction sites after being pumped into recipient cells (69). Another strategy is the selection of plasmid variants that lost restriction sites, as seems to happen in the case of plasmid RP4 (70). A combination of more than one antirestriction strategy is exemplified by the case of the *E. faecalis* Tn*916*-like conjugative transposons, which confer antimicrobial resistance to both Gram-positive and Gram-negative bacteria. Two reasons for Tn*916*'s broad host range are the presence within the element of *ardA* antirestriction systems and few restriction sites (71). This observation highlights the importance of antirestriction strategies to counteract RM systems of potential hosts, thus increasing the ability of conjugative elements to spread to a greater variability of bacteria.

Host Strategies: CRISPR-Cas

Additional defense systems, sometimes operating synergistically with RM systems, are CRISPR-Cas systems (72). Unlike RM systems, which provide a primitive innate immunity, CRISPR-Cas systems can be thought of as providing adaptive immunity, sequence-directed against foreign elements (73). CRISPR loci, present in 45% of bacterial and 84% of archaeal sequenced genomes (74), consist of an array of repetitive sequences of 30 to 40 bp, partially palindromic, and interspersed by equally short spacer sequences of viral or plasmid origin (75).

The CRISPR-Cas defense mechanism can be divided in two phases: immunization and immunity (76). In the immunization phase, also known as adaptation or spacer acquisition, sequences from the invading genome integrate into the CRISPR array. The acquisition of new spacers provides an efficient response against phages that escape immunity by mutating the target site (77). In the immunity phase, immunity is accomplished in two steps: guide RNA biogenesis, where a

TABLE 1 Antirestriction strategies

Mechanism	Antirestriction strategy	Examples	Reference(s)
Incoming genome modification	Reduction or reorientation of restriction sites	T3 or T7 phages, RP4 plasmid	70, 254, 255
	Incorporation of unusual bases or methylation	Mu or SPβ phages	256
Restriction site occlusion	Transient occlusion of restriction sites by proteins cotransported with the DNA	P1 phage DarA/DarB, IncW plasmids ArdC	69, 257
Host RM system alteration	MTase stimulation to modify incoming DNA	λ phage Ral protein	258
	Destruction of REase cofactors	T3 phage SAMase	259
REase inhibition	Direct inhibition of REases through mimicking DNA size, shape, and electric charge	T7 phage Ocr protein, IncN, IncF, and IncI plasmids ArdA/ArdB	68, 260

CRISPR array is transcribed and processed to generate small CRISPR RNAs (crRNAs); and targeting, in which the spacer in the crRNA serves as a guide to direct cleavage of the complementary sequence at the invading DNA (protospacer) by the Cas nucleases.

Bacteria must distinguish between protospacers of invading genomes and spacers of their CRISPR arrays to avoid cleavage of their own chromosome (78). CRISPR-Cas systems can be classified into three types, based on their Cas content, crRNA biogenesis mechanism, and targeting requirements (79). In type I and II systems, autoimmunity is prevented through a sequence called protospacer adjacent motif (PAM), only present in the invading DNA, upstream of the protospacer. The presence of this sequence is essential for foreign DNA cleavage by Cas nucleases (80). No PAM requirements have been described in type III systems, where autoimmunity inhibition is thought to occur through differential base pairing between crRNA and protospacer, preventing cleavage when full complementarity is detected (81). In addition, Chi sites (8-nucleotide motifs highly enriched in bacterial genomes) limit the acquisition of chromosomal fragments, favoring the acquisition of foreign elements, also more likely fragmented during replication (82). A failure in autoimmunity prevention leads to host death, a consequence that is being exploited for the use of CRISPR-Cas systems as genome-editing tools in both prokaryotes and eukaryotes (83, 84).

Among the numerous emerging applications of CRISPR-Cas systems (85), their ability to attack plasmid DNA during conjugation provides new weapons against AbR dissemination. In their first work, Marraffini and Sontheimer showed that a spacer from a clinical isolate of *Staphylococcus epidermidis*, which matched a region of the relaxase gene of staphylococcal conjugative plasmids, prevented transfer of plasmids containing this sequence by conjugation and transformation (78). Moreover, the CRISPR-Cas target was shown to be DNA instead of RNA by placing

a self-splicing intron in the relaxase target sequence. In this line of research, the analysis of CRISPR spacers related to conjugative plasmids revealed that protospacers are not randomly distributed but display a MOB family-dependent bias. Whereas MOB_P plasmids are usually targeted within the lagging regions, protospacers of the MOB_F family are mostly located in the leading region (the first plasmid section entering the recipient cell). Nevertheless, when conjugative transfer of the MOB_F plasmid F was inhibited using a type I CRISPR-Cas system, the level of protection was independent of the protospacer position and the DNA strand, suggesting that the observed bias depends either on the spacer acquisition phase or on the first regions becoming double-stranded (86). Additional studies demonstrate the conjugation-interfering role of CRISPR-Cas in different bacteria (87) and highlight the importance of these systems in preventing the acquisition of MGEs carrying AbR genes (88). In addition to plasmid transfer inhibition, spacers of plasmid origin could target AbR genes to induce plasmid loss (89) or even trigger AbR pathogen death (90, 91), among other interesting alternatives with countless possibilities.

Other Host Factors Involved in the Control of Conjugation

Recently discovered defense systems against phage infection and bacterial transformation might also be involved in protection against bacterial conjugation. This is the case for prokaryotic Argonaute proteins, homologs to the eukaryotic nucleases involved in RNA interference (92, 93), or bacteriophage exclusion, a mechanism that protects bacteria from phage replication (94, 95).

Besides the previously described defense barriers against incoming DNA, several studies aimed to find additional host barriers to conjugation or potential targets to control the process. Early studies demonstrated the contribution of the basic cellular machinery (replication, protein synthesis, or energy supply) in bacterial conjugation (96). In particular, DNA polymerase III was shown to be required in recipient cells for the synthesis of the transferred complementary strand (97), as well as in donors to replace the transferred strand (98). Another example is helicase PcrA of *Bacillus subtilis*, needed for ICE*Bs1* DNA unwinding after nicking (99). Although its *E. coli* homolog, UvrD, is not essential for growth, PcrA is a second helicase essential for *B. subtilis* viability (100). Nevertheless, targeting essential enzymes as a barrier to conjugation would kill the host, acting therefore like a conventional antibiotic (101). To avoid the selective pressure that increases the probability of AbR emergence, nonessential functions are preferred to control bacterial conjugation. This may be the case of the stationary-phase sigma factor RpoS, which regulates ICE*clc* excision in *Pseudomonas knackmussii* and is required for its conjugative transfer (102).

A mechanism potentially deleterious for conjugation as well as for recipient cell viability is the SOS response. The SOS response is stimulated by the appearance of ssDNA and its interaction with the RecA protein, which inactivates the LexA repressor, thereby inducing several genes involved in DNA repair, recombination, and mutagenesis (103). Some conjugative plasmids are adapted to counteract the SOS response through a plasmid SOS interference (*psi*) system that inhibits RecA binding to ssDNA (104). Similarly, the SOS response to DNA damage inactivates the LexA repressor homolog, present in several ICEs, that controls integrase expression and ICE propagation (105). Therefore, the SOS response can be a positive or a negative regulator of bacterial conjugation.

Host factors involved in regulation of bacterial conjugation are exemplified by the case of plasmid F, a narrow-host-range plasmid well adapted to *E. coli* (106). While broad-host-range plasmids regulate their transfer mostly through plasmid-encoded repressors (107), narrow-host-range plasmids rely on several host-encoded regulatory factors that act at DNA, RNA, or protein levels (Table 2).

The first systematic screening for host genes involved in conjugation was carried out by Pérez-Mendoza and de la Cruz (108) using two collections of *E. coli* mutants as recipient cells: the Keio collection of 3,908 single-gene deletion mutants and a collection of 20,000 random transposon insertion mutants, which covered >99% of the *E. coli* nonessential genome. They studied the transfer of the broad-host-range IncW plasmid R388 on solid media through an automated conjugation assay based on the emission of luminescence by transconjugant bacteria. The work indicated that no nonessential recipient genes play a crucial role in conjugation. Therefore, required genes can be either essential for cell growth or redundant. The latter could be the case for the *uvrD* mutant, which showed 41% of wild-type conjugative transfer. UvrD is DNA helicase II, involved in rolling-circle replication of many plasmids (109). Despite being an interesting candidate, its barely significant effect suggested the involvement of an alternative helicase. Besides *uvrD* mutation, only mutations in lipopolysaccharide (LPS) biosynthesis showed a significant but modest decrease in R388 transfer (6 to 32% of wild type). A more drastic effect was observed on F plasmid liquid transfer, suggesting a role for LPS in mating-pair stabilization. Accordingly, several mutants were described that affect membrane integrity and were defective in recipient ability while increasing susceptibility to antibiotics, detergents, or phages. Among them were particular mutants of LPS biosynthesis or the outer membrane protein OmpA (110–117). Other reports characterized the effect of *rfa* (LPS synthesis) and *ompA* mutants on conjugation, proposing an adhesin at the F pilus tip as the receptor of its specific LPS group (118). More recently, recipient LPS was established as the specific receptor for the PilV adhesin of IncI plasmid R64 during liquid conjugation (119), while

TABLE 2 Host-encoded factors involved in conjugative transfer of IncF plasmids

Level	Host factor	Regulatory function	Reference(s)
DNA	ArcA/ArcB	Two-component regulatory system that activates transfer in response to oxygen levels	261
	SdhABCD	Succinate dehydrogenase that has a repressive effect under aerobic conditions, probably by regulating transcription of the activator TraJ	261
	Dam	Methylase that modifies certain promoter regions, changing their sensitivity to binding of activators, such as the leucine regulator Lrp to *traJ* promoter	262
	H-NS	Global repressor that silences newly acquired DNA, including transfer genes	263
	RpoS/RpoH	Alternate sigma factors that stimulate transcription from H-NS silenced promoters	264, 265
	FIS	Activator or repressor, depending on whether it acts alone or in competition with H-NS	266
	IHF	Transcriptional activator of transfer genes, besides its primary role as part of the relaxosome architecture	35, 267
	CRP	The cyclic AMP receptor is also a positive regulator of *traJ* expression in response to glucose levels	268
	Unknown	Host-encoded regulator involved in F transfer repression during stationary phase	269
RNA	RNase E	Ribonuclease that cleaves the antisense RNA FinP (downregulates the translation of the activator TraJ)	139
	Hfq	Global regulator that binds *traJ* mRNA, promoting its degradation	270
Protein	HslV/HslU	Heat shock protease-chaperone pair involved in TraJ degradation mediated by the two-component system CpxAR in response to extracytoplasmic stress	271
	GroEL	Chaperonin that interacts with TraJ, promoting its proteolysis	272

OmpA was shown to interact with F plasmid TraN for mating-pair stabilization (120).

Additional approaches using transposon mutagenesis revealed the nitrogen-related phosphotransferase system as the responsible mechanism for conjugative transfer inhibition of IncP-9 naphthalene catabolic plasmid pNAH7 from *E. coli* to *Pseudomonas putida* (121). Besides, combining transposon mutagenesis and massive sequencing (122), Johnson and Grossman found that there were no nonessential genes crucial for *B. subtilis* ICE*Bs1* conjugation (123). Functions slightly affecting the process were associated with membrane composition, agreeing with previous reports.

Although this review focuses on conjugative plasmids from Gram-negative bacteria, Gram-positive hosts also provide useful data on conjugation control. Gram-negative bacteria display a complex T4SS spanning two membranes with a cell-surface-attached filamentous pilus. In contrast, Gram-positive systems display a simpler T4SS for ssDNA

translocation across their single cytoplasmic membrane, with a peptidoglycan hydrolase for local digestion of the cell wall, and adhesins that mediate cell contact (124). The signal for initiating conjugal transfer remains unknown in Gram-negative bacteria (125). On the contrary, many plasmids from Gram-positive bacteria rely on secreted signaling peptides called pheromones to initiate conjugation (for instance, *E. faecalis* plasmids pAD1 and pCF10). These pheromones, and the machinery needed for their processing and secretion, are encoded by the chromosome of recipient bacteria (126). The previously mentioned ICE*Bs1* from *B. subtilis* uses an opposite mechanism that requires the uptake of inhibitory peptides by recipient cells, using a host-encoded oligopeptide permease (127).

Plasmid Strategies: Exclusion

The exclusion phenomenon was first observed when exponentially growing cells harboring plasmid F acted as poor conjugation recipients (128). This phenotype, later called "superinfection immunity" (129), was the combination of two independent mechanisms, plasmid incompatibility and exclusion. Both phenomena refer to an interference between related sex factors, associated with replication and conjugation, respectively (130). Plasmid F contains two exclusion systems, surface exclusion and entry exclusion, later considered as prototypes for all others. Surface exclusion acts through the outer membrane protein TraT, by reducing the ability of recipient cells (~10-fold) to form stable mating aggregates, whereas entry exclusion involves the recipient inner membrane protein TraS, which inhibits DNA transfer (~100-fold) after mating pairs have stabilized (131, 132). The precise mechanism of action remains unclear in both cases. Some hypotheses proposed candidates for the TraT receptor in donor cells, including pilins, a hypothetical adhesin at the pilus tip, or the mating-pair stabilization protein TraN. However, none was confirmed (118, 133). The mechanism of TraS exclusion involves the inner membrane protein TraG in donor cells (134). TraG-TraS recognition was later confirmed, suggesting that TraG is translocated into recipient cells for transfer initiation, a process blocked by TraS (135). However, the interacting partner in conjugative plasmids not related to F is unknown, although TraG-VirB6 similarities point to VirB6 as the TraS counterpart (136).

All conjugative plasmids contain at least one exclusion gene, usually TraS-like, indicating their importance for the conjugative element. Exclusion systems may be used to prevent competition among identical plasmid backbones, for donor cells to avoid uneconomical excess of DNA transfer, or for recipient cells to prevent death by lethal zygosis (an excess of conjugative cell contacts causing membrane damage). Interestingly, only IncF and IncH plasmids, which produce pili that are firmly attached to the donor cell, encode both types of exclusion systems, while plasmids whose pili detach easily from the cell express only entry exclusion (136).

Plasmid Strategies: Fertility Inhibition

Fertility inhibition was discovered when certain plasmids carrying multiple AbR determinants were introduced in cells containing plasmid F (137). These R plasmids were IncFII plasmids that produced protein FinO. FinO reduced F transfer by increasing intracellular levels of the antisense RNA FinP (138). FinP RNA specifically downregulates *traJ* mRNA translation, whose product is a transcriptional activator of the transfer region. FinO binds FinP and *traJ* mRNA helping duplex formation, which triggers *traJ* mRNA cleavage by RNase III and protects FinP from degradation by RNase E (139, 140). The F plasmid is naturally derepressed due to *finO* insertional inactivation by insertion sequence IS*3*, resulting in low levels of FinP (141). Therefore, the FinOP system results in a small fraction of cells being transfer competent, contributing to regulate the balance between conjugative transfer and plasmid burden (including metabolic overhead of constitutive expression and vulnerability to pilus-specific phages) in IncF plasmids. The absence of FinOP regulation in early transconjugant cells produces a transient epidemic spread that ensures infection of the recipient cell population (106).

Besides the FinOP autoregulatory mechanism, which also affects other IncF plasmids due to FinO *trans* activity, additional fertility inhibition systems were identified that reduce conjugative transfer of unrelated coresident plasmids (142). These mechanisms may play a role as competition tools for colonization of new hosts (143). Eleven functions from different plasmid groups have been associated with fertility inhibition of IncF, IncW, IncP, and T-DNA of *A. tumefaciens* pTi plasmid, as schematized in Fig. 3.

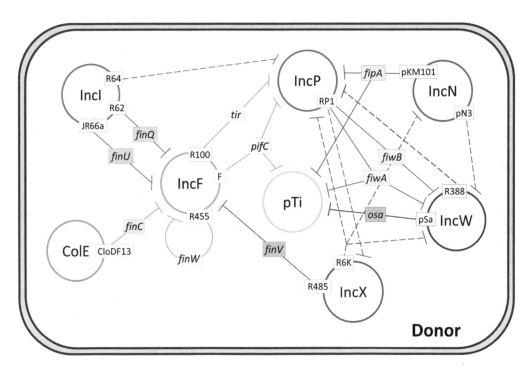

FIGURE 3 Network of interactions between conjugative plasmids that affects their conjugation capacity. Plasmid incompatibility groups are represented by colored circles. Continuous lines show fertility inhibition systems caused by genes in colored rectangles from plasmids in white boxes. Dashed lines show fertility inhibition systems caused by unidentified genes from plasmids in white boxes. See text for further details.

Transfer Inhibition of IncF Plasmids

Similar to the FinOP system, the FinQ and FinW systems act at the RNA level but independently of the main regulator TraJ. FinQ is encoded by IncI1 plasmids and acts via Rho-independent transcription termination at several sites of the *tra* operon (142–146). FinW is present in IncFI plasmids such as R455 and reduces transcription of TraM (142, 143, 145), a regulator activated by TraJ and essential for DNA processing during F transfer (147). FinC, FinU, and FinV fertility inhibition systems act posttranscriptionally. FinC is expressed by the mobilizable plasmid CloDF13 (which uses its own T4CP), probably to inhibit the function of the helper F T4CP during CloDF13 transfer (148). FinU and FinV are encoded by IncI1 plasmid JR66a and IncX plasmid R485, respectively. Since FinU inhibited both pilus assembly and entry exclusion,

it was suggested to affect transcription of the *tra* operon (143). Since transcription reduction was not proportional to the observed effect, the primary target of FinU was suggested to be the translation or function of one or more transfer proteins (145). FinV reduced pilus formation but did not produce an effect on surface exclusion (143). Therefore, it was suggested to act posttranscriptionally, affecting the activity of one of the proteins required for pilus assembly (145).

Transfer Inhibition of IncW Plasmids

The elements *fiwA* and *fiwB*, encoded by IncP1α plasmids such as RP1, inhibit transfer of IncW plasmids (149–151). When acting together, they reduce R388 conjugation 1 million times. While *fiwA* affects only R388 transferability, *fiwB* also affects pilus production, conferring resistance to PR4 bacteriophage (150). Unidentified genes in the IncX plasmid R6K also inhibited the fertility of IncW plasmid R388 (149) and IncN plasmid R46 (152). Similarly, IncP plasmid RP4 reduced conjugal transfer of the rhizobial plasmids pRmeGR4a and pRmeGR4b (153).

Transfer Inhibition of IncP Plasmids
IncP plasmids are targets of fertility inhibition as well. The IncI plasmid R64 encodes a function that inhibits IncP plasmid RP4 conjugative transfer up to 100-fold (154). IncX plasmid R6K and IncP plasmid RP1 showed reciprocal fertility inhibition through an unknown mechanism that resembled the FinOP regulation system (149). The first IncN plasmids reported to inhibit IncP plasmids' fertility were pN3 (149) and R390, which also inhibited transfer of IncW plasmid pSa (155). Fertility inhibition of IncP plasmids (or *fip*) was localized in IncN plasmid pKM101, which reduced RP1 transfer by 10,000-fold (156). The absence of effect in pilus synthesis or entry exclusion suggested that *fip* acted in a different way than the FinOP system. An apparently independent function was found in F plasmid that inhibits plasmid RP4 conjugative transfer 1,000-fold (157). It was identified as *pifC* (or *repC*), a gene involved in the initiation of F replication (158) and in the regulation of *pif* operon expression (phage interference function) (159). PifC inhibited both RP4 conjugation and RP4-assisted mobilization (160). As occurred with FipA of pKM101, PifC inhibition did not affect exclusion or pilus synthesis. A *pifC* functional homolog named *tir* (transfer inhibition of RP4) was discovered in the replication region of IncF plasmid R100 (161). The target of FipA and PifC in IncP plasmids was TraG, the T4CP that connects the relaxosome with the T4SS. Both proteins inhibited RSF1010 mobilization (which uses TraG of RP1), while CloDF13 mobilization (which codes for its own T4CP) was not affected. In addition, IncN-assisted RSF1010 mobilization enhanced by overexpression of *traG* was lost in the presence of *fipA* or *pifC* (162).

Transfer Inhibition of pTi Plasmid's T-DNA
IncW plasmid pSa abolished the plant tumor-inducing activity of the pTi's T-DNA of *A. tumefaciens* (163, 164). This suppressive activity was attributed to the *osa* gene (oncogenic suppression activity) (165). In contrast, the oncogenic suppression caused by IncQ mobilizable plasmids seemed to act by recruiting T-DNA's MPF for mobilization and competing for transfer more efficiently than T-DNA (166–169). Osa protein shows homology to FiwA from RP1 (170), responsible for IncW fertility inhibition (151), and was located at the bacterial inner membrane (171). Osa mode of action was related to export inhibition of VirE2 (172), a protein involved in T-DNA endonuclease protection and transport (173). Export of VirE3 and VirF virulence proteins was blocked by Osa (174). Afterwards, IncQ plasmid RSF1010 mobilization by T-DNA's transfer system was confirmed to be reduced by Osa (169). By the use of a transfer DNA immunoprecipitation assay, Cascales et al. (175) discovered that both IncQ mobilizable plasmids (which use the same pathway as T-DNA) and Osa fertility inhibitor suppressed plant tumorigenesis through inhibition of T-DNA and VirE2 binding to the T4CP (VirD4) receptor, blocking their passage through *A. tumefaciens* T4SS. In contrast to IncQ plasmids, which were proposed to block T-DNA's T4CP as a competing substrate with higher copy number and affinity for T4SS than T-DNA (167), Osa exerted its effects by modulating VirD4 receptor activity through direct protein-protein interaction. As occurred with FipA and PifC, Osa only inhibited mobilization of plasmids lacking their own T4CP (such as RSF1010), whereas mobilization of plasmids carrying their own T4CP (such as CloDF13) was not affected, thus confirming previous results (175). Recently, Osa crystal structure was solved

and shown to belong to the ParB/Srx super-family (176). ATPase and DNase activities were discovered within its active site, activities that were common to their homologs (fertility inhibition protein ICE1056Fin of *H. influenzae* ICEHin1056 and partition system elements KorB from IncP1α plasmid RK2 and ParB from bacteriophage P1). In addition, it was shown that T-DNA transfer was inhibited by Osa homologs ICE1056Fin and FiwA, and even by the unrelated fertility inhibition factors FipA and PifC. Immunoprecipitation and Western blot analysis showed Osa interaction with two other T4SS components, VirB4 and VirB11 ATPases. By *in vitro* reconstitution of a partial T4SS (comprising VirB4, VirB11, and Osa), degradation of T-DNA covalently bound to VirD2 relaxase was observed. This observation has placed Osa DNase activity as a key function of a fertility inhibition mechanistic model (176).

ARTIFICIAL STRATEGIES TO CONTROL CONJUGATION

Conjugation inhibitors (COINs) have been employed to target specific components of the conjugation machinery, such as conjugative relaxases or the pilus tip. Other compounds considered to be COINs inhibited conjugative transfer of several plasmids in different hosts either indirectly, by affecting bacterial growth, or directly, by targeting a common conjugative function, such as T4SS.

Relaxase Inhibitors

Garcillán-Barcia et al. obtained intracellular antibodies (intrabodies) able to inhibit conjugal transfer of plasmid R388 by blocking relaxase activity in recipient cells (42). After mice were immunized with TrwC relaxase, immunoglobulin variable sequences were PCR-amplified from mice mRNA, assembled as scFv (single-chain variable fragment) antibodies, and cloned into an M13 phagemid vector fused to pIII protein. The resulting library of phagemids was submitted to rounds of panning against the purified relaxase immobilized onto ELISA plates, to select antibodies that bind the relaxase more efficiently. The antibody with higher affinity for TrwC was expressed in an *E. coli* strain carrying mutations in the major disulfide bond reduction systems to allow intrabody folding and stability in the reducing cytoplasm of bacteria. It was used as a recipient in an R388 mating experiment, obtaining a 20-fold reduction in transfer frequency compared to a control expressing an unrelated intrabody. To search *in vivo* for more-potent intrabodies able to directly inhibit R388 conjugation, a second library from the first round of panning was expressed in recipient cells. The screening was performed by the use of a high-throughput conjugation assay that relies on the emission of luminescence in transconjugant cells (177). Several intrabodies inhibited R388 conjugation from 40- to 10,000-fold, confirming that R388 relaxase carried out an important function in recipient cells that could be blocked as a viable strategy to prevent plasmid transmission. When CloDF13 mobilization by R388 was tested, no change was detected, due to the usage of its own relaxase (MobC). An interesting broad-range intrabody was discovered that also reduced conjugative transfer of MOB$_F$ plasmids pKM101 and F, whose relaxase domains are 51 and 37% identical to TrwC, respectively. In addition, by mapping the epitopes recognized by one of the intrabodies, the R388 mechanism to terminate conjugative DNA processing was clarified, establishing the second catalytic tyrosine of the relaxase as an important player in this reaction. Although intrabodies are not the most suitable therapeutic candidates for conjugation control due to the pharmacokinetic problems of any macromolecule as a drug, the recognized epitopes of the relaxase could be targeted by other means in order to generate better applicable COINs.

Relaxase activity of F plasmid TraI was targeted *in vitro* by bisphosphonates, a set of small molecules that could apparently interfere with the relaxase active site by mimicking a covalent phosphotyrosine intermediate (178). Two of the most potent compounds were promising hits because they had already been approved for bone loss treatment, a fact that would facilitate their inclusion into the market. However, besides inhibition of F transfer *in vivo*, they also caused unexpected selective death of bacteria containing both a catalytically active TraI and F plasmid. Moreover, it was later concluded that bisphosphonates act as mere chelating agents that could affect any metal-dependent cellular process (179).

Pilus Blockers

Donor-recipient contact, the first step for plasmid conjugative transmission, can be inhibited by interfering with the function of the conjugative pilus (Fig. 4). The best-known inhibitors of conjugation by blocking conjugative pili are bacteriophages. Some DNA and RNA bacteriophages use conjugative pili as receptors to infect bacteria containing certain plasmids. The attachment of these phages to conjugative pili can obstruct potential donor-recipient contacts. This section will focus on COIN activity of male-specific bacteriophages without lytic activity, although phages inducing bacterial lysis possess high potential as antimicrobials against AbR bacteria. In fact, the male-specific phage PRD1, with lytic activity against bacteria containing IncP plasmids, was described as an effective plasmid-curing agent. It reduced the frequency of AbR bacteria even under selective pressure for plasmid maintenance, which promoted the emergence of conjugation-deficient mutants resistant to PRD1 (180, 181). Furthermore, lytic phages cause faster extinction of conjugative plasmids in bacterial populations, probably due to selection for phage resistance mutations that increase genetic burden, indirectly affecting plasmid stability (182). Although lytic phages have been

amply studied for their use in phage therapy, nonlytic bacteriophages infecting *Pseudomonas aeruginosa*, such as the filamentous Pf3 and Pf1 phages, could also be effective as antimicrobial adjuvants thanks to their ability to increase susceptibility to antibiotics (183). A similar effect was observed when Boeke et al. (184) expressed the pIII protein of F-specific filamentous phages, involved in pilus recognition. pIII causes pleiotropic effects in bacterial membranes, including increased sensitivity to detergents, antibiotics, and colicins and even a reduction in F conjugation and male-specific phage infection, probably by blocking pilus retraction.

The first report about the COIN activity of bacteriophages originates from an investigation on pilus function. After Brinton et al. (185) suggested an association between RNA phage receptors and transport of genetic material, Knolle (186) found that an inactivated RNA phage (called fr) interfered with F conjugation in the same way that mating partially prevented phage invasion. Similar results were obtained with phages f1 and f2 as mating inhibitors, which attach to the tip and the sides of the F pilus, respectively (187). F-specific DNA and RNA phages (M13 and R17) were employed by Novotny et al. (188) to prevent the formation of mating pairs, providing evidence that supports F pilus as the common element involved in an early step of both phage infection and conjugation. To discard nonspecific inhibition of bacterial growth caused by phages, transfer of IncF or IncI plasmids from the same donor cell was blocked by inactivated F- or I-specific bacteriophages, respectively (189). Using a cell counter to measure mating pairs, Ou (190) demonstrated that phage f1 inhibited MPF function completely, while MS2 did so only partially. Since the filamentous DNA phage f1 attaches to the F pilus tip while the RNA bacteriophage MS2 attaches laterally along the pilus, the pilus tip was established as the specific attachment mating site. Schreil and Christensen (191) confirmed that MS2 interfered with F con-

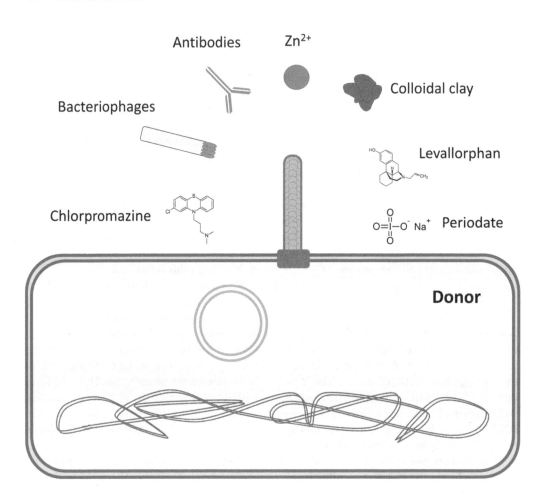

FIGURE 4 Artificial inhibitors of donor-recipient contact (pilus blockers). The tranquilizer chlorpromazine prevents plasmid conjugation and phage infection, possibly by modifying membrane topology. Male-specific bacteriophages bind the pilus tip through their pIII protein, blocking MPF and biofilm formation. Antibodies against conjugative pilus inhibit conjugation of specific plasmids. Zn^{2+} in the mating medium blocks F pilus contact with Zn^{2+}-containing receptor sites. Colloidal clay forms a coating on bacterial cells preventing liquid mating, phage infection, and predation. The opioid levallorphan inhibits MPF and adsorption of male-specific bacteriophages, probably by damaging pilus or bacterial membrane. Sodium periodate alters F pili, inhibiting donor fertility and bacteriophage infection. See the section on pilus blockers in the text for additional information.

jugation, but not due to competition for a common transport channel. Moreover, they disagreed with the reverse effect stated by Knolle (186), noticing that conjugation did not affect MS2 invasion.

A more recent study (192) revealed that M13 inhibition of F conjugation involved physical occlusion of the conjugative pilus by phage particles. Exogenous addition of pIII soluble fragment inhibited conjugation at nanomolar concentrations, whereas addition of the nonspecific protein bovine serum albumin did not. This result suggested that the effect was mediated by the phage coat protein pIII, known to interact with the F pilus (193). The concentration of pIII needed to inhibit F conjugation was 1,000-fold higher than the number of nonreplicating phage particles. The apparent higher affinity of phage particles when compared to isolated pIII protein could be due to cooperation between more than one pIII protein monomer to bind the pilus when they are attached to the phage structure, or to the irreversibility of the binding reaction in the case of phage particles. Lin et al. (192) also observed a 5-fold reduction in donor ability when bacteria were infected with replicating phages, probably due to decreased pilus elaboration. This effect could be important at low phage concentrations, when physical occlusion is less relevant. By constructing a chimeric phage in which the M13 N-terminal domain of pIII was substituted by the homologous sequence of If1 phage, M13 binding specificity was changed from F pilus to I pilus. Consequently, the chimeric phage inhibited conjugative transfer of IncI plasmids instead of F. They also presented a quantitative model for conjugation in the presence of phages that accurately described their COIN effect. Unlike other COINs, bacteriophages have the advantage of potential coevolution in case resistant bacteria appear.

A kinetic competition study between conjugation and M13 infection suggested that phage multiplicity of infection has to be high for the phages to act as effective antagonists to conjugation. At lower phage concentrations, conjugation persists despite phage inhibition, even in the absence of selective pressure (194). In spatially structured populations, such as surface-associated colonies and biofilms, M13 protein pIII effectively inhibited F conjugation. Moreover, spatial structure itself suppressed F conjugation due to isolation of donor and recipient populations, restricting conjugation to boundaries between them (195).

Besides conjugation and phage infection, conjugative pili are involved in the elaboration of biofilms, important targets in the battle against resistance (33). Therefore, bacteriophages affecting F conjugation could also prevent biofilm formation. Actually, male-specific filamentous DNA bacteriophage f1 prevented early biofilm formation by *E. coli* carrying F plasmid. Additionally, the fact that the RNA bacteriophage MS2 did not cause an inhibitory effect suggested that the pilus tip, not the sides, was important for early biofilm formation (196).

Antibodies directed against conjugative pili that are able to inhibit transfer of plasmids even more specifically than bacteriophages have been used to identify closely related resistance factors by analyzing the degree of inhibition (197). The results of this work agreed with previous serological analysis of sex pili detected through antigen-antibody reactions and observed by electron microscopy (198).

Other COINs could interfere with elaboration of mating pairs, either by blocking pilus tip in donors or pilus receptor in recipients or through nonspecific disorganization of bacterial membranes. A case in point is Zn^{2+}, which seemed contradictory at the start. First, Zn^{2+} prevented phage M13 adsorption to F pilus (199). Then, a reduction in F donor fertility was shown, probably by blocking pilus tip, thus inhibiting its interaction with recipient cells (200). Conversely, incubation with Zn^{2+} before mating enhanced the ability of recipients to form mating pairs (201). These paradoxical effects were explained by the use of the Zn^{2+} chelator orthophenanthroline (202). Zn^{2+} is probably involved in the formation of receptor sites on the recipient surface, and the initial contact could occur between the pilus tip and Zn^{2+} of receptor sites. Therefore, pretreatment of recipient cells increased their fertility through Zn^{2+} incorporation. However, an excess of Zn^{2+} in the mating medium would compete for the tips of F pili, hindering their access to receptor sites. The reduction of Zn^{2+} availability by the mentioned chelating agent drastically decreased conjugation, mainly acting during MPF.

Unlike Zn^{2+}, the effect caused by periodate in F donors was irreversible (203). After donor pretreatment, the number of transconjugant cells was greatly reduced, whereas treatment of recipient cells had no significant effect. Perborate and persulfate also decreased donor fertility, but to a lesser extent. The fact that addition of periodate to a mating in progress did not prevent conjugation between mating pairs already formed suggested an effect on MPF, probably by altering the surface of donor cells via polysaccharide oxidation. Consistent with this observation, Dettori et al. (204) showed that periodate also inhibits the adsorption of RNA bacteriophages to the sides of F pili. Consequently, an alteration of F pili seems to inhibit both donor fertility and bacteriophage infection (200).

The morphine derivative levallorphan, like Zn^{2+} and periodate, inhibited adsorption of phage MS2 to F pili (205). This inhibition was comparable to inhibition of MPF during R-factor transfer from *Proteus rettgeri* (now *Providencia rettgeri*) to *E. coli*, since both effects can be observed at the same concentration of levallorphan. Both inhibitory effects, on phage adsorption and conjugation, could be caused by damage of F pilus or the whole bacterial membrane (206). The tranquilizer chlorpromazine also reduced both IncF plasmid conjugative transfer and adsorption of male-specific bacteriophages (207). Since this is a cationic amphipathic molecule, it could act by modifying membrane topology through its insertion in the lipid bilayer. Another COIN probably affecting MPF is ammonium (153). It inhibited conjugative transfer of the rhizobial plasmid pRmeGR4a and pRmeGR4a-assisted mobilization of pRmeGR4b between *Rhizobium meliloti* strains. However, ammonium did not affect transmission of IncP plasmid RP4 or the rhizobial plasmids to *A. tumefaciens*. Thus, its effect seemed to take place on *R. meliloti* recipient cells, probably on their surface, but not on the transfer machinery.

An inert barrier between donors and recipients is an additional possibility to control bacterial conjugation. Colloidal clay, typically present in natural waters, prevented the transfer of IncF plasmid R1drd19 by forming a coating on bacterial cells (208). This clay envelope was also responsible for *E. coli*

protection from bacteriophage infection and bacterial predation (209, 210). In contrast, plasmids that promote conjugation less efficiently in liquid, such as IncP plasmid RP4, enhanced their transfer in water containing nanoalumina particles. In the presence of these particles, RP4 upregulated the expression of genes required for MPF (211). An unspecified component of *E. coli* cell wall was also described as an inhibitor of conjugal transfer. In this case, the inhibitory mechanism presumably involved competence between cell wall components and actual partners on the surface of cells, thereby preventing MPF (212, 213).

Nonspecific COINs

Bisphosphonates were first described as relaxase-specific inhibitors (178) but then reappraised as chelating agents (179). Similarly, other reported COINs were later revealed as inhibitors of different cellular processes. For instance, the ability of some plasmid-curing agents to inhibit conjugative transfer is easily attributable to their antiplasmid effect, which favors the growth of plasmid-free cells (214). The increased sensitivity of *E. coli* containing F plasmid to bile salts and SDS represents another example of this effect. While plasmid-free cells are resistant to these toxic detergents, cells with an active system for pilin secretion are more susceptible to their entry through the T4SS pore (215). A similar behavior was found by overexpressing RP4 genes, which caused enhanced cell permeability (216). Another interesting antiplasmid effect is mediated by the type VI secretion system (T6SS). T6SSs are produced by Gram-negative bacteria to kill prokaryotic and eukaryotic cells through contact-dependent delivery of toxic effectors (217). *P. aeruginosa* T6SS is assembled in response to T6SS attacks by competing bacteria in microbial communities (218). Besides T6SS, T4SS structural proteins of plasmid RP4 triggered *P. aeruginosa* attacks by T6SS (219). The work suggested that these donor-directed counterattacks are induced at MPF-mediated membrane perturbations in *P. aeruginosa* recipients to potentially block the acquisition of foreign DNA. Thus, T6SS would represent a new type of immune system against HGT, through a mechanism that indirectly inhibits conjugative transfer by killing donor cells.

Several antimicrobial drugs, even at subinhibitory concentrations, act as inhibitors of plasmid conjugative transfer. However, their lethal effects in donors and recipients, or the absence of COIN activity in nongrowing bacteria, suggested that these compounds interfere with essential bacterial functions rather than recognizing a specific plasmid target (220, 221). In fact, most of these antibiotics act on cellular functions, such as DNA replication, transcription, translation, or membrane integrity, which are also involved in conjugation (43). Similarly, COIN activity of other compounds could be related to their antibacterial activity. This is the case with nitrofurans (222) and pipemidic acid (223), which inhibited transfer of several plasmids in different hosts by interfering with DNA replication. Moreover, copper surfaces inhibit conjugal transfer indirectly (224), presumably by killing bacteria through DNA and membrane damage (225–227). Epigallocatechin gallate, an antimicrobial component of tea, inhibited conjugative transfer of plasmid R100 in *E. coli* (228). In addition, the phenolic compounds rottlerin and "the red compound" extracted from the plant *Mallotus philippensis* inhibit transfer of several plasmids at subinhibitory concentrations (229). Likewise, *Carica papaya* seed macerate, containing a previously detected antibacterial substance (230), was considered a COIN for a *Salmonella enterica* serovar Typhimurium conjugative plasmid in the mouse digestive tract at nonlethal concentrations (231). Another example could be sodium propionate, produced by intestinal bacteria and abundant in the large intestine. It was found to reduce the transfer frequency of IncF plasmid pSLT in the mouse

intestine (232). It also presented antibacterial properties against several microorganisms (233).

On the contrary, subinhibitory concentrations of certain antimicrobial agents can indirectly promote conjugation (234). For example, DNA damage caused by ciprofloxacin or mitomycin C induced SOS response, which is responsible for upregulating the excision and transfer of SXT ICE from *Vibrio cholerae* (235). In an SOS-independent manner, conjugative transposons from *Bacteroides* and *E. faecalis* increased their transfer when exposed to low concentrations of tetracycline (236, 237). Similarly, β-lactams stimulated the formation of bacterial aggregates, thus increasing conjugative transfer of a plasmid from *S. aureus* (238).

Unsaturated Fatty Acids

The first systematic search for COINs used conjugative plasmid R388 in *E. coli* as a model system (177). A luminescence-based high-throughput assay was used to measure R388 conjugation in the presence of >12,000 microbial extracts containing a variety of bioactive compounds. A control assay discarded compounds affecting bacterial growth, plasmid stability, or light emission. The first hits were oleic and linoleic acids, C_{18} unsaturated fatty acids (uFAs) containing one or two double bonds, respectively. The most potent compound was an atypical fatty acid named dehydrocrepenynic acid (DHCA), identified in an extract from the fungus *Sistotrema sernanderi*. DHCA is a C_{18} fatty acid with double bonds at positions 9 and 14 and a triple bond at position 12. Conjugation analysis using related compounds (including saturated fatty acids), suggested that a carboxylic group, a long carbon chain, and a double bond position were important features of COINs. Plasmids affected by linoleic acid and DHCA were R388 and pOX38, whereas RP4 or R6K were not. The fact that some plasmids were not affected argues against general metabolic disturbances as a cause. In addition, these results suggested that the inhibition target was involved in DNA processing (MOB), more similar between R388 and pOX38 than RP4 and R6K (239). However, the absence of effect on IncN plasmid pKM101, with a MOB module more similar to R388 and pOX38 than to RP4, weakened this hypothesis.

Recently, a novel set of natural COINs was discovered by analyzing a collection of bioactive compounds isolated from marine microorganisms (240). These compounds, called tanzawaic acids, are fungal polyketides more complex than uFAs. They are carboxylic acids with two aromatic rings at the end of an unsaturated aliphatic chain, thus confirming the importance of these two chemical characteristics for COIN activity.

2-Alkynoic Fatty Acids

A better understanding of COIN action in relevant conjugative systems is essential as a first step to treat complex environments. In order to chemically and biologically characterize the previously reported COIN activity, a set of 2-alkynoic fatty acids (2-AFAs) was synthesized (241). 2-Hexadecynoic acid (2-HDA) was identified as the most effective synthetic COIN, with similar potency to natural uFAs (177). A clinically representative set of conjugative plasmids was tested in the presence of 2-HDA to determine its activity range. Similarly to natural uFAs, 2-HDA inhibited transfer of IncF plasmids, the most common carriers of AbR genes in pathogenic *Enterobacteriaceae* (242). Transfer of IncW, IncF, and IncH plasmids was strongly inhibited by 2-HDA, while IncI, IncX, and IncL/M plasmid transfer was only moderately inhibited. On the other hand, IncN and IncP plasmids were resistant to COIN action. Also interesting for future applications was the fact that conjugation was inhibited irrespective of the bacterial host used as donor. The most remarkable result was obtained through a liquid mating experiment using the multiresistant plasmid R1drd19. In the ab-

sence of COINs, the IncF plasmid invaded the entire recipient population after just four generations. This was due to the high transmissibility of the plasmid, which caused plasmid dissemination even though plasmid-containing cells had slower growth rates than plasmid-free cells. Conversely, the presence of 2-HDA in the mating medium prevented plasmid conjugative transfer, flipping over the balance between plasmid transmission and burden, thus favoring colonization by plasmid-free cells. Consequently, 2-HDA was able to block plasmid invasiveness and reduce the prevalence of plasmid-containing cells in the bacterial population. Reversion from plasmid invasion to plasmid loss occurred at 50 μM 2-HDA, comparable to the observed 50% inhibitory concentration in R388 transfer. This suggested that 50% inhibition of conjugation was sufficient to prevent plasmid spread in the absence of selective pressure. These observations highlight the potential application of COINs to prevent AbR dissemination.

A recent study analyzed the activity of conjugative ATPases in the presence of uFAs (243). The component of R388 MPF system TrwD (VirB11 homolog), involved in pilus synthesis and DNA translocation (244, 245), was identified as the potential target. Conjugation frequency correlated with TrwD ATPase activity in the presence of different compounds, including saturated fatty acids, uFAs (177), synthetic AFAs, and AFA inactive analogs. Nevertheless, the absence of known TrwD homologs in IncF plasmids (246) still leaves unanswered questions. Given that transfer of mobilizable plasmids by IncF MPF is also affected by these COINs (241), the target in these plasmids, well adapted to *E. coli* after a long history of coevolution, could be an unidentified chromosomal ATPase involved in F conjugation and F-helped mobilization. Alternatively, another plasmid ATPase, such as the TrwK homolog TraC (VirB4), the only ATPase of plasmid F known to be required for MPF biogenesis (28), could be responsible.

T4SS Inhibitors Discovered by Biochemical Analysis

Other approaches to discover COINs take advantage of newly generated biochemical knowledge concerning related processes, such as T4SS-related virulence inhibition. For example, VirB11 ATPase was used as a target for the development of inhibitors, with the aim of preventing *Helicobacter pylori* virulence. The first described inhibitors targeted the *H. pylori* VirB11-type ATPase Cagα, blocking CagA toxin transport to host cells. The most active compound (CHIR-1, identified by a high-throughput screening that measured ATPase activity in the presence of small compound libraries) reduced *H. pylori* pathogenic effects in gastric cells and the ability of treated bacteria to colonize gastric mucosa in mice (247). Docking analysis using Cagα allowed the identification of a series of competitive inhibitors with potential as antibacterial agents (248). These antivirulence compounds could be tested in conjugative VirB11 homologs, such as TrwD of IncW plasmid R388.

Another example of how a T4SS inhibitor involved in protein secretion can extrapolate its activity to inhibit conjugative T4SS was reported by Shaffer et al. (249). They started from the structure of pilicides, small peptidomimetic molecules that target pilin chaperones and thereby inhibit assembly of type I pili, which mediate adhesion of uropathogenic *E. coli* (250). By screening a collection of pilicide derivatives with a central 2-pyridone scaffold, they found that compounds C10 and KSK85 disrupted *H. pylori cag* T4SS, thus inhibiting translocation of the oncogenic protein CagA and peptidoglycan to gastric cells. In addition, these molecules, in particular C10, effectively inhibited conjugative transfer of *A. tumefaciens* T-DNA to plant cells, and transmission of plasmids pKM101 and R1-16 between *E. coli* strains.

Type III secretion systems (T3SSs) of several pathogens were also targeted by new antivirulence drugs. They generally act as needles to inject virulence effectors into host cells (251). Several compounds were found to block T3SSs in different pathogenic bacteria (252). An interesting work developed a whole-cell high-throughput screening of T3SS inhibitors based in *S.* Typhimurium. A compound was identified that inhibited both T3SSs and T2SSs, probably by targeting an outer membrane component conserved between these two secretion systems (253). These results provide a proof of concept that compounds with a broad spectrum of activity against different bacterial secretion systems could be developed.

CONCLUSIONS

We have reviewed the multiple mechanisms by which conjugative transmission of plasmids can be affected. Given that conjugation is a sophisticated multistep process involving complexes of >15 proteins, it is reasonable that diverse mechanisms have been identified that disrupt one or more of the various steps. Up to now, the most efficient blocking mechanisms are the natural ones, such as RM, CRISPR, etc., that bacteria have used and perfected for millions of years to avoid "excessive" plasmid transmission. Artificial mechanisms found by scientific research are not yet as efficient but have the advantage over natural mechanisms of being less discriminating, which in our specific case is a valuable characteristic. The fight against AbR requires blocking mechanisms that impede its dissemination irrespective of the plasmid platform in which the resistance gene lies. Thus, COINs such as 2-HDA or other uFAs are broad-range inhibitors that can be used as lead compounds on which the pharmacological industry could work to obtain effective anticonjugation drugs. Alternative compounds and genetic devices have been reviewed that offer potentially different approaches to achieve the same goal. We hope that this review can inspire additional work that helps us win the fight against AbR transmission.

ACKNOWLEDGMENTS

Work at the F.D.L.C. laboratory was financed by the Spanish Ministry of Economy and Competitiveness (BFU2014-55534-C2-1-P and RTC-2015-3184-1), as well as by the European Seventh Framework Programme (612146/FP7-ICT-2013-10). M.G.'s work was supported by a Ph.D. fellowship from the University of Cantabria (Spain).

CITATION

Getino M, de la Cruz F. 2017. Natural and artificial strategies to control the conjugative transmission of plasmids. Microbiol Spectrum 6(1):MTBP-0015-2016.

REFERENCES

1. **Fleming A.** 1929. On the antibacterial action of cultures of a penicillium, with special reference to their use in the isolation of *B. Influenzae*. *Br J Exp Pathol* 10:226–236.
2. **D'Costa VM, McGrann KM, Hughes DW, Wright GD.** 2006. Sampling the antibiotic resistome. *Science* 311:374–377.
3. **Davies J, Davies D.** 2010. Origins and evolution of antibiotic resistance. *Microbiol Mol Biol Rev* 74:417–433.
4. **Clatworthy AE, Pierson E, Hung DT.** 2007. Targeting virulence: a new paradigm for antimicrobial therapy. *Nat Chem Biol* 3:541–548.
5. **Liu B, Pop M.** 2009. ARDB—Antibiotic Resistance Genes Database. *Nucleic Acids Res* 37 (Database issue):D443–D447.
6. **Cooper MA, Shlaes D.** 2011. Fix the antibiotics pipeline. *Nature* 472:32.
7. **O'Neill J.** 2014. *Antimicrobial Resistance: Tackling a Crisis for the Health and Wealth of Nations*. Review on Antimicrobial Resistance, London, United Kingdom. https://amr-review.org/sites/default/files/AMR%20Review%20Paper%20-%20Tackling%20a%20crisis%20for%20the%20health%20and%20wealth%20of%20nations_1.pdf.
8. **Heras B, Scanlon MJ, Martin JL.** 2015. Targeting virulence not viability in the search for future antibacterials. *Br J Clin Pharmacol* 79:208–215.
9. **Scully IL, Swanson K, Green L, Jansen KU, Anderson AS.** 2015. Anti-infective vaccination in the 21st century—new horizons for personal and public health. *Curr Opin Microbiol* 27:96–102.
10. **Nobrega FL, Costa AR, Kluskens LD, Azeredo J.** 2015. Revisiting phage therapy: new applications for old resources. *Trends Microbiol* 23:185–191.
11. **Dwidar M, Monnappa AK, Mitchell RJ.** 2012. The dual probiotic and antibiotic nature of *Bdellovibrio bacteriovorus*. *BMB Rep* 45:71–78.
12. **Williams JJ, Hergenrother PJ.** 2008. Exposing plasmids as the Achilles' heel of drug-resistant bacteria. *Curr Opin Chem Biol* 12:389–399.
13. **Thomas CM, Nielsen KM.** 2005. Mechanisms of, and barriers to, horizontal gene transfer between bacteria. *Nat Rev Microbiol* 3:711–721.
14. **Baquero F, Coque TM, de la Cruz F.** 2011. Ecology and evolution as targets: the need for novel eco-evo drugs and strategies to fight antibiotic resistance. *Antimicrob Agents Chemother* 55:3649–3660.
15. **Lawrence JG, Retchless AC.** 2009. The interplay of homologous recombination and horizontal gene transfer in bacterial speciation. *Methods Mol Biol* 532:29–53.
16. **Frost LS, Leplae R, Summers AO, Toussaint A.** 2005. Mobile genetic elements: the agents of open source evolution. *Nat Rev Microbiol* 3:722–732.
17. **Davison J.** 1999. Genetic exchange between bacteria in the environment. *Plasmid* 42:73–91.
18. **Halary S, Leigh JW, Cheaib B, Lopez P, Bapteste E.** 2010. Network analyses structure genetic diversity in independent genetic worlds. *Proc Natl Acad Sci U S A* 107:127–132.
19. **Amábile-Cuevas CF, Chicurel ME.** 1992. Bacterial plasmids and gene flux. *Cell* 70:189–199.
20. **Smillie C, Garcillán-Barcia MP, Francia MV, Rocha EP, de la Cruz F.** 2010. Mobility of plasmids. *Microbiol Mol Biol Rev* 74:434–452.
21. **Waters VL.** 1999. Conjugative transfer in the dissemination of beta-lactam and aminoglycoside resistance. *Front Biosci* 4:D433–D456.
22. **Norman A, Hansen LH, Sørensen SJ.** 2009. Conjugative plasmids: vessels of the communal gene pool. *Philos Trans R Soc Lond B Biol Sci* 364:2275–2289.
23. **Thoma L, Muth G.** 2015. The conjugative DNA-transfer apparatus of *Streptomyces*. *Int J Med Microbiol* 305:224–229.
24. **Fürste JP, Pansegrau W, Ziegelin G, Kröger M, Lanka E.** 1989. Conjugative transfer of promiscuous IncP plasmids: interaction of plasmid-encoded products with the transfer origin. *Proc Natl Acad Sci U S A* 86:1771–1775.

25. **Clark AJ, Adelberg EA.** 1962. Bacterial conjugation. *Annu Rev Microbiol* **16:**289–319.
26. **Christie PJ, Atmakuri K, Krishnamoorthy V, Jakubowski S, Cascales E.** 2005. Biogenesis, architecture, and function of bacterial type IV secretion systems. *Annu Rev Microbiol* **59:**451–485.
27. **Low HH, Gubellini F, Rivera-Calzada A, Braun N, Connery S, Dujeancourt A, Lu F, Redzej A, Fronzes R, Orlova EV, Waksman G.** 2014. Structure of a type IV secretion system. *Nature* **508:**550–553.
28. **Clarke M, Maddera L, Harris RL, Silverman PM.** 2008. F-pili dynamics by live-cell imaging. *Proc Natl Acad Sci U S A* **105:**17978–17981.
29. **Cabezón E, Ripoll-Rozada J, Peña A, de la Cruz F, Arechaga I.** 2015. Towards an integrated model of bacterial conjugation. *FEMS Microbiol Rev* **39:**81–95.
30. **Bradley DE.** 1980. Morphological and serological relationships of conjugative pili. *Plasmid* **4:**155–169.
31. **Bradley DE, Taylor DE, Cohen DR.** 1980. Specification of surface mating systems among conjugative drug resistance plasmids in *Escherichia coli* K-12. *J Bacteriol* **143:**1466–1470.
32. **del Solar G, Alonso JC, Espinosa M, Díaz-Orejas R.** 1996. Broad-host-range plasmid replication: an open question. *Mol Microbiol* **21:**661–666.
33. **Ghigo JM.** 2001. Natural conjugative plasmids induce bacterial biofilm development. *Nature* **412:**442–445.
34. **Garcillán-Barcia MP, Francia MV, de la Cruz F.** 2009. The diversity of conjugative relaxases and its application in plasmid classification. *FEMS Microbiol Rev* **33:**657–687.
35. **de la Cruz F, Frost LS, Meyer RJ, Zechner EL.** 2010. Conjugative DNA metabolism in Gram-negative bacteria. *FEMS Microbiol Rev* **34:**18–40.
36. **Byrd DR, Matson SW.** 1997. Nicking by transesterification: the reaction catalysed by a relaxase. *Mol Microbiol* **25:**1011–1022.
37. **Guasch A, Lucas M, Moncalián G, Cabezas M, Pérez-Luque R, Gomis-Rüth FX, de la Cruz F, Coll M.** 2003. Recognition and processing of the origin of transfer DNA by conjugative relaxase TrwC. *Nat Struct Biol* **10:**1002–1010.
38. **Llosa M, Grandoso G, Hernando MA, de la Cruz F.** 1996. Functional domains in protein TrwC of plasmid R388: dissected DNA strand transferase and DNA helicase activities reconstitute protein function. *J Mol Biol* **264:**56–67.
39. **Pansegrau W, Lanka E.** 1996. Mechanisms of initiation and termination reactions in conjugative DNA processing. Independence of tight

substrate binding and catalytic activity of relaxase (TraI) of IncPα plasmid RP4. *J Biol Chem* **271:**13068–13076.
40. **Llosa M, Gomis-Rüth FX, Coll M, de la Cruz Fd F.** 2002. Bacterial conjugation: a two-step mechanism for DNA transport. *Mol Microbiol* **45:**1–8.
41. **Draper O, César CE, Machón C, de la Cruz F, Llosa M.** 2005. Site-specific recombinase and integrase activities of a conjugative relaxase in recipient cells. *Proc Natl Acad Sci U S A* **102:** 16385–16390.
42. **Garcillán-Barcia MP, Jurado P, González-Pérez B, Moncalián G, Fernández LA, de la Cruz F.** 2007. Conjugative transfer can be inhibited by blocking relaxase activity within recipient cells with intrabodies. *Mol Microbiol* **63:**404–416.
43. **Viljanen P, Boratynski J.** 1991. The susceptibility of conjugative resistance transfer in gram-negative bacteria to physicochemical and biochemical agents. *FEMS Microbiol Rev* **8:**43–54.
44. **van Elsas JD, Fry JC, Hirsch P, Molin S.** 2000. Ecology of plasmid transfer and spread, p 175–206. *In* Thomas CM (ed), *The Horizontal Gene Pool: Bacterial Plasmids and Gene Spread.* Harwood Academic Publishers, Williston, VT.
45. **Aminov RI.** 2011. Horizontal gene exchange in environmental microbiota. *Front Microbiol* **2:**158.
46. **van Elsas JD, Bailey MJ.** 2002. The ecology of transfer of mobile genetic elements. *FEMS Microbiol Ecol* **42:**187–197.
47. **Koraimann G, Wagner MA.** 2014. Social behavior and decision making in bacterial conjugation. *Front Cell Infect Microbiol* **4:**54.
48. **Chatterjee A, Cook LC, Shu CC, Chen Y, Manias DA, Ramkrishna D, Dunny GM, Hu WS.** 2013. Antagonistic self-sensing and mate-sensing signaling controls antibiotic-resistance transfer. *Proc Natl Acad Sci U S A* **110:**7086–7090.
49. **Bertani G, Weigle JJ.** 1953. Host controlled variation in bacterial viruses. *J Bacteriol* **65:** 113–121.
50. **Roberts RJ, Vincze T, Posfai J, Macelis D.** 2015. REBAS—a database for DNA restriction and modification: enzymes, genes and genomes. *Nucleic Acids Res* **43**(D1):D298–D299.
51. **Vasu K, Nagaraja V.** 2013. Diverse functions of restriction-modification systems in addition to cellular defense. *Microbiol Mol Biol Rev* **77:** 53–72.
52. **Bickle TA.** 2004. Restricting restriction. *Mol Microbiol* **51:**3–5.
53. **Roberts RJ, Belfort M, Bestor T, Bhagwat AS, Bickle TA, Bitinaite J, Blumenthal RM, Degtyarev SK, Dryden DT, Dybvig K, Firman**

K, Gromova ES, Gumport RI, Halford SE, Hattman S, Heitman J, Hornby DP, Janulaitis A, Jeltsch A, Josephsen J, Kiss A, Klaenhammer TR, Kobayashi I, Kong H, Krüger DH, Lacks S, Marinus MG, Miyahara M, Morgan RD, Murray NE, Nagaraja V, Piekarowicz A, Pingoud A, Raleigh E, Rao DN, Reich N, Repin VE, Selker EU, Shaw PC, Stein DC, Stoddard BL, Szybalski W, Trautner TA, Van Etten JL, Vitor JM, Wilson GG, Xu SY. 2003. A nomenclature for restriction enzymes, DNA methyltransferases, homing endonucleases and their genes. *Nucleic Acids Res* **31**:1805–1812.

54. **Oliveira PH, Touchon M, Rocha EP.** 2014. The interplay of restriction-modification systems with mobile genetic elements and their prokaryotic hosts. *Nucleic Acids Res* **42**:10618–10631.

55. **Kobayashi I.** 2001. Behavior of restriction-modification systems as selfish mobile elements and their impact on genome evolution. *Nucleic Acids Res* **29**:3742–3756.

56. **Samson JE, Magadán AH, Sabri M, Moineau S.** 2013. Revenge of the phages: defeating bacterial defences. *Nat Rev Microbiol* **11**:675–687.

57. **Roer L, Aarestrup FM, Hasman H.** 2015. The *Eco*KI type I restriction-modification system in *Escherichia coli* affects but is not an absolute barrier for conjugation. *J Bacteriol* **197**:337–342.

58. **Waldron DE, Lindsay JA.** 2006. *Sau*1: a novel lineage-specific type I restriction-modification system that blocks horizontal gene transfer into *Staphylococcus aureus* and between *S. aureus* isolates of different lineages. *J Bacteriol* **188**:5578–5585.

59. **Pinedo CA, Smets BF.** 2005. Conjugal TOL transfer from *Pseudomonas putida* to *Pseudomonas aeruginosa*: effects of restriction proficiency, toxicant exposure, cell density ratios, and conjugation detection method on observed transfer efficiencies. *Appl Environ Microbiol* **71**:51–57.

60. **Geisenberger O, Ammendola A, Christensen BB, Molin S, Schleifer KH, Eberl L.** 1999. Monitoring the conjugal transfer of plasmid RP4 in activated sludge and in situ identification of the transconjugants. *FEMS Microbiol Lett* **174**:9–17.

61. **Schäfer A, Kalinowski J, Pühler A.** 1994. Increased fertility of *Corynebacterium glutamicum* recipients in intergeneric matings with *Escherichia coli* after stress exposure. *Appl Environ Microbiol* **60**:756–759.

62. **Trieu-Cuot P, Carlier C, Poyart-Salmeron C, Courvalin P.** 1991. Shuttle vectors containing a multiple cloning site and a *lacZα* gene for conjugal transfer of DNA from *Escherichia coli* to Gram-positive bacteria. *Gene* **102**:99–104.

63. **Zhou H, Wang Y, Yu Y, Bai T, Chen L, Liu P, Guo H, Zhu C, Tao M, Deng Z.** 2012. A non-restricting and non-methylating *Escherichia coli* strain for DNA cloning and high-throughput conjugation to *Streptomyces coelicolor*. *Curr Microbiol* **64**:185–190.

64. **Ohtani N, Sato M, Tomita M, Itaya M.** 2008. Restriction on conjugational transfer of pLS20 in *Bacillus subtilis* 168. *Biosci Biotechnol Biochem* **72**:2472–2475.

65. **Purdy D, O'Keeffe TA, Elmore M, Herbert M, McLeod A, Bokori-Brown M, Ostrowski A, Minton NP.** 2002. Conjugative transfer of clostridial shuttle vectors from *Escherichia coli* to *Clostridium difficile* through circumvention of the restriction barrier. *Mol Microbiol* **46**:439–452.

66. **Elhai J, Vepritskiy A, Muro-Pastor AM, Flores E, Wolk CP.** 1997. Reduction of conjugal transfer efficiency by three restriction activities of *Anabaena* sp. strain PCC 7120. *J Bacteriol* **179**:1998–2005.

67. **McMahon SA, Roberts GA, Johnson KA, Cooper LP, Liu H, White JH, Carter LG, Sanghvi B, Oke M, Walkinshaw MD, Blakely GW, Naismith JH, Dryden DT.** 2009. Extensive DNA mimicry by the ArdA anti-restriction protein and its role in the spread of antibiotic resistance. *Nucleic Acids Res* **37**:4887–4897.

68. **Wilkins BM.** 2002. Plasmid promiscuity: meeting the challenge of DNA immigration control. *Environ Microbiol* **4**:495–500.

69. **Belogurov AA, Delver EP, Agafonova OV, Belogurova NG, Lee LY, Kado CI.** 2000. Anti-restriction protein Ard (type C) encoded by IncW plasmid pSa has a high similarity to the "protein transport" domain of TraC1 primase of promiscuous plasmid RP4. *J Mol Biol* **296**:969–977.

70. **Wilkins BM, Chilley PM, Thomas AT, Pocklington MJ.** 1996. Distribution of restriction enzyme recognition sequences on broad host range plasmid RP4: molecular and evolutionary implications. *J Mol Biol* **258**:447–456.

71. **Clewell DB, Weaver KE, Dunny GM, Coque TM, Francia MV, Hayes F.** 2014. Extrachromosomal and mobile elements in enterococci: transmission, maintenance, and epidemiology, pp. 309–420. *In* Gilmore MS, Clewell DB, Ike Y, Shankar N (ed), *Enterococci: From Commensals to Leading Causes of Drug Resistant Infection.* Boston: Massachusetts Eye and Ear Infirmary.

72. **Dupuis ME, Villion M, Magadán AH, Moineau S.** 2013. CRISPR-Cas and restriction-modification systems are compatible and increase phage resistance. *Nat Commun* **4**:2087.

73. **Barrangou R, Fremaux C, Deveau H, Richards M, Boyaval P, Moineau S, Romero DA, Horvath P.** 2007. CRISPR provides acquired resistance against viruses in prokaryotes. *Science* **315:**1709–1712.

74. **Grissa I, Vergnaud G, Pourcel C.** 2007. The CRISPRdb database and tools to display CRISPRs and to generate dictionaries of spacers and repeats. *BMC Bioinformatics* **8:**172.

75. **Jansen R, Embden JD, Gaastra W, Schouls LM.** 2002. Identification of genes that are associated with DNA repeats in prokaryotes. *Mol Microbiol* **43:**1565–1575.

76. **Marraffini LA.** 2015. CRISPR-Cas immunity in prokaryotes. *Nature* **526:**55–61.

77. **Andersson AF, Banfield JF.** 2008. Virus population dynamics and acquired virus resistance in natural microbial communities. *Science* **320:**1047–1050.

78. **Marraffini LA, Sontheimer EJ.** 2008. CRISPR interference limits horizontal gene transfer in staphylococci by targeting DNA. *Science* **322:**1843–1845.

79. **Makarova KS, Haft DH, Barrangou R, Brouns SJ, Charpentier E, Horvath P, Moineau S, Mojica FJ, Wolf YI, Yakunin AF, van der Oost J, Koonin EV.** 2011. Evolution and classification of the CRISPR-Cas systems. *Nat Rev Microbiol* **9:**467–477.

80. **Sashital DG, Wiedenheft B, Doudna JA.** 2012. Mechanism of foreign DNA selection in a bacterial adaptive immune system. *Mol Cell* **46:**606–615.

81. **Marraffini LA, Sontheimer EJ.** 2010. Self versus non-self discrimination during CRISPR RNA-directed immunity. *Nature* **463:**568–571.

82. **Levy A, Goren MG, Yosef I, Auster O, Manor M, Amitai G, Edgar R, Qimron U, Sorek R.** 2015. CRISPR adaptation biases explain preference for acquisition of foreign DNA. *Nature* **520:**505–510.

83. **Sontheimer EJ, Barrangou R.** 2015. The bacterial origins of the CRISPR genome-editing revolution. *Hum Gene Ther* **26:**413–424.

84. **Jiang W, Bikard D, Cox D, Zhang F, Marraffini LA.** 2013. RNA-guided editing of bacterial genomes using CRISPR-Cas systems. *Nat Biotechnol* **31:**233–239.

85. **Pennisi E.** 2013. The CRISPR craze. *Science* **341:**833–836.

86. **Westra ER, Staals RH, Gort G, Høgh S, Neumann S, de la Cruz F, Fineran PC, Brouns SJ.** 2013. CRISPR-Cas systems preferentially target the leading regions of MOB_F conjugative plasmids. *RNA Biol* **10:**749–761.

87. **Samson JE, Magadan AH, Moineau S.** 2015. The CRISPR-Cas immune system and genetic transfers: reaching an equilibrium. *Microbiol Spectr* **3:**PLAS-0034-2014.

88. **Price VJ, Huo W, Sharifi A, Palmer KL.** 2016. CRISPR-Cas and restriction-modification act additively against conjugative antibiotic resistance plasmid transfer in *Enterococcus faecalis*. *mSphere* **1:**e00064-16.

89. **Garneau JE, Dupuis ME, Villion M, Romero DA, Barrangou R, Boyaval P, Fremaux C, Horvath P, Magadán AH, Moineau S.** 2010. The CRISPR/Cas bacterial immune system cleaves bacteriophage and plasmid DNA. *Nature* **468:**67–71.

90. **Bikard D, Euler CW, Jiang W, Nussenzweig PM, Goldberg GW, Duportet X, Fischetti VA, Marraffini LA.** 2014. Exploiting CRISPR-Cas nucleases to produce sequence-specific antimicrobials. *Nat Biotechnol* **32:**1146–1150.

91. **Yosef I, Manor M, Kiro R, Qimron U.** 2015. Temperate and lytic bacteriophages programmed to sensitize and kill antibiotic-resistant bacteria. *Proc Natl Acad Sci U S A* **112:**7267–7272.

92. **Makarova KS, Wolf YI, van der Oost J, Koonin EV.** 2009. Prokaryotic homologs of Argonaute proteins are predicted to function as key components of a novel system of defense against mobile genetic elements. *Biol Direct* **4:**29.

93. **Swarts DC, Jore MM, Westra ER, Zhu Y, Janssen JH, Snijders AP, Wang Y, Patel DJ, Berenguer J, Brouns SJ, van der Oost J.** 2014. DNA-guided DNA interference by a prokaryotic Argonaute. *Nature* **507:**258–261.

94. **Barrangou R, van der Oost J.** 2015. Bacteriophage exclusion, a new defense system. *EMBO J* **34:**134–135.

95. **Goldfarb T, Sberro H, Weinstock E, Cohen O, Doron S, Charpak-Amikam Y, Afik S, Ofir G, Sorek R.** 2015. BREX is a novel phage resistance system widespread in microbial genomes. *EMBO J* **34:**169–183.

96. **Curtiss R III, Charamella LJ, Stallions DR, Mays JA.** 1968. Parental functions during conjugation in *Escherichia coli* K-12. *Bacteriol Rev* **32:**320–348.

97. **Wilkins BM, Hollom SE.** 1974. Conjugational synthesis of F *lac*+ and Col I DNA in the presence of rifampicin and in *Escherichia coli* K12 mutants defective in DNA synthesis. *Mol Gen Genet* **134:**143–156.

98. **Kingsman A, Willetts N.** 1978. The requirements for conjugal DNA synthesis in the donor strain during F*lac* transfer. *J Mol Biol* **122:**287–300.

99. **Lee CA, Babic A, Grossman AD.** 2010. Autonomous plasmid-like replication of a conjugative transposon. *Mol Microbiol* **75:**268–279.

100. **Petit MA, Dervyn E, Rose M, Entian KD, McGovern S, Ehrlich SD, Bruand C.** 1998. PcrA is an essential DNA helicase of *Bacillus subtilis* fulfilling functions both in repair and rolling-circle replication. *Mol Microbiol* **29:**261–273.

101. **Tarantino PM Jr, Zhi C, Wright GE, Brown NC.** 1999. Inhibitors of DNA polymerase III as novel antimicrobial agents against gram-positive eubacteria. *Antimicrob Agents Chemother* **43:** 1982–1987.

102. **Miyazaki R, Minoia M, Pradervand N, Sulser S, Reinhard F, van der Meer JR.** 2012. Cellular variability of RpoS expression underlies subpopulation activation of an integrative and conjugative element. *PLoS Genet* **8:**e1002818.

103. **Roca AI, Cox MM.** 1997. RecA protein: structure, function, and role in recombinational DNA repair. *Prog Nucleic Acid Res Mol Biol* **56:**129–223.

104. **Petrova V, Chitteni-Pattu S, Drees JC, Inman RB, Cox MM.** 2009. An SOS inhibitor that binds to free RecA protein: the PsiB protein. *Mol Cell* **36:**121–130.

105. **Baharoglu Z, Bikard D, Mazel D.** 2010. Conjugative DNA transfer induces the bacterial SOS response and promotes antibiotic resistance development through integron activation. *PLoS Genet* **6:**e1001165.

106. **Frost LS, Koraimann G.** 2010. Regulation of bacterial conjugation: balancing opportunity with adversity. *Future Microbiol* **5:**1057–1071.

107. **Fernandez-Lopez R, Del Campo I, Revilla C, Cuevas A, de la Cruz F.** 2014. Negative feedback and transcriptional overshooting in a regulatory network for horizontal gene transfer. *PLoS Genet* **10:**e1004171.

108. **Pérez-Mendoza D, de la Cruz F.** 2009. *Escherichia coli* genes affecting recipient ability in plasmid conjugation: are there any? *BMC Genomics* **10:**71.

109. **Bruand C, Ehrlich SD.** 2000. UvrD-dependent replication of rolling-circle plasmids in *Escherichia coli*. *Mol Microbiol* **35:**204–210.

110. **Watanabe T, Arai T, Hattori T.** 1970. Effects of cell wall polysaccharide on the mating ability of *Salmonella typhimurium*. *Nature* **225:**70–71.

111. **Monner DA, Jonsson S, Boman HG.** 1971. Ampicillin-resistant mutants of *Escherichia coli* K-12 with lipopolysaccharide alterations affecting mating ability and susceptibility to sex-specific bacteriophages. *J Bacteriol* **107:**420–432.

112. **Skurray RA, Hancock RE, Reeves P.** 1974. Con⁻ mutants: class of mutants in *Escherichia coli* K-12 lacking a major cell wall protein and defective in conjugation and adsorption of a bacteriophage. *J Bacteriol* **119:**726–735.

113. **Havekes L, Tommassen J, Hoekstra W, Lugtenberg B.** 1977. Isolation and characterization of *Escherichia coli* K-12 F⁻ mutants defective in conjugation with an I-type donor. *J Bacteriol* **129:**1–8.

114. **Hoekstra WP, Havekes AM.** 1979. On the role of the recipient cell during conjugation in *Escherichia coli*. *Antonie van Leeuwenhoek* **45:**13–18.

115. **Sanderson KE, Janzer J, Head J.** 1981. Influence of lipopolysaccharide and protein in the cell envelope on recipient capacity in conjugation of *Salmonella typhimurium*. *J Bacteriol* **148:** 283–293.

116. **Manoil C, Rosenbusch JP.** 1982. Conjugation-deficient mutants of *Escherichia coli* distinguish classes of functions of the outer membrane OmpA protein. *Mol Gen Genet* **187:**148–156.

117. **Duke J, Guiney DG Jr.** 1983. The role of lipopolysaccharide structure in the recipient cell during plasmid-mediated bacterial conjugation. *Plasmid* **9:**222–226.

118. **Anthony KG, Sherburne C, Sherburne R, Frost LS.** 1994. The role of the pilus in recipient cell recognition during bacterial conjugation mediated by F-like plasmids. *Mol Microbiol* **13:**939–953.

119. **Ishiwa A, Komano T.** 2000. The lipopolysaccharide of recipient cells is a specific receptor for PilV proteins, selected by shufflon DNA rearrangement, in liquid matings with donors bearing the R64 plasmid. *Mol Gen Genet* **263:**159–164.

120. **Klimke WA, Rypien CD, Klinger B, Kennedy RA, Rodriguez-Maillard JM, Frost LS.** 2005. The mating pair stabilization protein, TraN, of the F plasmid is an outer-membrane protein with two regions that are important for its function in conjugation. *Microbiology* **151:**3527–3540.

121. **Inoue K, Miyazaki R, Ohtsubo Y, Nagata Y, Tsuda M.** 2013. Inhibitory effect of *Pseudomonas putida* nitrogen-related phosphotransferase system on conjugative transfer of IncP-9 plasmid from *Escherichia coli*. *FEMS Microbiol Lett* **345:**102–109.

122. **van Opijnen T, Camilli A.** 2013. Transposon insertion sequencing: a new tool for systems-level analysis of microorganisms. *Nat Rev Microbiol* **11:**435–442.

123. **Johnson CM, Grossman AD.** 2014. Identification of host genes that affect acquisition of an integrative and conjugative element in *Bacillus subtilis*. *Mol Microbiol* **93:**1284–1301.

124. **Bhatty M, Laverde Gomez JA, Christie PJ.** 2013. The expanding bacterial type IV secretion lexicon. *Res Microbiol* **164:**620–639.

125. **Lang S, Kirchberger PC, Gruber CJ, Redzej A, Raffl S, Zellnig G, Zangger K, Zechner EL.**

2011. An activation domain of plasmid R1 TraI protein delineates stages of gene transfer initiation. *Mol Microbiol* **82:**1071–1085.

126. **Dunny GM.** 2013. Enterococcal sex pheromones: signaling, social behavior, and evolution. *Annu Rev Genet* **47:**457–482.

127. **Auchtung JM, Lee CA, Monson RE, Lehman AP, Grossman AD.** 2005. Regulation of a *Bacillus subtilis* mobile genetic element by intercellular signaling and the global DNA damage response. *Proc Natl Acad Sci U S A* **102:**12554–12559.

128. **Lederberg J, Cavalli LL, Lederberg EM.** 1952. Sex compatibility in *Escherichia coli*. *Genetics* **37:**720–730.

129. **Watanabe T.** 1963. Infective heredity of multiple drug resistance in bacteria. *Bacteriol Rev* **27:**87–115.

130. **Novick RP.** 1969. Extrachromosomal inheritance in bacteria. *Bacteriol Rev* **33:**210–263.

131. **Achtman M, Kennedy N, Skurray R.** 1977. Cell–cell interactions in conjugating *Escherichia coli*: role of *traT* protein in surface exclusion. *Proc Natl Acad Sci U S A* **74:**5104–5108.

132. **Achtman M, Manning PA, Edelbluth C, Herrlich P.** 1979. Export without proteolytic processing of inner and outer membrane proteins encoded by F sex factor *tra* cistrons in *Escherichia coli* minicells. *Proc Natl Acad Sci U S A* **76:**4837–4841.

133. **Klimke WA, Frost LS.** 1998. Genetic analysis of the role of the transfer gene, *traN*, of the F and R100-1 plasmids in mating pair stabilization during conjugation. *J Bacteriol* **180:**4036–4043.

134. **Anthony KG, Klimke WA, Manchak J, Frost LS.** 1999. Comparison of proteins involved in pilus synthesis and mating pair stabilization from the related plasmids F and R100-1: insights into the mechanism of conjugation. *J Bacteriol* **181:**5149–5159.

135. **Audette GF, Manchak J, Beatty P, Klimke WA, Frost LS.** 2007. Entry exclusion in F-like plasmids requires intact TraG in the donor that recognizes its cognate TraS in the recipient. *Microbiology* **153:**442–451.

136. **Garcillán-Barcia MP, de la Cruz F.** 2008. Why is entry exclusion an essential feature of conjugative plasmids? *Plasmid* **60:**1–18.

137. **Watanabe T, Fukasawa T.** 1962. Episome-mediated transfer of drug resistance in Enterobacteriaceae. IV. Interactions between resistance transfer factor and F-factor in *Escherichia coli* K-12. *J Bacteriol* **83:**727–735.

138. **Koraimann G, Teferle K, Markolin G, Woger W, Högenauer G.** 1996. The FinOP repressor system of plasmid R1: analysis of the antisense RNA control of *traJ* expression and conjugative DNA transfer. *Mol Microbiol* **21:**811–821.

139. **Jerome LJ, van Biesen T, Frost LS.** 1999. Degradation of FinP antisense RNA from F-like plasmids: the RNA-binding protein, FinO, protects FinP from ribonuclease E. *J Mol Biol* **285:**1457–1473.

140. **Jerome LJ, Frost LS.** 1999. *In vitro* analysis of the interaction between the FinO protein and FinP antisense RNA of F-like conjugative plasmids. *J Biol Chem* **274:**10356–10362.

141. **Frost LS, Ippen-Ihler K, Skurray RA.** 1994. Analysis of the sequence and gene products of the transfer region of the F sex factor. *Microbiol Rev* **58:**162–210.

142. **Gasson MJ, Willetts NS.** 1977. Further characterization of the F fertility inhibition systems of "unusual" Fin⁺ plasmids. *J Bacteriol* **131:**413–420.

143. **Gasson MJ, Willetts NS.** 1975. Five control systems preventing transfer of *Escherichia coli* K-12 sex factor F. *J Bacteriol* **122:**518–525.

144. **Gasson M, Willetts N.** 1976. Transfer gene expression during fertility inhibition of the *Escherichia coli* K12 sex factor F by the I-like plasmid R62. *Mol Gen Genet* **149:**329–333.

145. **Gaffney D, Skurray R, Willetts N, Brenner S.** 1983. Regulation of the F conjugation genes studied by hybridization and *tra-lacZ* fusion. *J Mol Biol* **168:**103–122.

146. **Ham LM, Skurray R.** 1989. Molecular analysis and nucleotide sequence of *finQ*, a transcriptional inhibitor of the F plasmid transfer genes. *Mol Gen Genet* **216:**99–105.

147. **Penfold SS, Simon J, Frost LS.** 1996. Regulation of the expression of the *traM* gene of the F sex factor of *Escherichia coli*. *Mol Microbiol* **20:**549–558.

148. **Willetts N.** 1980. Interactions between the F conjugal transfer system and CloDF13::Tna plasmids. *Mol Gen Genet* **180:**213–217.

149. **Olsen RH, Shipley PL.** 1975. RP1 properties and fertility inhibition among P, N, W, and X incompatibility group plasmids. *J Bacteriol* **123:**28–35.

150. **Yusoff K, Stanisich VA.** 1984. Location of a function on RP1 that fertility inhibits Inc W plasmids. *Plasmid* **11:**178–181.

151. **Fong ST, Stanisich VA.** 1989. Location and characterization of two functions on RP1 that inhibit the fertility of the IncW plasmid R388. *J Gen Microbiol* **135:**499–502.

152. **Pinney RJ, Smith JT.** 1974. Fertility inhibition of an N group R factor by a group X R factor, R6K. *J Gen Microbiol* **82:**415–418.

153. **Herrera-Cervera JA, Olivares J, Sanjuan J.** 1996. Ammonia inhibition of plasmid pRmeGR4a conjugal transfer between *Rhizobium meliloti* strains. *Appl Environ Microbiol* **62:**1145–1150.

154. **Datta N, Hedges RW, Shaw EJ, Sykes RB, Richmond MH.** 1971. Properties of an R factor from *Pseudomonas aeruginosa. J Bacteriol* **108:** 1244–1249.

155. **Coetzee JN, Datta N, Hedges RW.** 1972. R factors from *Proteus rettgeri. J Gen Microbiol* **72:**543–552.

156. **Winans SC, Walker GC.** 1985. Fertility inhibition of RP1 by IncN plasmid pKM101. *J Bacteriol* **161:**425–427.

157. **Tanimoto K, Iino T.** 1983. Transfer inhibition of RP4 by F factor. *Mol Gen Genet* **192:**104–109.

158. **Tanimoto K, Iino T.** 1984. An essential gene for replication of the mini-F plasmid from origin I. *Mol Gen Genet* **196:**59–63.

159. **Miller JF, Malamy MH.** 1983. Identification of the *pifC* gene and its role in negative control of F factor *pif* gene expression. *J Bacteriol* **156:**338–347.

160. **Miller JF, Lanka E, Malamy MH.** 1985. F factor inhibition of conjugal transfer of broad-host-range plasmid RP4: requirement for the protein product of *pif* operon regulatory gene *pifC. J Bacteriol* **163:**1067–1073.

161. **Tanimoto K, Iino T, Ohtsubo H, Ohtsubo E.** 1985. Identification of a gene, *tir* of R100, functionally homologous to the *F3* gene of F in the inhibition of RP4 transfer. *Mol Gen Genet* **198:** 356–357.

162. **Santini JM, Stanisich VA.** 1998. Both the *fipA* gene of pKM101 and the *pifC* gene of F inhibit conjugal transfer of RP1 by an effect on *traG. J Bacteriol* **180:**4093–4101.

163. **Loper JE, Kado CI.** 1979. Host range conferred by the virulence-specifying plasmid of *Agrobacterium tumefaciens. J Bacteriol* **139:**591–596.

164. **Farrand S, Kado C, Ireland C.** 1981. Suppression of tumorigenicity by the IncW R plasmid pSa in *Agrobacterium tumefaciens. Mol Gen Genet* **181:**44–51.

165. **Close SM, Kado CI.** 1991. The *osa* gene of pSa encodes a 21.1-kilodalton protein that suppresses *Agrobacterium tumefaciens* oncogenicity. *J Bacteriol* **173:**5449–5456.

166. **Ward JE Jr, Dale EM, Binns AN.** 1991. Activity of the *Agrobacterium* T-DNA transfer machinery is affected by *virB* gene products. *Proc Natl Acad Sci U S A* **88:**9350–9354.

167. **Binns AN, Beaupré CE, Dale EM.** 1995. Inhibition of VirB-mediated transfer of diverse substrates from *Agrobacterium tumefaciens* by the IncQ plasmid RSF1010. *J Bacteriol* **177:** 4890–4899.

168. **Stahl LE, Jacobs A, Binns AN.** 1998. The conjugal intermediate of plasmid RSF1010 inhibits *Agrobacterium tumefaciens* virulence and VirB-dependent export of VirE2. *J Bacteriol* **180:** 3933–3939.

169. **Lee LY, Gelvin SB.** 2004. Osa protein constitutes a strong oncogenic suppression system that can block *vir*-dependent transfer of IncQ plasmids between *Agrobacterium* cells and the establishment of IncQ plasmids in plant cells. *J Bacteriol* **186:**7254–7261.

170. **Chen CY, Kado CI.** 1994. Inhibition of *Agrobacterium tumefaciens* oncogenicity by the *osa* gene of pSa. *J Bacteriol* **176:**5697–5703.

171. **Chen CY, Kado CI.** 1996. Osa protein encoded by plasmid pSa is located at the inner membrane but does not inhibit membrane association of VirB and VirD virulence proteins in *Agrobacterium tumefaciens. FEMS Microbiol Lett* **135:**85–92.

172. **Lee LY, Gelvin SB, Kado CI.** 1999. pSa causes oncogenic suppression of *Agrobacterium* by inhibiting VirE2 protein export. *J Bacteriol* **181:**186–196.

173. **Chumakov MI.** 2013. Protein apparatus for horizontal transfer of agrobacterial T-DNA to eukaryotic cells. *Biochemistry (Mosc)* **78:**1321–1332.

174. **Schrammeijer B, den Dulk-Ras A, Vergunst AC, Jurado Jácome E, Hooykaas PJ.** 2003. Analysis of Vir protein translocation from *Agrobacterium tumefaciens* using *Saccharomyces cerevisiae* as a model: evidence for transport of a novel effector protein VirE3. *Nucleic Acids Res* **31:**860–868.

175. **Cascales E, Atmakuri K, Liu Z, Binns AN, Christie PJ.** 2005. *Agrobacterium tumefaciens* oncogenic suppressors inhibit T-DNA and VirE2 protein substrate binding to the VirD4 coupling protein. *Mol Microbiol* **58:**565–579.

176. **Maindola P, Raina R, Goyal P, Atmakuri K, Ojha A, Gupta S, Christie PJ, Iyer LM, Aravind L, Arockiasamy A.** 2014. Multiple enzymatic activities of ParB/Srx superfamily mediate sexual conflict among conjugative plasmids. *Nat Commun* **5:**5322.

177. **Fernandez-Lopez R, Machón C, Longshaw CM, Martin S, Molin S, Zechner EL, Espinosa M, Lanka E, de la Cruz F.** 2005. Unsaturated fatty acids are inhibitors of bacterial conjugation. *Microbiology* **151:**3517–3526.

178. **Lujan SA, Guogas LM, Ragonese H, Matson SW, Redinbo MR.** 2007. Disrupting antibiotic resistance propagation by inhibiting the conjugative DNA relaxase. *Proc Natl Acad Sci U S A* **104:**12282–12287.

179. **Nash RP, McNamara DE, Ballentine WK III, Matson SW, Redinbo MR.** 2012. Investigating the impact of bisphosphonates and structurally related compounds on bacteria containing conjugative plasmids. *Biochem Biophys Res Commun* **424:**697–703.

180. **Jalasvuori M, Friman VP, Nieminen A, Bamford JK, Buckling A.** 2011. Bacteriophage selection against a plasmid-encoded sex apparatus leads to the loss of antibiotic-resistance plasmids. *Biol Lett* **7:**902–905.

181. **Ojala V, Laitalainen J, Jalasvuori M.** 2013. Fight evolution with evolution: plasmid-dependent phages with a wide host range prevent the spread of antibiotic resistance. *Evol Appl* **6:**925–932.

182. **Harrison E, Wood AJ, Dytham C, Pitchford JW, Truman J, Spiers A, Paterson S, Brockhurst MA.** 2015. Bacteriophages limit the existence conditions for conjugative plasmids. *mBio* **6:**e00586.

183. **Hagens S, Habel A, Bläsi U.** 2006. Augmentation of the antimicrobial efficacy of antibiotics by filamentous phage. *Microb Drug Resist* **12:**164–168.

184. **Boeke JD, Model P, Zinder ND.** 1982. Effects of bacteriophage f1 gene III protein on the host cell membrane. *Mol Gen Genet* **186:**185–192.

185. **Brinton CC Jr, Gemski P Jr, Carnahan J.** 1964. A new type of bacterial pilus genetically controlled by the fertility factor of *E. coli* K 12 and its role in chromosome transfer. *Proc Natl Acad Sci U S A* **52:**776–783.

186. **Knolle P.** 1967. Evidence for the identity of the mating-specific site of male cells of *Escherichia coli* with the receptor site of an RNA phage. *Biochem Biophys Res Commun* **27:**81–87.

187. **Ippen KA, Valentine RC.** 1967. The sex hair of *E. coli* as sensory fiber, conjugation tube, or mating arm? *Biochem Biophys Res Commun* **27:**674–680.

188. **Novotny C, Knight WS, Brinton CC Jr.** 1968. Inhibition of bacterial conjugation by ribonucleic acid and deoxyribonucleic acid male-specific bacteriophages. *J Bacteriol* **95:**314–326.

189. **Salzman TC.** 1971. Coordination of sex pili with their specifying R factors. *Nat New Biol* **230:**278–279.

190. **Ou JT.** 1973. Inhibition of formation of *Escherichia coli* mating pairs by f1 and MS2 bacteriophages as determined with a Coulter counter. *J Bacteriol* **114:**1108–1115.

191. **Schreil W, Christensen JR.** 1974. Conjugation and phage MS 2 infection with Hfr *Escherichia coli*. *Arch Mikrobiol* **95:**19–28.

192. **Lin A, Jimenez J, Derr J, Vera P, Manapat ML, Esvelt KM, Villanueva L, Liu DR, Chen IA.** 2011. Inhibition of bacterial conjugation by phage M13 and its protein g3p: quantitative analysis and model. *PLoS One* **6:**e19991.

193. **Lubkowski J, Hennecke F, Plückthun A, Wlodawer A.** 1999. Filamentous phage infection: crystal structure of g3p in complex with its coreceptor, the C-terminal domain of TolA. *Structure* **7:**711–722.

194. **Wan Z, Goddard NL.** 2012. Competition between conjugation and M13 phage infection in *Escherichia coli* in the absence of selection pressure: a kinetic study. *G3 (Bethesda)* **2:**1137–1144.

195. **Freese PD, Korolev KS, Jiménez JI, Chen IA.** 2014. Genetic drift suppresses bacterial conjugation in spatially structured populations. *Biophys J* **106:**944–954.

196. **May T, Tsuruta K, Okabe S.** 2011. Exposure of conjugative plasmid carrying *Escherichia coli* biofilms to male-specific bacteriophages. *ISME J* **5:**771–775.

197. **Harden V, Meynell E.** 1972. Inhibition of gene transfer by antiserum and identification of serotypes of sex pili. *J Bacteriol* **109:**1067–1074.

198. **Lawn AM, Meynell E.** 1970. Serotypes of sex pili. *J Hyg (Lond)* **68:**683–694.

199. **Tzagoloff H, Pratt D.** 1964. The initial steps in infection with coliphage M13. *Virology* **24:**372–380.

200. **Ou JT, Anderson TF.** 1972. Effect of Zn^{2+} on bacterial conjugation: inhibition of mating pair formation. *J Bacteriol* **111:**177–185.

201. **Ou JT.** 1973. Effect of Zn^{2+} on bacterial conjugation: increase in ability of F⁻ cells to form mating pairs. *J Bacteriol* **115:**648–654.

202. **Ou JT, Reim R.** 1976. Effect of 1,10-phenanthroline on bacterial conjugation in *Escherichia coli* K-12: inhibition of maturation from preliminary mates into effective mates. *J Bacteriol* **128:**363–371.

203. **Sneath PH, Lederberg J.** 1961. Inhibition by periodate of mating in *Escherichia coli* K-12. *Proc Natl Acad Sci U S A* **47:**86–90.

204. **Dettori R, Maccacaro G, Piccinin G.** 1961. Sex-specific bacteriophages of *Escherichia coli* K12. *G Microbiol* **9:**141–150.

205. **Raab C, Röschenthaler R.** 1970. Inhibition of adsorption and replication of the RNA-phage MS-2 in *Escherichia coli* C 3000 by levallorphan. *Biochem Biophys Res Commun* **41:**1429–1436.

206. **Löser R, Boquet PL, Röschenthaler R.** 1971. Inhibition of R-factor transfer by levallorphan. *Biochem Biophys Res Commun* **45:**204–211.

207. **Mándi Y, Molnár J.** 1981. Effect of chlorpromazine on conjugal plasmid transfer and sex pili. *Acta Microbiol Acad Sci Hung* **28:**205–210.

208. **Singleton P.** 1983. Colloidal clay inhibits conjugal transfer of R-plasmid R1*drd-19* in *Escherichia coli*. *Appl Environ Microbiol* **46:**756–757.

209. **Roper MM, Marshall KC.** 1977. Effects of a clay mineral on microbial predation and parasitism of *Escherichia coli*. *Microb Ecol* **4:**279–289.

210. **Roper MM, Marshall KC.** 1978. Effect of clay particle size on clay-*Escherichia coli*-

bacteriophage interactions. *Microbiology* **106**: 187–189.

211. **Qiu Z, Yu Y, Chen Z, Jin M, Yang D, Zhao Z, Wang J, Shen Z, Wang X, Qian D, Huang A, Zhang B, Li JW.** 2012. Nanoalumina promotes the horizontal transfer of multiresistance genes mediated by plasmids across genera. *Proc Natl Acad Sci U S A* **109**:4944–4949.

212. **Schwartz GH, Eiler D, Kern M.** 1965. Solubilization of the conjugation inhibitor from *Escherichia coli* cell wall. *J Bacteriol* **89**:89–94.

213. **Lancaster JH, Goldschmidt EP, Wyss O.** 1965. Characterization of conjugation factors in *Escherichia coli* cell walls. I. Inhibition of recombination by cell walls and cell extracts. *J Bacteriol* **89**:1478–1481.

214. **Spengler G, Molnár A, Schelz Z, Amaral L, Sharples D, Molnár J.** 2006. The mechanism of plasmid curing in bacteria. *Curr Drug Targets* **7**:823–841.

215. **Bidlack JE, Silverman PM.** 2004. An active type IV secretion system encoded by the F plasmid sensitizes *Escherichia coli* to bile salts. *J Bacteriol* **186**:5202–5209.

216. **Daugelavicius R, Bamford JK, Grahn AM, Lanka E, Bamford DH.** 1997. The IncP plasmid-encoded cell envelope-associated DNA transfer complex increases cell permeability. *J Bacteriol* **179**:5195–5202.

217. **Russell AB, Peterson SB, Mougous JD.** 2014. Type VI secretion system effectors: poisons with a purpose. *Nat Rev Microbiol* **12**: 137–148.

218. **Basler M, Ho BT, Mekalanos JJ.** 2013. Tit-for-tat: type VI secretion system counterattack during bacterial cell-cell interactions. *Cell* **152**:884–894.

219. **Ho BT, Basler M, Mekalanos JJ.** 2013. Type 6 secretion system-mediated immunity to type 4 secretion system-mediated gene transfer. *Science* **342**:250–253.

220. **Weisser J, Wiedemann B.** 1987. Inhibition of R-plasmid transfer in *Escherichia coli* by4-quinolones. *Antimicrob Agents Chemother* **31**: 531–534.

221. **Debbia EA, Massaro S, Campora U, Schito GC.** 1994. Inhibition of F'lac transfer by various antibacterial drugs in *Escherichia coli*. *New Microbiol* **17**:65–68.

222. **Michel-Briand Y, Laporte JM.** 1985. Inhibition of conjugal transfer of R plasmids by nitrofurans. *J Gen Microbiol* **131**:2281–2284.

223. **Nakamura S, Inoue S, Shimizu M, Iyobe S, Mitsuhashi S.** 1976. Inhibition of conjugal transfer of R plasmids by pipemidic acid and related compounds. *Antimicrob Agents Chemother* **10**: 779–785.

224. **Warnes SL, Highmore CJ, Keevil CW.** 2012. Horizontal transfer of antibiotic resistance genes on abiotic touch surfaces: implications for public health. *mBio* **3**:e00489-12.

225. **Warnes SL, Green SM, Michels HT, Keevil CW.** 2010. Biocidal efficacy of copper alloys against pathogenic enterococci involves degradation of genomic and plasmid DNAs. *Appl Environ Microbiol* **76**:5390–5401.

226. **Warnes SL, Caves V, Keevil CW.** 2012. Mechanism of copper surface toxicity in *Escherichia coli* O157:H7 and *Salmonella* involves immediate membrane depolarization followed by slower rate of DNA destruction which differs from that observed for Gram-positive bacteria. *Environ Microbiol* **14**:1730–1743.

227. **Hong R, Kang TY, Michels CA, Gadura N.** 2012. Membrane lipid peroxidation in copper alloy-mediated contact killing of *Escherichia coli*. *Appl Environ Microbiol* **78**:1776–1784.

228. **Zhao WH, Hu ZQ, Hara Y, Shimamura T.** 2001. Inhibition by epigallocatechin gallate (EGCg) of conjugative R plasmid transfer in *Escherichia coli*. *J Infect Chemother* **7**:195–197.

229. **Oyedemi BO, Shinde V, Shinde K, Kakalou D, Stapleton PD, Gibbons S.** 2016. Novel R-plasmid conjugal transfer inhibitory and antibacterial activities of phenolic compounds from *Mallotus philippensis* (Lam.) Mull. Arg. *J Glob Antimicrob Resist* **5**:15–21.

230. **Emeruwa AC.** 1982. Antibacterial substance from *Carica papaya* fruit extract. *J Nat Prod* **45**: 123–127.

231. **Leite AA, Nardi RM, Nicoli JR, Chartone-Souza E, Nascimento AM.** 2005. *Carica papaya* seed macerate as inhibitor of conjugative R plasmid transfer from *Salmonella typhimurium* to *Escherichia coli* in vitro and in the digestive tract of gnotobiotic mice. *J Gen Appl Microbiol* **51**:21–26.

232. **García-Quintanilla M, Ramos-Morales F, Casadesús J.** 2008. Conjugal transfer of the *Salmonella enterica* virulence plasmid in the mouse intestine. *J Bacteriol* **190**:1922–1927.

233. **Heseltine WW, Galloway LD.** 1951. Some antibacterial properties of sodium propionate. *J Pharm Pharmacol* **3**:581–585.

234. **Couce A, Blázquez J.** 2009. Side effects of antibiotics on genetic variability. *FEMS Microbiol Rev* **33**:531–538.

235. **Beaber JW, Hochhut B, Waldor MK.** 2004. SOS response promotes horizontal dissemination of antibiotic resistance genes. *Nature* **427**:72–74.

236. **Stevens AM, Shoemaker NB, Li LY, Salyers AA.** 1993. Tetracycline regulation of genes on *Bacteroides* conjugative transposons. *J Bacteriol* **175**:6134–6141.

237. **Torres OR, Korman RZ, Zahler SA, Dunny GM.** 1991. The conjugative transposon Tn*925*: enhancement of conjugal transfer by tetracycline in *Enterococcus faecalis* and mobilization of chromosomal genes in *Bacillus subtilis* and *E. faecalis*. *Mol Gen Genet* **225:**395–400.

238. **Barr V, Barr K, Millar MR, Lacey RW.** 1986. Beta-lactam antibiotics increase the frequency of plasmid transfer in *Staphylococcus aureus*. *J Antimicrob Chemother* **17:**409–413.

239. **Francia MV, Varsaki A, Garcillán-Barcia MP, Latorre A, Drainas C, de la Cruz F.** 2004. A classification scheme for mobilization regions of bacterial plasmids. *FEMS Microbiol Rev* **28:**79–100.

240. **Getino M, Fernández-López R, Palencia-Gándara C, Campos-Gómez J, Sánchez-López JM, Martínez M, Fernández A, de la Cruz F.** 2016. Tanzawaic acids, a chemically novel set of bacterial conjugation inhibitors. *PLoS One* **11:** e0148098.

241. **Getino M, Sanabria-Ríos DJ, Fernández-López R, Campos-Gómez J, Sánchez-López JM, Fernández A, Carballeira NM, de la Cruz F.** 2015. Synthetic fatty acids prevent plasmid-mediated horizontal gene transfer. *mBio* **6:** e01032-e15.

242. **Carattoli A.** 2009. Resistance plasmid families in *Enterobacteriaceae*. *Antimicrob Agents Chemother* **53:**2227–2238.

243. **Ripoll-Rozada J, García-Cazorla Y, Getino M, Machón C, Sanabria-Ríos D, de la Cruz F, Cabezón E, Arechaga I.** 2016. Type IV traffic ATPase TrwD as molecular target to inhibit bacterial conjugation. *Mol Microbiol* **100:**912–921.

244. **Kerr JE, Christie PJ.** 2010. Evidence for VirB4-mediated dislocation of membrane-integrated VirB2 pilin during biogenesis of the *Agrobacterium* VirB/VirD4 type IV secretion system. *J Bacteriol* **192:**4923–4934.

245. **Atmakuri K, Cascales E, Christie PJ.** 2004. Energetic components VirD4, VirB11 and VirB4 mediate early DNA transfer reactions required for bacterial type IV secretion. *Mol Microbiol* **54:**1199–1211.

246. **Guglielmini J, Néron B, Abby SS, Garcillán-Barcia MP, de la Cruz F, Rocha EP.** 2014. Key components of the eight classes of type IV secretion systems involved in bacterial conjugation or protein secretion. *Nucleic Acids Res* **42:** 5715–5727.

247. **Hilleringmann M, Pansegrau W, Doyle M, Kaufman S, MacKichan ML, Gianfaldoni C, Ruggiero P, Covacci A.** 2006. Inhibitors of *Helicobacter pylori* ATPase Cagα block CagA transport and *cag* virulence. *Microbiology* **152:** 2919–2930.

248. **Sayer JR, Walldén K, Pesnot T, Campbell F, Gane PJ, Simone M, Koss H, Buelens F, Boyle TP, Selwood DL, Waksman G, Tabor AB.** 2014. 2- and 3-substituted imidazo[1,2-a]pyrazines as inhibitors of bacterial type IV secretion. *Bioorg Med Chem* **22:**6459–6470.

249. **Shaffer CL, Good JA, Kumar S, Krishnan KS, Gaddy JA, Loh JT, Chappell J, Almqvist F, Cover TL, Hadjifrangiskou M.** 2016. Peptidomimetic small molecules disrupt type IV secretion system activity in diverse bacterial pathogens. *mBio* **7:**e00221-e16.

250. **Pinkner JS, Remaut H, Buelens F, Miller E, Aberg V, Pemberton N, Hedenström M, Larsson A, Seed P, Waksman G, Hultgren SJ, Almqvist F.** 2006. Rationally designed small compounds inhibit pilus biogenesis in uropathogenic bacteria. *Proc Natl Acad Sci U S A* **103:** 17897–17902.

251. **Galán JE, Lara-Tejero M, Marlovits TC, Wagner S.** 2014. Bacterial type III secretion systems: specialized nanomachines for protein delivery into target cells. *Annu Rev Microbiol* **68:**415–438.

252. **Charro N, Mota LJ.** 2015. Approaches targeting the type III secretion system to treat or prevent bacterial infections. *Expert Opin Drug Discov* **10:** 373–387.

253. **Felise HB, Nguyen HV, Pfuetzner RA, Barry KC, Jackson SR, Blanc MP, Bronstein PA, Kline T, Miller SI.** 2008. An inhibitor of Gram-negative bacterial virulence protein secretion. *Cell Host Microbe* **4:**325–336.

254. **Krüger DH, Barcak GJ, Reuter M, Smith HO.** 1988. *Eco*RII can be activated to cleave refractory DNA recognition sites. *Nucleic Acids Res* **16:**3997–4008.

255. **Meisel A, Bickle TA, Krüger DH, Schroeder C.** 1992. Type III restriction enzymes need two inversely oriented recognition sites for DNA cleavage. *Nature* **355:**467–469.

256. **Warren RA.** 1980. Modified bases in bacteriophage DNAs. *Annu Rev Microbiol* **34:**137–158.

257. **Iida S, Streiff MB, Bickle TA, Arber W.** 1987. Two DNA antirestriction systems of bacteriophage P1, *darA*, and *darB*: characterization of *darA*⁻ phages. *Virology* **157:**156–166.

258. **Zabeau M, Friedman S, Van Montagu M, Schell J.** 1980. The *ral* gene of phage lambda. I. Identification of a non-essential gene that modulates restriction and modification in *E. coli*. *Mol Gen Genet* **179:**63–73.

259. **Studier FW, Movva NR.** 1976. SAMase gene of bacteriophage T3 is responsible for overcoming host restriction. *J Virol* **19:**136–145.

260. **Walkinshaw MD, Taylor P, Sturrock SS, Atanasiu C, Berge T, Henderson RM, Edwardson**

JM, Dryden DT. 2002. Structure of Ocr from bacteriophage T7, a protein that mimics B-form DNA. *Mol Cell* **9**:187–194.

261. **Serna A, Espinosa E, Camacho EM, Casadesús J.** 2010. Regulation of bacterial conjugation in microaerobiosis by host-encoded functions ArcAB and sdhABCD. *Genetics* **184**:947–958.

262. **Camacho EM, Serna A, Casadesús J.** 2005. Regulation of conjugal transfer by Lrp and Dam methylation in plasmid R100. *Int Microbiol* **8**:279–285.

263. **Will WR, Lu J, Frost LS.** 2004. The role of H-NS in silencing F transfer gene expression during entry into stationary phase. *Mol Microbiol* **54**:769–782.

264. **Shin M, Song M, Rhee JH, Hong Y, Kim YJ, Seok YJ, Ha KS, Jung SH, Choy HE.** 2005. DNA looping-mediated repression by histone-like protein H-NS: specific requirement of $E\sigma^{70}$ as a cofactor for looping. *Genes Dev* **19**:2388–2398.

265. **Wada C, Imai M, Yura T.** 1987. Host control of plasmid replication: requirement for the σ factor σ^{32} in transcription of mini-F replication initiator gene. *Proc Natl Acad Sci U S A* **84**:8849–8853.

266. **Dorman CJ.** 2009. Nucleoid-associated proteins and bacterial physiology. *Adv Appl Microbiol* **67**:47–64.

267. **Gamas P, Caro L, Galas D, Chandler M.** 1987. Expression of F transfer functions depends on the *Escherichia coli* integration host factor. *Mol Gen Genet* **207**:302–305.

268. **Starcic M, Zgur-Bertok D, Jordi BJ, Wösten MM, Gaastra W, van Putten JP.** 2003. The cyclic AMP-cyclic AMP receptor protein complex regulates activity of the *traJ* promoter of the *Escherichia coli* conjugative plasmid pRK100. *J Bacteriol* **185**:1616–1623.

269. **Frost LS, Manchak J.** 1998. F⁻ phenocopies: characterization of expression of the F transfer region in stationary phase. *Microbiology* **144**:2579–2587.

270. **Will WR, Frost LS.** 2006. Hfq is a regulator of F-plasmid TraJ and TraM synthesis in *Escherichia coli*. *J Bacteriol* **188**:124–131.

271. **Lau-Wong IC, Locke T, Ellison MJ, Raivio TL, Frost LS.** 2008. Activation of the Cpx regulon destabilizes the F plasmid transfer activator, TraJ, via the HslVU protease in *Escherichia coli*. *Mol Microbiol* **67**:516–527.

272. **Zahrl D, Wagner A, Tscherner M, Koraimann G.** 2007. GroEL plays a central role in stress-induced negative regulation of bacterial conjugation by promoting proteolytic degradation of the activator protein TraJ. *J Bacteriol* **189**:5885–5894.

Fitness Costs of Plasmids: A Limit to Plasmid Transmission

4

ALVARO SAN MILLAN[1] and R. CRAIG MACLEAN[2]

INTRODUCTION

Horizontal gene transfer (HGT) is a key source of genetic diversity in bacteria (1), and plasmids are one of the main vehicles driving this process (2). Plasmids are widely distributed across prokaryotes, and help bacteria adapt to a myriad of different environments, conditions, and stresses (3, 4), playing a key role in bacterial ecology and evolution (5–7). The most vivid testimony to the power of plasmids as catalysts for bacterial adaptation is their role in the spread of antibiotic resistance among clinical pathogens (8), which has emerged as a major health problem over the past decades (9).

Despite the potential benefits conferred by plasmids, they also produce a burden (fitness cost) in the host, manifesting as a reduced growth rate and weakened competitiveness of plasmid-bearing strains under conditions that do not select for plasmid-encoded genes (10, 11). This fitness cost imposed by plasmids, coupled with the potential plasmid loss during bacterial cell division, hinders the survival of plasmids in bacterial communities. Moreover, any beneficial gene carried by the plasmid could eventually move to the chromosome (12), making it difficult to understand why plasmids persist (the

[1]Department of Microbiology, Hospital Universitario Ramon y Cajal (IRYCIS) and Centro de Investigacion Biomedica en Red (CIBERESP), Madrid, Spain; [2]Department of Zoology, University of Oxford, Oxford, United Kingdom.
Microbial Transmission in Biological Processes
Edited by Fernando Baquero, Emilio Bouza, J.A. Gutiérrez-Fuentes, and Teresa M. Coque
© 2018 American Society for Microbiology, Washington, DC
doi:10.1128/microbiolspec.MTBP-0016-2017

"plasmid paradox"). Several early studies investigated the consequences of the fitness costs of plasmids on their ability to survive in bacterial populations (13–18). These studies established the "existence conditions" for plasmids, which in general involved a relatively high rate of horizontal spread by conjugation, especially when plasmids acted as pure genetic parasites (in the absence of selection for plasmid-encoded traits). Most recently, Harrison and Brockhurst proposed that the plasmid paradox could be explained by compensatory evolution (19). The idea underlying this hypothesis is that even if plasmids produce a cost when they first arrive in a new bacterial host, this cost could be alleviated over time through compensatory mutations in the plasmid and/or the host chromosome (20). In recent years, several studies have analyzed the molecular basis of the cost and compensation of plasmids in bacterial populations (21–28), generating new models of the existence conditions of plasmids (22, 24). These studies evaluate a number of selection, transfer, and compensation regimes that could explain plasmid survival in bacterial populations, and have revealed new evidence about the molecular mechanisms underlying the cost of and adaptation to plasmids.

This review expands on previous reviews on the origins of HGT-related costs in light of new data available in the plasmid literature (10). Specifically, we analyze the potential fitness effects produced by plasmids during each step of their life cycle in the host bacterium, as well as the mechanisms that help bacteria and plasmids control these effects. Here, we focus on the effects of plasmids on the bacterial host, so, unless otherwise specified, when we talk about fitness (or fitness costs) we refer to the bacterium, which is not necessarily linked to plasmid fitness due to the potential for HGT of these genetic elements. Finally, we explore some of the main challenges and questions in the field of plasmid evolution.

DISSECTING THE FITNESS COSTS PRODUCED BY PLASMIDS

Infection by a plasmid usually entails a fitness cost that reduces the reproductive rate of the host bacterium (11). This fitness cost plays a key role in the population biology of plasmids by generating selection against plasmid-carrying strains. The origins of these costs are manifold (10), and we are only beginning to understand them. Deciphering the molecular mechanisms underlying plasmid fitness costs is essential for efforts to predict future plasmid-bacteria associations driving the evolution of antibiotic resistance. In this section, we dissect the costs produced by plasmids during the different phases of their biology in the host bacterium (Fig. 1). The actual cost of a plasmid likely emerges from the combination of and interactions among these effects; however, each of these factors is likely to make a different relative contribution to the overall fitness cost.

Plasmid Reception

The first step in plasmid acquisition by a new host is the physical arrival of the plasmid in the cell. Plasmids can be transmitted by any of the three HGT mechanisms: transformation (29, 30), phage-mediated transduction (31), and conjugation (3). Conjugation is considered the most important mechanism of plasmid transmission, and the conjugative process has been extensively studied (discussed below). During conjugation, the plasmid enters the new cell as single-stranded DNA (32), producing a transient activation of the SOS response (33). The SOS response is a bacterial stress response triggered by an increase in single-stranded DNA in the cell, which leads to a rise in mutation and recombination rates (34). Activation of the SOS regulon also results in inhibition of cell division, which by definition translates into a decrease in bacterial fitness in the short term (35). The potential impact of conjugation-

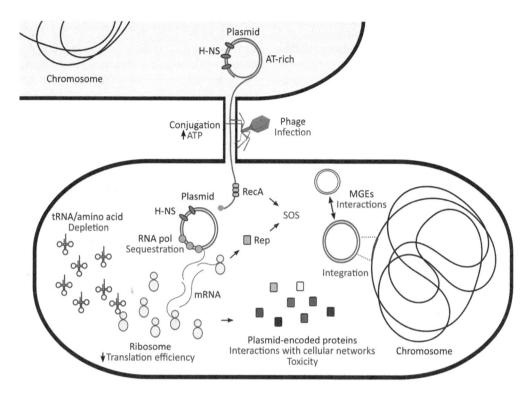

FIGURE 1 Fitness costs produced by plasmids. Potential fitness effects produced by plasmids during their life cycle in the bacterial host.

mediated SOS response activation on recipient cell fitness is indicated by the presence of anti-SOS genes, such as *psiB*, in conjugative plasmids (36). These factors are transferred as part of the plasmid-leading region and are expressed upon arrival of the plasmid in the new cell (37, 38). PsiB binds to the SOS regulon activator RecA, impeding the formation of RecA nucleoproteins that trigger the SOS response (33, 36). The SOS response can also be triggered by plasmid transformation and transduction (39, 40), so plasmid reception through these pathways will also produce a potential decrease in fitness.

Plasmid reception also entails a transient transcriptional overshooting of plasmid genes regulated by negative feedback loops (41, 42). Until the plasmid-encoded transcriptional repressors are expressed in the recipient cell, expensive plasmid functions such as conjugation will be derepressed, producing a transient elevation in the fitness cost produced by the plasmid. The effect of this cost is to reduce vertical plasmid transmission; however, the transient overexpression of conjugative genes helps the plasmid to rapidly spread horizontally in a bacterial population with available recipient cells (41).

Plasmid Integration

Following successful transfer to a recipient cell, certain plasmids can integrate into the chromosome of the host (43). Although the integration of a plasmid carrying adaptive genes on the chromosome may be potentially advantageous for the host, this process can also produce deleterious effects associated with the disruption of host genes (44). This is the case with integrative and conjugative elements (ICEs), which integrate into and excise from the host cell chromosome thanks to an ICE-encoded recombinase (43). Some ICE families target a single specific attachment site in the bacterial chromosome, usually in a tRNA gene (45), suggesting that these plasmids have evolved a strategy to avoid arbitrary disruption of the host genome during integration. However, other ICE families target multiple attachment sites (46), and some families, like Tn916, integrate almost randomly in the host chromosome (47). This nonspecific integration can disrupt protein coding or regulatory regions or can interfere in the expression of genes flanking the integration site, entailing fitness costs in the recipient bacterium.

Plasmid Replication

Plasmids usually produce only a small increase in the total amount of DNA in the bacterium. It is therefore widely accepted that the main fitness cost associated with plasmids comes not from replication but from downstream events such as expression of plasmid genes (10, 11). There is, nevertheless, evidence indicating that plasmid replication does incur a fitness cost for the bacterial host. A particularly interesting observation regarding replication-related fitness costs is that plasmid DNA is significantly richer in AT than the host chromosome (48, 49). This difference is also observed for other "intracellular parasites" such as endosymbionts or phages (48, 50). Rocha and Danchin proposed that this bias might reflect the higher energy cost of G and C and the lower availability of these nucleotides in the host cell compared with A and T/U (48). This hypothesis predicts that replication of plasmids with a higher GC content would produce a higher cost; however, testing this experimentally is difficult because AT-rich transcripts tend to produce a higher cost than GC-rich transcripts in bacteria (51), and this would produce a confounding effect. Indeed, this selective advantage of GC-rich genes has

been proposed as the cause of the wide variation in GC content in prokaryote genomes (51), despite mutation in bacteria being biased toward AT (52, 53). The AT bias in plasmids therefore remains intriguing, and an alternative explanation could be "xenogeneic silencing," discussed below under "Mechanisms for Minimizing Plasmid Costs" (54).

An important side effect of plasmid replication is the pleiotropic effects of plasmid-encoded replication initiation (Rep) proteins (23, 55). Plasmids usually encode their own Rep proteins, enabling auto control of plasmid copy number (56). These proteins subsequently recruit several other DNA polymerases and helicases from the bacterial host to proceed with plasmid replication (55). Overexpression of plasmid replication proteins can therefore lead to sequestration of the cellular DNA replication machinery, stalling chromosomal replication, inducing the SOS response, and inhibiting cell division (23, 55). The control of plasmid Rep protein expression can be altered when the plasmid arrives in a new bacterial host due to interactions with chromosomal-encoded genes (23). This deleterious effect has been observed in bacteria carrying small multicopy plasmids, such as pNUK73 in *Pseudomonas aeruginosa* or pSC101 in *Escherichia coli* (23, 55). Multicopy plasmids probably require a high level of Rep protein expression to maintain their high copy number, increasing the potential for this deleterious effect.

Conjugation

Plasmids can transfer directly between bacteria in a process known as conjugation (57). During the classical conjugation process in Gram-negative bacteria, plasmid DNA travels through a type IV secretion system (T4SS) between donor and recipient bacteria (58, 59). Conjugative plasmids carry all the genetic information required to synthetize the T4SS and the proteins needed to escort plasmid DNA to the new host (3). Conjugation provides plasmids with the opportunity to replicate horizontally, and, all else being equal, this should increase the relative frequency of the plasmid in the population. However, conjugation is energetically expensive (it requires three plasmid-encoded ATPases [58]) and entails a reduction in bacterial host fitness, thus reducing the rate of vertical plasmid transmission (60). The fitness cost associated with conjugation comes primarily from the high ATP demand for mating-channel formation and plasmid DNA translocation (58). To minimize this cost, plasmids tightly control the expression of conjugative systems (41, 61–63). The result is a general repression of conjugation genes, with only a few cells in the population expressing the conjugative machinery (63). Conjugation can, however, be derepressed, either through chemical signaling (61, 62) or through transcriptional overshooting of conjugative genes in new recipient cells (41, 42), enabling a wave of plasmid transfer when there are recipient bacteria available in the population.

Several reports pinpoint conjugation as a source of plasmid cost for the bacterial host (28, 64, 65). For example, the fitness cost associated with plasmids R1 and RP4 in *E. coli* is reduced after the conjugation rate is decreased or abolished by natural selection in an experimental setting (64). Also, the expression of plasmid R1 conjugation genes has been shown to activate stress responses in *E. coli* (65), although it is not clear if this is cause or consequence of the cost of plasmid carriage. Finally, in a recent analysis of the IncN antibiotic resistance plasmid pKP33, Porse and colleagues showed that the loss of the conjugation region reduced the burden associated with plasmid carriage in *E. coli* (28).

Another potentially deadly consequence of conjugation is bacteriophage infection. Certain phages use the conjugative T4SS as an attachment site for invading the bacterial cell (66, 67). T4SS-specific phages can therefore select against plasmid-carrying bacteria (68)

and have been proposed as an alternative approach to counteracting the plasmid-mediated spread of antibiotic resistance (69).

Expression of Plasmid-Encoded Genes

The main biosynthetic burden associated with plasmid carriage is likely the expression of plasmid-encoded genes. For example, it is well established that highly expressed genes are less likely to be transferred horizontally (70, 71), demonstrating that the cost of expressing newly acquired genes can have profound evolutionary consequences. The costs associated with gene expression can arise from gene transcription, translation, or subsequent interactions between plasmid-encoded proteins and cellular networks (explored in the next section). Transcription is not considered a major cost (51), and the cost of plasmid gene expression appears to be predominantly derived from the translation of protein-encoding plasmid genes (71). Nevertheless, a recent report showed that acquired AT-rich genes can produce toxic effects due to the sequestration of RNA polymerases (72).

The cost of translation is determined by the discrepancy between plasmid mRNA abundance and the availability of cellular tRNAs, amino acids, and ribosomes. In general, for highly expressed genes the principal source of translation-associated cost is thought to be the imbalance between codon usage by the foreign genes and the available tRNA pool in the recipient bacterium (73). Several reports show that HGT is favored when there is codon usage compatibility between foreign genes and the bacterial host (translational selection) (74, 75). Due to the general AT bias of plasmids, plasmid gene codon usage is very likely to differ from the optimal codon usage by chromosomal genes (73). This difference will affect the translation efficiency (initiation, speed, and accuracy) of plasmid genes (73), leading to inefficient ribosome allocation and ribosome pausing. These alterations will produce costly effects such as increased mRNA degradation, ribosome sequestration, protein mistranslation, and protein misfolding (76–79; reviewed in 73 and 80). The deleterious effects of low translation efficiency will increase with gene expression level. Since some plasmid genes are tightly repressed (e.g., conjugation genes) and others are highly expressed (e.g., integron cassettes), one might expect highly expressed plasmid genes to incur a heavier fitness cost than less expressed genes due to codon usage differences compared to chromosomal genes. Another possible deleterious effect of plasmid gene translation is the depletion of the host cell amino acid pool (81). Amino acid starvation reduces bacterial growth rate and activates the bacterial stringent response (82), leading to increased abundance of ribosomes and charged tRNAs (83, 84). This response serves to alleviate the amino acid depletion; however, the starvation-induced tRNA pools will alter the cellular balance between mRNA and tRNA, impacting host bacterium physiology and fitness.

The centrality of translation as the main plasmid fitness cost is exemplified by a recent study of pQBR103 (25). This mega plasmid from *Pseudomonas fluorescens* produces a major burden for the host cell due to the increased transcriptional demand imposed by the plasmid-encoded genes. This demand induces a marked increase in the expression of genes involved in protein production (25). Interestingly, bacteria are able to compensate this cost during experimental evolution by reducing cellular translational requirements. This reduction is achieved by mutations in the bacterial regulatory system *gacA/gacS*, which controls the biosynthesis of a wide range of secondary metabolites (25).

Effects of Plasmid-Encoded Proteins on Bacterial Physiology

Plasmids bring new proteins to the host bacteria, and the potential effects of these proteins on bacterial physiology are impossible to predict. The most prominent examples of plasmid-encoded proteins having a deleterious effect on the host cell are postsegregational killing systems (PSKSs) (85). PSKSs are plasmid addiction mechanisms, usually encoding a stable toxin and a labile cognate antitoxin. If the plasmid is lost during cell division, the plasmid-free cell will succumb to the vertically inherited toxin protein because there will be no antitoxin to counteract its effect. PSKSs thus ensure the stability of the plasmid in the host bacteria, and they are able to expand the plasmid host range (26). However, if the partitioning systems are not fine-tuned, PSKSs will kill many plasmid-free segregant cells. Similarly to PSKSs, plasmid-encoded bacteriocins that are secreted outside the cell will also promote plasmid maintenance, since immunity genes are carried by the plasmids as well (86).

Plasmid-encoded proteins can also cause fitness costs due to unwanted interactions with cellular networks or cytotoxic effects. At the end of last century, Jain and colleagues observed that genes encoding proteins involved in complex interactions with other proteins are horizontally transferred less frequently than those encoding proteins that form part of simpler systems with fewer interactions (87), and these authors developed the "complexity hypothesis" to explain this bias. More recently, Cohen et al. confirmed that protein connectivity (the number of protein-protein interactions) correlated negatively with the transferability of the coding genes (88). On the other hand, transferability is decreased by a lack of recipient cell proteins that physiologically couple with the acquired proteins, because the acquired protein is not in a hospitable metabolic context (89). Interactions between plasmid-encoded proteins and cellular networks thus appear to have the potential to produce a variety of deleterious effects that can influence plasmid transferability.

There are a handful of reports in the literature demonstrating major fitness costs as a consequence of cellular network alterations by specific plasmid-encoded proteins (23, 26, 55, 90). In most cases, the deleterious interactions involve the plasmid Rep protein. Rep proteins connect extensively with host protein networks because they need to recruit many cellular enzymes, such as DNA polymerases and helicases, in order for plasmid replication to proceed (91). These interactions can result in the sequestration of the cellular replication machinery, altering the replication network and activating stress responses (23, 55). Interestingly, host cell helicases appear to play a key role in Rep-induced costs (23, 26, 90). In *P. aeruginosa*, costly overexpression of the Rep protein encoded by the small plasmid pNUK73 is dependent on an accessory helicase, inactivation of which fully compensates the cost of the plasmid (23). Moreover, the cost of an IncP-1b minireplicon is compensated by mutations in chromosomal helicases in *Pseudomonas moraviensis* (26) and by mutations in the helicase-binding domain of the plasmid Rep protein in *Shewanella oneidensis* (90).

Fitness Effects Due to Interactions between Mobile Genetic Elements

Bacteria often carry multiple mobile genetic elements (MGEs), and interactions among MGEs can affect host fitness. These interactions are common; for example, plasmids can inhibit the conjugative transfer of other coresident plasmids in a process known as fertility inhibition (132). The coexistence of several plasmids in the same host can either potentiate or alleviate plasmid-mediated costs, as recently reported for *P. aeruginosa*, *E. coli*, and *Agrobacterium tumefaciens* (21, 92, 93). In addition to direct MGE interactions, MGEs can influence each other indirectly through their effects on host elements. For example, plasmid-mediated activation of the SOS response can trigger phage induction or mobilize genomic islands (94). MGE interactions may have originated through a shared coevolutionary history (95, 96) or simply be the result of accidental interactions (23). Acci-

dental interactions are a more likely explanation for costly interactions, because HGT brings together genes with different evolutionary histories, and interactions are unlikely to be mutually beneficial through chance alone.

Many types of MGE interactions have been reported, and most of them are likely to affect bacterial fitness. One of the most interesting cases is the cross talk between phages and pathogenicity islands in *Staphylococcus aureus*, in which phage genome and chromosomal island compete for packaging in the phage capsid in an ongoing arms race (95). Another example is the destabilizing interaction between partitioning proteins from a genomic island and an Inc-P7 plasmid in *Pseudomonas putida* (96). There are also specific examples of MGE interactions producing deleterious effects in the host. In *Enterococcus faecium*, the coexistence of Tn*5386* and Tn*916* ICEs produces genomic deletions in the host genome. In *P. aeruginosa*, interactions between proteins encoded by a phage, a small genomic island, and the plasmid pNUK73 produce a major reduction in bacterial fitness (23).

MECHANISMS FOR MINIMIZING PLASMID COSTS

In this section, we discuss the mechanisms aimed at reducing plasmid costs on the host once the plasmid has been acquired. However, for a detailed explanation on host and plasmid barriers to plasmid acquisition see (132). The fitness costs of plasmids limit their existence in bacterial populations, and plasmids are therefore under strong selection pressure to control these costs in order to maximize their vertical spread. The host bacterium also needs to adopt strategies to cope with the presence of plasmids once they are successfully established. The previous section outlines some of the mechanisms controlling the fitness costs of plasmids, such as the action of anti-SOS genes on conjugative plasmids or the tight control of the expression of conjugative systems. Most plasmid-associated costs arise upon the expression of plasmid-carried genes, and therefore transcriptional regulation is a key route to minimizing plasmids costs. This section briefly outlines some of the mechanisms that plasmids and host bacteria have evolved to control the expression of plasmid genes.

Plasmid gene expression can be controlled by a range of different nucleoid-associated proteins (97), such as H-NS (histone-like nucleoid structuring protein) from enterobacteria. These proteins act as transcriptional repressors that silence the expression of acquired genes, a phenomenon called xenogeneic silencing (98–100). Silencing of foreign DNA by H-NS is based on its ability to target sequences with a higher AT content than the host genome (99, 101), which it achieves by binding not to a specific target sequence but to a consensus curved DNA structure commonly associated with promoters (102, 103). H-NS thus enables plasmid acquisition by reducing both the potential deleterious effects of plasmid-encoded proteins (99) and the potential sequestration of RNA polymerases by AT-rich genes (72). H-NS-mediated repression is modulated by environmental conditions and multiple countersilencing mechanisms (54), so that plasmid genes are still expressed to a certain extent, providing potentially adaptive benefits to the host bacteria. Interestingly, conjugative plasmids can also carry H-NS-like genes that repress the expression of foreign genes, including their own (104–106). Plasmid-encoded H-NS-like genes have been proposed to help plasmid conjugation by reducing the cost of plasmid acquisition (105). This hypothesis is supported by the high prevalence of these genes in conjugative plasmids (104). Taken together, these pieces of evidence suggest that xenogeneic silencing could be beneficial both for plasmid, enabling plasmid propagation, and bacterium, providing new genes at low cost. Therefore, we argue that selection for xenogeneic silenc-

ing could be responsible for maintaining the general AT bias in plasmids and other MGEs compared to their host chromosomes.

Plasmids also use specific regulators to control the transcription of their own genes, especially those related to plasmid housekeeping processes. Genes involved in the energetically expensive conjugative process are tightly self-regulated (41), as is the expression of partition and replication genes (91, 107, 108). In contrast, the transcription of plasmid-encoded accessory genes (mediating bacterial adaptation to the environment) is not always fine-tuned, and represents an important potential source of fitness cost. These accessory genes are frequently encoded in genetic elements that generate high expression levels, such as integrons. Integrons are genetic platforms that acquire open reading frames, called cassettes, through the action of the integron integrase (109). These cassettes are expressed from a single strong promoter, creating a gradient of cassette transcription (110, 133). Integrons are very prevalent in plasmids and are generally related to antibiotic resistance (111). Transcriptional analysis has shown that integron cassettes are among the highest-expressed plasmid genes, representing an important potential source of fitness cost to host bacteria (112–114).

CHALLENGES IN THE FIELD

Antibiotic resistance in bacteria is a major health problem, and plasmids are essential vectors of the dissemination of antibiotic resistance to clinically relevant pathogens (8). Plasmids can promote bacterial survival in the presence of antibiotics, but, as we have seen, they can also impose a fitness cost when they enter a new bacterial host. The past few years have witnessed growing interest in the fitness effects of plasmids (21–28, 115), and some of the general principles underlying these effects are now beginning to be identified. However, we still are a long way from understanding the specific molecular basis of these costs or being able to predict plasmid fitness effects in a bacterial host. This final section discusses future research directions that may help to answer some of the outstanding questions about the fitness effects of plasmids and how they dictate the evolution of plasmid-mediated antibiotic resistance: What makes a bacterial-antibiotic resistance plasmid association successful? What is the molecular basis of the fitness effects of antibiotic resistance plasmids in clinical strains? Can we predict which plasmid-bacteria associations are likely to arise in the future?

Investigating Clinically Relevant Plasmid-Bacterium Combinations

One of the main challenges in the field is to develop experimental models of clinically relevant plasmid-bacterium combinations. Most studies of plasmid fitness costs have involved laboratory-adapted bacterial strains and plasmids of low clinical relevance. If we want to understand the evolution of plasmid-mediated antibiotic resistance, we will need to investigate the fitness effects of antibiotic resistance plasmids in high-risk pathogenic bacteria. Gram-negative pathogens, particularly enterobacteria such as *E. coli* and *Klebsiella pneumoniae*, are currently the most concerning cause of multiresistant infections in hospitals (116–118), and these bacterial strains acquire resistance to frontline antibiotics such as β-lactams primarily by plasmid transmission (8). Interestingly, associations between plasmid types and enterobacteria clones are not random. Rather, certain bacterial clones carry highly specific types of resistance plasmids (e.g., *E. coli* ST131 and IncF plasmids are often associated [119]) but not others, even when clone and plasmid coincide in time and space (e.g., *E. coli* ST131 and pOXA-48 are seldom associated [119, 120]). Studying the molecular basis of the effect of epidemic plasmids on clinically relevant enterobacteria strains may help to reveal why some plasmid-bacterium associations are especially successful. These

approaches could also improve our capacity to predict the evolution of plasmid-mediated antibiotic resistance in clinically relevant scenarios.

Expanding the Experimental Conditions

Another limitation of studies of the fitness effects of plasmids in bacteria is that they are usually carried out *in vitro*, using conditions very different from the natural environments of the bacterial hosts. Several experimental models can be used to measure fitness under conditions that more closely reproduce the natural habitat of the host bacteria. These range from *in vitro* systems, such as Biolog plates, that provide a variety of carbon sources (121, 122), through more-complex synthetic systems or *ex vivo* animal models (123, 124), all the way to *in vivo* analysis in nematodes (e.g., *Caenorhabditis elegans* [125]), insects (e.g., *Galleria mellonella* [126]), and mice or pigs (127, 128). Nevertheless, despite the evident differences between laboratory culture medium and the natural bacterial habitat, the overall fitness effects of plasmids measured *in vitro* correlate quite well with their effects measured in mouse models (11).

Exploring Interactions between MGEs

Previous studies revealed that interactions between MGEs play an important part in the fitness effects produced by these elements (21, 23, 92, 95). Moreover, interactions between plasmids and other MGEs can also alter the evolutionary trajectories of plasmid-carrying bacteria, as recently shown for a plasmid-phage combination in *P. fluorescens* (129). In natural microbial communities, bacteria are exposed to a wide range of MGEs, and understanding how interactions between these elements shape the fitness effects and evolution of MGE-bacteria associations is an exciting challenge. Understanding interactions between different plasmids and between plasmids and other MGEs may help to explain plasmid distribution in bacteria (21, 130).

High-Throughput Approaches

Predicting the fitness effects of specific plasmid types in specific bacterial clones is of paramount importance if we are to predict which plasmid-bacteria associations are likely to arise in the future and anticipate the evolution and epidemiology of plasmid-mediated antibiotic resistance. In a recent meta-analysis, Vogwill and MacLean analyzed available data on the fitness effects of 49 plasmids examined in 16 studies (11). Remarkably, these authors found that the same plasmid generally has a very different fitness cost in different hosts, and that the variation coefficient for fitness effects of a single plasmid in different hosts does not differ significantly from that for the fitness effects of different plasmids in the same host (11). These results highlight the impossibility of using the fitness cost of a plasmid measured in one bacterial host to predict the effects of the same plasmid in other bacterial clones. This question will therefore need to be addressed through high-throughput studies using factorial designs combining multiple plasmids and multiple bacterial clones. Such studies could provide insight into the general trends of the fitness effects of specific plasmid types on specific bacterial groups (genus, species, and high-risk clonal complexes). It will also be necessary to test not only initial plasmid costs but also the ability of compensatory evolution to reduce the cost of specific combinations. Understanding these general trends in fitness effects and the capacity for compensation may assist predictions of which plasmid-bacteria associations we are likely to encounter in real-life scenarios.

Integrative Analysis of Plasmid Costs

A full understanding of the origin of the costs produced by plasmids requires detailed knowledge of the molecular basis underlying them. To date, only a handful of studies have investigated the genetic basis of plasmid fitness costs (23, 25–28) or the transcriptional effects of plasmids on the bacterial host (23, 25, 113, 131). In our experience, the best way to investigate the molecular mechanisms underlying the fitness costs of plasmids is to first obtain a compensated clone from the parental plasmid-carrying strain (22, 23). One can then analyze and compare the plasmid-carrying and plasmid-free naive and compensated strains, obtaining a clearer picture of the basis of cost and compensation (23, 25). Most studies using this approach include the sequencing of the whole genome of the plasmid-carrying strains before and after compensatory adaptation, allowing the genetic basis of cost and compensation to be determined (23, 25, 26, 28). In two studies, the origins of the cost were further investigated using transcriptomic analysis of naive and compensated plasmid-carrying strains (23, 25). Because gene expression is such a key determinant of the cost of plasmid carriage, transcriptomic approaches are an essential tool in the investigation of the mechanisms underlying the cost of plasmid carriage. However, a major challenge in the field is the adoption of a more integrated approach to the analysis of plasmid fitness effects. Genomics and transcriptomics should therefore be complemented with metabolomic and proteomic analyses to yield a full picture of the origins of the costs of plasmids.

ACKNOWLEDGMENTS

This work was supported by the Instituto de Salud Carlos III (Plan Estatal de I+D+i 2013-2016). Grant CP15-00012, PI16-00860, and CIBER (CB06/02/0053) actions, cofinanced by the European Development Regional Fund "A way to achieve Europe" (ERDF). A.S.M. is supported by a Miguel Servet fellowship from the Instituto de Salud Carlos III (MS15/00012) cofinanced by the European

Social Fund "Investing in your future" (ESF) and ERDF.

CITATION

San Millan A, Maclean RC. 2017. Fitness costs of plasmids: a limit to plasmid transmission. Microbiol Spectrum 5(5):MTBP-0016-2017.

REFERENCES

1. **Wiedenbeck J, Cohan FM.** 2011. Origins of bacterial diversity through horizontal genetic transfer and adaptation to new ecological niches. *FEMS Microbiol Rev* **35:**957–976.
2. **Summers DK.** 1996. *The Biology of Plasmids.* Blackwell Science Ltd, Oxford, United Kingdom.
3. **Smillie C, Garcillán-Barcia MP, Francia MV, Rocha EP, de la Cruz F.** 2010. Mobility of plasmids. *Microbiol Mol Biol Rev* **74:**434–452.
4. **Smalla K, Jechalke S, Top EM.** 2015. Plasmid detection, characterization, and ecology. *Microbiol Spectr* **3:**PLAS-0038-2014.
5. **Ochman H, Lawrence JG, Groisman EA.** 2000. Lateral gene transfer and the nature of bacterial innovation. *Nature* **405:**299–304.
6. **Gogarten JP, Townsend JP.** 2005. Horizontal gene transfer, genome innovation and evolution. *Nat Rev Microbiol* **3:**679–687.
7. **San Millan A, Escudero JA, Gifford DR, Mazel D, MacLean RC.** 2016. Multicopy plasmids potentiate the evolution of antibiotic resistance in bacteria. *Nat Ecol Evol* **1:**10.
8. **Carattoli A.** 2013. Plasmids and the spread of resistance. *Int J Med Microbiol* **303:**298–304.
9. **Review on Antimicrobial Resistance.** 2016. *Tackling Drug-Resistant Infections Globally: Final Report and Recommendations.* Review on Antimicrobial Resistance, London, United Kingdom. https://amr-review.org/sites/default/files/160518_Final%20paper_with%20cover.pdf. Accessed date 12/01/2017.
10. **Baltrus DA.** 2013. Exploring the costs of horizontal gene transfer. *Trends Ecol Evol* **28:**489–495.
11. **Vogwill T, MacLean RC.** 2015. The genetic basis of the fitness costs of antimicrobial resistance: a meta-analysis approach. *Evol Appl* **8:**284–295.
12. **Hall JP, Wood AJ, Harrison E, Brockhurst MA.** 2016. Source-sink plasmid transfer dynamics maintain gene mobility in soil bacterial communities. *Proc Natl Acad Sci U S A* **113:**8260–8265.
13. **Stewart FM, Levin BR.** 1977. The population biology of bacterial plasmids: a priori conditions for the existence of conjugationally transmitted factors. *Genetics* **87:**209–228.
14. **Levin BR, Stewart FM.** 1980. The population biology of bacterial plasmids: a priori conditions for the existence of mobilizable nonconjugative factors. *Genetics* **94:**425–443.
15. **Simonsen L.** 1991. The existence conditions for bacterial plasmids: theory and reality. *Microb Ecol* **22:**187–205.
16. **Bergstrom CT, Lipsitch M, Levin BR.** 2000. Natural selection, infectious transfer and the existence conditions for bacterial plasmids. *Genetics* **155:**1505–1519.
17. **Lili LN, Britton NF, Feil EJ.** 2007. The persistence of parasitic plasmids. *Genetics* **177:**399–405.
18. **Krone SM, Lu R, Fox R, Suzuki H, Top EM.** 2007. Modelling the spatial dynamics of plasmid transfer and persistence. *Microbiology* **153:**2803–2816.
19. **Harrison E, Brockhurst MA.** 2012. Plasmid-mediated horizontal gene transfer is a coevolutionary process. *Trends Microbiol* **20:**262–267.
20. **Bouma JE, Lenski RE.** 1988. Evolution of a bacteria/plasmid association. *Nature* **335:**351–352.
21. **San Millan A, Heilbron K, MacLean RC.** 2014. Positive epistasis between co-infecting plasmids promotes plasmid survival in bacterial populations. *ISME J* **8:**601–612.
22. **San Millan A, Peña-Miller R, Toll-Riera M, Halbert ZV, McLean AR, Cooper BS, MacLean RC.** 2014. Positive selection and compensatory adaptation interact to stabilize non-transmissible plasmids. *Nat Commun* **5:**5208.
23. **San Millan A, Toll-Riera M, Qi Q, MacLean RC.** 2015. Interactions between horizontally acquired genes create a fitness cost in *Pseudomonas aeruginosa. Nat Commun* **6:**6845.
24. **Peña-Miller R, Rodríguez-González R, MacLean RC, San Millan A.** 2015. Evaluating the effect of horizontal transmission on the stability of plasmids under different selection regimes. *Mob Genet Elements* **5:**1–5.
25. **Harrison E, Guymer D, Spiers AJ, Paterson S, Brockhurst MA.** 2015. Parallel compensatory evolution stabilizes plasmids across the parasitism-mutualism continuum. *Curr Biol* **25:**2034–2039.
26. **Loftie-Eaton W, Yano H, Burleigh S, Simmons RS, Hughes JM, Rogers LM, Hunter SS, Settles ML, Forney LJ, Ponciano JM, Top EM.** 2016. Evolutionary paths that expand plasmid host-range: implications for spread of antibiotic resistance. *Mol Biol Evol* **33:**885–897.
27. **Yano H, Wegrzyn K, Loftie-Eaton W, Johnson J, Deckert GE, Rogers LM, Konieczny I, Top**

EM. 2016. Evolved plasmid-host interactions re-duce plasmid interference cost. *Mol Microbiol* **101:**743–756.

28. **Porse A, Schønning K, Munck C, Sommer MO.** 2016. Survival and evolution of a large multidrug resistance plasmid in new clinical bacterial hosts. *Mol Biol Evol* **33:**2860–2873.

29. **Lorenz MG, Wackernagel W.** 1994. Bacterial gene transfer by natural genetic transformation in the environment. *Microbiol Rev* **58:**563–602.

30. **Matsumoto A, Sekoguchi A, Imai J, Kondo K, Shibata Y, Maeda S.** 2016. Natural *Escherichia coli* strains undergo cell-to-cell plasmid trans-formation. *Biochem Biophys Res Commun* **481:**59–62.

31. **Quiles-Puchalt N, Martínez-Rubio R, Ram G, Lasa I, Penadés JR.** 2014. Unravelling bacte-riophage Φ11 requirements for packaging and transfer of mobile genetic elements in *Staphy-lococcus aureus. Mol Microbiol* **91:**423–437.

32. **Vielmetter W, Bonhoeffer F, Schütte A.** 1968. Genetic evidence for transfer of a single DNA strand during bacterial conjugation. *J Mol Biol* **37:**81–86.

33. **Baharoglu Z, Bikard D, Mazel D.** 2010. Conju-gative DNA transfer induces the bacterial SOS response and promotes antibiotic resistance de-velopment through integron activation. *PLoS Genet* **6:**e1001165.

34. **Baharoglu Z, Mazel D.** 2014. SOS, the formi-dable strategy of bacteria against aggressions. *FEMS Microbiol Rev* **38:**1126–1145.

35. **Jones C, Holland IB.** 1985. Role of the SulB (FtsZ) protein in division inhibition during the SOS response in *Escherichia coli*: FtsZ stabilizes the inhibitor SulA in maxicells. *Proc Natl Acad Sci U S A* **82:**6045–6049.

36. **Petrova V, Chitteni-Pattu S, Drees JC, Inman RB, Cox MM.** 2009. An SOS inhibitor that binds to free RecA protein: the PsiB protein. *Mol Cell* **36:**121–130.

37. **Jones AL, Barth PT, Wilkins BM.** 1992. Zygotic induction of plasmid *ssb* and *psiB* genes follow-ing conjugative transfer of Incl1 plasmid Collb-P9. *Mol Microbiol* **6:**605–613.

38. **Althorpe NJ, Chilley PM, Thomas AT, Brammar WJ, Wilkins BM.** 1999. Transient transcriptional activation of the Incl1 plasmid anti-restriction gene (*ardA*) and SOS inhibi-tion gene (*psiB*) early in conjugating recipient bacteria. *Mol Microbiol* **31:**133–142.

39. **Baharoglu Z, Krin E, Mazel D.** 2012. Con-necting environment and genome plasticity in the characterization of transformation-induced SOS regulation and carbon catabolite control of the *Vibrio cholerae* integron integrase. *J Bacte-riol* **194:**1659–1667.

40. **Campoy S, Hervàs A, Busquets N, Erill I, Teixidó L, Barbé J.** 2006. Induction of the SOS response by bacteriophage lytic development in *Salmonella enterica. Virology* **351:**360–367.

41. **Fernandez-Lopez R, Del Campo I, Revilla C, Cuevas A, de la Cruz F.** 2014. Negative feed-back and transcriptional overshooting in a regu-latory network for horizontal gene transfer. *PLoS Genet* **10:**e1004171.

42. **Fernandez-Lopez R, de la Cruz F.** 2015. Reboot-ing the genome: the role of negative feedback in horizontal gene transfer. *Mob Genet Elements* **4:** 1–6.

43. **Johnson CM, Grossman AD.** 2015. Integrative and conjugative elements (ICEs): what they do and how they work. *Annu Rev Genet* **49:** 577–601.

44. **León-Sampedro R, Novais C, Peixe L, Baquero F, Coque TM.** 2016. Diversity and evolution of the Tn*5801-tet*(M)-like integrative and conju-gative elements among *Enterococcus, Strepto-coccus,* and *Staphylococcus. Antimicrob Agents Chemother* **60:**1736–1746.

45. **Dimopoulou ID, Russell JE, Mohd-Zain Z, Herbert R, Crook DW.** 2002. Site-specific re-combination with the chromosomal tRNA^{Leu} gene by the large conjugative *Haemophilus* resis-tance plasmid. *Antimicrob Agents Chemother* **46:**1602–1603.

46. **Cheng Q, Paszkiet BJ, Shoemaker NB, Gardner JF, Salyers AA.** 2000. Integration and excision of a *Bacteroides* conjugative transposon, CTnDOT. *J Bacteriol* **182:**4035–4043.

47. **Roberts AP, Mullany P.** 2009. A modular mas-ter on the move: the Tn*916* family of mobile ge-netic elements. *Trends Microbiol* **17:**251–258.

48. **Rocha EP, Danchin A.** 2002. Base composition bias might result from competition for metabolic resources. *Trends Genet* **18:**291–294.

49. **Nishida H.** 2012. Comparative analyses of base compositions, DNA sizes, and dinucleotide fre-quency profiles in archaeal and bacterial chro-mosomes and plasmids. *Int J Evol Biol* **2012:** 342482.

50. **Wernegreen JJ.** 2015. Endosymbiont evolution: predictions from theory and surprises from ge-nomes. *Ann N Y Acad Sci* **1360:**16–35.

51. **Raghavan R, Kelkar YD, Ochman H.** 2012. A selective force favoring increased G+C content in bacterial genes. *Proc Natl Acad Sci U S A* **109:** 14504–14507.

52. **Hershberg R, Petrov DA.** 2010. Evidence that mutation is universally biased towards AT in bacteria. *PLoS Genet* **6:**e1001115.

53. **Hildebrand F, Meyer A, Eyre-Walker A.** 2010. Evidence of selection upon genomic GC-content in bacteria. *PLoS Genet* **6:**e1001107.

54. **Fang FC, Rimsky S.** 2008. New insights into transcriptional regulation by H-NS. *Curr Opin Microbiol* **11:**113–120.

55. **Ingmer H, Miller C, Cohen SN.** 2001. The RepA protein of plasmid pSC101 controls *Escherichia coli* cell division through the SOS response. *Mol Microbiol* **42:**519–526.

56. **del Solar G, Espinosa M.** 2000. Plasmid copy number control: an ever-growing story. *Mol Microbiol* **37:**492–500.

57. **Lederberg J, Tatum EL.** 1953. Sex in bacteria; genetic studies, 1945–1952. *Science* **118:**169–175.

58. **Ilangovan A, Connery S, Waksman G.** 2015. Structural biology of the Gram-negative bacterial conjugation systems. *Trends Microbiol* **23:** 301–310.

59. **Costa TR, Ilangovan A, Ukleja M, Redzej A, Santini JM, Smith TK, Egelman EH, Waksman G.** 2016. Structure of the bacterial sex F pilus reveals an assembly of a stoichiometric protein-phospholipid complex. *Cell* **166:**1436–1444.e10.

60. **Turner PE, Cooper VS, Lenski RE.** 1998. Trade-off between horizontal and vertical modes of transmission in bacterial plasmids. *Evolution* **52:** 315–329.

61. **Kozlowicz BK, Shi K, Gu ZY, Ohlendorf DH, Earhart CA, Dunny GM.** 2006. Molecular basis for control of conjugation by bacterial pheromone and inhibitor peptides. *Mol Microbiol* **62:** 958–969.

62. **McAnulla C, Edwards A, Sanchez-Contreras M, Sawers RG, Downie JA.** 2007. Quorum-sensing-regulated transcriptional initiation of plasmid transfer and replication genes in *Rhizobium leguminosarum* biovar *viciae*. *Microbiology* **153:**2074–2082.

63. **Koraimann G, Wagner MA.** 2014. Social behavior and decision making in bacterial conjugation. *Front Cell Infect Microbiol* **4:**54.

64. **Dahlberg C, Chao L.** 2003. Amelioration of the cost of conjugative plasmid carriage in *Escherichia coli* K12. *Genetics* **165:**1641–1649.

65. **Zahrl D, Wagner M, Bischof K, Koraimann G.** 2006. Expression and assembly of a functional type IV secretion system elicit extracytoplasmic and cytoplasmic stress responses in *Escherichia coli*. *J Bacteriol* **188:**6611–6621.

66. **Caro LG, Schnös M.** 1966. The attachment of the male-specific bacteriophage F1 to sensitive strains of *Escherichia coli*. *Proc Natl Acad Sci U S A* **56:**126–132.

67. **Novotny C, Knight WS, Brinton CC Jr.** 1968. Inhibition of bacterial conjugation by ribonucleic acid and deoxyribonucleic acid male-specific bacteriophages. *J Bacteriol* **95:**314–326.

68. **Jalasvuori M, Friman VP, Nieminen A, Bamford JK, Buckling A.** 2011. Bacteriophage selection against a plasmid-encoded sex apparatus leads to the loss of antibiotic-resistance plasmids. *Biol Lett* **7:**902–905.

69. **Ojala V, Laitalainen J, Jalasvuori M.** 2013. Fight evolution with evolution: plasmid-dependent phages with a wide host range prevent the spread of antibiotic resistance. *Evol Appl* **6:** 925–932.

70. **Park C, Zhang J.** 2012. High expression hampers horizontal gene transfer. *Genome Biol Evol* **4:**523–532.

71. **Sorek R, Zhu Y, Creevey CJ, Francino MP, Bork P, Rubin EM.** 2007. Genome-wide experimental determination of barriers to horizontal gene transfer. *Science* **318:**1449–1452.

72. **Lamberte LE, Baniulyte G, Singh SS, Stringer AM, Bonocora RP, Stracy M, Kapanidis AN, Wade JT, Grainger DC.** 2017. Horizontally acquired AT-rich genes in *Escherichia coli* cause toxicity by sequestering RNA polymerase. *Nat Microbiol* **2:**16249.

73. **Plotkin JB, Kudla G.** 2011. Synonymous but not the same: the causes and consequences of codon bias. *Nat Rev Genet* **12:**32–42.

74. **Tuller T, Girshovich Y, Sella Y, Kreimer A, Freilich S, Kupiec M, Gophna U, Ruppin E.** 2011. Association between translation efficiency and horizontal gene transfer within microbial communities. *Nucleic Acids Res* **39:**4743–4755.

75. **Medrano-Soto A, Moreno-Hagelsieb G, Vinuesa P, Christen JA, Collado-Vides J.** 2004. Successful lateral transfer requires codon usage compatibility between foreign genes and recipient genomes. *Mol Biol Evol* **21:**1884–1894.

76. **Komar AA, Lesnik T, Reiss C.** 1999. Synonymous codon substitutions affect ribosome traffic and protein folding during in vitro translation. *FEBS Lett* **462:**387–391.

77. **Kudla G, Murray AW, Tollervey D, Plotkin JB.** 2009. Coding-sequence determinants of gene expression in *Escherichia coli*. *Science* **324:** 255–258.

78. **Cortazzo P, Cerveñansky C, Marín M, Reiss C, Ehrlich R, Deana A.** 2002. Silent mutations affect in vivo protein folding in *Escherichia coli*. *Biochem Biophys Res Commun* **293:**537–541.

79. **Drummond DA, Wilke CO.** 2008. Mistranslation-induced protein misfolding as a dominant constraint on coding-sequence evolution. *Cell* **134:** 341–352.

80. **Ling J, O'Donoghue P, Söll D.** 2015. Genetic code flexibility in microorganisms: novel mechanisms and impact on physiology. *Nat Rev Microbiol* **13:**707–721.

81. **Bonomo J, Gill RT.** 2005. Amino acid content of recombinant proteins influences the metabolic burden response. *Biotechnol Bioeng* **90:**116–126.

82. **Shachrai I, Zaslaver A, Alon U, Dekel E.** 2010. Cost of unneeded proteins in *E. coli* is reduced after several generations in exponential growth. *Mol Cell* **38:**758–767.

83. **Dittmar KA, Sørensen MA, Elf J, Ehrenberg M, Pan T.** 2005. Selective charging of tRNA isoacceptors induced by amino-acid starvation. *EMBO Rep* **6:**151–157.

84. **Elf J, Nilsson D, Tenson T, Ehrenberg M.** 2003. Selective charging of tRNA isoacceptors explains patterns of codon usage. *Science* **300:**1718–1722.

85. **Hernández-Arriaga AM, Chan WT, Espinosa M, Díaz-Orejas R.** 2014. Conditional activation of toxin-antitoxin systems: postsegregational killing and beyond. *Microbiol Spectr* **2:**2.

86. **San Millan JL, Hernandez-Chico C, Pereda P, Moreno F.** 1985. Cloning and mapping of the genetic determinants for microcin B17 production and immunity. *J Bacteriol* **163:**275–281.

87. **Jain R, Rivera MC, Lake JA.** 1999. Horizontal gene transfer among genomes: the complexity hypothesis. *Proc Natl Acad Sci U S A* **96:**3801–3806.

88. **Cohen O, Gophna U, Pupko T.** 2011. The complexity hypothesis revisited: connectivity rather than function constitutes a barrier to horizontal gene transfer. *Mol Biol Evol* **28:**1481–1489.

89. **Pál C, Papp B, Lercher MJ.** 2005. Horizontal gene transfer depends on gene content of the host. *Bioinformatics* **21**(Suppl 2):ii222–ii223.

90. **Sota M, Yano H, Hughes JM, Daughdrill GW, Abdo Z, Forney LJ, Top EM.** 2010. Shifts in the host range of a promiscuous plasmid through parallel evolution of its replication initiation protein. *ISME J* **4:**1568–1580.

91. **del Solar G, Giraldo R, Ruiz-Echevarría MJ, Espinosa M, Díaz-Orejas R.** 1998. Replication and control of circular bacterial plasmids. *Microbiol Mol Biol Rev* **62:**434–464.

92. **Silva RF, Mendonça SC, Carvalho LM, Reis AM, Gordo I, Trindade S, Dionisio F.** 2011. Pervasive sign epistasis between conjugative plasmids and drug-resistance chromosomal mutations. *PLoS Genet* **7:**e1002181.

93. **Morton ER, Platt TG, Fuqua C, Bever JD.** 2014. Non-additive costs and interactions alter the competitive dynamics of co-occurring ecologically distinct plasmids. *Proc Biol Sci* **281:**20132173.

94. **Fornelos N, Browning DF, Butala M.** 2016. The use and abuse of LexA by mobile genetic elements. *Trends Microbiol* **24:**391–401.

95. **Penadés JR, Christie GE.** 2015. The phage-inducible chromosomal islands: a family of highly evolved molecular parasites. *Annu Rev Virol* **2:**181–201.

96. **Miyakoshi M, Shintani M, Inoue K, Terabayashi T, Sai F, Ohkuma M, Nojiri H,** Nagata Y, Tsuda M. 2012. ParI, an orphan ParA family protein from *Pseudomonas putida* KT2440-specific genomic island, interferes with the partition system of IncP-7 plasmids. *Environ Microbiol* **14:**2946–2959.

97. **Shintani M, Suzuki-Minakuchi C, Nojiri H.** 2015. Nucleoid-associated proteins encoded on plasmids: occurrence and mode of function. *Plasmid* **80:**32–44.

98. **Baños RC, Vivero A, Aznar S, García J, Pons M, Madrid C, Juárez A.** 2009. Differential regulation of horizontally acquired and core genome genes by the bacterial modulator H-NS. *PLoS Genet* **5:**e1000513.

99. **Navarre WW, Porwollik S, Wang Y, McClelland M, Rosen H, Libby SJ, Fang FC.** 2006. Selective silencing of foreign DNA with low GC content by the H-NS protein in *Salmonella. Science* **313:**236–238.

100. **Ali SS, Soo J, Rao C, Leung AS, Ngai DH, Ensminger AW, Navarre WW.** 2014. Silencing by H-NS potentiated the evolution of *Salmonella. PLoS Pathog* **10:**e1004500.

101. **Gordon BR, Li Y, Cote A, Weirauch MT, Ding P, Hughes TR, Navarre WW, Xia B, Liu J.** 2011. Structural basis for recognition of AT-rich DNA by unrelated xenogeneic silencing proteins. *Proc Natl Acad Sci U S A* **108:**10690–10695.

102. **Yamada H, Yoshida T, Tanaka K, Sasakawa C, Mizuno T.** 1991. Molecular analysis of the *Escherichia coli hns* gene encoding a DNA-binding protein, which preferentially recognizes curved DNA sequences. *Mol Gen Genet* **230:**332–336.

103. **Jáuregui R, Abreu-Goodger C, Moreno-Hagelsieb G, Collado-Vides J, Merino E.** 2003. Conservation of DNA curvature signals in regulatory regions of prokaryotic genes. *Nucleic Acids Res* **31:**6770–6777.

104. **Takeda T, Yun CS, Shintani M, Yamane H, Nojiri H.** 2011. Distribution of genes encoding nucleoid-associated protein homologs in plasmids. *Int J Evol Biol* **2011:**685015.

105. **Doyle M, Fookes M, Ivens A, Mangan MW, Wain J, Dorman CJ.** 2007. An H-NS-like stealth protein aids horizontal DNA transmission in bacteria. *Science* **315:**251–252.

106. **Lang KS, Johnson TJ.** 2016. Characterization of Acr2, an H-NS-like protein encoded on A/C2-type plasmids. *Plasmid* **87-88:**17–27.

107. **Friedman SA, Austin SJ.** 1988. The P1 plasmid-partition system synthesizes two essential proteins from an autoregulated operon. *Plasmid* **19:**103–112.

108. **Bingle LE, Thomas CM.** 2001. Regulatory circuits for plasmid survival. *Curr Opin Microbiol* **4:**194–200.

109. **Escudero JA, Loot C, Nivina A, Mazel D.** 2015. The integron: adaptation on demand. *Microbiol Spectr* **3**:MDNA3-0019-2014.

110. **Collis CM, Hall RM.** 1995. Expression of antibiotic resistance genes in the integrated cassettes of integrons. *Antimicrob Agents Chemother* **39:** 155–162.

111. **Bennett PM.** 2008. Plasmid encoded antibiotic resistance: acquisition and transfer of antibiotic resistance genes in bacteria. *Br J Pharmacol* **153** (Suppl 1):S347–S357.

112. **Lang KS, Johnson TJ.** 2015. Transcriptome modulations due to A/C2 plasmid acquisition. *Plasmid* **80**:83–89.

113. **Lang KS, Danzeisen JL, Xu W, Johnson TJ.** 2012. Transcriptome mapping of pAR060302, a *bla*CMY-2-positive broad-host-range IncA/C plasmid. *Appl Environ Microbiol* **78**:3379–3386.

114. **Lacotte Y, Ploy MC, Raherison S.** 2017. Class 1 integrons are low-cost structures in *Escherichia coli*. *ISME J* **11**:1535–1544.

115. **Dougherty K, Smith BA, Moore AF, Maitland S, Fanger C, Murillo R, Baltrus DA.** 2014. Multiple phenotypic changes associated with large-scale horizontal gene transfer. *PLoS One* **9**:e102170.

116. **Brusselaers N, Vogelaers D, Blot S.** 2011. The rising problem of antimicrobial resistance in the intensive care unit. *Ann Intensive Care* **1**:47.

117. **Boucher HW, Talbot GH, Bradley JS, Edwards JE, Gilbert D, Rice LB, Scheld M, Spellberg B, Bartlett J.** 2009. Bad bugs, no drugs: no ESKAPE! An update from the Infectious Diseases Society of America. *Clin Infect Dis* **48**:1–12.

118. **European Centre for Disease Prevention and Control.** 2015. *Antimicrobial Resistance Surveillance in Europe 2014.* European Centre for Disease Prevention and Control, Stockholm, Sweden. http://ecdc.europa.eu/en/publications/Publications/antimicrobial-resistance-europe-2014.pdf. Accessed date 17/12/2016.

119. **Stoesser N, Sheppard AE, Pankhurst L, De Maio N, Moore CE, Sebra R, Turner P, Anson LW, Kasarskis A, Batty EM, Kos V, Wilson DJ, Phetsouvanh R, Wyllie D, Sokurenko E, Manges AR, Johnson TJ, Price LB, Peto TE, Johnson JR, Didelot X, Walker AS, Crook DW, Modernizing Medical Microbiology Informatics Group (MMMIG).** 2016. Evolutionary history of the global emergence of the *Escherichia coli* epidemic clone ST131. *mBio* **7**: e02162.

120. **Dimou V, Dhanji H, Pike R, Livermore DM, Woodford N.** 2012. Characterization of *Enterobacteriaceae* producing OXA-48-like carbapenemases in the UK. *J Antimicrob Chemother* **67**:1660–1665.

121. **Toll-Riera M, San Millan A, Wagner A, MacLean RC.** 2016. The genomic basis of evolutionary innovation in *Pseudomonas aeruginosa*. *PLoS Genet* **12**:e1006005.

122. **Gifford DR, Moss E, MacLean RC.** 2016. Environmental variation alters the fitness effects of rifampicin resistance mutations in *Pseudomonas aeruginosa*. *Evolution* **70**:725–730.

123. **Turner KH, Wessel AK, Palmer GC, Murray JL, Whiteley M.** 2015. Essential genome of *Pseudomonas aeruginosa* in cystic fibrosis sputum. *Proc Natl Acad Sci U S A* **112**:4110–4115.

124. **Harrison F, Diggle SP.** 2016. An *ex vivo* lung model to study bronchioles infected with *Pseudomonas aeruginosa* biofilms. *Microbiology* **162**: 1755–1760.

125. **Paulander W, Pennhag A, Andersson DI, Maisnier-Patin S.** 2007. *Caenorhabditis elegans* as a model to determine fitness of antibiotic-resistant *Salmonella enterica* serovar Typhimurium. *Antimicrob Agents Chemother* **51**:766–769.

126. **Ramarao N, Nielsen-Leroux C, Lereclus D.** 2012. The insect *Galleria mellonella* as a powerful infection model to investigate bacterial pathogenesis. *J Vis Exp* (70):e4392.

127. **Ubeda C, Bucci V, Caballero S, Djukovic A, Toussaint NC, Equinda M, Lipuma L, Ling L, Gobourne A, No D, Taur Y, Jenq RR, van den Brink MR, Xavier JB, Pamer EG.** 2013. Intestinal microbiota containing *Barnesiella* species cures vancomycin-resistant *Enterococcus faecium* colonization. *Infect Immun* **81**:965–973.

128. **Græsbøll K, Nielsen SS, Toft N, Christiansen LE.** 2014. How fitness reduced, antimicrobial resistant bacteria survive and spread: a multiple pig-multiple bacterial strain model. *PLoS One* **9**:e100458.

129. **Harrison E, Truman J, Wright R, Spiers AJ, Paterson S, Brockhurst MA.** 2015. Plasmid carriage can limit bacteria-phage coevolution. *Biol Lett* **11**:11.

130. **Medaney F, Ellis RJ, Raymond B.** 2016. Ecological and genetic determinants of plasmid distribution in *Escherichia coli*. *Environ Microbiol* **18**:4230–4239.

131. **Shintani M, Takahashi Y, Tokumaru H, Kadota K, Hara H, Miyakoshi M, Naito K, Yamane H, Nishida H, Nojiri H.** 2010. Response of the *Pseudomonas* host chromosomal transcriptome to carriage of the IncP-7 plasmid pCAR1. *Environ Microbiol* **12**:1413–1426.

132. **Getino M, de la Cruz F.** 2017. Natural and artificial strategies to control the conjugative transmission of plasmids. *Microbiol Spectr* In press.

133. **Lacotte Y, Ploy MC, Raherison S.** 2017. Class 1 integrons are low-cost structures in *Escherichia coli*. *ISME J* **11**:1535–1544.

Basic Processes in *Salmonella*-Host Interactions: Within-Host Evolution and the Transmission of the Virulent Genotype

5

MÉDÉRIC DIARD[1] and WOLF-DIETRICH HARDT[1]

INTRODUCTION

In line with Koch's postulates, studying virulence typically translates into identifying and characterizing the molecular determinants that underlie colonization of a host by a pathogen and the subsequent appearance of symptoms (1). In this conceptual framework, the presence of pathogens implies damage to the host whose intensity is proportional to the virulence of the pathogen. This approach is based on the observation that damage is often related to the expression of specific features of the pathogen, i.e., the virulence factors (2).

It has also become clear that the role of the host in defining virulence of pathogens is absolutely central. The degree of sensitivity of the host is thought to determine (to a large extent) whether pathogenic organisms are effectively virulent or if they remain innocuous upon colonization. Indeed, such innocuous behavior can often be observed in cases of virulence factor-studded pathogens (3) (for examples, see Table 1). One should therefore consider virulence as a probabilistic property of organisms in given hosts and virulence factors as genetic determinants that increase the chance to cause damage. This also means that transmission of virulence does not necessarily rely on triggering symptoms. This is of importance for the vast majority of pathogens and their evolution.

[1]Institute of Microbiology, Department of Biology, ETH Zurich, Zurich, Switzerland.
Microbial Transmission in Biological Processes
Edited by Fernando Baquero, Emilio Bouza, J.A. Gutiérrez-Fuentes, and Teresa M. Coque
© 2018 American Society for Microbiology, Washington, DC
doi:10.1128/microbiolspec.MTBP-0012-2016

TABLE 1 Asymptomatic carriage of bona fide pathogenic bacteria in humans

Pathogen	Asymptomatic carriage[a]	Disease	Disease incidence	Reference(s)
Mycobacterium tuberculosis	10%[b]	Tuberculosis	10->500 per 100,000[b]	4
Nontyphoidal *Salmonella* spp.	≈1%	Diarrhea	~400 per 100,000	5
Neisseria meningitidis	5–10%	Meningitis	0.3–0.5 per 100,000	6, 7
Chlamydia trachomatis	3.8%[c]	Sexually transmitted diseases	426 per 100,000	8
Staphylococcus aureus	≈30%	Bacteremia[d]	10–30 per 100,000[e]	9, 10

[a]In the entire "healthy" population.
[b]TB incidence is particularly high in developing countries; here, up to 80% of the population can test positive in the tuberculin test.
[c]In men aged 18 to 26.
[d]*S. aureus* can also cause numerous other diseases.
[e]*S. aureus* bacteremia.

The dual nature of virulence, depending on one side on a pathogen that may express or encode but not express (or successfully deploy) virulence factors, and on the other side on the sensitivity of the host to the presence of the pathogen, implies that its evolutionary dynamics is particularly challenging to generalize. Nevertheless, understanding virulence beyond its purely mechanistic aspects should not be overlooked. Determining why and in which circumstances the virulence of a pathogen can be an adaptive trait should ultimately allow us to predict and to control its evolution.

In order to achieve such a goal, one should ideally consider the complete life cycles of pathogens, including within-host growth, survival in the environment, and modes of transmission to new hosts. The impact of virulence on the reproductive success of pathogens, meaning their ability to repeat their life cycles host after host, should be precisely addressed (11). In this respect, adaptive virulence is synonymous with maintenance and efficient transmission of the virulent genotype from one host to the other.

Experimental attempts to tackle this problem remain scarce for multiple reasons. Considering, for instance, pathogens infecting humans, animal models do not always exist, and when they do, they do not necessarily allow reconstitution of all the infection steps. Moreover, the full life cycle of a pathogen can be complex and often includes phases in various environments or in more than one type of

host. And lastly, our knowledge of pathogen life cycles is most of the time incomplete and strong selective pressures in favor of or against virulence could remain concealed.

In this chapter, we discuss recent advances in addressing the adaptive value of virulence of the archetypal enteropathogenic bacterium *Salmonella enterica* serovar Typhimurium, a pathogen well characterized in laboratory model hosts such as mice. Rodents are natural hosts for *S.* Typhimurium and tractable surrogates in which the progression of the disease mimics pathogenesis in humans (12). Please note that most of experimental results described here were obtained by making use of the antibiotic-pretreated mouse model. The antibiotic pretreatment opens the intestinal niche for *S.* Typhimurium, which is otherwise occupied by the host's microbiota. This allows very reproducible colonization but comes at the price of abrogating the initial competition between *Salmonella* and the microbiota, which certainly plays a role in the evolution of the pathogen.

S. Typhimurium infects hosts via the fecal-oral route by the uptake of contaminated food or water. In immunocompetent humans, *S.* Typhimurium causes a self-limiting diarrhea that lasts for 5 to 7 days. The diarrhea is accompanied by inflammation that is thought to provide an advantage to *Salmonella* over the protective microbiota (13). However, within-host growth seems to have a negative impact on the evolution of virulence (14). This paradox will be addressed in this chapter. We will also discuss processes that may help to maintain virulence.

Evidence for direct transmission from person to person is rare, and this route of transmission seems restricted to situations of intense contact, such as between hospitalized patients and staff members (15). Patients can asymptomatically carry nontyphoidal *Salmonella* (NTS) for years with sporadic relapses, which could favor spreading of *Salmonella* in the environment and subsequent transmission (16). As described below, *Salmonella* spp. are facultative intracellular pathogens that are able to invade the host tissues, where they could remain dormant, making the disease chronic. However, in immunocompromised hosts, such as HIV-infected patients, unrestricted intracellular bacteria can spread and cause life-threatening bacteremia requiring antibiotic treatment (17).

The reservoirs for NTS are mainly domesticated birds, swine, and cattle, but also wild rodents and plants (18). *S.* Typhimurium is therefore able to colonize a wide variety of hosts and environments in which functions such as virulence factors could have dissimilar adaptive values (19). Consequently, the regulation of gene expression by environmental cues is key to ensure the maintenance of virulence (20). Due to the broad range of hosts that can serve as reservoirs, utilization of "uniform" environmental cues that are present in equivalent sites within the different hosts would seem essential for regulation. This point will be discussed in more detail later below.

SALMONELLA IN THE GUT LUMEN: WITHIN-HOST SELECTION FOR ATTENUATED DEFECTORS

The Competition for the Gut

To initiate host colonization right after ingestion, *S.* Typhimurium must survive the acidic pH of the stomach. This requires the acid response, while virulence factors are not needed. Then the bacteria are faced with a high density of physical and chemical host defenses and a very dense microbiota population, which deplete nutrients, produce inhibitors, and occupy mucosal binding sites, thereby effectively prohibiting *S.* Typhimurium growth, a phenomenon called colonization resistance (CR).

We recently discovered how *S.* Typhimurium can profit from metabolic intermediates of the microbiota metabolism (i.e., molecular H_2 released by microbiota fermentation) to fuel the initial growth in this niche (*hyb* H_2 hydrogenase and fumarate reductase are two key gut colonization factors [21, 22]). The archetypical symptoms that seem to promote the selection for virulence of this pathogen are only triggered once the bacteria have reached sufficiently high densities in the gut lumen (~10^8 CFU per g of stool) (23). Beyond this threshold, pathogen invasion into intestinal epithelial cells is frequent enough to elicit the acute mucosal innate immune response (i.e., gut inflammation), which fosters the growth of *S.* Typhimurium (13) (Fig. 1).

Work from the past few years has provided initial insights into why *S.* Typhimurium growth is enhanced in the lumen of the inflamed gut, supporting the view that this pathogen constructs its niche by triggering the host innate immune defenses. The gut inflammation represents a major ecological perturbation (for a review, see reference 24): antimicrobial proteins that preferentially inhibit the growth of *Salmonella* competitors are secreted (e.g., RegIIIb and lipocalin-2); high-energy nutrients sensed by the chemotactic receptors of *Salmonella* are released (e.g., galactose-rich glycoconjugates [25]); and an alternative electron acceptor (tetrathionate) is formed from endogenous thiosulfate by reactive oxygen species mainly generated by neutrophils massively recruited in the gut lumen (26). *S.* Typhimurium growth is further fueled by ethanolamine that is massively released into the lumen of the inflamed gut (27).

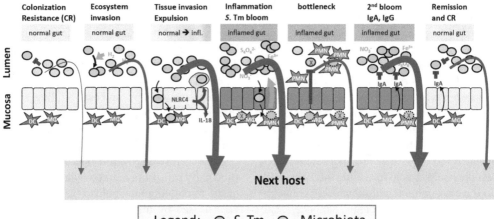

FIGURE 1 The different steps of the gut infection cycle by *Salmonella* Typhimurium. Red arrows depict the potential for *S.* Typhimurium (*S.* Tm) transmission to the next host during each step. Blue- and red-colored cells depict healthy and inflamed guts, respectively. PMN, polymorphonuclear neutrophils; DC, dendritic cells; MΦ, macrophages; IgA/G, immunoglobulin A/G produced as part of the host's adaptive immune response 2 weeks postinfection—this follows the regrowth of *Salmonella* (2nd bloom) after a population bottleneck inflicted by the innate immune response (at day 2 postinfection); IL-18, interleukin-18; Casp-1, caspase-1.

The link between gut inflammation and efficient gut luminal pathogen growth is quite striking. In the absence of inflammation, *S.* Typhimurium fails to sustain the colonization of conventional mice. This was demonstrated by making use of antibiotic-pretreated mice in which the intestinal microbiota and CR are transiently disrupted. In these conditions, *S.* Typhimurium strains resistant to the antibiotic reach in a few hours a population size of 10^9 CFU/g of stool. Thanks to gut inflammation, virulent wild-type strains can maintain themselves for 2 to 3 weeks, provided that the mouse does not die from systemic infection (e.g., in resistant Nramp$^{+/+}$ mice) (28, 29). In contrast, avirulent strains unable to elicit inflammation are excluded from the intestine by the regrowing microbiota already by 3 to 4 days post-antibiotic treatment (13). Moreover, mice carrying a simplified microbiota (e.g., the altered Schaedler flora) can durably shed high loads of avirulent strains of *Salmonella* (30), and introducing additional microbiota strains can fortify CR in such models (31). This clearly demonstrates the

protective role of the intestinal microbiota against enteropathogens as well as the adaptive value of enteric virulence.

Of note, the pronounced inflammation triggered by fully virulent *S.* Typhimurium strains leads to a strong mucosal defense that transiently reduced the pathogen load in the gut lumen from 10^9 CFU/g at day 1 to $<10^4$ CFU/g of stool at day 2 postinfection (32). Attenuated strains do not provoke such a stark decimation. The underlying mechanisms will be an interesting topic for future work, and this shows that gut inflammation has two sides: it benefits *Salmonella* over all but remains costly (Fig. 1).

The niche construction strategy could be a general property of enteropathogenic bacteria, maximizing their transmission. Besides *S.* Typhimurium, *Citrobacter rodentium* is a second experimentally validated case of an enteropathogen able to profit from inflammation, which provides evidence of convergent evolution. *C. rodentium* was discovered in the 1960s after outbreaks in laboratory mouse colonies in the United States and

Japan (33, 34). This pathogen is a model for the study of human pathogens that induce intestinal attaching-and-effacing lesions, e.g., enteropathogenic (EPEC) and enterohemorrhagic *Escherichia coli* (EHEC) (35). The major virulence determinants of *C. rodentium* are located at the locus of enterocyte effacement (LEE), which is conserved in EPEC and EHEC and encodes a type 3 secretion system (TTSS) and secreted effectors. Effectors are injected via the TTSS into epithelial cells, and provoke the formation of an actin pedestal on the apical side of the host cell where the bacteria are attached. The infection by *C. rodentium* is self-limiting, as bacteria stop expressing *ler*, the main positive regulator of LEE expression, after a few days (36). Inflammation then resolves, and the regrowing microbiota eventually excludes *C. rodentium*.

Similarities with *S.* Typhimurium are striking also with regard to the molecular mechanisms that underlie the triggering and exploitation of gut inflammation to compete against the protective host microbiota. Just like *C. rodentium, S.* Typhimurium expresses a TTSS, the *Salmonella* pathogenicity island 1 (SPI-1)-encoded TTSS-1, and injects proinflammatory effector proteins into the cytosol of enterocytes. This provokes cytoskeletal rearrangements and allows the entry of *Salmonella* into these nonphagocytic cells (37–41). From the enterocytes, *Salmonella* can translocate into the lamina propria, get phagocytized by monocytes and possibly also infect other cell types (42), and reach systemic organs (lymph nodes, spleen, and liver) (40). The intracellular niche plays an important role in transmission of *Salmonella*, which will be discussed in the sections below.

At the end of the acute phase of the disease, the host's adaptive immune system mounts a protective secretory immunoglobulin A (sIgA) antibody response. After 10 to 15 days, the antibodies can thereby promote remission and the regrowth of a normal microbiota (29). Thus, the pathogen elimination from the gut at the end of an infection is attributable to the tipping of a delicate balance between the pathogen's virulence, the microbiota, and the host response (Fig. 1).

Microevolution of *S.* Typhimurium in the Gut

In a favorable intestinal niche, *Enterobacteriaceae* such as *S.* Typhimurium can grow quickly (25-min to 2-h doubling time) (43) and maintain high densities (10^9 bacteria/g of intestinal content) for several days. This is particularly true in the antibiotic-pretreated mouse model but also in conventional mice provided that *S.* Typhimurium manages to trigger intestinal inflammation (13). Consequently, within-host microevolution of the pathogen occurs at observable rates, allowing us to experimentally address dynamics of horizontal gene transfer (HGT) and mutation accumulation and their impact on the transmission of virulence.

Population density, inflammation, sIgA, and HGT

Horizontal transfer of mobile genetic elements is a major driving force of virulence evolution (44). The murine model of *S.* Typhimurium infection provides a potent model to study the dynamics of HGT *in vivo*.

It is demonstrated that the conjugative plasmid pColIB9 is efficiently transmitted from *S.* Typhimurium SL1344 to strains of *E. coli* that are able to bloom in the inflamed gut (45). The conjugative transfer of the derepressed pColIB9 being only contact dependent, the role of the inflammation is nevertheless indirect. Indeed, in antibiotic-pretreated mice, avirulent strains of *S.* Typhimurium are equally able to exchange pColIB9 in absence of gut inflammation (46), the limiting factor being the population densities of donor and recipient strains.

On the other hand, the inflammation directly stimulates temperate bacteriophage transfer (lysogenic conversion) between strains of *S.* Typhimurium in the gut (46). Several lines of evidence suggest that stresses encountered by *S.* Typhimurium SL1344 within the inflamed gut trigger the SOS response, which controls the expression of the lytic cycle genes of the SopEΦ prophage. Thereby, the host's innate immune defense increases the amounts of free virions in the gut and the acquisition of the bacteriophage by a coinfecting recipient strain (*S.* Typhimurium 14028S) (46).

We were able to limit both conjugation and lysogenic conversion by vaccinating the mice against *S.* Typhimurium (43, 46). Mice treated with dead *S.* Typhimurium 4 weeks before infection can be highly colonized by virulent strains while not showing any sign of intestinal inflammation (47). The presence of specific sIgA in the gut lumen enchains the rapidly dividing *Salmonella*, which therefore form monoclonal clumps (43). This enchained growth prevents triggering of

inflammation and thereby the transfer of SopEΦ. Moreover, the monoclonal nature of the *S.* Typhimurium clumps renders contact-dependent conjugative transfer less frequent (43).

The rise of defectors

Among key features that make *Salmonella* such a successful pathogen are the TTSS-1 and effector proteins that are injected into the cytosol of host cells, where they manipulate host-cellular responses and eventually trigger gut inflammation (12, 48). As described above, inflammation is a shared resource that helps *S.* Typhimurium to outcompete the microbiota and to maximize the transmission to new hosts via the fecal-oral route (13) (Fig. 2). On the other hand, the expression of TTSS-1 and the induction of inflammation represent a sig-

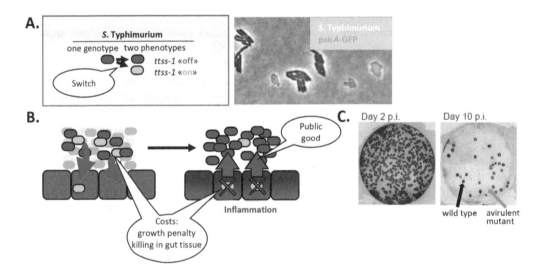

FIGURE 2 The division of labor and the rise of defectors. (A) (Left) Bimodal expression of *ttss-1*. The population of *S.* Typhimurium is divided into cells that express *ttss-1* and cells that do not. (Right) Microscopy picture showing microcolonies on an agar pad of slow-growing *ttss-1* "on" cells (expressing green fluorescent protein [GFP] under the control of P*sicA*, the promoter controlling the SPI-1 operon *sicAsipBCDA*) and fast-growing "off" cells. Reproduced with permission from reference 49. (B) The *ttss-1* "on" cells enter into the mucosa and trigger inflammation. Most of these cells are killed by the mucosal innate immune response. Moreover, *ttss-1* expression correlates with a substantial growth retardation. The *ttss-1* "off" cells grow quickly in the lumen, ensuring the transmission of the virulent genotype. The inflammation is a public good shared among all cells in the lumen. (C) Colony blot obtained and described in reference 14. Within-host evolution of *S.* Typhimurium leads to the rise of avirulent mutants (defectors), which are clones that do not express *ttss-1*. The frequency of defectors was increasing between day 2 and day 10 postinfection (p.i.).

nificant fitness burden for *Salmonella*, namely, (i) strong growth retardation (14, 49) and (ii) killing by the innate immune system when the bacteria invade the host tissues (50). Bacteria that express TTSS-1 are growing only half as fast as *S*. Typhimurium cells that do not express it (14, 49), and 90% of the bacteria that reach the intracellular niche are eliminated by the host innate immune response (50) (Fig. 2B). Thus, the elicitation of gut inflammation (a "public good") is associated with high costs to the TTSS-1-expressing bacteria. We analyzed if such a strategy is sustainable in the long run, as the costly production of public goods could be unstable. Indeed, we found that within-host evolution of *S*. Typhimurium results in the evolution of avirulent mutants (Fig. 2C). In other words, the virulence of *S*. Typhimurium is a cooperative trait that is prone to the selection of defectors, i.e., clones that profit from a public good without contributing to its production (14, 51). In this case, defectors are mutants with a defect in a central positive regulator (*hilD*) of *ttss-1* expression. Thus, the defectors have lost the ability to express TTSS-1 and therefore profit from the inflammation without paying any fitness cost (growth defect or intracellular killing). Within-host competition drives the evolution of *S*. Typhimurium, and therefore defectors increase in frequency during long-term infections. When the frequency of defectors becomes too high, the inflammation cannot be sustained and the whole *Salmonella* population drops (presumably by microbiota regrowth), thus further accelerating the recovery of the host. The rise of the defectors turns out to be detrimental to the long-term colonization of the host.

All isolated defectors carried point mutations in the *hilD* gene, which encodes the main positive regulator of TTSS-1 expression. When coinoculated with an isogenic virulent wild-type clone of *S*. Typhimurium, a synthetic *hilD* deletion mutant wins the competition and protects the host from full-blown inflammation. We hypothesized *hilD* mutants to grow faster than wild-type strains, as up to 40% of the wild-type population experience the growth defect associated with virulence expression (14). However, the HilD regulon comprises numerous functions (52), and alternative explanations, such as a reduced death rate or a better-adapted metabolism, are still open to investigation. In any case, defectors could potentially be used as probiotics in order to competitively exclude virulent strains of *Salmonella*. This could be a good alternative to less and less efficient antibiotics against NTS (53, 54).

The selection for attenuated clones carrying mutations in transcriptional regulators of virulence, as observed in laboratory mice, was recently reported in patients persistently infected by NTS (16). Mutations were discovered, for instance, in *hilD* and *barA*, both positively regulating the expression of TTSS-1. This suggests that the fitness costs associated with virulence expression are a constraint on its evolution in a wide range of ecological contexts (i.e., *in vitro*, in mice, and in human hosts).

Phenotypic Variability as an Adaptive Trait: the Division of Labor Theory

In spite of the inherent instability of *S*. Typhimurium virulence, most patient isolates express TTSS-1. This raises the question of how defectors are kept at bay in nature. Intriguingly, in isogenic populations of *S*. Typhimurium and upon homogeneous inducing conditions, not all bacterial cells express TTSS-1 (14, 50). The expression of *Salmonella* virulence is tightly regulated and *ttss-1* is expressed in a bimodal fashion (Fig. 2). Yet poorly understood regulatory mechanisms allow the coexistence of cells expressing TTSS-1 (TTSS-1 "on") with a pool of phenotypically avirulent cells (TTSS-1 "off"). The "off" cells carry the virulent genotype as well as the "on" cells and are able to switch on the expression of *ttss-1* stochastically when encountering inducing cues from the environment. As mentioned before, the "on" cells grow just half as fast as the "off" cells (14, 49). The reason for the growth defect is still unclear although probably multifactorial, as many genes are coregulated with TTSS-1 (i.e., the HilD regulon) (52, 55).

Accordingly, a mathematical model of *S.* Typhimurium population dynamics predicted that decreasing the initial proportion of TTSS-1 "off" cells, by manipulating the regulation of *ttss-1* expression, should lead to faster fixation of mutants that never switch on the expression of *ttss-1* (TTSS-1 locked "off" defectors) (14). This model was simulating competitions between populations of wild-type *S.* Typhimurium (TTSS-1 "on" or "off"), defectors (locked "off"), and the microbiota in the gut. In this model, the inflammation was triggered above a certain population size of *ttss-1*-expressing cells, as observed *in vivo* (14, 49). Varying the frequency of TTSS-1 "on" versus "off" cells in the wild-type population revealed an optimum that allows *S.* Typhimurium on one hand to trigger inflammation and to outcompete the microbiota and on the other hand to limit the rise of defectors. This optimal theoretical TTSS-1 "on" frequency was ~35%, very close to the frequency observed in the wild-type population in inducing conditions (14).

Predictions from this model were experimentally verified by following the evolution of an *S.* Typhimurium mutant that formed a reduced proportion of TTSS-1 "off" cells (higher TTSS-1 "on" frequency) at the beginning of the experiment. The mutant was a knockout of *hilE*, a gene encoding a negative regulator of *ttss-1* expression. Thus, *hilE* mutants do form populations with increased fractions of "on" cells. As predicted by the model, *hilD* mutants (TTSS-1 locked "off" defectors) were increasing in frequency much faster in the *hilE* mutant background than in the wild-type background during within-host growth. This demonstrated that the avirulent phenotype indeed serves to slow down the rise of defectors, probably by occupying the same ecological niche (14).

These results suggested that fine-tuned bimodal gene expression could be adaptive. We hypothesized that it could allow division of labor between two subpopulations of *Salmonella*: the TTSS-1 "on" cells express virulence factors and trigger inflammation, while the TTSS-1 "off" cells compete with fast-growing defector mutants, thus ensuring the transmission of the virulent genotype.

S. TYPHIMURIUM IN THE TISSUES, A HETEROGENEOUS RESERVOIR FOR THE VIRULENT GENOTYPE

S. Typhimurium can invade the epithelium using its flagella, the SiiE adhesin, and the SPI-1-encoded TTSS-1 (12, 56–58). This invasion is balanced by a swift innate host defense that reduces epithelial pathogen loads in an NLRC4 (NOD-like receptor subfamily C 4) inflammasome-dependent fashion (NLRC4-inflammasome driven expulsion of infected enterocytes) (41). The exact mechanisms driving the pathogen's expulsion from this site remain poorly understood.

Within host cells, *S.* Typhimurium resides in the *Salmonella*-containing vacuole (SCV) and expresses the SPI-2-encoded TTSS-2. Thirty different effector proteins are then secreted through the membrane of the SCV into the host cell cytosol (for a review about their functions, see reference 59). This process is driven by the conditions inside the SCV, i.e., low nutrients and low pH. TTSS-2 is essential to ensure the systemic survival of *S.* Typhimurium and full virulence. Although the importance of SPI-2 effectors in intraepithelial growth in mice seems rather limited (58; B. Felmy, personal communication), they play a significant role in survival and division inside macrophages (60).

Depending on the host cell type, various proportions of intracellular bacteria can escape the SCV and divide in the cytosol (a phenomenon reviewed in reference 61). Transient coexpression of TTSS-1 and TTSS-2 upon entry could favor destabilization of the nascent SCV by TTSS-1 (62–64). Once in the cytosol, *S.* Typhimurium expresses TTSS-1 and the flagella. Luminal release of epithelial cells loaded with bacteria that are primed to reinvade the mucosa is thought to help intestinal spreading and sustaining of the gut inflammation (64, 65).

The heterogeneity in *S.* Typhimurium physiological states and death rates tends to further increase with the multiplicity of cell types hosting the bacteria within systemic organs such as the spleen (66, 67). This aspect of the infection process in *Salmonella* spp. is a fairly general feature of intracellular pathogens, e.g., *Yersinia pseudotuberculosis* (68) or *Mycobacterium tuberculosis* (69) (reviewed in reference 70). Such heterogeneity may promote chronic infections and impair the efficacy of antibiotics in treating diseases, with implications for the evolution of virulence. Mouse-to-mouse experimental transmissions of clones isolated from spleen or liver have demonstrated that growth conditions within host tissues select for increased virulence (71) and pathoadaptive mutations (72). As discussed in the next section, systemic dissemination of NTS is not (always) an evolutionary dead end. During prolonged infections in hosts able to contain systemic spread, extraintestinal sites represent a reservoir for virulent genotypes. Sporadic reseeding of the gut from the tissues (i.e., in relapses) can also promote the fecal shedding of virulent NTS and their natural transmission to new hosts.

IMPACT OF ANTIBIOTICS ON THE TRANSMISSION OF THE VIRULENT GENOTYPE

The cooperative virulence of *S.* Typhimurium is inherently unstable in the gut lumen, from where the pathogen is excreted into the environment and can reach new hosts. Within this niche, avirulent defector mutants evolve. When the frequency of defectors is high enough, they can eventually impair the

transmission of virulent genotypes to the next host (73) (Fig. 3). This happens particularly in the absence of ecological disturbance in the gut lumen, where competition for resources favors defectors, although different selection regimes in variable environments can influence the rate of defector fixation (74).

One of the strongest disturbances that can occur in the ecological niche of a pathogen is the presence of antibiotics. In the gut lumen, pathogen cells are growing and are highly sensitive to and efficiently killed by antibiotics. However, in systemic organs as well as in the cells of the intestinal mucosa, it was

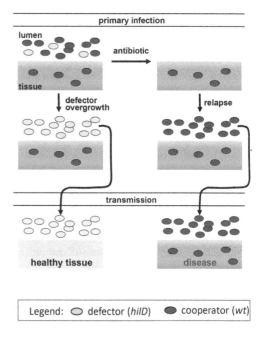

Legend: ○ defector (*hilD*)   ● cooperator (*wt*)

FIGURE 3 Antibiotic treatments select for virulent clones of *S.* Typhimurium able to form persisters in the host tissues. **(Left)** In the absence of antibiotics, defectors can reach fixation and their transmission to the next host prevents disease. **(Right)** Antibiotics kill all cells in the lumen: defectors (*hilD* mutants) and virulent wild-type (*wt*) cooperators. However, *wt* cells survive in the tissues and can reseed the lumen upon antibiotic withdrawal. This leads to successful transmission of the virulent genotype to the next hosts. Reproduced with permission from reference 73.

observed that *S.* Typhimurium is relatively tolerant to antibiotics (67, 75). In infected mice treated with the fluoroquinolone ciprofloxacin, the gut luminal population of *S.* Typhimurium SL1344 drops below the detection limit within a few hours after the onset of the therapy, while a substantial population remains viable in the intestinal mucosa (73) (Fig. 3) and other systemic organs (e.g., in the mesenteric lymph nodes) (75). These pathogen cells can survive for at least 10 days under continuous ciprofloxacin therapy. The ciprofloxacin is able to diffuse systemically and penetrate host cells. This means that intracellular *Salmonella* is indeed exposed to this antibiotic. The observed resistance is due not to mutation but rather to the expression of a transient tolerant phenotype called "persister" (76), which seems linked here to the slow replication rate of a subset of intracellular bacteria (67, 75, 77). Persisters can be isolated from the host's tissues and normally cultivated *in vitro*. The reisolated clones present a sensitivity to ciprofloxacin that is identical to that of the ancestor clone, before passage in mice and exposure to the antibiotic. This indicates that ciprofloxacin survival is due to phenotypic adaptation, not to selection of genetically resistant mutants.

Upon clearance of the antibiotic, fully virulent clones of *S.* Typhimurium were able to reseed the gut lumen directly from the mucosa and to reestablish acute inflammation. Moreover, when transmitted to naive mice, the reseeding population was able to trigger colitis, while a population invaded by defectors (i.e., stool from untreated mice) was incapable of causing any symptoms (Fig. 3).

This demonstrates that in the presence of antibiotics, tissue invasion represents a potent selective advantage that offsets the fitness cost associated with TTSS-1 expression. In other words, antibiotic treatments can artificially inflict a cost of cheating (which was absent in our original experiments where we detected the upgrowth of defectors in the gut luminal pathogen population) that is higher than the benefit from not expressing virulence. This observation revealed two important aspects of the pathogen-host interaction: first, an important detrimental effect of antibiotic-based therapies against NTS, namely the selection for virulence; and second, a possible role of the persister phenotype in the evolution of facultative intracellular pathogens.

PERSPECTIVES: CAN THE PROCESS OF TRANSMISSION IN ITSELF MAINTAIN A VIRULENT GENOTYPE?

The life cycle of enteropathogens is not limited to within-host growth. It also includes transmission steps often associated with passages through harsh extrahost environments that can dramatically alter the structure of the pathogen population, a factor influencing the emergence of cooperation in general (78) and of cooperative virulence in particular (79). Transmission events often imply random sampling of bacteria reaching the next host (population bottleneck). This reduces the genetic variability previously generated within the donor host and can favor clones that are not necessarily more adapted (genetic drift) (80). The impact of population bottlenecks depends on the size of these bottlenecks (i.e., the effective population size reaching the next host) and on the genetic diversity of the population when they occur. Transmission could therefore help maintain virulence when virulent clones are overrepresented in the donor and have a higher chance to pass through the bottleneck without defectors. Once released into the environment, defectors could also be more or less efficient than virulent clones in reaching new hosts. In the most extreme case, i.e., clonal transmission, defectors have no chance to trigger inflammation by themselves, a scenario that should strongly favor the evolution (or maintenance) of virulence. Further investigations are required to understand the evolutionary dynamics of NTS virulence after successive passages from hosts to hosts.

CITATION

Diard M, Hardt WD. 2017. Basic processes in *Salmonella*-host interactions: within-host evolution and the transmission of the virulent genotype. Microbiol Spectrum 5(5):MTBP-0012-2016.

REFERENCES

1. **Falkow S.** 1988. Molecular Koch's postulates applied to microbial pathogenicity. *Rev Infect Dis* **10**(Suppl 2):S274–S276.
2. **Isberg RR, Falkow S.** 1985. A single genetic locus encoded by *Yersinia pseudotuberculosis* permits invasion of cultured animal cells by *Escherichia coli* K-12. *Nature* **317**:262–264.
3. **Casadevall A, Pirofski LA.** 2003. The damage-response framework of microbial pathogenesis. *Nat Rev Microbiol* **1**:17–24.
4. **World Health Organization.** 2016. *Global Tuberculosis Report 2016.* World Health Organization, Geneva, Switzerland.
5. **Centers for Disease Control and Prevention.** 2012. *Pathogens causing US foodborne illnesses, hospitalizations, and deaths, 2000–2008.* http://www.cdc.gov/foodborneburden/PDFs/pathogens-complete-list-01-12.pdf. Accessed 03.20.2017
6. **Cohn AC, MacNeil JR, Harrison LH, Hatcher C, Theodore J, Schmidt M, Pondo T, Arnold KE, Baumbach J, Bennett N, Craig AS, Farley M, Gershman K, Petit S, Lynfield R, Reingold A, Schaffner W, Shutt KA, Zell ER, Mayer LW, Clark T, Stephens D, Messonnier NE.** 2010. Changes in *Neisseria meningitidis* disease epidemiology in the United States, 1998–2007: implications for prevention of meningococcal disease. *Clin Infect Dis* **50**:184–191.
7. **MacNeil J, Cohn A.** 2011. Meningococcal disease, p 01–11. *In* Centers for Disease Control and Prevention (ed), *VPD Surveillance Manual*, 5th ed. Centers for Disease Control and Prevention, Atlanta, GA.
8. **Mishori R, McClaskey EL, WinklerPrins VJ.** 2012. Chlamydia trachomatis infections: screening, diagnosis, and management. *Am Fam Physician* **86**:1127–1132.
9. **Wertheim HF, Melles DC, Vos MC, van Leeuwen W, van Belkum A, Verbrugh HA, Nouwen JL.** 2005. The role of nasal carriage in *Staphylococcus aureus* infections. *Lancet Infect Dis* **5**:751–762.
10. **Tong SY, Davis JS, Eichenberger E, Holland TL, Fowler VG Jr.** 2015. *Staphylococcus aureus* infections: epidemiology, pathophysiology, clinical manifestations, and management. *Clin Microbiol Rev* **28**:603–661.
11. **Alizon S, Michalakis Y.** 2015. Adaptive virulence evolution: the good old fitness-based approach. *Trends Ecol Evol* **30**:248–254.
12. **Kaiser P, Diard M, Stecher B, Hardt WD.** 2012. The streptomycin mouse model for *Salmonella* diarrhea: functional analysis of the microbiota, the pathogen's virulence factors, and the host's mucosal immune response. *Immunol Rev* **245**:56–83.
13. **Stecher B, Robbiani R, Walker AW, Westendorf AM, Barthel M, Kremer M, Chaffron S, Macpherson AJ, Buer J, Parkhill J, Dougan G, von Mering C, Hardt WD.** 2007. *Salmonella enterica* serovar Typhimurium exploits inflammation to compete with the intestinal microbiota. *PLoS Biol* **5**:2177–2189.
14. **Diard M, Garcia V, Maier L, Remus-Emsermann MN, Regoes RR, Ackermann M, Hardt WD.** 2013. Stabilization of cooperative virulence by the expression of an avirulent phenotype. *Nature* **494**:353–356.
15. **Steere AC, Hall WJ III, Wells JG, Craven PJ, Leotsakis N, Farmer JJ III, Gangarosa EJ.** 1975. Person-to-person spread of *Salmonella* Typhimurium after a hospital common-source outbreak. *Lancet* **1**:319–322.
16. **Marzel A, Desai PT, Goren A, Schorr YI, Nissan I, Porwollik S, Valinsky L, McClelland M, Rahav G, Gal-Mor O.** 2016. Persistent infections by nontyphoidal *Salmonella* in humans: epidemiology and genetics. *Clin Infect Dis* **62**:879–886.
17. **Dhanoa A, Fatt QK.** 2009. Non-typhoidal *Salmonella* bacteraemia: epidemiology, clinical characteristics and its' association with severe immunosuppression. *Ann Clin Microbiol Antimicrob* **8**:15.
18. **Rabsch W, Fruth A, Simon S, Szabo I, Malorny B.** 2014. The zoonotic agent *Salmonella*, p 179–211. *In* Sing A (ed), *Zoonoses—Infections Affecting Humans and Animals.* Springer, Dordrecht, The Netherlands.
19. **Chaudhuri RR, Morgan E, Peters SE, Pleasance SJ, Hudson DL, Davies HM, Wang J, van Diemen PM, Buckley AM, Bowen AJ, Pullinger GD, Turner DJ, Langridge GC, Turner AK, Parkhill J, Charles IG, Maskell DJ, Stevens MP.** 2013. Comprehensive assignment of roles for *Salmonella* Typhimurium genes in intestinal colonization of food-producing animals. *PLoS Genet* **9**:e1003456.
20. **Porcheron G, Schouler C, Dozois CM.** 2016. Survival games at the dinner table: regulation of enterobacterial virulence through nutrient sensing and acquisition. *Curr Opin Microbiol* **30**:98–106.
21. **Maier L, Vyas R, Cordova CD, Lindsay H, Schmidt TS, Brugiroux S, Periaswamy B,**

Bauer R, Sturm A, Schreiber F, von Mering C, Robinson MD, Stecher B, Hardt WD. 2013. Microbiota-derived hydrogen fuels *Salmonella* Typhimurium invasion of the gut ecosystem. *Cell Host Microbe* 14:641–651.

22. **Maier L, Barthel M, Stecher B, Maier RJ, Gunn JS, Hardt WD. 2014.** *Salmonella* Typhimurium strain ATCC14028 requires H2-hydrogenases for growth in the gut, but not at systemic sites. *PLoS One* 9:e110187.

23. **Barthel M, Hapfelmeier S, Quintanilla-Martínez L, Kremer M, Rohde M, Hogardt M, Pfeffer K, Rüssmann H, Hardt WD. 2003.** Pretreatment of mice with streptomycin provides a *Salmonella* enterica serovar Typhimurium colitis model that allows analysis of both pathogen and host. *Infect Immun* 71:2839–2858.

24. **Faber F, Bäumler AJ. 2014.** The impact of intestinal inflammation on the nutritional environment of the gut microbiota. *Immunol Lett* 162 (2 Pt A):48–53.

25. **Stecher B, Barthel M, Schlumberger MC, Haberli L, Rabsch W, Kremer M, Hardt WD. 2008.** Motility allows *S.* Typhimurium to benefit from the mucosal defence. *Cell Microbiol* 10:1166–1180.

26. **Winter SE, Thiennimitr P, Winter MG, Butler BP, Huseby DL, Crawford RW, Russell JM, Bevins CL, Adams LG, Tsolis RM, Roth JR, Bäumler AJ. 2010.** Gut inflammation provides a respiratory electron acceptor for *Salmonella*. *Nature* 467:426–429.

27. **Thiennimitr P, Winter SE, Bäumler AJ. 2012.** *Salmonella*, the host and its microbiota. *Curr Opin Microbiol* 15:108–114.

28. **Stecher B, Paesold G, Barthel M, Kremer M, Jantsch J, Stallmach T, Heikenwalder M, Hardt WD. 2006.** Chronic *Salmonella enterica* serovar Typhimurium-induced colitis and cholangitis in streptomycin-pretreated *Nramp1*$^{+/+}$ mice. *Infect Immun* 74:5047–5057.

29. **Endt K, Stecher B, Chaffron S, Slack E, Tchitchek N, Benecke A, Van Maele L, Sirard JC, Mueller AJ, Heikenwalder M, Macpherson AJ, Strugnell R, von Mering C, Hardt WD. 2010.** The microbiota mediates pathogen clearance from the gut lumen after non-typhoidal *Salmonella* diarrhea. *PLoS Pathog* 6:e1001097.

30. **Stecher B, Chaffron S, Käppeli R, Hapfelmeier S, Freedrich S, Weber TC, Kirundi J, Suar M, McCoy KD, von Mering C, Macpherson AJ, Hardt WD. 2010.** Like will to like: abundances of closely related species can predict susceptibility to intestinal colonization by pathogenic and commensal bacteria. *PLoS Pathog* 6: e1000711.

31. **Brugiroux S, Beutler M, Pfann C, Garzetti D, Ruscheweyh HJ, Ring D, Diehl M, Herp S, Lötscher Y, Hussain S, Bunk B, Pukall R, Huson DH, Münch PC, McHardy AC, McCoy KD, Macpherson AJ, Loy A, Clavel T, Berry D, Stecher B. 2016.** Genome-guided design of a defined mouse microbiota that confers colonization resistance against *Salmonella enterica* serovar Typhimurium. *Nat Microbiol* 2:16215.

32. **Maier L, Diard M, Sellin ME, Chouffane ES, Trautwein-Weidner K, Periaswamy B, Slack E, Dolowschiak T, Stecher B, Loverdo C, Regoes RR, Hardt WD. 2014.** Granulocytes impose a tight bottleneck upon the gut luminal pathogen population during *Salmonella* Typhimurium colitis. *PLoS Pathog* 10:e1004557.

33. **Brennan PC, Fritz TE, Flynn RJ, Poole CM. 1965.** *Citrobacter freundii* associated with diarrhea in a laboratory mice. *Lab Anim Care* 15: 266–275.

34. **Muto T, Nakagawa M, Isobe Y, Saito M, Nakano T, Imaizumi K. 1969.** Infectious megaenteron of mice. I. Manifestation and pathological observation. *Jpn J Med Sci Biol* 22:363–374.

35. **Mundy R, MacDonald TT, Dougan G, Frankel G, Wiles S. 2005.** *Citrobacter rodentium* of mice and man. *Cell Microbiol* 7:1697–1706.

36. **Kamada N, Kim YG, Sham HP, Vallance BA, Puente JL, Martens EC, Núñez G. 2012.** Regulated virulence controls the ability of a pathogen to compete with the gut microbiota. *Science* 336: 1325–1329.

37. **Schlumberger MC, Hardt WD. 2006.** *Salmonella* type III secretion effectors: pulling the host cell's strings. *Curr Opin Microbiol* 9:46–54.

38. **Hapfelmeier S, Hardt WD. 2005.** A mouse model for *S. typhimurium*-induced enterocolitis. *Trends Microbiol* 13:497–503.

39. **Müller AJ, Hoffmann C, Galle M, Van Den Broeke A, Heikenwalder M, Falter L, Misselwitz B, Kremer M, Beyaert R, Hardt WD. 2009.** The *S.* Typhimurium effector SopE induces caspase-1 activation in stromal cells to initiate gut inflammation. *Cell Host Microbe* 6:125–136.

40. **Müller AJ, Kaiser P, Dittmar KE, Weber TC, Haueter S, Endt K, Songhet P, Zellweger C, Kremer M, Fehling HJ, Hardt WD. 2012.** *Salmonella* gut invasion involves TTSS-2-dependent epithelial traversal, basolateral exit, and uptake by epithelium-sampling lamina propria phagocytes. *Cell Host Microbe* 11: 19–32.

41. **Sellin ME, Müller AA, Felmy B, Dolowschiak T, Diard M, Tardivel A, Maslowski KM, Hardt WD. 2014.** Epithelium-intrinsic NAIP/NLRC4

inflammasome drives infected enterocyte expulsion to restrict *Salmonella* replication in the intestinal mucosa. *Cell Host Microbe* **16**:237–248.

42. **Núñez-Hernández C, Tierrez A, Ortega AD, Pucciarelli MG, Godoy M, Eisman B, Casadesús J, García-del Portillo F.** 2013. Genome expression analysis of nonproliferating intracellular *Salmonella enterica* serovar Typhimurium unravels an acid pH-dependent PhoP-PhoQ response essential for dormancy. *Infect Immun* **81:**154–165.

43. **Moor K, Diard M, Sellin ME, Felmy B, Wotzka SY, Toska A, Bakkeren E, Arnoldini M, Bansept F, Co AD, Völler T, Minola A, Fernandez-Rodriguez B, Agatic G, Barbieri S, Piccoli L, Casiraghi C, Corti D, Lanzavecchia A, Regoes RR, Loverdo C, Stocker R, Brumley DR, Hardt WD, Slack E.** 2017. High-avidity IgA protects the intestine by enchaining growing bacteria. *Nature* **544:**498–502.

44. **Pallen MJ, Wren BW.** 2007. Bacterial pathogenomics. *Nature* **449:**835–842.

45. **Stecher B, Denzler R, Maier L, Bernet F, Sanders MJ, Pickard DJ, Barthel M, Westendorf AM, Krogfelt KA, Walker AW, Ackermann M, Dobrindt U, Thomson NR, Hardt WD.** 2012. Gut inflammation can boost horizontal gene transfer between pathogenic and commensal *Enterobacteriaceae. Proc Natl Acad Sci U S A* **109:**1269–1274.

46. **Diard M, Bakkeren E, Cornuault JK, Moor K, Hausmann A, Sellin ME, Loverdo C, Aertsen A, Ackermann M, De Paepe M, Slack E, Hardt WD.** 2017. Inflammation boosts bacteriophage transfer between *Salmonella* spp. *Science* **355:**1211–1215.

47. **Moor K, Wotzka SY, Toska A, Diard M, Hapfelmeier S, Slack E.** 2016. Peracetic acid treatment generates potent inactivated oral vaccines from a broad range of culturable bacterial species. *Front Immunol* **7:**34.

48. **van der Heijden J, Finlay BB.** 2012. Type III effector-mediated processes in *Salmonella* infection. *Future Microbiol* **7:**685–703.

49. **Sturm A, Heinemann M, Arnoldini M, Benecke A, Ackermann M, Benz M, Dormann J, Hardt WD.** 2011. The cost of virulence: retarded growth of *Salmonella* Typhimurium cells expressing type III secretion system 1. *PLoS Pathog* **7:**e1002143.

50. **Ackermann M, Stecher B, Freed NE, Songhet P, Hardt WD, Doebeli M.** 2008. Self-destructive cooperation mediated by phenotypic noise. *Nature* **454:**987–990.

51. **West SA, Griffin AS, Gardner A, Diggle SP.** 2006. Social evolution theory for microorganisms. *Nat Rev Microbiol* **4:**597–607.

52. **Petrone BL, Stringer AM, Wade JT.** 2014. Identification of HilD-regulated genes in *Salmonella enterica* serovar Typhimurium. *J Bacteriol* **196:**1094–1101.

53. **Bush K, Courvalin P, Dantas G, Davies J, Eisenstein B, Huovinen P, Jacoby GA, Kishony R, Kreiswirth BN, Kutter E, Lerner SA, Levy S, Lewis K, Lomovskaya O, Miller JH, Mobashery S, Piddock LJ, Projan S, Thomas CM, Tomasz A, Tulkens PM, Walsh TR, Watson JD, Witkowski J, Witte W, Wright G, Yeh P, Zgurskaya HI.** 2011. Tackling antibiotic resistance. *Nat Rev Microbiol* **9:**894–896.

54. **World Health Organization.** 2012. *The Evolving Threat of Antimicrobial Resistance: Options for Action.* World Health Organization, Geneva, Switzerland.

55. **Colgan AM, Kröger C, Diard M, Hardt WD, Puente JL, Sivasankaran SK, Hokamp K, Hinton JC.** 2016. The impact of 18 ancestral and horizontally-acquired regulatory proteins upon the transcriptome and sRNA landscape of *Salmonella enterica* serovar Typhimurium. *PLoS Genet* **12:**e1006258.

56. **Stecher B, Hapfelmeier S, Müller C, Kremer M, Stallmach T, Hardt WD.** 2004. Flagella and chemotaxis are required for efficient induction of *Salmonella enterica* serovar Typhimurium colitis in streptomycin-pretreated mice. *Infect Immun* **72:**4138–4150.

57. **Gerlach RG, Cláudio N, Rohde M, Jäckel D, Wagner C, Hensel M.** 2008. Cooperation of *Salmonella* pathogenicity islands 1 and 4 is required to breach epithelial barriers. *Cell Microbiol* **10:**2364–2376.

58. **Hapfelmeier S, Stecher B, Barthel M, Kremer M, Müller AJ, Heikenwalder M, Stallmach T, Hensel M, Pfeffer K, Akira S, Hardt WD.** 2005. The Salmonella pathogenicity island (SPI)-2 and SPI-1 type III secretion systems allow *Salmonella* serovar *typhimurium* to trigger colitis via MyD88-dependent and MyD88-independent mechanisms. *J Immunol* **174:**1675–1685.

59. **Figueira R, Holden DW.** 2012. Functions of the *Salmonella* pathogenicity island 2 (SPI-2) type III secretion system effectors. *Microbiology* **158:**1147–1161.

60. **Salcedo SP, Noursadeghi M, Cohen J, Holden DW.** 2001. Intracellular replication of *Salmonella typhimurium* strains in specific subsets of splenic macrophages *in vivo. Cell Microbiol* **3:**587–597.

61. **Knodler LA.** 2015. *Salmonella enterica*: living a double life in epithelial cells. *Curr Opin Microbiol* **23:**23–31.

62. **Vonaesch P, Sellin ME, Cardini S, Singh V, Barthel M, Hardt WD.** 2014. The *Salmonella*

Typhimurium effector protein SopE transiently localizes to the early SCV and contributes to intracellular replication. *Cell Microbiol* **16:**1723–1735.

63. Hautefort I, Thompson A, Eriksson-Ygberg S, Parker ML, Lucchini S, Danino V, Bongaerts RJ, Ahmad N, Rhen M, Hinton JC. 2008. During infection of epithelial cells *Salmonella enterica* serovar Typhimurium undergoes a time-dependent transcriptional adaptation that results in simultaneous expression of three type 3 secretion systems. *Cell Microbiol* **10:**958–984.

64. Laughlin RC, Knodler LA, Barhoumi R, Payne HR, Wu J, Gomez G, Pugh R, Lawhon SD, Bäumler AJ, Steele-Mortimer O, Adams LG. 2014. Spatial segregation of virulence gene expression during acute enteric infection with *Salmonella enterica* serovar Typhimurium. *mBio* **5:**e00946-e13.

65. Knodler LA, Vallance BA, Celli J, Winfree S, Hansen B, Montero M, Steele-Mortimer O. 2010. Dissemination of invasive *Salmonella* via bacterial-induced extrusion of mucosal epithelia. *Proc Natl Acad Sci U S A* **107:**17733–17738.

66. Burton NA, Schürmann N, Casse O, Steeb AK, Claudi B, Zankl J, Schmidt A, Bumann D. 2014. Disparate impact of oxidative host defenses determines the fate of *Salmonella* during systemic infection in mice. *Cell Host Microbe* **15:**72–83.

67. Claudi B, Spröte P, Chirkova A, Personnic N, Zankl J, Schürmann N, Schmidt A, Bumann D. 2014. Phenotypic variation of *Salmonella* in host tissues delays eradication by antimicrobial chemotherapy. *Cell* **158:**722–733.

68. Davis KM, Mohammadi S, Isberg RR. 2015. Community behavior and spatial regulation within a bacterial microcolony in deep tissue sites serves to protect against host attack. *Cell Host Microbe* **17:**21–31.

69. Tan S, Sukumar N, Abramovitch RB, Parish T, Russell DG. 2013. *Mycobacterium tuberculosis* responds to chloride and pH as synergistic cues to the immune status of its host cell. *PLoS Pathog* **9:**e1003282.

70. Bumann D. 2015. Heterogeneous host-pathogen encounters: act locally, think globally. *Cell Host Microbe* **17:**13–19.

71. Zelle MR. 1942. Genetic constitutions of host and pathogen in mouse typhoid. *J Infect Dis* **71:** 131–152.

72. Nilsson AI, Kugelberg E, Berg OG, Andersson DI. 2004. Experimental adaptation of *Salmonella typhimurium* to mice. *Genetics* **168:**1119–1130.

73. Diard M, Sellin ME, Dolowschiak T, Arnoldini M, Ackermann M, Hardt WD. 2014. Antibiotic treatment selects for cooperative virulence of *Salmonella* Typhimurium. *Curr Biol* **24:**2000–2005.

74. Brockhurst MA, Buckling A, Gardner A. 2007. Cooperation peaks at intermediate disturbance. *Curr Biol* **17:**761–765.

75. Kaiser P, Regoes RR, Dolowschiak T, Wotzka SY, Lengefeld J, Slack E, Grant AJ, Ackermann M, Hardt WD. 2014. Cecum lymph node dendritic cells harbor slow-growing bacteria phenotypically tolerant to antibiotic treatment. *PLoS Biol* **12:**e1001793.

76. Balaban NQ, Gerdes K, Lewis K, McKinney JD. 2013. A problem of persistence: still more questions than answers? *Nat Rev Microbiol* **11:** 587–591.

77. Helaine S, Cheverton AM, Watson KG, Faure LM, Matthews SA, Holden DW. 2014. Internalization of *Salmonella* by macrophages induces formation of nonreplicating persisters. *Science* **343:**204–208.

78. Nowak MA, May RM. 1992. Evolutionary games and spatial chaos. *Nature* **359:**826–829.

79. Griffin AS, West SA, Buckling A. 2004. Cooperation and competition in pathogenic bacteria. *Nature* **430:**1024–1027.

80. Kimura M. 1984. *The Neutral Theory of Molecular Evolution.* Cambridge University Press, Cambridge, United Kingdom.

Salmonella Intracellular Lifestyles and Their Impact on Host-to-Host Transmission

6

M. GRACIELA PUCCIARELLI[1,2] and FRANCISCO GARCÍA-DEL PORTILLO[1]

INTRODUCTION

The bacterial species *Salmonella enterica* comprises Gram-negative pathogenic microorganisms that cause infections in humans and livestock. *S. enterica* is subdivided into six subspecies, with subspecies I responsible for infections in warm-blooded vertebrates, including mammals and birds (1, 2). To date, >2,500 serovars have been reported in subspecies I. Some of these serovars are host adapted, whereas others infect a broad range of hosts. Host-adapted serovars cause systemic infections that result in typhoid (paratyphoid) fever and bacteremia. Among these serovars are Typhi, Paratyphi A, Paratyphi C (humans), Cholerasuis (swine), Dublin (cow), and Gallinarum (fowl). Non-typhoidal serovars normally cause self-limiting gastroenteritis, although the severity of the infection varies depending on the immune defense status of the host and/or a unique genetic makeup that may render the clone highly invasive. An example is the recently characterized invasive serovar Typhimurium isolates that cause systemic disease in HIV-infected individuals of sub-Saharan African countries (3, 4) and Latin America (5). Importantly, high

[1]Laboratory of Intracellular Bacterial Pathogens, Departamento de Biotecnología Microbiana, Centro Nacional de Biotecnología-Consejo Superior de Investigaciones Científicas (CNB-CSIC), Madrid, Spain; [2]Centro de Biología Molecular Severo Ochoa (CBMSO-CSIC), Departamento de Biología Molecular, Universidad Autónoma de Madrid, Madrid, Spain.

Microbial Transmission in Biological Processes
Edited by Fernando Baquero, Emilio Bouza, J.A. Gutiérrez-Fuentes, and Teresa M. Coque
© 2018 American Society for Microbiology, Washington, DC
doi:10.1128/microbiolspec.MTBP-0009-2016

transmissibility has been reported for all serovars, especially in those areas in which hygiene conditions in water and food are poor. The ability of all *S. enterica* serovars to cause persistent asymptomatic infections, especially following infection by host-adapted serovars, imposes more difficulties on control of transmission (6, 7). This capacity to persist in the host without causing pathology has attracted physicians and microbiologists for more than a century, given its undoubtable negative impact on pathogen eradication. The reader is directed to the pioneering book *The Carrier Problem in Infectious Diseases* by Ledingham and Arkwright, which in 1912 exhaustively compiled all existing information about cases of asymptomatic carriers and their impact on pathogen transmission (8). These authors focused on six diseases known at that time to have high transmission rates, including typhoid and paratyphoid fever, diphtheria, epidemic cerebrospinal meningitis, dysentery, and cholera (8). Studies performed in mouse asymptomatic chronic infection models using the serovar Typhimurium have identified pathogen genes required to persist in the animal for long periods of time (weeks to a few months) (9, 10). These studies also showed that serovar Typhimurium evolves during a chronic infection in the host and that this condition selects for adaptive mutations (9). This is an intense and fascinating area of research that will certainly aid to combat *Salmonella* transmissibility among individuals. We also refer to the chapter in this book by Wolf-Dietrich Hardt and colleagues, which addresses within-host evolution in *Salmonella* and the transmission of the virulent genotype in populations differentially affected by antibiotic treatments.

S. enterica is one of the bacterial pathogens in which the ability to invade eukaryotic cells was first reported. Using a guinea pig model in which the animals were challenged with serovar Typhimurium, Takeuchi demonstrated that bacteria transiently disrupted the brush border during the penetration of enterocytes, to later be confined within membrane-bound vacuoles (11). These pioneering observations were later confirmed *in vitro* using cultured cell lines such as human epithelial HeLa cells (12, 13). Subsequent cell biology studies focused on defining the intracellular trafficking route of the phagosomal compartment harboring serovar Typhimurium, coined the *Salmonella*-containing vacuole (SCV) in the initial studies (14). Current data support a variety of SCV "prototypes" with disparate biogenesis routes depending on the infected host cell type (15). This disparity may reflect differences between host cell defenses responding to the intruder microbe and the survival strategies used by the pathogen. In most cases, these different SCV types and pathogen-host interactions are observed even in the same tissue or organ (Fig. 1). The bacterial strains and host cells used, ranging from established phagocytic and nonphagocytic cell lines of tumor or nontumor origin to primary cultures and organoids (16–18), are also variables that affect SCV biogenesis. For example, entry of serovar Typhimurium into macrophages selects for a subpopulation of persistent intracellular bacteria (19). This observation denotes that the transition to the intracellular niche of phagocytic cells can promote persistence and, as a result, transmissibility.

Much recent data also sustain the capacity of serovar Typhimurium to break the SCV membrane and reach the cytosol of epithelial cells (20, 21), a favorable microenvironment thought to favor massive pathogen proliferation. On the other hand, there is accumulating evidence about distinct strategies used by this pathogen to limit proliferation and persist inside the infected host cell. In this chapter, we evaluate what is known about the intraphagosomal and cytosolic lifestyles of *Salmonella* and their potential relationships with two phenomena known to enhance host-to-host transmissibility: (i) localized intestinal inflammation with massive loss of bacteria in the stool and (ii) the establishment of chronic persistent infections. Both conditions predispose to abrupt or periodic shedding of

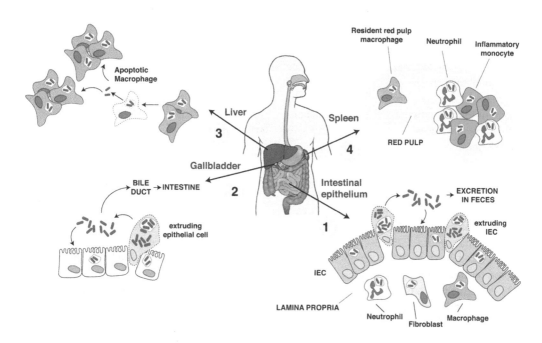

FIGURE 1 Distinct intracellular lifestyles of *S. enterica* serovar Typhimurium reported in various host locations during local inflammation of the intestine or acute systemic disease. (1) Limited proliferation of serovar Typhimurium in intestinal epithelial cells (IECs) during penetration of the intestinal barrier. The pathogen proliferates actively in a few IECs, which are rapidly extruded by a mechanism that depends on the inflammasome proteins NAIP/NLRC4. This proliferation was reported to occur within phagosomes and in the cytosol. Bacteria have also been observed in phagocytic (neutrophils, macrophages) and nonphagocytic cells (fibroblasts) in the underlying lamina propria. (2) Extrusion of heavily infected epithelial cells observed in the epithelium lining the gallbladder. As in the IECs, there is also evidence for replication of intracellular cytosolic serovar Typhimurium cells. (3) Serovar Typhimurium targets mainly macrophages in the liver. The most-accepted models support an increase in infection foci due to subsequent episodes of macrophage infection, a few rounds of intracellular replication of the pathogen, and reinfection of nearby macrophages. The intracellular lifestyle in these macrophages is entirely intraphagosomal. (4) Serovar Typhimurium colonizes distinct types of phagocytes in the red pulp of the spleen. The infection is highly contained by inflammatory monocytes and neutrophils, although some bacteria colonize and persist in resident macrophages. Note that the proliferation detected in the few epithelial cells that extrude in the intestinal epithelium and gallbladder ultimately favors shedding of the pathogen outside the host. Although not shown, serovar Typhimurium has also been shown to persist in macrophages present in mesenteric lymph nodes.

bacteria to the external (outside the host) environment.

SALMONELLA TRANSITION TO THE INTRACELLULAR NICHE IN THE EUKARYOTIC CELL

Typhoidal and nontyphoidal *S. enterica* serovars invade eukaryotic cells using effector proteins translocated by specialized type III secretion apparatuses encoded in the *Salmonella* pathogenicity islands 1 (SPI-1) and 2 (SPI-2) (2, 22, 23). Hereinafter, we refer to these systems as T1 and T2, respectively. Invasion of nonphagocytic cells has been extensively studied in immortal cultured epithelial cell lines such as HeLa, derived from human cervical cancer cells. Entry into the epithelial cell is of paramount importance for *Salmonella* pathogenesis since it allows the pathogen to penetrate the intestinal barrier. At the mechanistic level, translocated T1 effectors alter cytoskeleton dynamics to recruit actin to the site of bacterial contact and to obtain in this manner the required mechanical force for bacterial ingestion. This mode of entry, known as "trigger," is accompanied by massive reorganization of the actin cytoskeleton and the formation of membrane ruffles that capture the invading bacterium to culminate in its efficient ingestion (24). T1 effectors involved in this process include SopB, SopE, and SopE2, which contribute to bacterial invasion and biogenesis of the early SCV compartment (2, 25). SopB function has been linked to (i) actin rearrangement promoted by the small GTPase Rho; (ii) annexin A2 recruitment, which facilitates actin accumulation; and (iii) the generation of phosphatidylinositol 3-phosphate by recruiting the small GTPase Rab5 and the phosphatidylinositol 3-kinase Vps34 (2). The T1 effectors SopE and SopE2 act as guanine nucleotide exchange factors of the small GTPases Rac1 and Cdc42. Activation of these two GTPases leads to actin reorganization promoted by stimulation of actin nucleation factors of the Wiskott-Aldrich syndrome protein (WASP) family (26). SipA and SipC, which promote actin bundling, are additional T1 effectors required for invasion. Following bacterial internalization, SptP, another T1 effector, reverses the alterations to the cell cytoskeleton by inactivating the Rho GTPase (2, 25, 27).

The nontyphoidal serovars Typhimurium and Enteritidis can also invade nonphagocytic cells by T1-independent mechanisms that mimic the zipper-like mode of entry (Table 1) (28–31). This entry process is driven essentially by adhesin-receptor interactions. The pathogen surface proteins Rck and PagN have been implicated in this process (29, 30). T1-independent entry mediated by the pathogen occurs in fibroblast and epithelial cell lines (28, 31). Of note, the nontyphoidal serovar Typhimurium can cause infections in chicken, bovine, and murine animal models independently of a functional T1 system (29). Similar observations were reported

for the serovar Enteritidis (32, 33) and the host-adapted serovar Gallinarum (Table 1) (34). Thus, *Salmonella* could exploit multiple entry mechanisms of nonphagocytic cells (29), with preferable usage in specific hosts and with probable benefit for host-to-host transmission.

Internalization of *Salmonella* serovars into professional phagocytic cells such as macrophages or dendritic cells has also been studied in detail. Alternative modes of entry can occur depending on whether the entry is triggered by the pathogen (e.g., via T1-translocated effectors) or driven by the phagocyte using dedicated receptors that promote phagocytosis. Early reports using serovar Typhimurium suggested that the phagosomal compartments harboring wild-type and isogenic T1-defective strains were indistinguishable (35). However, later studies in macrophages showed marked differences. Thus, the phagosomal compartment formed after T1-induced entry or the uptake of complement-opsonized serovar Typhimurium was permissive for growth, whereas IgG-opsonized or nonopsonized bacteria were killed in the phagosome (36). The fate of serovar Typhimurium inside macrophages, the preferred cell type targeted by this pathogen *in vivo* (Fig. 1), can be therefore highly variable depending on the mode of entry (37).

BIOGENESIS AND MATURATION OF THE SCV

Early studies in the 1980s showed that serovar Typhimurium survival inside macrophages was a requisite for causing disease in mice (38). This observation paved the way to analyze this phagosomal compartment in more detail. As mentioned above, this compartment is now generically known as the *Salmonella*-containing vacuole in both phagocytic and nonphagocytic cells (20, 39–42). A hallmark of the SCV is its pronounced dynamics in spatial and temporal terms involving interactions with various organelles of the

TABLE 1 *Salmonella* and host responses discussed in this chapter with probable impact on host-to-host transmission of the pathogen

Host and/or pathogen response	Pathogen functions or effectors involved[a]	*S. enterica* serovar(s) in which it has been investigated	Reference(s)
Selection of persister bacteria inside macrophages	toxin-antitoxin (TA) loci	Typhimurium	19
Selection of small-colony variants in persistent infections of fibroblasts	*hemL*, *lpd*, and *aroD* (inactivating mutations)	Typhimurium	75
Production of toxins by the pathogen to restrain growth	TA loci (suspected in host) and TacT toxin	Typhimurium	19, 135
Pathogen proliferation in cytosol of epithelial cells	SPI-1 (T1), YdgT, CorA, and RecA	Typhimurium	20, 21, 141
Attenuation of pathogen proliferation inside fibroblasts	PhoP-PhoQ, RpoS, SlyA, IgaA	Typhimurium	65
SPI-1-mediated invasiveness	SPI-1 (T1) and dedicated effectors (SopB, SopE, SopE2, SipA, SipB, and SptP)	Typhimurium, Typhi, Enteritidis, and many other serovars	142
SPI-1-independent invasion and pathogenicity in animal models	RcsK and PagN; other?	Typhimurium, Enteritidis, and Gallinarum	29, 34, 143
Modulation of intracellular proliferation rate due to the presence or absence of defined Rab GTPases (Rab29, Rab32) in the SCV	GtgE (a T1/T2 effector)	Typhimurium and Typhi (ectopic expression of GtgE)	50, 51
Sifs supporting intracellular bacterial growth	SifA, SseJ (T2 effectors), and PLEKHM1 (host protein)	Typhimurium and Typhi	53, 56
Selective autophagy of a subpopulation of intracellular bacteria triggered by a membranous aggresome	SPI-2	Typhimurium	57
Inflammasome activation in intestinal epithelial cells	NAIP/NLRC4 and caspase-1 (host proteins)	Typhimurium	63
Uptake of distinct carbon sources (polysaccharides?) by intracellular bacteria in chronically infected hosts	KdgR (proposed enhanced activity of this regulator)	Typhimurium	77
Uptake of nutrients (e.g., amino acids) via the Sif tubular membranous extensions	SPI-2 effectors involved in Sif formation; dedicated pathogen transporters?	Typhimurium	78
Active proliferation in the host (acute infection)	SPI-2; ubiquinone synthesis	Typhimurium	82
Persistence in host tissues and organs	FabB (β-ketoacyl-ACP synthase I): synthesis of unsaturated fatty acids and cyclopropane	Typhimurium	82
Sequestration of substrate to host enzyme, generating toxic compounds	DalS (pathogen D-Ala transporter), DAO (host enzyme generating toxic compounds from D-Ala)	Typhimurium	111
Maintenance of integrity of SCV membrane; increased ubiquitination of cytosolic bacteria	TBK1 (host protein)	Typhimurium	109, 110
Modulation of the inflammatory status of the pathogen (M1/M2) by intracellular bacteria	Unknown (response associated to bacterial load)	Typhimurium	115
High proliferation in a low percentage of infected cells in gallbladder and intestinal epithelia	Unknown	Typhimurium	60, 63

[a]SPI-1, *Salmonella*-pathogenicity island.

infected cell, including early and late endosomes and the Golgi apparatus (43, 44). Intracellular trafficking of the SCV has been intensively examined *in vitro* in cultured cell lines. These studies demonstrated the intervention of protein effectors translocated by the T1 and T2 systems. T1 effectors participate in the early stages of SCV maturation, while T2 effectors act a few hours later (2- to 3-h postinfection) to model the intracellular replicative or survival niche. The literature on *Salmonella* T1 and T2 effectors linked to SCV biogenesis is abundant. We refer to excellent reviews that summarize the action of translocated pathogen effector proteins that engage fundamental processes in the infected cell, including cytoskeleton dynamics, vesicular trafficking, and cytokinesis (2, 22, 23, 43, 45–47). Some of the activities demonstrated for T1 and T2 effectors include chemical modification of eukaryotic targets with activities such as acetyltransferase, ADP-ribosyltransferase, tyrosine phosphatase, E3 ubiquitin ligase, deubiquitinase phosphothreonine-ligase, cysteine protease, or glycerophospholipid cholesterol acyltransferase (2, 22, 46). Other *Salmonella* effectors act as enzymes altering certain metabolite pools in the host cell (e.g., phosphoinositide phosphate) or mimicking host proteins that regulate nucleotide exchange in GTPases of the Rho and Rab families (26, 48–50).

The presence or absence of defined sets of effectors can contribute to host specificity. In human macrophages, the SCV containing serovar Typhi is decorated with the GTPase Rab29, which correlates to a state of survival and low proliferation rate for intracellular bacteria (51). However, ectopic expression in serovar Typhi of the T1/T2 effector GtgE, absent in this serovar, results in Rab29 proteolysis and augmented growth in human macrophages (Fig. 2A) (51). This observation links the intracellular survival and persistence of serovar Typhi to a defined repertoire of type III effectors. Based on these findings, it is tempting to speculate that the absence or presence of certain T1 or T2 effectors could direct the maturation of the SCV to either a persistence-promoting environment or a permissive niche for rapid growth. GtgE, encoded by genomes of nontyphoidal serovars, also targets the GTPase Rab32, and this process facilitates proliferation of nontyphoidal serovars such as Typhimurium. Mouse macrophages, which normally restrict serovar Typhi intracellular growth, become permissive for recombinant serovar Typhi strains expressing GtgE, similarly to how they behave when infected with broad-range nontyphoidal serovars such as Typhimurium (Fig. 2A) (50).

The characterization of the SCV trafficking route led to the identification of membrane extensions emanating from the phagosomal compartment, known as *Salmonella*-induced filaments (Sifs) (52). This tubular network is enriched in lysosomal membrane glycoproteins and its mechanism of formation has been deciphered in detail (47, 53). Sif formation is driven by the T2 effector SifA, which links the adaptor protein SKIP and kinesin to the SCV and the microtubule network to induce endosome tubulation (53). Other T2 effectors such as SseJ, which modifies lipid content of the SCV by increasing the amount of cholesterol esters, are required for Sif formation (2). Sifs are a type of structure not observed in uninfected cells, as was reported further for other tubular networks associated with serovar Typhimurium infection (47, 53). The ultimate benefit of this elaborated membranous network is at present unknown, although recent studies favor a role in nutrient acquisition by the pathogen (47). The lack of T2 effectors involved in the generation of these tubular structures results in attenuation of serovar Typhimurium in the mouse model (54, 55), which supports a relevant role for this structure in *Salmonella* pathogenesis. A host protein that contributes to the biogenesis of the SCV and to the connection of this compartment with Sifs is the lysosomal adaptor named Pleckstrin homology domain-containing protein family member 1 (PLEKHM1) (56). This protein interacts with

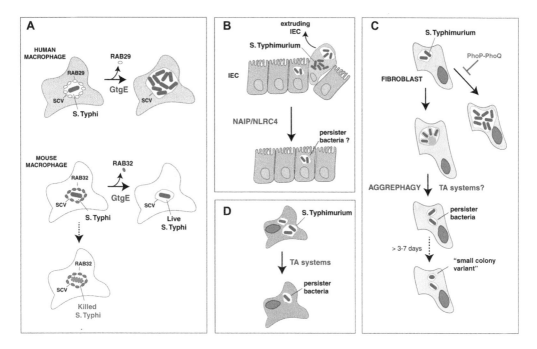

FIGURE 2 Representative conditions reported to control intracellular growth of serovars Typhimurium and Typhi favoring persistence inside the infected cell. These examples include (A) the production by intracellular serovar Typhi of defined type III effector proteins targeting Rab proteins (see text for details); (B) inflammasome intervention in IECs to exclude cells heavily infected with serovar Typhimurium; and (C) attenuation of intracellular growth in fibroblasts linked to changes in yet undefined functions of intracellular serovar Typhimurium regulated by the two-component regulatory system PhoP-PhoQ or other regulators (SlyA, RpoS). This process could be either followed by or occur concomitantly with selective autophagy attack (aggrephagy). Formation of small-colony serovar Typhimurium variants has also been shown to occur in fibroblasts at long postinfection times. (D) The actions of toxins encoded in TA loci contribute to the selection of serovar Typhimurium persisters following ingestion by macrophages.

the T2 effector SifA, the host GTPase Rab7, and the HOPS complex, a multisubunit homotypic fusion and vacuole protein sorting platform. Lack of PLEKHM1 leads to the formation of abnormal vacuoles containing serovar Typhimurium, to the absence of Sifs, and to a lower intracellular bacterial load in epithelial cells and fibroblasts (56). A slightly decreased bacterial load in mice lacking PLEKHM1 was also claimed *in vivo* (56). These data are relevant since they unequivocally link to the capacity of serovar Typhimurium to modify the SCV compartment, as observed in *in vitro* cultured cell lines, to proliferation in the animal organs. Future studies should address whether the observed

changes in bacterial load observed *in vivo* are manifested at the single-cell level.

A recent report describes another example of host membrane manipulation by serovar Typhimurium with direct consequences for the progeny of intracellular bacteria. During infection of fibroblasts, serovar Typhimurium induces the formation of Sif-like structures that do not evolve into an intricate network. Instead, these Sif-like tubular endosomes collapse into a membranous aggregate (aggresome) that recruits autophagy machinery (57). The autophagosome formed in response to the aggregate digests this extraneous body as well as those nearby bacteria captured in the autophagosomal compartment (57).

Intracellular bacteria located far from the aggresome are not attacked by the autophagy machinery and remain alive. This strategy allows bacteria to "self-control" their progeny within the infected cell. These persistently infected cells could favor host-to-host transmissibility by periodic release of intracellular bacteria.

INTRAPHAGOSOMAL VERSUS CYTOSOLIC INTRACELLULAR LIFESTYLE

A large body of evidence has shown that serovar Typhimurium can actively lyse the membrane of the nascent SCV, resulting in colonization of the host cell cytosol (20). This phenotype has been observed mainly in epithelial cells, both in vitro in distinct epithelial cell lines (58) and in vivo (59) (Fig. 1). Of much interest, cytosolic bacteria "hyper-replicate" (58), leading to destruction of the infected epithelial cell. Unlike intraphagosomal bacteria, cytosolic bacteria express flagella and have a functional T1 secretion system (59). In the gallbladder epithelium, the hyperreplication of cytosolic bacteria results in the extrusion of infected cells harboring a large progeny of intracellular bacteria (59, 60) (Fig. 1). The phenomenon is also observed in polarized intestinal epithelial cells (59). This pathogen-induced "exfoliation" resembles that taking place during natural turnover of the intestinal epithelium. However, a major difference is that the epithelial cell infected with serovar Typhimurium undergoes inflammatory cell lysis (pyroptosis), induced by activation of caspase-1 (59), which leads to the release of proinflammatory cytokines such as interleukin-18 (IL-18). These data highlight a new concept in pathogen biology: as was previously shown for macrophages and other phagocytic and immune cells such as dendritic cells and neutrophils, epithelial cells harbor inflammasomes that respond to Salmonella infection (61, 62). Inflammasomes are cytoplasmic signaling complexes that recognize pathogen components such as lipopolysaccharide (LPS), flagellin or proteins of the T1 secretion apparatus and induce the inflammatory caspase-1 and caspase-11 (61, 62). Caspase activation is the key step required for production of inflammatory cytokines (IL-1α, IL-1β, and IL-18), which is followed by their release concomitant to the cell death (61, 62). Are inflammasomes an important host factor affecting or promoting Salmonella transmissibility? A recent study focused on the role of inflammasomes in restricting Salmonella proliferation in intestinal epithelial cells. Two main components of the inflammasome platform that is active in epithelial cells, NAIP/NLRC4 (neuronal apoptosis inhibitor protein/NOD-like receptor subfamily C 4) and caspase-1, contribute to extrusion of heavily infected epithelial cells (Fig. 2B) (59, 63). This phenomenon, however, does not guarantee bacterial clearance. In wild-type mice, serovar Typhimurium persists for 36 h—the last time point measured in the study—in intestinal epithelial cells harboring a low average number (2 to 3 cells) of intracellular bacteria (63). These data suggest that inflammasomes may become active at early infection times to control the burst of intracellular replication occurring in a few epithelial cells of the intestinal barrier. This situation presents a striking parallelism with the control of an early replication burst taking place in fibroblasts, which is aborted following aggrephagy of an endosomal membranous aggregate (Fig. 2C) (57).

Based on these observations, we could speculate on an exploitation of the inflammasome machinery by serovar Typhimurium to "self-control" and to attenuate intracellular growth. This condition could certainly preserve integrity of the infected cell and ensure transmissibility. On the pathogen side, extrusion of heavily infected cells together with persistence in some other cells of the epithelial barrier (both in intestine and gallbladder) seems doubly beneficial. Thus, such strategy results in release of many bacteria to the intestinal or gallbladder lumen, increasing the probability of reinfection and spreading to the external environment (Fig. 1). Whether there is a potential pathogen reservoir remaining after the control of the initial growth burst by the NAIP/NLRC4 inflammasome axis (63) has not yet been investigated. Comparable long-term studies at the cellular level in the gallbladder are also lacking.

Strong evidence supporting the role of inflammasomes in control of serovar Typhimurium proliferation comes from the exacerbated bacterial growth in intestinal epithelial cells and increased colonization of lymph nodes noted in mice lacking components of this host defense (63). This has serious consequences for the host since the pathogen can then rapidly spread to deeper tissues. Still intriguing is the interplay between extrusion of heavily infected cells and the simultaneous presence of epithelial cells having low numbers of intracellular bacteria, which could act as reservoir. Noteworthy, there is also evidence of serovar Typhimurium targeting nonphagocytic stromal cells located in the intestinal lamina propria, in which the pathogen actively restrains growth (64). This response is driven by, among others, the master virulence two-component regulatory system PhoP-PhoQ (Fig. 2C) (65). The persistent infection of stromal cells by serovar Typhimurium indicates that other potential niches for intracellular persistence may exist at the level of the intestine, which could be explored in future studies.

The interaction of cytosolic bacteria with inflammasome components remains to be further clarified. Epithelial cells utilize caspase-11, responsible for inducing IL-18 expression, to respond to LPS located in the cytosol, but the exact source of this envelope component *in vivo* remains unknown. For serovar Typhimurium infection of epithelial cells, it was shown that intraphagosomal bacteria release LPS embedded in vesicles (66). Whether caspase-11 recognizes the LPS produced by intraphagosomal bacteria and/or LPS released by actively growing cytosolic bacteria has yet to be determined.

THE SCV AS A SUITABLE NICHE TO PROLONG HOST INFECTION IN A NONGROWING STATE

Most studies focused on host-to-host transmissibility of *Salmonella* have exploited *in vivo* chronic infection models, especially those involving serovar Typhimurium and 129X1/SvJ inbred mice (6, 67). In this model, a subset of the chronically infected mice often behave as "supershedders" ($>10^8$ CFU/g), and this phenomenon correlates with high numbers of bacteria in the lumen of the colon (68). This behavior probably reflects a failure in the capacity of the endogenous intestinal microbiota to control pathogen proliferation. The 129X1/SvJ inbred mouse model allowed detection of potential niches for long-term infections such as macrophages located in mesenteric lymph nodes (69) and anti-inflammatory M2-type macrophages (70). The model also been exploited to identify pathogen functions required for these chronic infections, including, among others, T1 and T2 effector proteins, fimbrial proteins, regulatory proteins involved in outer membrane homeostasis, and proteins encoded in pathogenicity islands (10). In addition to these studies, clinical and epidemiological data show the gallbladder as another niche in which typhoidal and nontyphoidal *Salmonella* serovars could persist in chronic and asymptomatic infections, therefore ensuring host-to-host transmissibility (71, 72). As mentioned above, the gallbladder epithelium is permissive for intracellular replication of serovar Typhimurium, but this phenomenon has been reported in acute infection models (59, 60). A comparative analysis in the gallbladder of chronically infected mice has not been performed to date. Besides the potential intracellular reservoir in the epithelial cells lining the gallbladder, biofilms formed on gallstones may contribute to pathogen transmissibility during asymptomatic and chronic infections (73, 74). The capacity of serovar Typhimurium to form biofilms in this niche has been demonstrated to require functions that ensure survival in the presence of high doses of bile salts as well as type 1 fimbriae, these latter involved in attachment to and persistence in gallstone surfaces (74).

Despite this valuable information on the modes and functions that distinct *Salmonella* serovars exploit to persist in the host, no study has formally linked a defined intracellular lifestyle with long-term infection of the host. Indeed, we are still far from understanding how this pathogen adapts to live within the SCV phagosome in a nongrowing state. Some studies, however, provide clues supporting a unique lifestyle linked to persistence. Viable serovar Typhimurium has been isolated from cultured fibroblasts—in which bacteria show limited intracellular proliferation—as long as 21 days after entering into these cells (75). Many of the isolates rescued after such persistent infection of the fibroblast harbored mutations in the *hemL*, *lpd*, and *aroD* genes. Two of these mutations, *hemL* and *lpd*, impact respiratory rates, leading to a less oxidative environment and, as a consequence, to a less toxic environment (75). The same applies to *aroD*, which decreases bacterial growth rate. These mutations confer a "small-colony variant" phenotype, which resembles the type of variants isolated from chronic infections caused by other important pathogens such *Staphylococcus aureus* (76). These small-colony variants in serovar Typhimurium, as in *S. aureus*, maintain a stable phenotype outside the eukaryotic cells and do not revert to fast-growing bacteria. The mechanisms by which a long residence inside the fibroblast selects for these types of mutations should be addressed in future studies. It is also important to note that these serovar Typhimurium variants become resistant to some specific classes of antibiotics, such as aminoglycosides (75), and that these isolates persist at higher rates than wild-type bacteria inside the fibroblast. This latter observation indicates that the adaptation to nongrowing intracellular state inside the SCV may be an advantage to persistence within the infected cell.

In line with these observations, recent studies have shown that serovar Typhimurium evolves *in vivo* during a long-term chronic infection of mice (9). Individually tagged bacteria were used to challenge 129X1/SvJ mice in the chronic infection model. Point mutations that increased fitness in animal organs were selected in some dominant clones along the chronic infection. One of these mutations mapped to *kdgR* (9), a transcriptional regulator that modulates uptake of distinct carbon sources. Intriguingly, the KdgR regulon favors persistence of serovar Typhimurium in vegetable soft rots in association with defined phytopathogens such as *Pectobacterium carotovorum* (77). This role in persistence was linked to increased uptake of carbon sources derived from pectin degradation and utilization of the Entner-Doudoroff pathway, both regulated by KdgR (77). Mammalian cells do not produce pectin, so it is tempting to speculate that the action of KdgR in intracellular serovar Typhimurium is related to the hydrolysis and product utilization of some yet unknown polysaccharide. Since KdgR variants with point mutations confer selective advantage in the mouse chronic infection model, it would be interesting to discern whether such a phenotype correlates with alterations in the intracellular lifestyle of the pathogen in distinct host cell types. Future studies will be valuable to obtain proof of concept relating physiological status of serovar Typhimurium in the SCV (or the cytosol) to preference for a defined outcome of the infection, in terms of chronic/asymptomatic or acute infection.

The nutritional status of serovar Typhimurium within the SCV has been recently addressed in macrophages and epithelial cells using a large collection of auxotrophic mutants in essential amino acids (78). This approach identified amino acids that are provided by the infected cell versus those that must be synthetized by the pathogen and, therefore, showed which metabolic pathways are preferentially used by actively growing bacteria. As an example, alanine is provided by the infected macrophage to the SCV, while that is the case of asparagine in the SCV of epithelial cells (78). These data imply distinct metabolic status of intracellular serovar Typhimurium depending on the host cell type. Interestingly, growth of defined auxotrophic mutants is restored in epithelial cells by supplementation of the corresponding amino acid only if intracellular bacteria induce Sif formation. This means that these endomembrane tubular extensions could facilitate nutrition acquisition by the pathogen. Such an assumption also correlates with the above-mentioned phenotype in fibroblasts, in which bacteria persist inside the SCV in the absence of stable Sifs (57).

Proteomic studies and phenotypic assays in metabolic mutants have also shown that fatty acids and glycerol are major energy sources used by serovar Typhimurium *in vivo* during acute infection of mice (79). Of interest, this study speculates about a marked flexibility in the pathways that the pathogen uses to metabolize host nutrients, ensuring in this manner an efficient metabolic flux even if some of the nutrients become scarce under specific conditions. Additional data obtained in cultured macrophages and epithelial cells pointed to glucose as a preferred energy source for intracellular replication (80, 81). Mutants defective for glycolysis from glucose are also impaired for successful colonization of mice (80). Thus, serovar Typhimurium does not use a single type of nutrient as an energy source. This metabolic flexibility represents a clear obstacle for the host to control the infection.

Chronic infection models following challenge of mice with serovar Typhimurium *purA ssaGH* mutants, unable to proliferate in organs, have shown metabolic differences for bacteria in acute versus persistent infections (82). Mutations in metabolic functions required for acute infection, like some mapped to the *ubiC* gene, have no effect on the persistence established by the *purA ssaGH* mutant. The *ubiC* mutation prevents ubiquinone synthesis and, as result, proliferation of wild-type bacteria. However, it has no effect on the *purA ssaGH* persistent mutant. As an exception, a mutation in *fabB*, which encodes β-ketoacyl-acyl carrier protein (ACP) synthase I, required for biosynthesis of unsaturated fatty acids and cyclopropane, decreases substantially the persistence of the *purA ssaGH* double mutant (82). Intriguingly, small-colony variants appeared at high rate in the *purA ssaGH fabB* mutants when isolated from chronically infected mice, a phenomenon resembling that discussed in fibroblasts.

THE BATTLE FOR INTRACELLULAR SURVIVAL: A BALANCE BETWEEN HOST DEFENSES AND THE COUNTERACTING STRATEGIES OF THE PATHOGEN

Host-to-host transmission of typhoidal and nontyphoidal *Salmonella* serovars is influenced by the rate of access to the intestinal lumen and proliferation of the pathogen. This ensures rapid exit outside the host via the intestinal tract. In addition, the maintenance of the pathogen in intracellular niches could potentially favor a periodic colonization of the intestine, allowing transmission of the pathogen to the external environment. The second mechanism implies a delicate balance between host defenses and strategies of the pathogen to remain alive in intracellular locations. Of note, recent data obtained in serovar Typhimurium support its capacity to intentionally establish a persistence state. Below, we discuss evidence sustaining this view.

The innate immune system controls intracellular infections by limiting nutrients to the intruder, producing antimicrobial peptides, releasing oxygen- and nitrogen-derived reactive species, or acidifying the compartment containing the pathogen (83). Another process equally important in this respect is autophagy (84, 85). However, autophagy is subverted by certain pathogens to acquire nutrient and membrane material for their own benefit (86, 87). Important intracellular bacterial pathogens such as *Coxiella burnetii,* *Francisella tularensis,* or *Brucella* spp. divert nutrients from the autophagosomal compartment or even fuse and proliferate inside this specialized organelle (87). For serovar Typhimurium, contrasting data have been reported. These studies have shown (i) autophagy actively killing cytosolic serovar Typhimurium or bacteria contained in damaged SCV membranes (88–90), (ii) exploitation of autophagy to promote proliferation (91), and (iii) eradication of part of the progeny facilitating the establishment of perdurable persistent infections (57).

Models involving transgenic mice deficient in these innate defense mechanisms illustrate their role in controlling intracellular growth of serovar Typhimurium. Some examples are mice deficient in (i) the Nramp1 transporter, which imposes nutritional stress on the pathogen by removing essential divalent cations from the phagosomal compartment (92, 93); (ii) the NAPDH oxidase, responsible for the oxidative burst in phagocytes by producing reactive oxygen species (94); (iii) the nitric oxide synthase, which generates reactive nitrogen species (95); (iv) key elements of the inflammasome such as NLRP3 (NOD-like receptor family pyrin domain containing 3) and NLRC4, or the pyroptosis-inducing caspase-1 (63, 96–99); (v) components of the autophagy machinery such as Atg5 (100–102); and (vi) proinflammatory cytokines (tumor necrosis factor α and gamma interferon). Increased susceptibility to serovar Typhimurium infection and augmented intracellular replication rates linked to the lack of these defenses have been demonstrated in macrophages or embryonic fibroblasts obtained from these knockout transgenic mice (63, 99, 100, 103, 104). Collectively, these data show the important balance existing between host defenses and survival strategies of the pathogen that may result in a defined intracellular lifestyle. Fortunately, the number of studies addressing these changes in susceptibility to *Salmonella* infection from the host side is continuously increasing. Genome-wide asso-

ciation studies represent a nonbiased method to identify pathways related to human diseases, and this information can be exploited to identify important host proteins that can control *Salmonella* growth. A recent study focused on an allele (T300A) in an autophagy protein, ATG16L1, previously identified as one of the 140 risk loci linked to Crohn's disease (105). Transcriptome analyses in cells obtained from wild-type and *ATG16L1-T330A* cells exposed to pathogen-derived compounds identified a set of genes differentially expressed. One of them, CLEC12A, was associated with autophagy proteins. *In vitro* and *in vivo* infection models revealed that CLEC12A modulates autophagy of serovar Typhimurium and that mice lacking this protein are more susceptible to the infection (105). Thus, from genome-wide association analyses it is possible to unravel new host functions that control the intracellular lifestyle of serovar Typhimurium (106) and, as a consequence, have impact on host-to-host transmission.

Studies based on RNA interference targeting the human kinome have also led to the identification of host factors involved in restricting serovar Typhimurium intracellular proliferation, including kinases interacting with Akt1/protein kinase B (107). Another kinase, TANK-binding kinase 1 (TBK1), recruits autophagy proteins to ubiquitinated cytosolic serovar Typhimurium (108, 109). TBK1 has been shown to maintain the integrity of the SCV membrane, preventing access to the cytosol (110). Therefore, TBK1 seems to play a dual role, as a defense mechanism favoring serovar Typhimurium intravacuolar persistence or, alternatively, stimulating autophagy of cytosolic bacteria that escape from the SCV.

DalS, a transporter used by intracellular serovar Typhimurium to capture D-alanine and required for virulence (111), also exemplifies the interplay existing between host defense mechanisms and pathogen strategies to survive and persist in the intracellular environment. D-Alanine is a substrate of the eukaryotic enzyme D-amino acid oxidase (DAO), which generates reactive oxygen molecules from this D-amino acid. The DalS-mediated import of D-alanine by intracellular serovar Typhimurium contributes to its survival within neutrophils during the early stage of the infection by decreasing availability of this substrate to DAO. This strategy has been proposed as a step crucial for the pathogen to withstand host defenses, allowing the infection of more-permissive host cells (112).

Novel transcriptomic sequencing technologies involving dual RNA-seq have generated much information about regulatory RNAs and genes that are up- and downregulated in both serovar Typhimurium and the host cell (113). These data, obtained in the growth-permissive intracellular environment of HeLa epithelial cells, provide a valuable insight into host and pathogen functions modulating bacterial load, activity of signaling pathways, and production of proinflammatory cytokines at various times postinfection (113). These robust technologies could also be applied to examine the pathogen-host interplay in conditions that impede massive pathogen intracellular growth (i.e., activated macrophages or fibroblasts). The possibility of analyzing gene expression at the single-cell level (114) should certainly provide new clues on how bacteria interact with a defined host cell type and how such cross talk evolves over time. A recent single-cell RNA-seq study proves this postulate, demonstrating that the physiological status of macrophages bearing either high or low amounts of serovar Typhimurium cells differs substantially (115). Macrophages harboring persistent nongrowing bacteria display an M1 proinflammatory status, whereas those with a large number of fast-growing bacteria show an M2 anti-inflammatory state (115).

HETEROGENEITY OF *SALMONELLA* INFECTIONS AND ITS PROBABLE IMPACT ON HOST-TO-HOST TRANSMISSIBILITY

In vivo studies reveal a plethora of encounters taking place between invading bacteria and distinct host cell types in distinct anatomical sites (116, 117). Early studies showed a preference of serovar Typhimurium to target macrophages in target organs such as liver and spleen (118, 119). Other host cell types such as neutrophils, dendritic cells, and nonphagocytic stromal cells are also infected. Mathematical modeling and real-time video microscopy indicate that host cells repeatedly encounter bacteria and that these contacts translate to infection in a relatively low number of the cases. About 5% of the macrophages contacted are ultimately infected (117). Moreover, the number of intracellular serovar Typhimurium bacteria per infected macrophage remains low (3 to 4 bacteria/cell). This latter observation involves a scenario based on relatively low rounds of pathogen replication followed by lysis of the infected cells and reinfection of neighboring cells. This strategy has been proposed to be responsible for the increase in infection foci and pathogen dissemination through the organ (120). These *in vivo* data occasionally remain underappreciated when using *in vitro* infection models, in which often high intracellular proliferation rates are detected, especially in established cell lines of tumor origin (58). Nonetheless, high intracellular replication rates have been observed for serovar Typhimurium *in vivo* in defined sites, as epithelial cells of the gallbladder (59, 60) and intestinal epithelia (63) (Fig. 1). Interestingly, only a relatively small fraction of infected epithelial cells supports exacerbated intracellular proliferation of bacteria (see Fig. 1 of reference 63). This evidence supports a tight control of serovar Typhimurium intracellular replication that might be effective when host defenses and pathogen counterattack intersect.

Powerful microscopy technologies, including real-time imaging of live cells in culture and in the whole animal together with fluorescent growth rate-based reporters, have shown that these encounter episodes of different nature occur concomitantly in a reduced surface area of the infected tissue.

Heterogeneous subsets of slow- and fast-growing serovar Typhimurium in intracellular locations are observed in these studies (121). Bacteria either displaying slow growth or that are nondividing were shown to survive better following an antimicrobial challenge (121). Disparate rates of pathogen death were also found in populations of infected macrophages, polymorphonuclear cells, or inflammatory monocytes that occupy the spleen red pulp in the first days postinfection (122). Of interest, reactive oxygen species produced by neutrophils and inflammatory macrophages reduce bacterial burden, although they are unable to eradicate the pathogen. This partial control of the primary infection facilitates transmission of bacteria to more permissive cells of the spleen red pulp such as resident macrophages (Fig. 1). In conclusion, the available data support the idea that, at least for the case of colonization of deeper tissues by serovar Typhimurium, there are subsets of bacteria that occupy various tissue microenvironments (123). This heterogeneity may reflect differences in the genetic makeup and the immune or polarization status of the invaded host cell, as is shown in the above-mentioned recent RNA-seq study of macrophages harboring either nongrowing or fast-growing bacteria (115). Stochastic phenomena affecting the expression of host defenses and/or survival strategies of the pathogen after host encounter may also contribute to these heterogeneous responses.

"SELF-DEFENSE" MECHANISMS ACTING IN INTRACELLULAR *SALMONELLA*

The formation of persister cells ("persisters") has been shown to increase following the ingestion of serovar Typhimurium by macrophages (19). The persistent state is illustrated by tolerance to antibiotics in cells that remain viable upon exposure to these compounds while staying nonreplicative. Persisters are present in populations of exponentially growing cells and differ from antibiotic-resistant bacteria. Thus, once persisters resume growth in the absence of the antibiotic pressure, they are equally affected if subjected to new rounds of treatment with these compounds (124). In these terms, persistence represents a transient physiological state in which bacteria are positively selected when confronting the stress if they have a reduced growth rate. Such a situation is exemplified when bacterial cultures are exposed to antibiotics that act on fast-replicating bacteria such as β-lactams, quinonoles, or aminoglycosides. As mentioned above, the persistent phenotype can also be favored in pathogens inside eukaryotic cells following exposure to the intracellular environment of macrophages (19). This situation should, however, be distinguished from the selection of small-colony variants of serovar Typhimurium resistant to aminoglycosides, which are selected with stable mutations after a long residence (>72 h) in the intracellular niche of fibroblasts (75). At first glance, both persistence strategies increase residence in the host and constitute positive factors that promote pathogen transmissibility.

Do bacteria restrain growth intentionally to reach a persistent state? Many of the mechanisms known were first characterized in *Escherichia coli*, in which elevated levels of the alarmone ppGpp accumulating in response to nutritional stress play an important role (125, 126). The fact that bacteria use specific mechanisms to reach this state favors the idea of persistence as a programmed, epigenetic phenomenon with a genetic basis (127, 128).

Much work has been accumulated in recent years regarding the involvement of toxin-antitoxin (TA) modules in bacterial persistence and virulence (126, 129–131). Most TA loci encode two antagonistic proteins, the toxin involved in inhibiting growth and the antitoxin that regulates toxin activity. The first mutation associated with increased persistence rates in *E. coli* was mapped to the *hipAB* TA locus, which coded for the HipA serine kinase that is partially phosphorylated *in vivo*. HipA kinase activity is required for persister formation in defined conditions (132). Recent studies show that HipA phosphorylates tRNA synthetase GltX (133), leading to inhibition of protein synthesis. This situation favors accumulation of the ppGpp alarmone following increased levels of uncharged tRNAs, a condition that stimulates the ppGpp-producing enzymes RelA and SpoT (126). Other toxins encoded in TA loci act as RNases that recognize and cleave 23S rRNA, tRNAs, and either free or ribosome-bound mRNA; kinases that target elongation factor EF-Tu; or as inhibitors of DNA replication by targeting of DNA gyrase (126).

The fact that TA modules arrest bacterial growth makes them attractive candidates to contribute to pathogen persistence during infection (Table 1) (129, 130). Under these conditions, pathogen-host coexistence increases, and as a result, so does transmissibility. An increased rate of persisters in serovar Typhimurium-infected macrophages was associated with the activity in the pathogen of as many as 14 TA loci (19). A recent study in fibroblasts demonstrated the production by nongrowing intracellular serovar Typhimurium of a series of toxins encoded by TA loci (134). This work also showed distinct responses of certain TA loci in permissive (epithelial) and nonpermissive (fibroblasts) nonphagocytic cells regarding pathogen proliferation (134). These observations suggest that the nongrowing persistence state reached by serovar Typhimurium inside fibroblasts may require the intervention of a subset of TA loci (Fig. 2D). The usage by the pathogen of multiple TA loci may reflect a "safeguard" strategy to ensure rapid arrest of growth before defenses of the infected host cell irreversibly inactivate essential pathogen functions. A recent study revealed that serovar Typhimurium can arrest growth by using an enzyme encoded in a TA system, named TacT, which acetylates amino groups of amino acids charged on tRNA molecules, having a strong effect on translation (135). This study also identified a deactylase, CobB, which removes the acetyl group to resume growth. Whether TacT and/or CobB are active in intracellular bacteria has not yet been determined.

The role played by TA loci in persistence of serovar Typhimurium and other pathogens (129) supports the widely accepted model of a programmed phenomenon. It is worth noting that early studies in serovar Typhimurium also provided evidence for a genetic program involved in attenuating intracellular growth inside fibroblasts (65). This program is orchestrated by defined regulators, including the two-component regulatory system PhoP-PhoQ (Fig. 2C), involved in maintenance of envelope homeostasis, and the alternative sigma factor RpoS, among others (65). Mutants lacking these regulatory proteins "overgrow" inside the infected fibroblasts when compared to the parental wild-type bacteria, a response that also occurs *in vivo* in stromal nonphagocytic cells and in primary intestinal fibroblasts (41, 64). Whether the growth-attenuating response directed by these regulators correlates to the intervention of some specific TA loci is at present unknown.

CONCLUSIONS AND FUTURE PERSPECTIVES

Epidemiological data point to typhoidal and nontyphoidal *Salmonella* serovars as pathogens that are highly transmitted from host to host. Modern *in vivo* technologies are providing new insights into the behavior of these bacteria in distinct host cell types, at various infection times, and in diverse tissues/organs. The bulk of new data obtained point to an unsuspected complexity and heterogeneity in the type of encounters that occur when the pathogen attacks the intestinal epithelium or when, in the case of acute infections, it disseminates to deep organs. This complexity is now registered at the single-cell level in several *in vitro* and *in vivo* infection models and needs to be integrated with the intrinsic variability in genome content among different *Salmonella* species, subspecies, and serovars, and even among isolates belonging to the same serovar. Most of the studies to date have focused on serovar Typhimurium, with relatively few comparable analyses in other serovars (Table 1).

Fortunately, recent studies pinpoint for the first time mutations in defined genes that alter pathogen behavior regarding persistence in the host and the ability to colonize the intestine or extraintestinal sites (136). Genome-wide expression data also exist for the colonization by intracellular serovar Typhimurium of distinct host cell types such as macrophages, epithelial cells, and fibroblasts (64, 137, 138), and these data should be exploited at the functional level. Comparative genomics is also a powerful resource, and there is now evidence of mutations causing the emergence in immunocompromised hosts of highly adapted clones in serovars normally infecting a broad range of hosts (139). Some studies also reported mutations in defined "invasive" serovar Typhimurium clones that associate with immune-deficient and immune-competent hosts and infect with high mortality rate, especially in the sub-Saharan Africa (140).

We are therefore facing a scenario in which new molecular and cellular data are rapidly generated with modern techniques in apparently simplified models (e.g., cultured cell lines), which nonetheless exhibit marked heterogeneity. A major future goal will be to understand the basis of this heterogeneity so as to further extrapolate such knowledge to the genomic and epidemiological data. This is certainly challenging, as revealed by the still limited number of studies that attempt to join the cellular/molecular and epidemiological landscapes. Filling this gap is essential to increase our knowledge on evolution of typhoidal and nontyphoidal *Salmonella* serovars as intracellular bacterial pathogens, their adaptation to multiple lifestyles inside the eukaryotic cell, and how these lifestyles impact host-to-host transmissibility.

ACKNOWLEDGMENTS

We apologize for those studies that could not be cited due to space limitations. Work in our laboratories is supported by grants BIO2014-55238-R (to M.G.P.) and BIO2013-46281-P, PCIN-2016-082, and BIO2016-77639-P (MINECO/FEDER) (to F.G.-dP.) from the Spanish Ministry of Economy and Competitiveness and European Regional Development Fund.

CITATION

Pucciarelli MG, García-Del Portillo F. 2017. *Salmonella* intracellular lifestyles and their impact on host-to-host transmission. Microbiol Spectrum 5(4):MTBP-0009-2016.

REFERENCES

1. **Rivera-Chávez F, Bäumler AJ.** 2015. The pyromaniac inside you: *Salmonella* metabolism in the host gut. *Annu Rev Microbiol* **69:**31–48.
2. **LaRock DL, Chaudhary A, Miller SI.** 2015. Salmonellae interactions with host processes. *Nat Rev Microbiol* **13:**191–205.
3. **de Jong HK, Parry CM, van der Poll T, Wiersinga WJ.** 2012. Host-pathogen interaction in invasive salmonellosis. *PLoS Pathog* **8:** e1002933.
4. **Graham SM.** 2010. Nontyphoidal salmonellosis in Africa. *Curr Opin Infect Dis* **23:**409–414.
5. **Wiesner M, Calva JJ, Bustamante VH, Pérez-Morales D, Fernández-Mora M, Calva E, Silva C.** 2016. A multi-drug resistant *Salmonella* Typhimurium ST213 human-invasive strain (33676) containing the *bla*$_{CMY-2}$ gene on an IncF plasmid is attenuated for virulence in BALB/c mice. *BMC Microbiol* **16:**18.
6. **Monack DM.** 2012. *Salmonella* persistence and transmission strategies. *Curr Opin Microbiol* **15:**100–107.
7. **Gopinath S, Carden S, Monack D.** 2012. Shedding light on *Salmonella* carriers. *Trends Microbiol* **20:**320–327.
8. **Ledingham JCG, Arkwright JA.** 1912. *The Carrier Problem in Infectious Diseases.* Edward Arnold, London, United Kingdom.
9. **Søndberg E, Jelsbak L.** 2016. *Salmonella* Typhimurium undergoes distinct genetic adaption during chronic infections of mice. *BMC Microbiol* **16:**30.

10. **Lawley TD, Chan K, Thompson LJ, Kim CC, Govoni GR, Monack DM.** 2006. Genome-wide screen for *Salmonella* genes required for long-term systemic infection of the mouse. *PLoS Pathog* 2:e11.

11. **Takeuchi A.** 1967. Electron microscope studies of experimental Salmonella infection. I. Penetration into the intestinal epithelium by *Salmonella typhimurium*. *Am J Pathol* 50:109–136.

12. **Kihlström E, Edebo L.** 1976. Association of viable and inactivated *Salmonella typhimurium* 395 MS and MR 10 with HeLa cells. *Infect Immun* 14:851–857.

13. **Giannella RA, Washington O, Gemski P, Formal SB.** 1973. Invasion of HeLa cells by *Salmonella typhimurium*: a model for study of invasiveness of Salmonella. *J Infect Dis* 128:69–75.

14. **Garcia-del Portillo F, Finlay BB.** 1995. Targeting of *Salmonella typhimurium* to vesicles containing lysosomal membrane glycoproteins bypasses compartments with mannose 6-phosphate receptors. *J Cell Biol* 129:81–97.

15. **Brumell JH, Perrin AJ, Goosney DL, Finlay BB.** 2002. Microbial pathogenesis: new niches for *Salmonella*. *Curr Biol* 12:R15–R17.

16. **Scanu T, Spaapen RM, Bakker JM, Pratap CB, Wu LE, Hofland I, Broeks A, Shukla VK, Kumar M, Janssen H, Song JY, Neefjes-Borst EA, te Riele H, Holden DW, Nath G, Neefjes J.** 2015. *Salmonella* manipulation of host signaling pathways provokes cellular transformation associated with gallbladder carcinoma. *Cell Host Microbe* 17:763–774.

17. **Forbester JL, Goulding D, Vallier L, Hannan N, Hale C, Pickard D, Mukhopadhyay S, Dougan G.** 2015. Interaction of *Salmonella enterica* serovar Typhimurium with intestinal organoids derived from human induced pluripotent stem cells. *Infect Immun* 83:2926–2934.

18. **Zhang YG, Wu S, Xia Y, Sun J.** 2014. *Salmonella*-infected crypt-derived intestinal organoid culture system for host-bacterial interactions. *Physiol Rep* 2:e12147.

19. **Helaine S, Cheverton AM, Watson KG, Faure LM, Matthews SA, Holden DW.** 2014. Internalization of *Salmonella* by macrophages induces formation of nonreplicating persisters. *Science* 343:204–208.

20. **Knodler LA.** 2015. *Salmonella enterica*: living a double life in epithelial cells. *Curr Opin Microbiol* 23:23–31.

21. **Malik-Kale P, Winfree S, Steele-Mortimer O.** 2012. The bimodal lifestyle of intracellular *Salmonella* in epithelial cells: replication in the cytosol obscures defects in vacuolar replication. *PLoS One* 7:e38732.

22. **Figueira R, Holden DW.** 2012. Functions of the *Salmonella* pathogenicity island 2 (SPI-2) type III secretion system effectors. *Microbiology* 158:1147–1161.

23. **Moest TP, Méresse S.** 2013. *Salmonella* T3SSs: successful mission of the secret(ion) agents. *Curr Opin Microbiol* 16:38–44.

24. **Galán JE, Wolf-Watz H.** 2006. Protein delivery into eukaryotic cells by type III secretion machines. *Nature* 444:567–573.

25. **Patel JC, Galán JE.** 2005. Manipulation of the host actin cytoskeleton by *Salmonella*—all in the name of entry. *Curr Opin Microbiol* 8:10–15.

26. **Schlumberger MC, Hardt WD.** 2005. Triggered phagocytosis by *Salmonella*: bacterial molecular mimicry of RhoGTPase activation/deactivation. *Curr Top Microbiol Immunol* 291:29–42.

27. **Agbor TA, McCormick BA.** 2011. *Salmonella* effectors: important players modulating host cell function during infection. *Cell Microbiol* 13:1858–1869.

28. **Aiastui A, Pucciarelli MG, García-del Portillo F.** 2010. *Salmonella enterica* serovar Typhimurium invades fibroblasts by multiple routes differing from the entry into epithelial cells. *Infect Immun* 78:2700–2713.

29. **Velge P, Wiedemann A, Rosselin M, Abed N, Boumart Z, Chaussé AM, Grépinet O, Namdari F, Roche SM, Rossignol A, Virlogeux-Payant I.** 2012. Multiplicity of *Salmonella* entry mechanisms, a new paradigm for *Salmonella* pathogenesis. *MicrobiologyOpen* 1:243–258.

30. **Mijouin L, Rosselin M, Bottreau E, Pizarro-Cerda J, Cossart P, Velge P, Wiedemann A.** 2012. *Salmonella enteritidis* Rck-mediated invasion requires activation of Rac1, which is dependent on the class I PI 3-kinases-Akt signaling pathway. *FASEB J* 26:1569–1581.

31. **Rosselin M, Abed N, Virlogeux-Payant I, Bottreau E, Sizaret PY, Velge P, Wiedemann A.** 2011. Heterogeneity of type III secretion system (T3SS)-1-independent entry mechanisms used by *Salmonella* Enteritidis to invade different cell types. *Microbiology* 157:839–847.

32. **Desin TS, Lam PK, Koch B, Mickael C, Berberov E, Wisner AL, Townsend HG, Potter AA, Köster W.** 2009. *Salmonella enterica* serovar Enteritidis pathogenicity island 1 is not essential for but facilitates rapid systemic spread in chickens. *Infect Immun* 77:2866–2875.

33. **Rychlik I, Karasova D, Sebkova A, Volf J, Sisak F, Havlickova H, Kummer V, Imre A, Szmolka A, Nagy B.** 2009. Virulence potential of five major pathogenicity islands (SPI-1 to SPI-5) of *Salmonella enterica* serovar Enteritidis for chickens. *BMC Microbiol* 9:268.

34. **Jones MA, Wigley P, Page KL, Hulme SD, Barrow PA.** 2001. *Salmonella enterica* serovar Gallinarum requires the *Salmonella* pathogenicity island 2 type III secretion system but not the *Salmonella* pathogenicity island 1 type III secretion system for virulence in chickens. *Infect Immun* **69:**5471–5476.

35. **Rathman M, Barker LP, Falkow S.** 1997. The unique trafficking pattern of *Salmonella typhimurium*-containing phagosomes in murine macrophages is independent of the mechanism of bacterial entry. *Infect Immun* **65:**1475–1485.

36. **Drecktrah D, Knodler LA, Ireland R, Steele-Mortimer O.** 2006. The mechanism of *Salmonella* entry determines the vacuolar environment and intracellular gene expression. *Traffic* **7:**39–51.

37. **Valdez Y, Ferreira RB, Finlay BB.** 2009. Molecular mechanisms of *Salmonella* virulence and host resistance. *Curr Top Microbiol Immunol* **337:**93–127.

38. **Fields PI, Swanson RV, Haidaris CG, Heffron F.** 1986. Mutants of *Salmonella typhimurium* that cannot survive within the macrophage are avirulent. *Proc Natl Acad Sci U S A* **83:**5189–5193.

39. **Malik-Kale P, Jolly CE, Lathrop S, Winfree S, Luterbach C, Steele-Mortimer O.** 2011. *Salmonella*—at home in the host cell. *Front Microbiol* **2:**125.

40. **Bakowski MA, Braun V, Brumell JH.** 2008. *Salmonella*-containing vacuoles: directing traffic and nesting to grow. *Traffic* **9:**2022–2031.

41. **García-del Portillo F, Núñez-Hernández C, Eisman B, Ramos-Vivas J.** 2008. Growth control in the *Salmonella*-containing vacuole. *Curr Opin Microbiol* **11:**46–52.

42. **Holden DW.** 2002. Trafficking of the *Salmonella* vacuole in macrophages. *Traffic* **3:**161–169.

43. **Steele-Mortimer O.** 2008. The *Salmonella*-containing vacuole: moving with the times. *Curr Opin Microbiol* **11:**38–45.

44. **Ramsden AE, Holden DW, Mota LJ.** 2007. Membrane dynamics and spatial distribution of *Salmonella*-containing vacuoles. *Trends Microbiol* **15:**516–524.

45. **Zhao Y, Gorvel JP, Méresse S.** 2016. Effector proteins support the asymmetric apportioning of *Salmonella* during cytokinesis. *Virulence* **7:**669–678.

46. **van der Heijden J, Finlay BB.** 2012. Type III effector-mediated processes in *Salmonella* infection. *Future Microbiol* **7:**685–703.

47. **Liss V, Hensel M.** 2015. Take the tube: remodelling of the endosomal system by intracellular *Salmonella enterica*. *Cell Microbiol* **17:**639–647.

48. **Jackson LK, Nawabi P, Hentea C, Roark EA, Haldar K.** 2008. The *Salmonella* virulence protein SifA is a G protein antagonist. *Proc Natl Acad Sci U S A* **105:**14141–14146.

49. **D'Costa VM, Braun V, Landekic M, Shi R, Proteau A, McDonald L, Cygler M, Grinstein S, Brumell JH.** 2015. *Salmonella* disrupts host endocytic trafficking by SopD2-mediated inhibition of Rab7. *Cell Rep* **12:**1508–1518.

50. **Spanò S, Galán JE.** 2012. A Rab32-dependent pathway contributes to *Salmonella typhi* host restriction. *Science* **338:**960–963.

51. **Spanò S, Liu X, Galán JE.** 2011. Proteolytic targeting of Rab29 by an effector protein distinguishes the intracellular compartments of human-adapted and broad-host *Salmonella*. *Proc Natl Acad Sci U S A* **108:**18418–18423.

52. **Garcia-del Portillo F, Zwick MB, Leung KY, Finlay BB.** 1993. *Salmonella* induces the formation of filamentous structures containing lysosomal membrane glycoproteins in epithelial cells. *Proc Natl Acad Sci U S A* **90:**10544–10548.

53. **Schroeder N, Mota LJ, Méresse S.** 2011. *Salmonella*-induced tubular networks. *Trends Microbiol* **19:**268–277.

54. **Stein MA, Leung KY, Zwick M, Garcia-del Portillo F, Finlay BB.** 1996. Identification of a *Salmonella* virulence gene required for formation of filamentous structures containing lysosomal membrane glycoproteins within epithelial cells. *Mol Microbiol* **20:**151–164.

55. **Freeman JA, Ohl ME, Miller SI.** 2003. The *Salmonella enterica* serovar Typhimurium translocated effectors SseJ and SifB are targeted to the *Salmonella*-containing vacuole. *Infect Immun* **71:**418–427.

56. **McEwan DG, Richter B, Claudi B, Wigge C, Wild P, Farhan H, McGourty K, Coxon FP, Franz-Wachtel M, Perdu B, Akutsu M, Habermann A, Kirchof A, Helfrich MH, Odgren PR, Van Hul W, Frangakis AS, Rajalingam K, Macek B, Holden DW, Bumann D, Dikic I.** 2015. PLEKHM1 regulates *Salmonella*-containing vacuole biogenesis and infection. *Cell Host Microbe* **17:**58–71.

57. **López-Montero N, Ramos-Marquès E, Risco C, García-Del Portillo F.** 2016. Intracellular *Salmonella* induces aggrephagy of host endomembranes in persistent infections. *Autophagy* **12:**1886–1901.

58. **Knodler LA, Nair V, Steele-Mortimer O.** 2014. Quantitative assessment of cytosolic *Salmonella* in epithelial cells. *PLoS One* **9:**e84681.

59. **Knodler LA, Vallance BA, Celli J, Winfree S, Hansen B, Montero M, Steele-Mortimer O.** 2010. Dissemination of invasive *Salmonella* via bacterial-induced extrusion of mucosal epithelia. *Proc Natl Acad Sci U S A* **107:**17733–17738.

60. **Menendez A, Arena ET, Guttman JA, Thorson L, Vallance BA, Vogl W, Finlay BB.** 2009. *Salmonella* infection of gallbladder epithelial cells drives local inflammation and injury in a model of acute typhoid fever. *J Infect Dis* **200:**1703–1713.

61. **Crowley SM, Knodler LA, Vallance BA.** 2016. *Salmonella* and the inflammasome: battle for intracellular dominance. *Curr Top Microbiol Immunol* **397:**43–67.

62. **Sellin ME, Maslowski KM, Maloy KJ, Hardt WD.** 2015. Inflammasomes of the intestinal epithelium. *Trends Immunol* **36:**442–450.

63. **Sellin ME, Müller AA, Felmy B, Dolowschiak T, Diard M, Tardivel A, Maslowski KM, Hardt WD.** 2014. Epithelium-intrinsic NAIP/NLRC4 inflammasome drives infected enterocyte expulsion to restrict *Salmonella* replication in the intestinal mucosa. *Cell Host Microbe* **16:** 237–248.

64. **Núñez-Hernández C, Tierrez A, Ortega AD, Pucciarelli MG, Godoy M, Eisman B, Casadesús J, García-del Portillo F.** 2013. Genome expression analysis of nonproliferating intracellular *Salmonella enterica* serovar Typhimurium unravels an acid pH-dependent PhoP-PhoQ response essential for dormancy. *Infect Immun* **81:** 154–165.

65. **Cano DA, Martínez-Moya M, Pucciarelli MG, Groisman EA, Casadesús J, García-Del Portillo F.** 2001. *Salmonella enterica* serovar Typhimurium response involved in attenuation of pathogen intracellular proliferation. *Infect Immun* **69:**6463–6474.

66. **Garcia-del Portillo F, Stein MA, Finlay BB.** 1997. Release of lipopolysaccharide from intracellular compartments containing *Salmonella typhimurium* to vesicles of the host epithelial cell. *Infect Immun* **65:**24–34.

67. **Ruby T, McLaughlin L, Gopinath S, Monack D.** 2012. *Salmonella*'s long-term relationship with its host. *FEMS Microbiol Rev* **36:**600–615.

68. **Lawley TD, Bouley DM, Hoy YE, Gerke C, Relman DA, Monack DM.** 2008. Host transmission of *Salmonella enterica* serovar Typhimurium is controlled by virulence factors and indigenous intestinal microbiota. *Infect Immun* **76:**403–416.

69. **Monack DM, Bouley DM, Falkow S.** 2004. *Salmonella typhimurium* persists within macrophages in the mesenteric lymph nodes of chronically infected *Nramp1*$^{+/+}$ mice and can be reactivated by IFNγ neutralization. *J Exp Med* **199:**231–241.

70. **Eisele NA, Ruby T, Jacobson A, Manzanillo PS, Cox JS, Lam L, Mukundan L, Chawla A, Monack DM.** 2013. *Salmonella* require the fatty acid regulator PPARδ for the establishment of a metabolic environment essential for long-term persistence. *Cell Host Microbe* **14:**171–182.

71. **Gonzalez-Escobedo G, Gunn JS.** 2013. Gallbladder epithelium as a niche for chronic *Salmonella* carriage. *Infect Immun* **81:**2920–2930.

72. **Gunn JS, Marshall JM, Baker S, Dongol S, Charles RC, Ryan ET.** 2014. *Salmonella* chronic carriage: epidemiology, diagnosis, and gallbladder persistence. *Trends Microbiol* **22:**648–655.

73. **Bäumler AJ, Winter SE, Thiennimitr P, Casadesús J.** 2011. Intestinal and chronic infections: *Salmonella* lifestyles in hostile environments. *Environ Microbiol Rep* **3:**508–517.

74. **Gonzalez-Escobedo G, Gunn JS.** 2013. Identification of *Salmonella enterica* serovar Typhimurium genes regulated during biofilm formation on cholesterol gallstone surfaces. *Infect Immun* **81:**3770–3780.

75. **Cano DA, Pucciarelli MG, Martínez-Moya M, Casadesús J, García-del Portillo F.** 2003. Selection of small-colony variants of *Salmonella enterica* serovar Typhimurium in nonphagocytic eucaryotic cells. *Infect Immun* **71:**3690–3698.

76. **Proctor RA, Kriegeskorte A, Kahl BC, Becker K, Löffler B, Peters G.** 2014. *Staphylococcus aureus* small colony variants (SCVs): a road map for the metabolic pathways involved in persistent infections. *Front Cell Infect Microbiol* **4:**99.

77. **George AS, Salas González I, Lorca GL, Teplitski M.** 2015. Contribution of the *Salmonella enterica* KdgR regulon to persistence of the pathogen in vegetable soft rots. *Appl Environ Microbiol* **82:**1353–1360.

78. **Popp J, Noster J, Busch K, Kehl A, Zur Hellen G, Hensel M.** 2015. Role of host cell-derived amino acids in nutrition of intracellular *Salmonella enterica*. *Infect Immun* **83:**4466–4475.

79. **Steeb B, Claudi B, Burton NA, Tienz P, Schmidt A, Farhan H, Mazé A, Bumann D.** 2013. Parallel exploitation of diverse host nutrients enhances *Salmonella* virulence. *PLoS Pathog* **9:**e1003301.

80. **Bowden SD, Rowley G, Hinton JC, Thompson A.** 2009. Glucose and glycolysis are required for the successful infection of macrophages and mice by *Salmonella enterica* serovar Typhimurium. *Infect Immun* **77:**3117–3126.

81. **Bowden SD, Hopper-Chidlaw AC, Rice CJ, Ramachandran VK, Kelly DJ, Thompson A.** 2014. Nutritional and metabolic requirements for the infection of HeLa cells by *Salmonella enterica* serovar Typhimurium. *PLoS One* **9:**e96266.

82. **Barat S, Steeb B, Mazé A, Bumann D.** 2012. Extensive in vivo resilience of persistent *Salmonella*. *PLoS One* **7:**e42007.

83. **Fang FC, Frawley ER, Tapscott T, Vázquez-Torres A.** 2016. Bacterial stress responses during host infection. *Cell Host Microbe* **20:**133–143.

84. **Wileman T.** 2013. Autophagy as a defence against intracellular pathogens. *Essays Biochem* **55:**153–163.

85. **Jo EK, Yuk JM, Shin DM, Sasakawa C.** 2013. Roles of autophagy in elimination of intracellular bacterial pathogens. *Front Immunol* **4:**97.

86. **Steele S, Brunton J, Kawula T.** 2015. The role of autophagy in intracellular pathogen nutrient acquisition. *Front Cell Infect Microbiol* **5:**51.

87. **Winchell CG, Steele S, Kawula T, Voth DE.** 2016. Dining in: intracellular bacterial pathogen interplay with autophagy. *Curr Opin Microbiol* **29:**9–14.

88. **Birmingham CL, Brumell JH.** 2006. Autophagy recognizes intracellular *Salmonella enterica* serovar Typhimurium in damaged vacuoles. *Autophagy* **2:**156–158.

89. **Huett A, Heath RJ, Begun J, Sassi SO, Baxt LA, Vyas JM, Goldberg MB, Xavier RJ.** 2012. The LRR and RING domain protein LRSAM1 is an E3 ligase crucial for ubiquitin-dependent autophagy of intracellular *Salmonella* Typhimurium. *Cell Host Microbe* **12:**778–790.

90. **Spinnenhirn V, Farhan H, Basler M, Aichem A, Canaan A, Groettrup M.** 2014. The ubiquitin-like modifier FAT10 decorates autophagy-targeted *Salmonella* and contributes to *Salmonella* resistance in mice. *J Cell Sci* **127:**4883–4893.

91. **Yu HB, Croxen MA, Marchiando AM, Ferreira RB, Cadwell K, Foster LJ, Finlay BB.** 2014. Autophagy facilitates *Salmonella* replication in HeLa cells. *mBio* **5:**e00865-e14.

92. **Wessling-Resnick M.** 2015. Nramp1 and other transporters involved in metal withholding during infection. *J Biol Chem* **290:**18984–18990.

93. **Vassiloyanakopoulos AP, Okamoto S, Fierer J.** 1998. The crucial role of polymorphonuclear leukocytes in resistance to *Salmonella dublin* infections in genetically susceptible and resistant mice. *Proc Natl Acad Sci U S A* **95:**7676–7681.

94. **Segal BH, Grimm MJ, Khan AN, Han W, Blackwell TS.** 2012. Regulation of innate immunity by NADPH oxidase. *Free Radic Biol Med* **53:**72–80.

95. **Bogdan C.** 2015. Nitric oxide synthase in innate and adaptive immunity: an update. *Trends Immunol* **36:**161–178.

96. **Puri AW, Broz P, Shen A, Monack DM, Bogyo M.** 2012. Caspase-1 activity is required to bypass macrophage apoptosis upon *Salmonella* infection. *Nat Chem Biol* **8:**745–747.

97. **Lara-Tejero M, Sutterwala FS, Ogura Y, Grant EP, Bertin J, Coyle AJ, Flavell RA, Galán JE.** 2006. Role of the caspase-1 inflammasome in *Salmonella typhimurium* pathogenesis. *J Exp Med* **203:**1407–1412.

98. **Miao EA, Rajan JV.** 2011. *Salmonella* and caspase-1: a complex interplay of detection and evasion. *Front Microbiol* **2:**85.

99. **Broz P, Newton K, Lamkanfi M, Mariathasan S, Dixit VM, Monack DM.** 2010. Redundant roles for inflammasome receptors NLRP3 and NLRC4 in host defense against *Salmonella*. *J Exp Med* **207:**1745–1755.

100. **Birmingham CL, Smith AC, Bakowski MA, Yoshimori T, Brumell JH.** 2006. Autophagy controls *Salmonella* infection in response to damage to the *Salmonella*-containing vacuole. *J Biol Chem* **281:**11374–11383.

101. **Kreibich S, Emmenlauer M, Fredlund J, Rämö P, Münz C, Dehio C, Enninga J, Hardt WD.** 2015. Autophagy proteins promote repair of endosomal membranes damaged by the *Salmonella* type three secretion system 1. *Cell Host Microbe* **18:**527–537.

102. **Benjamin JL, Sumpter R Jr, Levine B, Hooper LV.** 2013. Intestinal epithelial autophagy is essential for host defense against invasive bacteria. *Cell Host Microbe* **13:**723–734.

103. **Shiloh MU, MacMicking JD, Nicholson S, Brause JE, Potter S, Marino M, Fang F, Dinauer M, Nathan C.** 1999. Phenotype of mice and macrophages deficient in both phagocyte oxidase and inducible nitric oxide synthase. *Immunity* **10:**29–38.

104. **Boyle KB, Randow F.** 2013. The role of 'eat-me' signals and autophagy cargo receptors in innate immunity. *Curr Opin Microbiol* **16:**339–348.

105. **Begun J, Lassen KG, Jijon HB, Baxt LA, Goel G, Heath RJ, Ng A, Tam JM, Kuo SY, Villablanca EJ, Fagbami L, Oosting M, Kumar V, Schenone M, Carr SA, Joosten LA, Vyas JM, Daly MJ, Netea MG, Brown GD, Wijmenga C, Xavier RJ.** 2015. Integrated genomics of Crohn's disease risk variant identifies a role for CLEC12A in antibacterial autophagy. *Cell Rep* **11:**1905–1918.

106. **Miller SI, Chaudhary A.** 2016. A cellular GWAS approach to define human variation in cellular pathways important to inflammation. *Pathogens* **5:**E39.

107. **Kuijl C, Savage ND, Marsman M, Tuin AW, Janssen L, Egan DA, Ketema M, van den Nieuwendijk R, van den Eeden SJ, Geluk A, Poot A, van der Marel G, Beijersbergen RL, Overkleeft H, Ottenhoff TH, Neefjes J.** 2007. Intracellular bacterial growth is controlled by a kinase network around PKB/AKT1. *Nature* **450:**725–730.

108. **Wild P, Farhan H, McEwan DG, Wagner S, Rogov VV, Brady NR, Richter B, Korac J, Waidmann O, Choudhary C, Dötsch V, Bumann D, Dikic I.** 2011. Phosphorylation of the

autophagy receptor optineurin restricts *Salmonella* growth. *Science* **333**:228–233.

109. **Thurston TL, Boyle KB, Allen M, Ravenhill BJ, Karpiyevich M, Bloor S, Kaul A, Noad J, Foeglein A, Matthews SA, Komander D, Bycroft M, Randow F.** 2016. Recruitment of TBK1 to cytosol-invading *Salmonella* induces WIPI2-dependent antibacterial autophagy. *EMBO J* **35**:1779–1792.

110. **Radtke AL, Delbridge LM, Balachandran S, Barber GN, O'Riordan MX.** 2007. TBK1 protects vacuolar integrity during intracellular bacterial infection. *PLoS Pathog* **3**:e29.

111. **Osborne SE, Tuinema BR, Mok MC, Lau PS, Bui NK, Tomljenovic-Berube AM, Vollmer W, Zhang K, Junop M, Coombes BK.** 2012. Characterization of DalS, an ATP-binding cassette transporter for D-alanine, and its role in pathogenesis in *Salmonella enterica*. *J Biol Chem* **287**:15242–15250.

112. **Tuinema BR, Reid-Yu SA, Coombes BK.** 2014. *Salmonella* evades D-amino acid oxidase to promote infection in neutrophils. *mBio* **5**:e01886.

113. **Westermann AJ, Förstner KU, Amman F, Barquist L, Chao Y, Schulte LN, Müller L, Reinhardt R, Stadler PF, Vogel J.** 2016. Dual RNA-seq unveils noncoding RNA functions in host-pathogen interactions. *Nature* **529**:496–501.

114. **Saliba AE, Westermann AJ, Gorski SA, Vogel J.** 2014. Single-cell RNA-seq: advances and future challenges. *Nucleic Acids Res* **42**:8845–8860.

115. **Saliba AE, Li L, Westermann AJ, Appenzeller S, Stapels DA, Schulte LN, Helaine S, Vogel J.** 2016. Single-cell RNA-seq ties macrophage polarization to growth rate of intracellular *Salmonella*. *Nat Microbiol* **2**:16206.

116. **Watson KG, Holden DW.** 2010. Dynamics of growth and dissemination of *Salmonella* in vivo. *Cell Microbiol* **12**:1389–1397.

117. **Gog JR, Murcia A, Osterman N, Restif O, McKinley TJ, Sheppard M, Achouri S, Wei B, Mastroeni P, Wood JL, Maskell DJ, Cicuta P, Bryant CE.** 2012. Dynamics of *Salmonella* infection of macrophages at the single cell level. *J R Soc Interface* **9**:2696–2707.

118. **Richter-Dahlfors A, Buchan AM, Finlay BB.** 1997. Murine salmonellosis studied by confocal microscopy: *Salmonella typhimurium* resides intracellularly inside macrophages and exerts a cytotoxic effect on phagocytes in vivo. *J Exp Med* **186**:569–580.

119. **Salcedo SP, Noursadeghi M, Cohen J, Holden DW.** 2001. Intracellular replication of *Salmonella typhimurium* strains in specific subsets of splenic macrophages in vivo. *Cell Microbiol* **3**:587–597.

120. **Mastroeni P, Grant A, Restif O, Maskell D.** 2009. A dynamic view of the spread and intracellular distribution of *Salmonella enterica*. *Nat Rev Microbiol* **7**:73–80.

121. **Claudi B, Spröte P, Chirkova A, Personnic N, Zankl J, Schürmann N, Schmidt A, Bumann D.** 2014. Phenotypic variation of *Salmonella* in host tissues delays eradication by antimicrobial chemotherapy. *Cell* **158**:722–733.

122. **Burton NA, Schürmann N, Casse O, Steeb AK, Claudi B, Zankl J, Schmidt A, Bumann D.** 2014. Disparate impact of oxidative host defenses determines the fate of *Salmonella* during systemic infection in mice. *Cell Host Microbe* **15**:72–83.

123. **Bumann D.** 2015. Heterogeneous host-pathogen encounters: act locally, think globally. *Cell Host Microbe* **17**:13–19.

124. **Gerdes K, Maisonneuve E.** 2012. Bacterial persistence and toxin-antitoxin loci. *Annu Rev Microbiol* **66**:103–123.

125. **Hauryliuk V, Atkinson GC, Murakami KS, Tenson T, Gerdes K.** 2015. Recent functional insights into the role of (p)ppGpp in bacterial physiology. *Nat Rev Microbiol* **13**:298–309.

126. **Maisonneuve E, Gerdes K.** 2014. Molecular mechanisms underlying bacterial persisters. *Cell* **157**:539–548.

127. **Kussell E, Leibler S.** 2005. Phenotypic diversity, population growth, and information in fluctuating environments. *Science* **309**:2075–2078.

128. **Kussell E, Kishony R, Balaban NQ, Leibler S.** 2005. Bacterial persistence: a model of survival in changing environments. *Genetics* **169**:1807–1814.

129. **Lobato-Márquez D, Díaz-Orejas R, García-Del Portillo F.** 2016. Toxin-antitoxins and bacterial virulence. *FEMS Microbiol Rev* **40**:592–609.

130. **Helaine S, Kugelberg E.** 2014. Bacterial persisters: formation, eradication, and experimental systems. *Trends Microbiol* **22**:417–424.

131. **Page R, Peti W.** 2016. Toxin-antitoxin systems in bacterial growth arrest and persistence. *Nat Chem Biol* **12**:208–214.

132. **Correia FF, D'Onofrio A, Rejtar T, Li L, Karger BL, Makarova K, Koonin EV, Lewis K.** 2006. Kinase activity of overexpressed HipA is required for growth arrest and multidrug tolerance in *Escherichia coli*. *J Bacteriol* **188**:8360–8367.

133. **Germain E, Castro-Roa D, Zenkin N, Gerdes K.** 2013. Molecular mechanism of bacterial persistence by HipA. *Mol Cell* **52**:248–254.

134. **Lobato-Márquez D, Moreno-Córdoba I, Figueroa V, Díaz-Orejas R, García-del Portillo F.** 2015. Distinct type I and type II toxin-antitoxin modules control *Salmonella* lifestyle inside eukaryotic cells. *Sci Rep* **5**:9374.

135. **Cheverton AM, Gollan B, Przydacz M, Wong CT, Mylona A, Hare SA, Helaine S.** 2016. A *Salmonella* toxin promotes persister formation through acetylation of tRNA. *Mol Cell* **63:**86–96.

136. **Nuccio SP, Bäumler AJ.** 2014. Comparative analysis of *Salmonella* genomes identifies a metabolic network for escalating growth in the inflamed gut. *mBio* **5:**e00929-e14.

137. **Srikumar S, Kröger C, Hébrard M, Colgan A, Owen SV, Sivasankaran SK, Cameron AD, Hokamp K, Hinton JC.** 2015. RNA-seq brings new insights to the intra-macrophage transcriptome of *Salmonella* Typhimurium. *PLoS Pathog* **11:**e1005262.

138. **Hautefort I, Thompson A, Eriksson-Ygberg S, Parker ML, Lucchini S, Danino V, Bongaerts RJ, Ahmad N, Rhen M, Hinton JC.** 2008. During infection of epithelial cells *Salmonella enterica* serovar Typhimurium undergoes a time-dependent transcriptional adaptation that results in simultaneous expression of three type 3 secretion systems. *Cell Microbiol* **10:**958–984.

139. **Klemm EJ, Gkrania-Klotsas E, Hadfield J, Forbester JL, Harris SR, Hale C, Heath JN, Wileman T, Clare S, Kane L, Goulding D, Otto TD, Kay S, Doffinger R, Cooke FJ, Carmichael A, Lever AML, Parkhill J, MacLennan CA,** Kumararatne D, Dougan G, Kingsley RA. 2016. Emergence of host-adapted *Salmonella* Enteritidis through rapid evolution in an immunocompromised host. *Nat Microbiol* **1:**15023.

140. **Okoro CK, Barquist L, Connor TR, Harris SR, Clare S, Stevens MP, Arends MJ, Hale C, Kane L, Pickard DJ, Hill J, Harcourt K, Parkhill J, Dougan G, Kingsley RA.** 2015. Signatures of adaptation in human invasive *Salmonella* Typhimurium ST313 populations tfrom sub-Saharan Africa. *PLoS Negl Trop Dis* **9:**e0003611.

141. **Wrande M, Andrews-Polymenis H, Twedt DJ, Steele-Mortimer O, Porwollik S, McClelland M, Knodler LA.** 2016. Genetic determinants of *Salmonella enterica* serovar Typhimurium proliferation in the cytosol of epithelial cells. *Infect Immun* **84:**3517–3526.

142. **Schlumberger MC, Hardt WD.** 2006. *Salmonella* type III secretion effectors: pulling the host cell's strings. *Curr Opin Microbiol* **9:**46–54.

143. **Rosselin M, Virlogeux-Payant I, Roy C, Bottreau E, Sizaret PY, Mijouin L, Germon P, Caron E, Velge P, Wiedemann A.** 2010. Rck of *Salmonella enterica*, subspecies enterica serovar Enteritidis, mediates Zipper-like internalization. *Cell Res* **20:**647–664.

Selection and Transmission of Antibiotic-Resistant Bacteria

7

DAN I. ANDERSSON[1] and DIARMAID HUGHES[1]

INTRODUCTION AND SCOPE

Antibiotics are compounds that inhibit (bacteriostatic drugs) or kill (bactericidal drugs) bacteria by a specific interaction with a specific target in the bacterial cell, and they are arguably the most important medical intervention introduced by humans. Ever since antibiotics were introduced on large scale in the late 1940s to treat human bacterial infectious diseases, there has been a steady selection and increase in the frequency of antibiotic-resistant bacteria, generating a very problematic situation (1–3). Resistance evolution is a complex process that is driven by the interaction between a number of biotic and abiotic factors. Fundamental factors underlying this dynamic are the rates of emergence and persistence of resistant bacterial clones; time and space gradients of antibiotics and other xenobiotics; and transmission rates within human populations and between humans and various other sources, including animals, the environment, food, etc. Furthermore, with the realization that antibiotic resistance has become a serious medical problem, human attempts to reduce transmission of infectious bacteria in general, and resistant ones in particular, by hygienic measures, vaccination, reduced antibiotic pressures, etc., has also influenced this dynamic.

[1]Department of Medical Biochemistry and Microbiology, Uppsala University, Uppsala, Sweden.
Microbial Transmission in Biological Processes
Edited by Fernando Baquero, Emilio Bouza, J.A. Gutiérrez-Fuentes, and Teresa M. Coque
© 2018 American Society for Microbiology, Washington, DC
doi:10.1128/microbiolspec.MTBP-0013-2016

Here we will describe some of the factors that influence the selection and transmission of resistant bacteria and discuss the options available to prevent these processes and reduce the rate of resistance evolution and/or transmission. In this description, we will follow the outline shown in Fig. 1, where we track the initial emergence of resistance in environmental bacteria, its transfer into pathogenic bacteria, and the subsequent transmission of these bacteria between different compartments and environments.

WHERE DID RESISTANCE GENES ORIGINATE AND WHY?

The majority of medically relevant antibiotics originate in nature and are synthesized by a variety of species, in particular soil-dwelling bacteria in the genus *Streptomyces* (4, 5). Both antibiotics and resistance genes are thought to be ancient and far predate the existence of humans. This has been inferred from phylogenetic studies suggesting that class A β-lactamases evolved billions of years ago and were transferred into the Gram-

positive bacteria about 800 million years ago and that the progenitors of β-lactamases, like CTX-M's, diverged 200 million to 300 million years ago (6). Further evidence that resistance genes are old is their presence in environments that have been untouched by humans (7–9), including in isolated caves (>4 million years), Beringian permafrost (30,000 years), and Siberian permafrost (15,000 to 40,000 years old).

The benefits of antibiotics for microbial producers is not entirely clear, but the standard explanation is that the producers use them as ecological weapons to inhibit neighboring competitors in the environment (10, 11). However, they might also have a more benevolent function as signals for cell-to-cell communication in microbial communities. A recent study that distinguished between these hypotheses provided strong evidence that antibiotics are weapons but that their expression is influenced by social interactions between competing strains and species (12). It is expected that the biosynthesis and release of antibiotics in various natural environments will expose many bacteria (both the producers and bystanders) to antibiot-

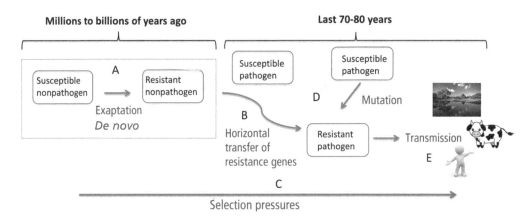

FIGURE 1 Schematic view of the evolution of antibiotic resistance. Key questions in understanding the emergence and transmission include: (A) What are the origins of resistance genes? (B) Where do resistant pathogens emerge? (C) Which are the most significant selective pressures driving resistance evolution? (D) Which are the biological factors that influence rates of resistance development? (E) What are the routes, directions, and magnitudes of flow of pathogens between humans, animals, and the environment?

ics and, as a consequence, select for the evolution of resistance mechanisms to protect against self-destruction (in antibiotic producers), to defend against antibiotics produced by other species, and/or to modulate intermicrobe communication.

Another hypothesis is that resistance genes originally performed metabolic functions unrelated to antibiotics and that they had weak secondary promiscuous activities that conferred a low-level resistance that was exapted and further evolved to become bona fide antibiotic resistance functions. For example, aminoglycoside acetylate-modifying enzymes could originally have been involved in sugar metabolism and modification of complex sugars. Similarly, the plasmid-borne, dual-activity fluoroquinolone acetylate-modifying enzyme AAC(6′)-Ib-cr (13–15) belongs to the GNAT (GCN5-related *N*-acetyltransferase) superfamily, with 10,000 known enzymes that perform a variety of coenzyme A-dependent acetylation reactions (16). Considering the low activity of this enzyme on fluoroquinolones (only a fewfold increase in MIC of fluoroquinolones), it is likely that this represents a weak promiscuous activity. Another example is the class A, C, and D (Ser-OH) β-lactamases that have been suggested to originate from penicillin-binding proteins (PBPs) by acquiring the capability to hydrolyze the acyl-enzyme bond between the β-lactam ring and the hydroxyl group of the PBP's active-site serine (17, 18). This notion is supported by experimental data showing that PBPs can evolve weak β-lactamase activity after mutagenesis (19–21). A final example of where a function might have been coopted is the TetX enzyme, a flavin-dependent monooxygenase that inactivates all known tetracyclines, including tigecycline. This enzyme belongs to the flavoprotein monooxygenase group, whose native metabolic function is in the hydroxylation and degradation of phenolic compounds (22).

Our possibilities to interfere with and slow down the rate by which novel resistance mechanisms evolve in nonpathogenic bacteria (e.g., *Streptomyces*) are at present nonexistent, but this type of knowledge is still useful since it provides the tools that allow us to explore the intrinsic potential of a bacterium to acquire a high-level resistance mechanism to a novel antibiotic by evolving an existing weak promiscuous activity into a more efficient enzyme. For example, by directed *in vitro* evolution of a suspected candidate enzyme or an adaptive evolution experiment with whole cells, one can explore the likelihood and efficiency of such a process (23).

TRANSFER FROM NONPATHOGENS TO PATHOGENS

Antibiotic resistance can propagate and transmit through either vertical transfer, whereby mutations or resistance genes are transfered to the offspring, or horizontal gene transfer (HGT), whereby antibiotic resistance genes are acquired from close relatives or other species and subsequently propagated to the offspring. The comprehensive genomic characterization of human pathogens during the last decades shows that horizontal transfer of preexisting genes contributes to the majority of current resistance problems generated by our use of antibiotics (24). The vast pool of existing resistance determinants present in the biosphere, known as the resistome, provides an evolutionary toolbox of ready-made genes that has the potential to be transferred within and between species and to confer resistance to any antibiotic that might be used against human and animal pathogens. Transfer mechanisms include conjugative transfer of plasmids and conjugative transposons, transduction via bacteriophages, and transformation of naked DNA taken up from the environment (discussed further in "Transmission of Resistance Genes," below). Apart from HGT, resistance can also arise by mutations (including point mutations, gene rearrangements, and amplification) of native resident genes.

Many horizontally transferred resistance genes are thought to have their origin in various environmental bacteria (25, 26). For example, the widespread and clinically relevant *CTX-M* class of genes was probably imported to pathogens from the chromosome of different species of the environmental genus *Kluyvera* (27–29). This particular case is especially interesting since it illustrates the importance of a transposable genetic element (insertion sequence IS*Ecp1*). This element facilitated selection and transfer by allowing both expression (by providing a promoter) and transposition of the progenitor resistance gene from *Kluyvera* into other species (30). Furthermore, the plasmid-encoded *qnrA* gene was most likely transferred from marine and freshwater *Shewanella algae* into various *Enterobacteriaceae* species, emphasizing the role of aquatic environments as resistance reservoirs (31). Similarly, *Shewanella oneidensis* is the natural reservoir of OXA-48, a plasmid-encoded, carbapenem-hydrolyzing β-lactamase gene found in *Klebsiella pneumoniae*, further indicating gene exchange between *Shewanella* spp. and *Enterobacteriaceae* (32). Another more recent example is provided by the *tetX* gene, which has been found in obligate anaerobes such as *Bacteroides* (33–37), in the soil bacterium *Sphingobacterium* sp. (38), and in manure-treated soil (39) and activated sludge from sewage treatment plants (40). TetX has been suggested to have its immediate origin in *Bacteroides fragilis*, where it was found to be located in two different transposons (34, 35). Up until very recently the *tetX* gene had not been found in human pathogens, but a study in a Sierra Leone hospital from 2013 showed that 21% of Gram-negative bacteria (e.g., *Escherichia coli*, *K. pneumoniae*, and *Enterobacter* sp.) isolated from urine carried the *tetX* gene, demonstrating that this particular resistance gene had rapidly entered into significant human pathogens from other bacteria (41). That this recent acquisition of resistance genes in human pathogens is driven by anthropogenic use of antibiotics is substantiated

by, for example, the demonstration that in agricultural soil the frequency of resistance genes (in particular genes conferring resistance to β-lactams and tetracycline) increased significantly from the 1940s (pre-antibiotics) to 2008 (42). Similarly, plasmids isolated before antibiotics were used by humans lacked resistance genes, indicating that mobilization of resistance genes to plasmids is a recent event (43).

These findings show that many resistance genes have their origins in environmental bacteria and that they have been mobilized by transposons and plasmids for transfer into pathogens. A key question with regard to our ability to influence and reduce these types of HGT events is where these transfer events from environmental bacteria to pathogens occurred. Unfortunately, we do not have any solid data regarding this question, but potential environments include sewage treatment plants, manure tanks, and manure-treated soils. In all these environments, one would expect both environmental bacteria and pathogens (in particular *Enterobacteriaceae*) to be present at high densities, at favorable temperatures (at least in sewage plants and manure tanks), and with weak antibiotic selective pressures present, all conditions that would be conducive to selection of rare HGT events of, for example, resistance plasmids. Several experimental studies have indeed shown that horizontal transfer of antibiotic resistance genes is a common occurrence in such environments (for reviews, see references 44 to 48). Another potential environment could be in humans and animals where environmental bacteria could transiently (e.g., via ingestion of food contaminated with environmental bacteria or mixed wound infections) be physically near pathogens for transfer. Demonstration that HGT can occur is a first step in demonstrating their role, but even with experimental demonstration of transfer it is still difficult to extrapolate from such data to assess which environments are the most relevant and where to make potential interventions. Apart from generally reducing the selective pressures provided by antibiotics and other potential selectors (biocides, heavy metals) to reduce enrichment for rare HGT events in these types of environments, it would also be possible to break potential transmission pathways by, for example, treating the water exiting from sewage plants with ozone or similar oxidative compounds (49, 50). This would have several beneficial effects in that it would reduce the levels of antibiotics (and other pharmaceuticals) released and also kill off most types of microorganisms present in the outgoing water.

THE ROLE OF SELECTIVE PRESSURES

Antimicrobial Drugs as Selectors

The rate of fixation of a neutral HGT event or a mutation = HGT/mutation rate, and classical theoretical work suggests the fixation time to be $4N_e$ generations (where N_e is the effective population size) (51). N_e in bacterial populations (e.g., *E. coli*) is estimated to be in the range of 10^5 to 10^9 (52, 53), implying that the fixation of a neutral resistance mutation/gene is unlikely and will take a very long time without selection. Also, most resistance mutations/genes are deleterious in the absence of antibiotics (reviewed in reference 54), which will further reduce the likelihood of their fixation. Thus, a selective pressure(s) must have driven the rise in antibiotic resistance over the last century. Obviously, human use of antibiotics in various settings has been the main driver for the rise in the frequency of resistant bacteria, and it is clear from studies at different geographic levels (e.g., county and country) that the frequency of resistant bacteria is positively correlated with the antibiotic pressure, i.e., the amount of antibiotic used (55–57). Antibiotics are present in humans, animals, and the environments at varying concentrations, and traditionally it has been assumed that selection of resistant bacteria only occurs at antibiotic concentrations between the MIC of the sus-

ceptible wild-type population (MIC_{susc}) and that of the resistant population (MIC_{res}), as outlined in the mutant selective window hypothesis (58). Recent studies have examined the selective potential of sub-MIC antibiotic concentrations and shown that drug concentrations several hundredfold below the MIC_{susc} can in fact be selective (59–62). Thus, the determined minimal selective concentrations (MSCs) were in the range of nanograms to picograms per milliliter for certain antibiotics (e.g., fluoroquinolones and tetracyclines), showing that the selective window is much wider than previously thought and expands far below the MIC_{susc} (reviewed in reference 63).

Apart from antibiotics, other potential selectors for antibiotic resistance include biocides (including heavy metals) that are widespread and extensively used in numerous types of settings (64, 65). Biocides could select for antibiotic resistance in at least three different ways: (i) by cross-resistance, where a biocide resistance mechanism confers resistance to an antibiotic, e.g., via upregulation of an efflux pump (66) or a specific target modification (67, 68); (ii) by coselection, where genetic colocalization (e.g., on a plasmid or in a clone) of biocide and antibiotic resistance determinants drives indirect enrichment of antibiotic resistance genes by virtue of biocide selection (69); and (iii) by the ability of biocides to reduce the MSC of antibiotics. With regard to the latter, it has been shown that certain heavy metals (e.g., silver) can strongly potentiate the selective effect of certain antibiotics and thereby cause a significant reduction in the MSC (L. M. Albrecht and D. I. Andersson, unpublished data). Such interactive (synergistic or antagonistic) effects on selection of combinations of different agents (antibiotics and biocides) present at sub-MIC levels are largely unexplored, but as suggested by recent experiments (Albrecht and Andersson, unpublished), the synergistic effects can be considerable. Thus, mixes of up to seven different selectors (antibiotics and heavy metals) reduced the MSC of each individual compound at least 4-fold. As natural environments (e.g., wastewater, soils) do generally contain complex mixes of different selectors, it is of great importance to determine how common and strong such interactions (in particular synergistic) are to correctly assess their selective potential.

Over all, these results indicate that, apart from exposure in treated humans and animals, selection can occur in many *ex vivo* environments where bacteria are exposed to sub-MIC levels of combinations of antimicrobial drugs due to their excretion from treated subjects (for example, effluent from hospitals), the use of antimicrobials in farming and aquaculture, the natural presence of heavy metals in soils, and pollution from antimicrobial production plants. Thus, it is likely that common weak selection pressures are important contributors to resistance selection and enrichment. However, at present we cannot estimate their relative importance as compared to that of the usually (above MIC) strong selection pressures reached in humans and animals that are treated for infections. Furthermore, with the introduction of MSC determinations as a tool to measure the selection potential of antibiotics, it might also be prudent to reexamine the maximum residue limits (MRLs) set for antibiotics in food. Based on the MSCs, our calculations for fluoroquinolones and tetracyclines (59) and the MRLs set for meat (70) suggest that a normal (100-g) daily consumption of meat that is contaminated with these particular antibiotic residues just below the MRL would still be high enough to cause selection for resistant bacteria (Andersson, unpublished data), implying that these MRLs ought to be reduced.

Other Selectors

Apart from different antimicrobials, there are other mechanisms that could enrich for and maintain resistance in a bacterial population. With regard to plasmids they might encode, apart from antibiotic resistances, virulence factors or growth-promoting factors. In addition, many plasmids have stability systems that ensure plasmid maintenance even without direct selection. The successful epidemic plasmids associated with the widespread clones of *E. coli* ST131 and *K. pneumoniae* ST258 appear to owe their success partly to the presence of highly stable (due to multiple partitioning and postsegregational killing systems) IncF-type plasmids encoding several antibiotic resistance genes and virulence factors (71). Furthermore, even though generally plasmids will reduce bacterial fitness in the absence of antibiotics, it has also been demonstrated that certain plasmids might enhance host fitness (growth rate) even in the absence of a selective pressure (72), indicating that plasmids can be maintained and enriched also without direct selection (73–77). At present, the mechanisms of such fitness increases are unclear.

Reducing Selection

With regard to our possibilities to reduce the emergence and frequency of resistance, a reduction in the selective pressure is our most effective and realistic approach. Considering the unwise way antibiotics have been and still are being used, there is considerable room for improvement when it comes to antibiotic stewardship. The required changes are manyfold and are, for example, associated with reducing economic incentives for antibiotic use, educating prescribers and patients, tightening regulation of antibiotic prescriptions, and discontinuing the use of antibiotics as growth promoters in animal farming. Similarly, the potential impact of biocides on enrichment of antibiotic resistance needs much further study and evaluation, which possibly might result in reduced biocide use.

Reduced antibiotic use will reduce the rate of emergence and enrichment of antibiotic-resistant bacteria, but whether the already existing problem of frequent resistance is reversible is questionable. As has been discussed in many papers, we find it likely that once a resistance problem has emerged the rate of reversibility will generally be slow after discontinued/reduced antibiotic use and that a reversibility strategy is unlikely to succeed (for a review, see reference 54).

FACTORS INFLUENCING THE RATE OF EMERGENCE AND SUCCESS OF RESISTANT CLONES

At a given selective pressure, the rate of emergence of resistant mutants, the steady-state frequency of resistance, and the potential for reversibility will be determined by a complex interplay between a number of biological parameters that are intrinsic to the specific combination of bacterial species and antibiotic. Thus, mutation/HGT rates, population sizes, fitness costs of resistance, the rate and efficiency of compensatory evolution, and potential epistatic interactions between drugs and/or combinations of resistance mutations all affect resistance evolution. As several recent reviews have covered this subject, we will not discuss this further here (54, 63, 78) except for a few brief comments on how we could potentially utilize these factors to our benefit.

One general conclusion is that the emergence of resistance in a population is predicted to be slowed by high fitness costs of resistance, especially if compensatory evolution is inefficient. Unfortunately, our ability to influence these parameters is limited, except during drug development, where one could specifically focus on drugs and drug targets in which the above requirements are fulfilled. At present, it is not possible to predict which types of targets are the least prone to resistance evolution, so identification of such targets and drugs remains a purely experimental question. However, a few generalities have emerged from such studies, suggesting that drugs with multiple targets, targets that are encoded by several identical genes (e.g., rRNA), and targets that when mutated show reduced fitness due to

pleiotropic physiological effects are less prone to resistance evolution (79). Furthermore, drugs that target complex essential metabolites (e.g., vancomycin, which targets a precursor of peptidoglycans) are expected to be less prone to resistance development because of the difficulties for the cell to mutationally alter the target while maintaining functionality (but obviously resistance could still appear by drug inactivation, reduced uptake, increased efflux, etc.). Thus, an interesting avenue for drug development would be to specifically search for novel drugs that target metabolites outside of the inner membrane (e.g., metabolites involved in lipopolysaccharide, teichoic acid, outer membrane, and peptidoglycan synthesis) since problems with cellular uptake (no need for uptake over the inner membrane) would be less and the propensity for resistance probably lower.

Other possible strategies could be to (i) identify drugs that reduce mutation rates, for example, by inhibiting the SOS response (80–82); (ii) identify drugs that reduce conjugation rates (82, 83); or (iii) use drug combinations during treatment and in particular to utilize the concept of collateral sensitivity. In our opinion, it is unlikely that drug developers will have the luxury of choosing between alternative development candidates with different effects on mutation rate, or that drugs inhibiting bacterial conjugation would significantly contribute to breaking resistance transmission. Hovever, the third possibility, drug combinations, has precedent in clinical treatment of, for example, tuberculosis and HIV to suppress the rate of resistance evolution. Of particular interest is collateral sensitivity, in which resistance to one drug confers increased susceptibility to a second drug (84–86), allowing two (or more) drugs to be alternated to select against resistance to either drug. Experimental data suggest that this approach can slow the rate of resistance development (84, 85), but until it has been shown in treated patients to reduce resistance evolution, the concept remains hypothetical.

TRANSMISSION OF RESISTANCE GENES

Many of the most problematic resistance problems today are directly associated with HGT of resistance genes. Examples include plasmid-borne resistance to β-lactams, macrolides, aminoglycosides, and fluoroquinolones (87), and most recently plasmid-borne resistance to colistin (88). In addition, HGT is the cause of resistant mosaic genes in pneumococci and *Neisseria* species (89, 90), and the source of most of the virulence genes found on pathogenicity islands (91). In this section, we discuss how antibiotics influence rates of HGT, and ongoing efforts to discover small-molecule inhibitors of HGT.

Mechanisms of HGT of Antibiotic Resistance Genes

The various mechanisms of HGT of resistance genes (24, 92) and the importance of HGT for mobilizing different reservoirs of resistance genes (26) have been extensively reviewed by others and are only outlined here. Briefly, the process of HGT involves two stages: firstly, getting resistance genes into a recipient cell, and secondly, ensuring

that they can be stably maintained. Selection is expected to act at several levels of HGT (Fig. 2). The actual DNA transfer process can occur by direct cell-to-cell contact, for example, involving conjugative plasmids or conjugative transposons that mediate the transfer resistance genes from one bacterial cell into another, including across species boundaries. HGT of resistance genes can also be mediated in the absence of direct cell-to-cell contact, with bacteriophages acting as vectors, or the DNA can be taken up directly from the environment (e.g., after release from dead cells) by transformation into a recipient cell. The rates of transfer in the case of conjugation and transformation are expected to be strongly influenced by the population density of donor and recipient cells. Thus, bacteria that, for example, share a common environment such as the human intestine or nasal passages are potentially much more likely to share DNA by processes involving direct contact than bacteria that normally live in, for example, marine environments. In such enclosed environments conjugation (and transformation) are likely to be the dominant mechanisms of HGT. Bacteriophages, however, may play a more important

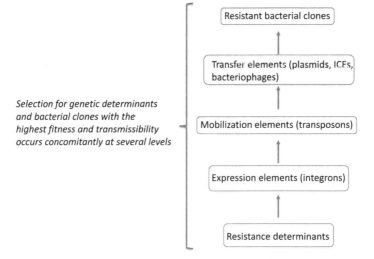

Selection for genetic determinants and bacterial clones with the highest fitness and transmissibility occurs concomitantly at several levels

Resistant bacterial clones

↑

Transfer elements (plasmids, ICEs, bacteriophages)

↑

Mobilization elements (transposons)

↑

Expression elements (integrons)

↑

Resistance determinants

FIGURE 2 **Selection for antibiotic resistance occurs at several levels of complexity to generate a successful resistant clone.**

role in mediating the transfer of DNA between bacterial species that occupy different environmental niches, because they are by their nature more widely spread and the DNA they contain is more likely to survive long periods than naked DNA in the environment. Thus, depending on the particular environment and the source of the genetic material involved, each of these mechanisms may play an important role in the HGT of resistance genes.

The second stage of HGT, ensuring the maintenance of the acquired genes, is equally important. HGT by plasmids is the most efficient because conjugative plasmids typically have inbuilt mechanisms to ensure their stable maintenance in a recipient bacterial cell. Genes that enter a recipient genome after transfer on a conjugative transposon typically depend on the recombination activity of an encoded integrase enzyme. DNA that enters a recipient by bacteriophage transduction or by transformation could also be recombined into the chromosome by an integrase enzyme if one is encoded on the transferred DNA, but otherwise will depend on homologous recombination. The ability of plasmids to replicate independently of the host chromosome (not depending on recombination to ensure maintenance) explains their very close relationship with HGT resistance genes. The contribution of bacteriophages was thought to be limited by the requirement that they attach to a specific host surface receptor to deliver DNA into a recipient, but recent evidence suggests that many bacteriophages may actually have very broad host range. The other factor that restricts the relative contribution of bacteriophages and transformation to HGT is the requirement that the delivered DNA can be successfully integrated into the recipient genome. This requirement explains the observed close connection between HGT and genes encoding integrases, but in some clinically important examples of resistance (e.g., penicillin resistance in streptococci and neisseriae), the integration of foreign DNA is primarily by homologous recombinations because donor and recipient are related species living in close proximity (89).

Antibiotics Can Influence Rates of HGT

As described above, factors such as the concentration and physical proximity of donor and recipient cells or DNA, the recipient spectrum of transducing phages, and the probability that an integrase enzyme successfully recombines foreign DNA into a genome are each expected to have a significant impact on the overall probability of HGT of antibiotic resistance genes. In addition to these factors, exposure of bacteria to antibiotics can in itself influence the rate of HGT by several mechanisms connected with induction of the SOS response (Fig. 3). The SOS system is a set of bacterial genes involved in the repair of

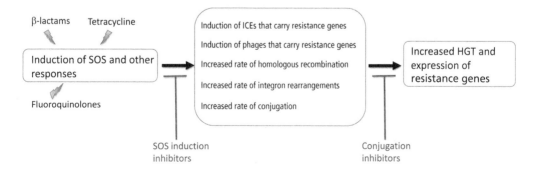

FIGURE 3 **Effects of antibiotics on HGT and potential inhibition points.**

DNA damage. The genes of the SOS system are coregulated by a repressor protein, LexA, and the system is induced in response to DNA damage when activated RecA protein interacts with LexA, catalyzing autocleavage and relieving repression (93). Exposure of bacteria to sublethal doses of several important classes of antibiotics, including fluoroquinolones such as ciprofloxacin (94), β-lactams such as ampicillin (95), and trimethoprim (96), has been shown to induce the SOS system (97). Antibiotic-induced induction of SOS is associated with several downstream effects that promote HGT of antibiotic resistance genes and genes encoding virulence factors. Examples include induction of integrating conjugative elements (ICEs) such as SXT in *Vibrio cholerae*, which encodes resistance to chloramphenicol, sulfamethoxazole, trimethoprim, and streptomycin (98); induction of several different temperate phages that package and transfer a pathogenicity island encoding virulence factors in staphylococci (99, 100); induction of a prophage encoding Shiga toxin in *E. coli* (101); and induction of phages that package and transduce an antibiotic resistance plasmid from *Salmonella* (102). There are also reported examples where sublethal antibiotic exposure promotes HGT of conjugative transposons (103, 104) and plasmids (105), independently of SOS induction. Another example of an SOS-independent effect on HGT involves transcriptional activation of the *com* regulon by of sublethal antibiotic exposure in *Streptococcus pneumoniae*, resulting in an increased frequency of transformation (106).

Besides increasing rates of HGT as described above, sublethal exposure of bacteria to antibiotics has also been shown to increase the rate of homologous recombination between divergent sequences (107), increasing the probability of successfully recombining HGT genes into a recipient genome. SOS induction by antibiotic exposure has also been shown to increase cassette rearrangements within integrons (108), and in one case an antibiotic-induced rearrangement was shown

to result in increased expression of a β-lactamase in a clinical isolate of *Pseudomonas aeruginosa* (109).

Efforts To Interfere with HGT of Resistance Genes

In the sections above we have presented evidence that a major source of antibiotic resistance is through acquisition of resistance genes in HGT events, sometimes stimulated by the presence of antibiotics in the environment. This raises the question of whether it is possible to interfere with HGT rates, and if so, how and where this should be done. Different antiresistance drug strategies have been suggested, some directed against plasmid-borne resistance and others aimed at developing drugs to suppress the SOS response. The direct antiplasmid approach includes the discovery of small molecules that interfere with plasmid replication, that activate plasmid-borne toxin genes, or that interfere with plasmid-mediated conjugation (110, 111). The heterogeneity of plasmid replication systems and of toxin-antitoxin systems argues that it might be very difficult to identify drugs with a useful spectrum of activity against these targets. Currently there is ongoing research into small-molecule drugs or antibodies that can interfere with plasmid conjugation systems. Unsaturated fatty acids (oleic and linoleic acids) were discovered to inhibit bacterial conjugation, acting on a clinically interesting range of Gram-negative bacteria including *Escherichia*, *Salmonella*, *Pseudomonas*, and *Acinetobacter* species (83, 112), by targeting a type IV secretion traffic ATPase (113). Recently, after screening a library of bioactive compounds from aquatic organisms, tanzawaic acids (fungal polyketides) were identified as inhibitors of IncW and IncFII conjugation systems (114). Because each of these conjugation-inhibiting compounds is a relatively nontoxic natural product, they may have uses in natural environments to reduce conjugation frequencies, or in therapy in combination with antibiotics. A very interesting recent finding is that bacterial conjugation efficiency is reduced by coculture with human intestinal cells, with the data suggesting that a secreted protein or peptide is responsible for the effect (115). This discovery opens up the possibility that a drug therapy could be developed to modulate conjugation of multidrug resistance plasmids in the human gut.

The second approach to control HGT of resistance genes is to investigate the possibility of developing drugs that reduce induction of the bacterial SOS response. It was previously shown that the accumulation of chromosomal mutations conferring resistance to fluoroquinolones or rifampin in *E. coli* in an *in vivo* infection model was strongly dependent on the bacteria having an active SOS response (116). This suggested that drugs capable of altering the bacterial SOS response would be generally useful in reducing the evolution of resistance because they could reduce mutation rates to resistance, reduce rates of HGT of resistance genes, and possibly act as adjuvants to DNA-damaging antibiotics (117). Screening programs have already identified several small-molecule inhibitors that prevent or reduce the ciprofloxacin-induced SOS response in *E. coli* (118), *Staphylococcus aureus* (119), or *Mycobacterium tuberculosis* (120), raising the hope that some compounds might be developed further into clinically useful drugs.

TRANSMISSION OF RESISTANT CLONES

In the previous section, we discussed HGT of resistance genes. However, for a resistant gene to be a clinical problem it must be associated with a genome that is successful in terms of its ability to promote bacterial transmission from the environment to a human host, or from host to host. In this section, we discuss some of the important routes and modes of transmission and the role played by successful epidemic clones in spreading multidrug resistance globally. Finally, we discuss

some of the measures that might be implemented to reduce rates of transmission.

Reservoirs of Resistant Bacteria and Modes of Transmission

In recent years several reviews have been published describing and discussing the ecological resevoirs of resistance genes and resistant bacterial pathogens, as well as the major routes of transmission (46, 121–125). The most important conclusion from these reviews is that there is currently very little evidence to quantify either the magnitude or the direction of transmission of resistance genes or pathogens between humans and any of these reservoirs. Here we limit ourselves to briefly summarizing some of the main points and conclusions from these reviews, before considering in more detail the significance of successful bacterial clones in the global dissemination of multidrug resistance. There is a great need for systematic, well-designed, long-term research, using metagenomic sequencing techniques, to map and quantify the routes and directions of transmission of both mobile resistance genes and resistant bacterial pathogens. At the moment, the only robust conclusion that can be made is that the anthropogenic use of antibiotics has almost certainly led to the contamination of many environments with antibiotic-resistant bacteria. What is not clear is the degree to which this contamination is responsible for the resistance problems within human populations. Acquiring high-quality information to quantitatively answer this question, using molecular typing on human, animal, and other environmental isolates, is essential for designing appropriate intervention strategies in the future.

The Role of Successful (Epidemic) Clones

Antibiotic resistance, whether arising due to mutation or by HGT, could in principle be selected in any of the bacteria within a pathogen population. However, whether a particular resistant clone subsequently becomes the founder of a bacterial population that causes a significant clinical problem depends on many factors, in particular its relative fitness in a range of appropriate environments and its transmissibility (Fig. 4). With the increasing use of whole-genome sequencing to analyze antibiotic-resistant bacterial pathogens, it has become clear that many of the major resistance problems are associated with a few successful bacterial clones within a species. Here we shall examine the evidence for clonal success, focusing on two of the most problematic multidrug-resistant Gram-negative pathogens, *E. coli* ST131 and *K. pneumoniae* ST258.

E. coli ST131

Although *E. coli* lives as a commensal of the gastrointestinal tract of humans and other animals, some genetic variants have developed into extraintestinal pathogens (126). Within the past 20 years a clone of the sequence type ST131 has become the predominant multidrug-resistant extraintestinal *E. coli* human pathogen globally (127). Its phenotype includes resistance to fluoroquinolones and extended-spectrum cephalosporins, primarily associated with CTX-M-15 (128, 129). Genome-wide sequence analysis of historical isolates by several groups has provided evidence supporting the hypothesis that ST131 is clonal and delineating its recent evolutionary history. An allele of *fimH* (encoding the type I fimbrial adhesin gene), designated *fimH30*, was identified as a signature of the globally dominant clone of ST131 (130). Fluoroquinolone resistance apparently evolved in the early 2000s, in a single ancestor within the *H30* lineage of ST131, referred to as *H30*-R

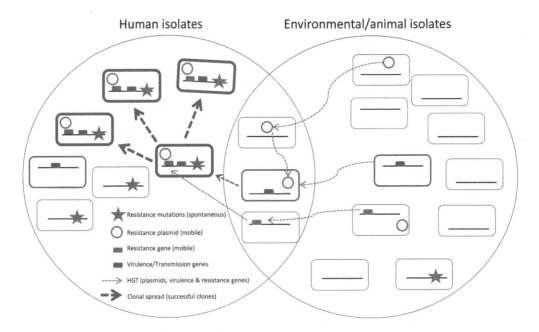

Human isolates   Environmental/animal isolates

Resistance mutations (spontaneous)

Resistance plasmid (mobile)

Resistance gene (mobile)

Virulence/Transmission genes

HGT (plasmids, virulence & resistance genes)

Clonal spread (successful clones)

FIGURE 4 Generic scheme for the creation and spread of globally successful antibiotic-resistant clones. In all environments (human, animal, and the wider environment), there are bacterial variants with resistance plasmids, resistance mutations, resistance genes, virulence genes, genes that increase transmission, etc. The mechanisms of HGT, coupled with selection by use of antibiotics, can select for combinations of these elements in one clone. When a clone arises that combines clinical resistance with high fitness and transmissibility, such a clone can spread through the global human population and become a dominant successful clone such as ST131 or ST258.

(131). ST131 isolates can carry plasmids with different β-lactamase genes, but most frequently carry CTX-M-15 (127, 132–137). More than 90% of the CTX-M-15-producing isolates of ST131 form a single-ancestor subclone (associated with three additional single nucleotide polymorphisms) within the fluoroquinolone resistance *H30* lineage, referred to as *H30*-Rx (138). Together these data strongly support the hypothesis that ST131 is a successsful multidrug-resistant clone that has spread globally in the recent past, raising the question of which features make ST131 such a successful pathogen. It is apparently associated with a high level of host-to-host transmissibility within household and hospital settings (137, 139, 140) and is more virulent than non-*H30* ST131 isolates (141), but the responsible virulence factors have not yet been identified (127). Recent comprehensive genomic analysis of ST131 isolates from varied sources provides strong evidence that not only are there multiple subtypes of ST131 circulating but that a key feature of their success has been the accumulation of compensatory mutations in regulatory regions in response to acquisition of multidrug resistance plasmids (72). ST131 has apparently not reached the end of its drug resistance evolutionary trajectory because there are increasingly frequent reports of carbapenemase resistance in ST131 isolates from around the world (142–149).

K. pneumoniae ST258

K. pneumoniae is a major cause of hospital-acquired pneumonias and bloodstream infections. Antibiotic resistance is a major problem, and it has become much worse in recent years as resistance to carbapenems, the preferred last-resort agents, has increased globally (150). Resistance to carbapenems in *K. pneumoniae* is due to plasmid-borne carbapenemases, KPC-2 and KPC-3 (151, 152), mainly associated with a global pandemic strain, ST258 (71). ST258 (clade II) originated after a major recombination event between the chromosomes of two different *K. pneu-*

moniae strains, ST11 and ST442, together with acquisition of an ICE (ICEKp258.2) encoding a type IV pilus and a type III restriction-modification system (153). In a subsequent recombination event, the capsular polysaccharide region of the chromosome was replaced with the equivalent region from *K. pneumoniae* strain ST42 to create ST258 (clade I) (153). The success of both ST258 clades may be closely connected with the presence of ICEKp258.2, which facilitates the carriage of KPC genes on narrow-host-range IncF plasmids (154). In contrast, its ancestor ST11 (which lacks ICEKp258.2) is associated with different carbapenemases carried on broad-host-range plasmids (155, 156).

Comparing *E. coli* ST131 and *K. pneumoniae* ST258 can provide some insights into how globally successful clones can originate. ST131 may be an example of an accident waiting to happen: a preexisting successful clone (with good virulence properties) that was initially selected to global prominence by exposure to fluoroquinolones (spontaneous resistance mutations), and capable of acquiring and maintaining IncF plasmids encoding CTX-M β-lactamases, providing resistance to cephalosporins (157). It has been speculated that the fluoroquinolone resistance mutations might also contribute by reducing the carriage cost of IncF CTX-M plasmids (71), although recent evidence suggests that a very important role was played by the accumulation of compensatory mutations affecting gene regulation (72). Accordingly, ST131 emerged from a favorable genotype in a series of relatively high-probability steps under selection by human use of antibiotics. In contrast to ST131, ST258 had its origin in a chromosomal recombination event, which together with the integration of ICEKp258.2 into the chromosome created a unique hybrid strain (153). Because we don't know how unlikely this series of recombination events is, it is difficult to say whether the creation of ST258 was a very unfortunate accident or a frequent event waiting to be selected. This creation of the chromosomal recombinant provided a suitable environment for the acquisition and maintenance of multi-drug-resistant IncF plasmids that also carry KPC-2 or KPC-3 enzymes (154). Whether, or which, additional features of the ST258 genome are critical for its global success is not currently known. ST131 and ST258 are not the only examples of successful antibiotic-resistant clones. Other high-risk resistant clones include *Salmonella enterica* serovar Typhimurium DT104, whose creation involved acquisition of the *Salmonella* genomic island I (158); *P. aeruginosa* ST146, which is highly transmissible in cystic fibrosis patients (159, 160); penicillin-nonsuseptible vaccine-escape strains of *S. pneumoniae* (161, 162); and the M1T1 clonal serotype of *Streptococcus pyogenes*, which evolved by multiple acquisitions of DNA encoding virulence factors (163).

Strategies To Reduce Transmission

Although the rapid evolution and global spread of ST131, ST258, and these other clones is alarming, their very clonality holds out the hope that a deep understanding of the genetics of these individual strains might provide clues for the design of targeted interventions, leading, for example, to the application of novel antivirulence drugs or vaccines that, if successful, would significantly reduce the burden on health care systems globally (157, 162, 164). Additional research and investment is required to understand more fully the epidemiology of these successful clones to determine which measures should be implemented to most successfully reduce transmission. Several obvious strategies are frequently suggested to reduce the reservoirs of antibiotic resistance and the transmission of resistance genes or resistant bacteria. Such measures include reducing the release of antibiotics into the environment, reducing unnecessary antibiotic use in medicine, reducing antibiotic use in animal husbandry and aquaculture, treating wastewater plants to destroy antibiotic residues, improving hospital hygiene, increasing patient

isolation for particular indications, and developing vaccine treatments to replace antibiotic use where possible (121–124). Information is available on the frequencies of clinically relevant pathogens in environments as varied as wastewater treatment plants, sewage sludge, and farm animals. However, there is very little data on the rates and directions of transmission of these resistant bacteria and genes between humans and any of these environments (121, 123, 125). What is required to tackle the transmission problem is a well-planned and long-term surveillance program. Without such a program there is a real danger that the major investment required could be misdirected. The surveillance must be based on detailed genetic and genomic analysis to identify bacterial variants and genes with the aim of quantifying accurately and in detail the major sources and directions of transmission of resistance genes and resistant bacteria between different environmental and biological compartments. Only with this information will it be possible to evaluate the effectiveness of alternative measures designed to reduce the burden of resistance on human health care.

CITATION

Andersson DI, Hughes D. 2017. Selection and transmission of antibiotic-resistant bacteria. Microbiol Spectrum 5(4):MTBP-0013-2016.

REFERENCES

1. **Carlet J, Jarlier V, Harbarth S, Voss A, Goossens H, Pittet D, Participants of the 3rd World Healthcare-Associated Infections Forum.** 2012. Ready for a world without antibiotics? The Pensières Antibiotic Resistance Call to Action. *Antimicrob Resist Infect Control* 1:11.
2. **Wittekamp BH, Bonten MJ.** 2012. Antibiotic prophylaxis in the era of multidrug-resistant bacteria. *Expert Opin Investig Drugs* 21:767–772.
3. **Woodford N, Livermore DM.** 2009. Infections caused by Gram-positive bacteria: a review of the global challenge. *J Infect* 59(Suppl 1):S4–S16.

4. **Procópio RE, Silva IR, Martins MK, Azevedo JL, Araújo JM.** 2012. Antibiotics produced by *Streptomyces*. *Braz J Infect Dis* **16:**466–471.

5. **Hasani A, Kariminik A, Issazadeh K.** 2014. Streptomycetes: characteristics and their antimicrobial activities. *Int J Adv Biol Biomed Res* **2:**63–75.

6. **Hall BG, Barlow M.** 2004. Evolution of the serine β-lactamases: past, present and future. *Drug Resist Updat* **7:**111–123.

7. **Bhullar K, Waglechner N, Pawlowski A, Koteva K, Banks ED, Johnston MD, Barton HA, Wright GD.** 2012. Antibiotic resistance is prevalent in an isolated cave microbiome. *PLoS One* **7:**e34953.

8. **D'Costa VM, King CE, Kalan L, Morar M, Sung WW, Schwarz C, Froese D, Zazula G, Calmels F, Debruyne R, Golding GB, Poinar HN, Wright GD.** 2011. Antibiotic resistance is ancient. *Nature* **477:**457–461.

9. **Petrova M, Gorlenko Z, Mindlin S.** 2011. Tn*5045*, a novel integron-containing antibiotic and chromate resistance transposon isolated from a permafrost bacterium. *Res Microbiol* **162:**337–345.

10. **Waksman SA, Woodruff HB.** 1940. The soil as a source of microorganisms antagonistic to disease-producing bacteria. *J Bacteriol* **40:**581–600.

11. **Martinez JL, Fajardo A, Garmendia L, Hernandez A, Linares JF, Martínez-Solano L, Sánchez MB.** 2009. A global view of antibiotic resistance. *FEMS Microbiol Rev* **33:**44–65.

12. **Abrudan MI, Smakman F, Grimbergen AJ, Westhoff S, Miller EL, van Wezel GP, Rozen DE.** 2015. Socially mediated induction and suppression of antibiosis during bacterial coexistence. *Proc Natl Acad Sci U S A* **112:**11054–11059.

13. **Ruiz J, Pons MJ, Gomes C.** 2012. Transferable mechanisms of quinolone resistance. *Int J Antimicrob Agents* **40:**196–203.

14. **Robicsek A, Jacoby GA, Hooper DC.** 2006. The worldwide emergence of plasmid-mediated quinolone resistance. *Lancet Infect Dis* **6:**629–640.

15. **Robicsek A, Strahilevitz J, Jacoby GA, Macielag M, Abbanat D, Park CH, Bush K, Hooper DC.** 2006. Fluoroquinolone-modifying enzyme: a new adaptation of a common aminoglycoside acetyltransferase. *Nat Med* **12:**83–88.

16. **Favrot L, Blanchard JS, Vergnolle O.** 2016. Bacterial GCN5-related *N*-acetyltransferases: from resistance to regulation. *Biochemistry* **55:**989–1002.

17. **Kelly JA, Dideberg O, Charlier P, Wery JP, Libert M, Moews PC, Knox JR, Duez C, Fraipont C, Joris B, Dusart J, Frere JM, Ghuysen JM.** 1986. On the origin of bacterial resistance to penicillin: comparison of a beta-lactamase and a penicillin target. *Science* **231:**1429–1431.

18. **Massova I, Mobashery S.** 1998. Kinship and diversification of bacterial penicillin-binding proteins and β-lactamases. *Antimicrob Agents Chemother* **42:**1–17.

19. **Chesnel L, Zapun A, Mouz N, Dideberg O, Vernet T.** 2002. Increase of the deacylation rate of PBP2x from *Streptococcus pneumoniae* by single point mutations mimicking the class A β-lactamases. *Eur J Biochem* **269:**1678–1683.

20. **Peimbert M, Segovia L.** 2003. Evolutionary engineering of a β-lactamase activity on a D-Ala D-Ala transpeptidase fold. *Protein Eng* **16:**27–35.

21. **Sun S, Selmer M, Andersson DI.** 2014. Resistance to β-lactam antibiotics conferred by point mutations in penicillin-binding proteins PBP3, PBP4 and PBP6 in *Salmonella enterica*. *PLoS One* **9:**e97202.

22. **Yang W, Moore IF, Koteva KP, Bareich DC, Hughes DW, Wright GD.** 2004. TetX is a flavin-dependent monooxygenase conferring resistance to tetracycline antibiotics. *J Biol Chem* **279:**52346–52352.

23. **Linkevicius M, Sandegren L, Andersson DI.** 2015. Potential of tetracycline resistance proteins to evolve tigecycline resistance. *Antimicrob Agents Chemother* **60:**789–796.

24. **Soucy SM, Huang J, Gogarten JP.** 2015. Horizontal gene transfer: building the web of life. *Nat Rev Genet* **16:**472–482.

25. **Wright GD.** 2010. Antibiotic resistance in the environment: a link to the clinic? *Curr Opin Microbiol* **13:**589–594.

26. **Perry JA, Westman EL, Wright GD.** 2014. The antibiotic resistome: what's new? *Curr Opin Microbiol* **21:**45–50.

27. **Poirel L, Kämpfer P, Nordmann P.** 2002. Chromosome-encoded Ambler class A β-lactamase of *Kluyvera georgiana*, a probable progenitor of a subgroup of CTX-M extended-spectrum β-lactamases. *Antimicrob Agents Chemother* **46:**4038–4040.

28. **Humeniuk C, Arlet G, Gautier V, Grimont P, Labia R, Philippon A.** 2002. β-Lactamases of *Kluyvera ascorbata*, probable progenitors of some plasmid-encoded CTX-M types. *Antimicrob Agents Chemother* **46:**3045–3049.

29. **Decoussier JW, Poirel L, Nordmann P.** 2001. Characterization of a chromosomally encoded extended-spectrum class A β-lactamase from *Kluyvera cryocrescens*. *Antimicrob Agents Chemother* **45:**3595–3598.

30. **Poirel L, Lartigue MF, Decousser JW, Nordmann P.** 2005. IS*Ecp1B*-mediated transposition of *bla*CTX-M in *Escherichia coli*. *Antimicrob Agents Chemother* **49:**447–450.

31. **Poirel L, Rodriguez-Martinez JM, Mammeri H, Liard A, Nordmann P.** 2005. Origin of plasmid-mediated quinolone resistance determinant QnrA. *Antimicrob Agents Chemother* **49:**3523–3525.

32. **Poirel L, Héritier C, Nordmann P.** 2004. Chromosome-encoded Ambler class D β-lactamase of *Shewanella oneidensis* as a progenitor of carbapenem-hydrolyzing oxacillinase. *Antimicrob Agents Chemother* **48:**348–351.

33. **Guiney DG Jr, Hasegawa P, Davis CE.** 1984. Expression in *Escherichia coli* of cryptic tetracycline resistance genes from bacteroides R plasmids. *Plasmid* **11:**248–252.

34. **Park BH, Levy SB.** 1988. The cryptic tetracycline resistance determinant on Tn*4400* mediates tetracycline degradation as well as tetracycline efflux. *Antimicrob Agents Chemother* **32:**1797–1800.

35. **Speer BS, Salyers AA.** 1988. Characterization of a novel tetracycline resistance that functions only in aerobically grown *Escherichia coli*. *J Bacteriol* **170:**1423–1429.

36. **Bartha NA, Sóki J, Urbán E, Nagy E.** 2011. Investigation of the prevalence of *tetQ*, *tetX* and *tetX1* genes in *Bacteroides* strains with elevated tigecycline minimum inhibitory concentrations. *Int J Antimicrob Agents* **38:**522–525.

37. **de Vries LE, Vallès Y, Agersø Y, Vaishampayan PA, García-Montaner A, Kuehl JV, Christensen H, Barlow M, Francino MP.** 2011. The gut as reservoir of antibiotic resistance: microbial diversity of tetracycline resistance in mother and infant. *PLoS One* **6:**e21644.

38. **Ghosh S, Sadowsky MJ, Roberts MC, Gralnick JA, LaPara TM.** 2009. *Sphingobacterium* sp. strain PM2-P1-29 harbours a functional *tet*(X) gene encoding for the degradation of tetracycline. *J Appl Microbiol* **106:**1336–1342.

39. **Heuer H, Kopmann C, Binh CTT, Top EM, Smalla K.** 2009. Spreading antibiotic resistance through spread manure: characteristics of a novel plasmid type with low %G+C content. *Environ Microbiol* **11:**937–949.

40. **Zhang XX, Zhang T.** 2011. Occurrence, abundance, and diversity of tetracycline resistance genes in 15 sewage treatment plants across China and other global locations. *Environ Sci Technol* **45:**2598–2604.

41. **Leski TA, Bangura U, Jimmy DH, Ansumana R, Lizewski SE, Stenger DA, Taitt CR, Vora GJ.** 2013. Multidrug-resistant *tet*(X)-containing hospital isolates in Sierra Leone. *Int J Antimicrob Agents* **42:**83–86.

42. **Knapp CW, Dolfing J, Ehlert PAI, Graham DW.** 2010. Evidence of increasing antibiotic resistance gene abundances in archived soils since 1940. *Environ Sci Technol* **44:**580–587.

43. **Hughes VM, Datta N.** 1983. Conjugative plasmids in bacteria of the 'pre-antibiotic' era. *Nature* **302:** 725–726.

44. **Bellanger X, Guilloteau H, Bonot S, Merlin C.** 2014. Demonstrating plasmid-based horizontal gene transfer in complex environmental matrices: a practical approach for a critical review. *Sci Total Environ* **493:**872–882.

45. **Michael I, Rizzo L, McArdell CS, Manaia CM, Merlin C, Schwartz T, Dagot C, Fatta-Kassinos D.** 2013. Urban wastewater treatment plants as hotspots for the release of antibiotics in the environment: a review. *Water Res* **47:**957–995.

46. **Marti E, Variatza E, Balcazar JL.** 2014. The role of aquatic ecosystems as reservoirs of antibiotic resistance. *Trends Microbiol* **22:**36–41.

47. **Bouki C, Venieri D, Diamadopoulos E.** 2013. Detection and fate of antibiotic resistant bacteria in wastewater treatment plants: a review. *Ecotoxicol Environ Saf* **91:**1–9.

48. **Zhang XX, Zhang T, Fang HH.** 2009. Antibiotic resistance genes in water environment. *Appl Microbiol Biotechnol* **82:**397–414.

49. **Pei J, Yao H, Wang H, Ren J, Yu X.** 2016. Comparison of ozone and thermal hydrolysis combined with anaerobic digestion for municipal and pharmaceutical waste sludge with tetracycline resistance genes. *Water Res* **99:**122–128.

50. **Oh J, Salcedo DE, Medriano CA, Kim S.** 2014. Comparison of different disinfection processes in the effective removal of antibiotic-resistant bacteria and genes. *J Environ Sci (China)* **26:**1238–1242.

51. **Kimura M, Ohta T.** 1969. The average number of generations until fixation of a mutant gene in a finite population. *Genetics* **61:**763–771.

52. **Charlesworth B.** 2009. Fundamental concepts in genetics: effective population size and patterns of molecular evolution and variation. *Nat Rev Genet* **10:**195–205.

53. **Berg OG.** 1996. Selection intensity for codon bias and the effective population size of *Escherichia coli*. *Genetics* **142:**1379–1382.

54. **Andersson DI, Hughes D.** 2011. Persistence of antibiotic resistance in bacterial populations. *FEMS Microbiol Rev* **35:**901–911.

55. **van de Sande-Bruinsma N, Grundmann H, Verloo D, Tiemersma E, Monen J, Goossens H, Ferech M, European Antimicrobial Resistance Surveillance System Group, European Surveillance of Antimicrobial Consumption Project Group.** 2008. Antimicrobial drug use and resistance in Europe. *Emerg Infect Dis* **14:**1722–1730.

56. **Bergman M, Nyberg ST, Huovinen P, Paakkari P, Hakanen AJ, Finnish Study Group for Antimicrobial Resistance.** 2009. Association between antimicrobial consumption and resistance in *Escherichia coli*. *Antimicrob Agents Chemother* **53:**912–917.

57. **Goossens H.** 2009. Antibiotic consumption and link to resistance. *Clin Microbiol Infect* **15**(Suppl 3): 12–15.

58. **Drlica K, Zhao X.** 2007. Mutant selection window hypothesis updated. *Clin Infect Dis* **44:**681–688.

59. **Gullberg E, Cao S, Berg OG, Ilbäck C, Sandegren L, Hughes D, Andersson DI.** 2011. Selection of resistant bacteria at very low antibiotic concentrations. *PLoS Pathog* **7:**e1002158.

60. **Liu A, Fong A, Becket E, Yuan J, Tamae C, Medrano L, Maiz M, Wahba C, Lee C, Lee K, Tran KP, Yang H, Hoffman RM, Salih A, Miller JH.** 2011. Selective advantage of resistant strains at trace levels of antibiotics: a simple and ultrasensitive color test for detection of antibiotics and genotoxic agents. *Antimicrob Agents Chemother* **55:**1204–1210.

61. **Gullberg E, Albrecht LM, Karlsson C, Sandegren L, Andersson DI.** 2014. Selection of a multidrug resistance plasmid by sublethal levels of antibiotics and heavy metals. *mBio* **5:** e01918-e14.

62. **Baquero F, Coque TM.** 2014. Widening the spaces of selection: evolution along sublethal antimicrobial gradients. *mBio* **5:**e02270.

63. **Andersson DI, Hughes D.** 2014. Microbiological effects of sublethal levels of antibiotics. *Nat Rev Microbiol* **12:**465–478.

64. **Scientific Committee on Emerging and Newly Identified Health Risks (SCENHIR).** 2009. *Assessment of the Antibiotic Resistance Effects of Biocides.* European Union, Brussels, Belgium. http://ec.europa.eu/health/ph_risk/committees/04_scenihr/docs/scenihr_o_021.pdf. Accessed 19 July 2017.

65. **European Chemicals Agency (ECHA).** *Biocidal Products Regulation.* ECHA, Helsinki, Finland. https://echa.europa.eu/regulations/biocidal-products-regulation. Accessed 19 July 2017.

66. **Webber MA, Whitehead RN, Mount M, Loman NJ, Pallen MJ, Piddock LJ.** 2015. Parallel evolutionary pathways to antibiotic resistance selected by biocide exposure. *J Antimicrob Chemother* **70:**2241–2248.

67. **Webber MA, Randall LP, Cooles S, Woodward MJ, Piddock LJ.** 2008. Triclosan resistance in *Salmonella enterica* serovar Typhimurium. *J Antimicrob Chemother* **62:**83–91.

68. **Sivaraman S, Zwahlen J, Bell AF, Hedstrom L, Tonge PJ.** 2003. Structure-activity studies of the inhibition of FabI, the enoyl reductase from *Escherichia coli*, by triclosan: kinetic analysis of mutant FabIs. *Biochemistry* **42:**4406–4413.

69. **Pal C, Bengtsson-Palme J, Kristiansson E, Larsson DG.** 2015. Co-occurrence of resistance genes to antibiotics, biocides and metals reveals novel insights into their co-selection potential. *BMC Genomics* **16:**964.

70. **U.S. Department of Agriculture (USDA).** *Maximum Residue Limits (MRL) Database.* USDA, Washington, DC. http://www.fas.usda.gov/maximum-residue-limits-mrl-database. Accessed 19 July 2017.

71. **Mathers AJ, Peirano G, Pitout JD.** 2015. The role of epidemic resistance plasmids and international high-risk clones in the spread of multidrug-resistant *Enterobacteriaceae*. *Clin Microbiol Rev* **28:**565–591.

72. **McNally A, Oren Y, Kelly D, Pascoe B, Dunn S, Sreecharan T, Vehkala M, Välimäki N, Prentice MB, Ashour A, Avram O, Pupko T, Dobrindt U, Literak I, Guenther S, Schaufler K, Wieler LH, Zhiyong Z, Sheppard SK, McInerney JO, Corander J.** 2016. Combined analysis of variation in core, accessory and regulatory genome regions provides a super-resolution view into the evolution of bacterial populations. *PLoS Genet* **12:** e1006280.

73. **Enne VI, Bennett PM, Livermore DM, Hall LM.** 2004. Enhancement of host fitness by the *sul2*-coding plasmid p9123 in the absence of selective pressure. *J Antimicrob Chemother* **53:** 958–963.

74. **Dionisio F, Conceição IC, Marques AC, Fernandes L, Gordo I.** 2005. The evolution of a conjugative plasmid and its ability to increase bacterial fitness. *Biol Lett* **1:**250–252.

75. **Yates CM, Shaw DJ, Roe AJ, Woolhouse ME, Amyes SG.** 2006. Enhancement of bacterial competitive fitness by apramycin resistance plasmids from non-pathogenic *Escherichia coli*. *Biol Lett* **2:**463–465.

76. **Bouma JE, Lenski RE.** 1988. Evolution of a bacteria/plasmid association. *Nature* **335:**351–352.

77. **Starikova I, Al-Haroni M, Werner G, Roberts AP, Sørum V, Nielsen KM, Johnsen PJ.** 2013. Fitness costs of various mobile genetic elements in *Enterococcus faecium* and *Enterococcus faecalis*. *J Antimicrob Chemother* **68:**2755–2765.

78. **Andersson DI, Hughes D.** 2010. Antibiotic resistance and its cost: is it possible to reverse resistance? *Nat Rev Microbiol* **8:**260–271.

79. **Hughes D, Andersson DI.** 2015. Evolutionary consequences of drug resistance: shared principles across diverse targets and organisms. *Nat Rev Genet* **16:**459–471.

80. **Cirz RT, Romesberg FE.** 2006. Induction and inhibition of ciprofloxacin resistance-conferring mutations in hypermutator bacteria. *Antimicrob Agents Chemother* **50:**220–225.

81. **Alam MK, Alhhazmi A, DeCoteau JF, Luo Y, Geyer CR.** 2016. RecA inhibitors potentiate antibiotic activity and block evolution of antibiotic resistance. *Cell Chem Biol* **23:**381–391.

82. **Culyba MJ, Mo CY, Kohli RM.** 2015. Targets for combating the evolution of acquired antibiotic resistance. *Biochemistry* **54:**3573–3582.

83. **Getino M, Sanabria-Ríos DJ, Fernández-López R, Campos-Gómez J, Sánchez-López JM, Fernández A, Carballeira NM, de la Cruz F.** 2015. Synthetic fatty acids prevent plasmid-mediated horizontal gene transfer. *mBio* **6:** e01032-e15.

84. **Kim S, Lieberman TD, Kishony R.** 2014. Alternating antibiotic treatments constrain evolutionary paths to multidrug resistance. *Proc Natl Acad Sci U S A* **111:**14494–14499.

85. **Imamovic L, Sommer MO.** 2013. Use of collateral sensitivity networks to design drug cycling protocols that avoid resistance development. *Sci Transl Med* **5:**204ra132.

86. **Lázár V, Nagy I, Spohn R, Csörgő B, Györkei Á, Nyerges Á, Horváth B, Vörös A, Busa-Fekete R, Hrtyan M, Bogos B, Méhi O, Fekete G, Szappanos B, Kégl B, Papp B, Pál C.** 2014. Genome-wide analysis captures the determinants of the antibiotic cross-resistance interaction network. *Nat Commun* **5:**4352.

87. **Blair JM, Webber MA, Baylay AJ, Ogbolu DO, Piddock LJ.** 2015. Molecular mechanisms of antibiotic resistance. *Nat Rev Microbiol* **13:**42–51.

88. **Liu YY, Wang Y, Walsh TR, Yi LX, Zhang R, Spencer J, Doi Y, Tian G, Dong B, Huang X, Yu LF, Gu D, Ren H, Chen X, Lv L, He D, Zhou H, Liang Z, Liu JH, Shen J.** 2016. Emergence of plasmid-mediated colistin resistance mechanism MCR-1 in animals and human beings in China: a microbiological and molecular biological study. *Lancet Infect Dis* **16:**161–168.

89. **Hakenbeck R, Brückner R, Denapaite D, Maurer P.** 2012. Molecular mechanisms of β-lactam resistance in *Streptococcus pneumoniae*. *Future Microbiol* **7:**395–410.

90. **Tapsall JW.** 2009. *Neisseria gonorrhoeae* and emerging resistance to extended spectrum cephalosporins. *Curr Opin Infect Dis* **22:**87–91.

91. **Finlay BB, Falkow S.** 1997. Common themes in microbial pathogenicity revisited. *Microbiol Mol Biol Rev* **61:**136–169.

92. **von Wintersdorff CJ, Penders J, van Niekerk JM, Mills ND, Majumder S, van Alphen LB, Savelkoul PH, Wolffs PF.** 2016. Dissemination of antimicrobial resistance in microbial ecosystems through horizontal gene transfer. *Front Microbiol* **7:**173.

93. **Butala M, Zgur-Bertok D, Busby SJ.** 2009. The bacterial LexA transcriptional repressor. *Cell Mol Life Sci* **66:**82–93.

94. **Drlica K, Zhao X.** 1997. DNA gyrase, topoisomerase IV, and the 4-quinolones. *Microbiol Mol Biol Rev* **61:**377–392.

95. **Maiques E, Ubeda C, Campoy S, Salvador N, Lasa I, Novick RP, Barbé J, Penadés JR.** 2006. β-Lactam antibiotics induce the SOS response and horizontal transfer of virulence factors in *Staphylococcus aureus*. *J Bacteriol* **188:** 2726–2729.

96. **Lewin CS, Amyes SG.** 1991. The role of the SOS response in bacteria exposed to zidovudine or trimethoprim. *J Med Microbiol* **34:**329–332.

97. **Baharoglu Z, Mazel D.** 2011. *Vibrio cholerae* triggers SOS and mutagenesis in response to a wide range of antibiotics: a route towards multiresistance. *Antimicrob Agents Chemother* **55:**2438–2441.

98. **Beaber JW, Hochhut B, Waldor MK.** 2004. SOS response promotes horizontal dissemination of antibiotic resistance genes. *Nature* **427:**72–74.

99. **Ubeda C, Maiques E, Knecht E, Lasa I, Novick RP, Penadés JR.** 2005. Antibiotic-induced SOS response promotes horizontal dissemination of pathogenicity island-encoded virulence factors in staphylococci. *Mol Microbiol* **56:**836–844.

100. **Chen J, Novick RP.** 2009. Phage-mediated intergeneric transfer of toxin genes. *Science* **323:** 139–141.

101. **Zhang X, McDaniel AD, Wolf LE, Keusch GT, Waldor MK, Acheson DW.** 2000. Quinolone antibiotics induce Shiga toxin-encoding bacteriophages, toxin production, and death in mice. *J Infect Dis* **181:**664–670.

102. **Bearson BL, Brunelle BW.** 2015. Fluoroquinolone induction of phage-mediated gene transfer in multidrug-resistant *Salmonella*. *Int J Antimicrob Agents* **46:**201–204.

103. **Torres OR, Korman RZ, Zahler SA, Dunny GM.** 1991. The conjugative transposon Tn*925*: enhancement of conjugal transfer by tetracycline in *Enterococcus faecalis* and mobilization of chromosomal genes in *Bacillus subtilis* and E. *faecalis*. *Mol Gen Genet* **225:**395–400.

104. **Stevens AM, Shoemaker NB, Li LY, Salyers AA.** 1993. Tetracycline regulation of genes on *Bacteroides* conjugative transposons. *J Bacteriol* **175:**6134–6141.

105. **Barr V, Barr K, Millar MR, Lacey RW.** 1986. Beta-lactam antibiotics increase the frequency of plasmid transfer in *Staphylococcus aureus*. *J Antimicrob Chemother* **17:**409–413.

106. **Prudhomme M, Attaiech L, Sanchez G, Martin B, Claverys JP.** 2006. Antibiotic stress induces genetic transformability in the human pathogen *Streptococcus pneumoniae*. *Science* **313:**89–92.

107. **López E, Elez M, Matic I, Blázquez J.** 2007. Antibiotic-mediated recombination: ciprofloxacin stimulates SOS-independent recombination of divergent sequences in *Escherichia coli*. *Mol Microbiol* **64:**83–93.

108. **Guerin E, Cambray G, Sanchez-Alberola N, Campoy S, Erill I, Da Re S, Gonzalez-Zorn B, Barbé J, Ploy MC, Mazel D.** 2009. The SOS response controls integron recombination. *Science* **324:**1034.

109. **Hocquet D, Llanes C, Thouverez M, Kulasekara HD, Bertrand X, Plésiat P, Mazel D, Miller SI.** 2012. Evidence for induction of integron-based antibiotic resistance by the SOS response in a clinical setting. *PLoS Pathog* **8:**e1002778.

110. **Williams JJ, Hergenrother PJ.** 2008. Exposing plasmids as the Achilles' heel of drug-resistant bacteria. *Curr Opin Chem Biol* **12:**389–399.

111. **Spengler G, Molnár A, Schelz Z, Amaral L, Sharples D, Molnár J.** 2006. The mechanism of plasmid curing in bacteria. *Curr Drug Targets* **7:**823–841.

112. **Fernandez-Lopez R, Machón C, Longshaw CM, Martin S, Molin S, Zechner EL, Espinosa M, Lanka E, de la Cruz F.** 2005. Unsaturated fatty acids are inhibitors of bacterial conjugation. *Microbiology* **151:**3517–3526.

113. **Ripoll-Rozada J, García-Cazorla Y, Getino M, Machón C, Sanabria-Ríos D, de la Cruz F, Cabezón E, Arechaga I.** 2016. Type IV traffic ATPase TrwD as molecular target to inhibit bacterial conjugation. *Mol Microbiol* **100:**912–921.

114. **Getino M, Fernández-López R, Palencia-Gándara C, Campos-Gómez J, Sánchez-López JM, Martínez M, Fernández A, de la Cruz F.** 2016. Tanzawaic acids, a chemically novel set of bacterial conjugation inhibitors. *PLoS One* **11:** e0148098.

115. **Machado AM, Sommer MO.** 2014. Human intestinal cells modulate conjugational transfer of multidrug resistance plasmids between clinical *Escherichia coli* isolates. *PLoS One* **9:**e100739.

116. **Cirz RT, Chin JK, Andes DR, de Crécy-Lagard V, Craig WA, Romesberg FE.** 2005. Inhibition of mutation and combating the evolution of antibiotic resistance. *PLoS Biol* **3:**e176.

117. **Mo CY, Manning SA, Roggiani M, Culyba MJ, Samuels AN, Sniegowski PD, Goulian M, Kohli RM.** 2016. Systematically altering bacterial SOS activity under stress reveals therapeutic strategies for potentiating antibiotics. *mSphere* **1:**e00163-16.

118. **Wigle TJ, Sexton JZ, Gromova AV, Hadimani MB, Hughes MA, Smith GR, Yeh LA, Singleton SF.** 2009. Inhibitors of RecA activity discovered by high-throughput screening: cell-permeable small molecules attenuate the SOS response in *Escherichia coli. J Biomol Screen* **14:**1092–1101.

119. **Peng Q, Zhou S, Yao F, Hou B, Huang Y, Hua D, Zheng Y, Qian Y.** 2011. Baicalein suppresses the SOS response system of *Staphylococcus aureus* induced by ciprofloxacin. *Cell Physiol Biochem* **28:**1045–1050.

120. **Nautiyal A, Patil KN, Muniyappa K.** 2014. Suramin is a potent and selective inhibitor of *Mycobacterium tuberculosis* RecA protein and the SOS response: RecA as a potential target for antibacterial drug discovery. *J Antimicrob Chemother* **69:**1834–1843.

121. **Holmes AH, Moore LS, Sundsfjord A, Steinbakk M, Regmi S, Karkey A, Guerin PJ, Piddock LJ.** 2016. Understanding the mechanisms and drivers of antimicrobial resistance. *Lancet* **387:**176–187.

122. **Yates TA, Khan PY, Knight GM, Taylor JG, McHugh TD, Lipman M, White RG, Cohen T, Cobelens FG, Wood R, Moore DA, Abubakar I.** 2016. The transmission of *Mycobacterium tuberculosis* in high burden settings. *Lancet Infect Dis* **16:**227–238.

123. **Aarestrup FM.** 2015. The livestock reservoir for antimicrobial resistance: a personal view on changing patterns of risks, effects of interventions and the way forward. *Philos Trans R Soc Lond B Biol Sci* **370:**20140085.

124. **Huijbers PM, Blaak H, de Jong MC, Graat EA, Vandenbroucke-Grauls CM, de Roda Husman AM.** 2015. Role of the environment in the transmission of antimicrobial resistance to humans: a review. *Environ Sci Technol* **49:**11993–12004.

125. **Arnold KE, Williams NJ, Bennett M.** 2016. 'Disperse abroad in the land': the role of wildlife in the dissemination of antimicrobial resistance. *Biol Lett* **12:**12.

126. **Croxen MA, Finlay BB.** 2010. Molecular mechanisms of *Escherichia coli* pathogenicity. *Nat Rev Microbiol* **8:**26–38.

127. **Nicolas-Chanoine MH, Bertrand X, Madec JY.** 2014. *Escherichia coli* ST131, an intriguing clonal group. *Clin Microbiol Rev* **27:**543–574.

128. **Nicolas-Chanoine MH, Blanco J, Leflon-Guibout V, Demarty R, Alonso MP, Caniça MM, Park YJ, Lavigne JP, Pitout J, Johnson JR.** 2008. Intercontinental emergence of *Escherichia coli* clone O25:H4-ST131 producing CTX-M-15. *J Antimicrob Chemother* **61:**273–281.

129. **Coque TM, Novais A, Carattoli A, Poirel L, Pitout J, Peixe L, Baquero F, Cantón R, Nordmann P.** 2008. Dissemination of clonally related *Escherichia coli* strains expressing extended-spectrum β-lactamase CTX-M-15. *Emerg Infect Dis* **14:**195–200.

130. **Johnson JR, Tchesnokova V, Johnston B, Clabots C, Roberts PL, Billig M, Riddell K, Rogers P, Qin X, Butler-Wu S, Price LB, Aziz M, Nicolas-Chanoine MH, Debroy C, Robicsek A, Hansen G, Urban C, Platell J, Trott DJ, Zhanel G, Weissman SJ, Cookson BT, Fang FC, Limaye AP, Scholes D, Chattopadhyay S, Hooper DC, Sokurenko EV.** 2013. Abrupt emergence of a single dominant multidrug-

resistant strain of *Escherichia coli*. *J Infect Dis* **207**:919–928.

131. **Price LB, Johnson JR, Aziz M, Clabots C, Johnston B, Tchesnokova V, Nordstrom L, Billig M, Chattopadhyay S, Stegger M, Andersen PS, Pearson T, Riddell K, Rogers P, Scholes D, Kahl B, Keim P, Sokurenko EV.** 2013. The epidemic of extended-spectrum-β-lactamase-producing *Escherichia coli* ST131 is driven by a single highly pathogenic subclone, H30-Rx. *mBio* **4**:e00377-e13.

132. **Woodford N, Carattoli A, Karisik E, Underwood A, Ellington MJ, Livermore DM.** 2009. Complete nucleotide sequences of plasmids pEK204, pEK499, and pEK516, encoding CTX-M enzymes in three major *Escherichia coli* lineages from the United Kingdom, all belonging to the international O25:H4-ST131 clone. *Antimicrob Agents Chemother* **53**:4472–4482.

133. **Naseer U, Haldorsen B, Tofteland S, Hegstad K, Scheutz F, Simonsen GS, Sundsfjord A, Norwegian ESBL Study Group.** 2009. Molecular characterization of CTX-M-15-producing clinical isolates of *Escherichia coli* reveals the spread of multidrug-resistant ST131 (O25:H4) and ST964 (O102:H6) strains in Norway. *APMIS* **117**:526–536.

134. **Novais Â, Viana D, Baquero F, Martínez-Botas J, Cantón R, Coque TM.** 2012. Contribution of IncFII and broad-host IncA/C and IncN plasmids to the local expansion and diversification of phylogroup B2 *Escherichia coli* ST131 clones carrying bla$_{CTX-M-15}$ and qnrS1 genes. *Antimicrob Agents Chemother* **56**:2763–2766.

135. **Partridge SR, Ellem JA, Tetu SG, Zong Z, Paulsen IT, Iredell JR.** 2011. Complete sequence of pJIE143, a *pir*-type plasmid carrying ISEcp1-bla$_{CTX-M-15}$ from an *Escherichia coli* ST131 isolate. *Antimicrob Agents Chemother* **55**:5933–5935.

136. **Bonnin RA, Poirel L, Carattoli A, Nordmann P.** 2012. Characterization of an IncFII plasmid encoding NDM-1 from *Escherichia coli* ST131. *PLoS One* **7**:e34752.

137. **Mathers AJ, Peirano G, Pitout JD.** 2015. *Escherichia coli* ST131: the quintessential example of an international multiresistant high-risk clone. *Adv Appl Microbiol* **90**:109–154.

138. **Banerjee R, Johnson JR.** 2014. A new clone sweeps clean: the enigmatic emergence of *Escherichia coli* sequence type 131. *Antimicrob Agents Chemother* **58**:4997–5004.

139. **Hilty M, Betsch BY, Bögli-Stuber K, Heiniger N, Stadler M, Küffer M, Kronenberg A, Rohrer C, Aebi S, Endimiani A, Droz S, Mühlemann K.** 2012. Transmission dynamics of extended-spectrum β-lactamase-producing Enterobacte-riaceae in the tertiary care hospital and the household setting. *Clin Infect Dis* **55**:967–975.

140. **Johnson JR, Miller S, Johnston B, Clabots C, Debroy C.** 2009. Sharing of *Escherichia coli* sequence type ST131 and other multidrug-resistant and urovirulent *E. coli* strains among dogs and cats within a household. *J Clin Microbiol* **47**:3721–3725.

141. **Banerjee R, Robicsek A, Kuskowski MA, Porter S, Johnston BD, Sokurenko E, Tchesnokova V, Price LB, Johnson JR.** 2013. Molecular epidemiology of *Escherichia coli* sequence type 131 and its H30 and H30-Rx subclones among extended-spectrum-β-lactamase-positive and -negative *E. coli* clinical isolates from the Chicago region, 2007 to 2010. *Antimicrob Agents Chemother* **57**:6385–6388.

142. **Johnson TJ, Hargreaves M, Shaw K, Snippes P, Lynfield R, Aziz M, Price LB.** 2015. Complete genome sequence of a carbapenem-resistant extraintestinal pathogenic *Escherichia coli* strain belonging to the sequence type 131 H30R subclade. *Genome Announc* **3**:e00272-15.

143. **Accogli M, Giani T, Monaco M, Giufrè M, García-Fernández A, Conte V, D'Ancona F, Pantosti A, Rossolini GM, Cerquetti M.** 2014. Emergence of *Escherichia coli* ST131 sub-clone H30 producing VIM-1 and KPC-3 carbapenemases, Italy. *J Antimicrob Chemother* **69**:2293–2296.

144. **Cai JC, Zhang R, Hu YY, Zhou HW, Chen GX.** 2014. Emergence of *Escherichia coli* sequence type 131 isolates producing KPC-2 carbapenemase in China. *Antimicrob Agents Chemother* **58**:1146–1152.

145. **Naas T, Cuzon G, Gaillot O, Courcol R, Nordmann P.** 2011. When carbapenem-hydrolyzing β-lactamase Kpc meets *Escherichia coli* ST131 in France. *Antimicrob Agents Chemother* **55**:4933–4934.

146. **Stoesser N, Sheppard AE, Peirano G, Sebra RP, Lynch T, Anson LW, Kasarskis A, Motyl MR, Crook DW, Pitout JD.** 2016. First report of bla$_{IMP-14}$ on a plasmid harboring multiple drug resistance genes in *Escherichia coli* sequence type 131. *Antimicrob Agents Chemother* **60**:5068–5071.

147. **Ortega A, Sáez D, Bautista V, Fernández-Romero S, Lara N, Aracil B, Pérez-Vázquez M, Campos J, Oteo J, Spanish Collaborating Group for the Antibiotic Resistance Surveillance Programme.** 2016. Carbapenemase-producing *Escherichia coli* is becoming more prevalent in Spain mainly because of the polyclonal dissemination of OXA-48. *J Antimicrob Chemother* **71**:2131–2138.

148. **O'Hara JA, Hu F, Ahn C, Nelson J, Rivera JI, Pasculle AW, Doi Y.** 2014. Molecular epi-

demiology of KPC-producing *Escherichia coli*: occurrence of ST131-*fimH30* subclone harboring pKpQIL-like IncFIIk plasmid. *Antimicrob Agents Chemother* **58**:4234–4237.

149. **Peirano G, Bradford PA, Kazmierczak KM, Badal RE, Hackel M, Hoban DJ, Pitout JD.** 2014. Global incidence of carbapenemase-producing *Escherichia coli* ST131. *Emerg Infect Dis* **20**:1928–1931.

150. **World Health Organization (WHO).** 2014. *Antimicrobial Resistance: Global Report on Surveillance 2014*. WHO, Geneva, Switzerland.

151. **Walther-Rasmussen J, Høiby N.** 2007. Class A carbapenemases. *J Antimicrob Chemother* **60**: 470–482.

152. **Nordmann P, Cuzon G, Naas T.** 2009. The real threat of *Klebsiella pneumoniae* carbapenemase-producing bacteria. *Lancet Infect Dis* **9**:228–236.

153. **Chen L, Mathema B, Pitout JD, DeLeo FR, Kreiswirth BN.** 2014. Epidemic *Klebsiella pneumoniae* ST258 is a hybrid strain. *mBio* **5**:e01355-e14.

154. **Chen L, Mathema B, Chavda KD, DeLeo FR, Bonomo RA, Kreiswirth BN.** 2014. Carbapenemase-producing *Klebsiella pneumoniae*: molecular and genetic decoding. *Trends Microbiol* **22**:686–696.

155. **Liu Y, Wan LG, Deng Q, Cao XW, Yu Y, Xu QF.** 2015. First description of NDM-1-, KPC-2-, VIM-2- and IMP-4-producing *Klebsiella pneumoniae* strains in a single Chinese teaching hospital. *Epidemiol Infect* **143**:376–384.

156. **Voulgari E, Gartzonika C, Vrioni G, Politi L, Priavali E, Levidiotou-Stefanou S, Tsakris A.** 2014. The Balkan region: NDM-1-producing *Klebsiella pneumoniae* ST11 clonal strain causing outbreaks in Greece. *J Antimicrob Chemother* **69**: 2091–2097.

157. **Stoesser N, Sheppard AE, Pankhurst L, De Maio N, Moore CE, Sebra R, Turner P, Anson LW, Kasarskis A, Batty EM, Kos V, Wilson DJ, Phetsouvanh R, Wyllie D, Sokurenko E, Manges AR, Johnson TJ, Price LB, Peto TE,** Johnson JR, Didelot X, Walker AS, Crook DW, Modernizing Medical Microbiology Informatics Group (MMMIG). 2016. Evolutionary history of the global emergence of the *Escherichia coli* epidemic clone ST131. *mBio* **7**:e02162.

158. **Leekitcharoenphon P, Hendriksen RS, Le Hello S, Weill FX, Baggesen DL, Jun SR, Ussery DW, Lund O, Crook DW, Wilson DJ, Aarestrup FM.** 2016. Global genomic epidemiology of *Salmonella enterica* serovar Typhimurium DT104. *Appl Environ Microbiol* **82**:2516–2526.

159. **Fothergill JL, Walshaw MJ, Winstanley C.** 2012. Transmissible strains of *Pseudomonas aeruginosa* in cystic fibrosis lung infections. *Eur Respir J* **40**: 227–238.

160. **McCallum SJ, Gallagher MJ, Corkill JE, Hart CA, Ledson MJ, Walshaw MJ.** 2002. Spread of an epidemic *Pseudomonas aeruginosa* strain from a patient with cystic fibrosis (CF) to non-CF relatives. *Thorax* **57**:559–560.

161. **Brueggemann AB, Pai R, Crook DW, Beall B.** 2007. Vaccine escape recombinants emerge after pneumococcal vaccination in the United States. *PLoS Pathog* **3**:e168.

162. **Henriques-Normark B, Blomberg C, Dagerhamn J, Bättig P, Normark S.** 2008. The rise and fall of bacterial clones: *Streptococcus pneumoniae*. *Nat Rev Microbiol* **6**:827–837.

163. **Nasser W, Beres SB, Olsen RJ, Dean MA, Rice KA, Long SW, Kristinsson KG, Gottfredsson M, Vuopio J, Raisanen K, Caugant DA, Steinbakk M, Low DE, McGeer A, Darenberg J, Henriques-Normark B, Van Beneden CA, Hoffmann S, Musser JM.** 2014. Evolutionary pathway to increased virulence and epidemic group A *Streptococcus* disease derived from 3,615 genome sequences. *Proc Natl Acad Sci U S A* **111**: E1768–E1776.

164. **Ruer S, Pinotsis N, Steadman D, Waksman G, Remaut H.** 2015. Virulence-targeted antibacterials: concept, promise, and susceptibility to resistance mechanisms. *Chem Biol Drug Des* **86**: 379–399.

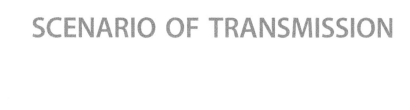

SCENARIO OF TRANSMISSION

Ecology and Evolution of Chromosomal Gene Transfer between Environmental Microorganisms and Pathogens

8

JOSÉ LUIS MARTÍNEZ[1]

INTRODUCTION

The evolution of living beings is a complex process, with a large degree of serendipity, in which the offspring displace the ancestors. Indeed, what we find in the current multicellular world, and more specifically in the animal world, are the last members of an evolutionary process; all other members in the same branch of the phylogenetic tree have disappeared. In this regard, most multicellular organisms can be considered as newcomers on Earth, which have appeared quite recently in evolutionary terms. Although there are still some progenitors that stand after the evolution of their siblings, the most common scenario for multicellular organisms is that ancestors disappear once the evolved progeny displace them (see the evolution of *Homo sapiens*). This type of recent evolution followed by extinction is not so frequent in the case of bacterial species, although it may have happened on some occasions (see the example of *Yersinia* described below). Indeed, the origin of different pathogens has been tracked to more than 100 million years ago, long before the human being (or an ancestor) was present on Earth (1). Despite this extremely long evolutionary time, which should have allowed for large diversification with the loss of ancestors, bacterial core genomes are remarkably

[1]Centro Nacional de Biotecnología, Consejo Superior de Investigaciones Científicas, Madrid, Spain.
Microbial Transmission in Biological Processes
Edited by Fernando Baquero, Emilio Bouza, J.A. Gutiérrez-Fuentes, and Teresa M. Coque
© 2018 American Society for Microbiology, Washington, DC
doi:10.1128/microbiolspec.MTBP-0006-2016

stable. It could be expected that the allelic variants of bacterial genes should cover nearly the entire potential spectrum of synonymous mutations and even those non-synonymous mutations without substantial associated fitness costs. However, today we can use multilocus sequence typing for distinguishing among different clones in bacterial populations, under the assumption that, at least for several of the core genome genes, fixation of mutations is not a frequent event (2). It then seems that, unless there is a major change in habitat, mutation-driven evolution is not the most important process in the speciation of bacteria in general, and in particular in the case of bacterial pathogens. A major force in such evolution, however, would be the acquisition of genetic elements (3–5), what has been dubbed evolution in quantum leaps (6). These acquired genes constitute the accessory genome of an organism and the pangenome of a given species (7).

If speciation is driven by the acquisition of novel genetic material, a full understanding of this process requires deciphering which is the origin of these elements, in particular those involved in antibiotic resistance and bacterial virulence; which are the bottlenecks involved in their transmission; and which are the consequences of the bacterial physiology of acquiring novel, adaptive traits through horizontal gene transfer (HGT).

If we take into consideration that most bacterial species evolved before the emergence of multicellularity and that the main process in their evolution is the shuffling from one bacterium to another of preexisting genes, a suitable conclusion would be that bacterial genes evolved in a unicellular world. In other words, elements that are dubbed virulence determinants or antibiotic resistance genes must have important functions besides those that they can play in human pathogens (8–12). These functions must be associated with the habitat of their original hosts, from which they have been transferred to the bacterial pathogens. Taking into

consideration the ancient origin of bacterial genes, which track to long before the emergence of human beings, the functions of these determinants should have ecological value in nonclinical, environmental ecosystems where the donors of virulence determinants and antibiotic resistance elements have evolved.

DIFFERENCES IN BACTERIAL SPECIES: GENERALISTS, SPECIALISTS, AND MULTISPECIALISTS

The recent capability of exploring a large number of genomes of different isolates belonging to the same bacterial species allows determination of which parts of the genome are shared by all (or most) members of such species and which parts are specific for a subset of members of the species and thus constitute the accessory genome (13–15). In principle, this may allow us to establish different categories of microorganisms. There are species whose members present large core genomes that allow them to colonize different ecosystems. Among such ecosystems, one of them can be the human host, and because of this some opportunistic pathogens, such as *Pseudomonas aeruginosa* or *Stenotrophomonas maltophilia*, are environmental bacteria that can infect immuno-compromised or debilitated patients using a set of virulence factors that are present in all members of the species (16). Indeed, it has been shown that environmental and clinical *P. aeruginosa* isolates are genetically and physiologically equivalent, indicating that this species does not present two phylogenetic branches, one composed of environmental microorganisms and another formed by virulent isolates (17–19). In addition, it has been shown that this microorganism can use the same virulence determinants for infecting different hosts, from plants to humans (20–22). Although some virulence determinants, such as the exotoxin ExoU, may have been acquired through HGT in *P. aeruginosa* (23) and HGT-acquired resistance genes are present in antibiotic-resistant isolates of this species (24, 25), most of its virulence and antibiotic resistance repertoire belongs to its core genome and is not derived from HGT-driven evolution.

Another category of pathogens is the specialists. This group comprises species in which most if not all members of the species are virulent for a few or specific hosts. Here it is worth distinguishing two groups. One is formed by pathogens, usually intracellular, presenting small genomes and for which HGT is not a major force in their evolution. Examples of this category are *Mycobacterium tuberculosis* and *Mycobacterium leprae*; these types of pathogens frequently colonize a single habitat (such as the mammal cell) and, as happens with endosymbionts (26–29), their pathway of evolution is genome reduction more than acquisition of novel traits. These microorganisms are well-adapted pathogens that have coevolved with their human hosts (30, 31). Whether or not this speciation process may end in commensalist or endosymbiotic behavior is beyond our current knowledge.

A different situation occurs with pathogens such as *Yersenia pestis*, which has evolved toward virulence from a nonvirulent ancestor by means of a pathway in which HGT has played a major role (32–38). Nevertheless, all members of the species contain the same HGT-acquired elements, which can be considered as belonging to the core genome of the microorganism, despite the fact that its current structure and the arrangement of genes within is the consequence of different HGT events. In addition, as in the case for the aforementioned intracellular pathogens, the evolution of this species toward infection has produced deadaptation for growing in other habitats, with the consequence that *Y. pestis* is a specialist, able to colonize just a small subset of different habitats, the most important ones being the different hosts involved in the transmission of and infection by this pathogen (see below).

Classical professional pathogens such as *Brucella melitensis* and *M. tuberculosis* that do not present a clear habitat outside their hosts are also likely within this category.

A final category may consist of the multispecialists. This category would include species that present ecotypes each capable of colonizing a subset of habitats. One of them is *Escherichia coli*; this bacterial species is formed by different clonal complexes, some of them commensals (of human or animals), others virulent, and some with an environmental habitat (39–46). Each of the groups has acquired its specific properties (for instance, virulence or capability of colonizing a specific host) through the incorporation of novel traits by means of HGT. Even more, in the case of pathogenic *E. coli* strains, there exist different clonal complexes producing different categories of infections in different hosts, each presenting a specific repertoire of virulence determinants (47). In this case, while the species as a whole can colonize a large number of habitats, each clonal complex presents specific ecological characteristics (niche specialization), and hence the species can be considered as a multispecialist. It is worth discussing whether some of these specific clonal complexes should be considered as independent species (such as the specialist *Shigella* when compared with some [likely also specialist] *E. coli* clonal complexes) themselves or, alternatively, whether their genomic structure and ecological behavior suggests they are in the route of speciation.

Based on their ecological behavior, there are then two broad categories of bacteria: those able to colonize a small range of habitats (specialists) and those with an ample distribution among ecosystems. For the latter, two categories emerge. If all members of the species can colonize all (or most) habitats, these bacteria are generalists. However, if the species presents different ecotypes, each able to differentially colonize a small range of habitats, I propose that these bacteria should be considered as multispecialists.

SPECIATION AND SHORT-SIGHTED EVOLUTION

Evolution is frequently supposed to work as an arrow in time, where each of the selected steps is consolidated and serves for further evolution toward diversification, which leads to the emergence of novel species. This classical view of gradual evolution does not usually fit well with the evolution of bacterial pathogens (and of microorganisms in general). For this category of living beings, the most important process in speciation is HGT, a mechanism by which bacteria acquire as a whole the required traits to colonize a novel habitat (15). This evolution in quantum leaps (48) is possible only in organisms, such as bacterial pathogens, where HGT is a frequent, or at least a selectable, event. However, the fact that the development of virulence, and in several cases of antibiotic resistance, involves the acquisition of foreign DNA does not mean that mutation and intragenomic recombination are not relevant for the evolution of pathogens. As we will describe in more detail later, the acquisition by HGT of elements that allow the colonization of a novel habitat is usually followed by the selection of mutants presenting a metabolism better fitted to the characteristics of the new environment. In addition, genome reduction is expected in the case of specialized pathogens that do not require all the traits required for colonizing a large number of different niches. The speciation process in bacterial pathogens should then usually include a first HGT event that allows the pathogen to enter and colonize the new host, followed by further acquisition of novel genes and fine-tuning of the bacterial physiology by means of mutation and genome reduction (49).

It is important, however, to mention that the evolution of pathogens does not always lead to a speciation process. On several occasions, instead of an arrow, the evolution of microorganisms follows a circle in which bacteria acquire very similar mutations (or even mobile elements) when confronted with a

new habitat/injury, but this adapted branch disappears when selection disappears as well (8, 50, 51). This scenario, which has been named short-sighted evolution (Fig. 1), is a frequent evolutionary pattern for generalist pathogens that can colonize different habitats as well as for pathogens confronted with strong (deadly) selective pressures such as the presence of antibiotics. They are able to evolve under the new situation, but when they return to their original habitat, they can be outcompeted by the nonevolved remaining population.

An example of this is the evolution of *P. aeruginosa* during long-term chronic infections in cystic fibrosis and chronic obstructive pulmonary disease patients. Different studies have shown that these patients are infected by a bacterial clone that evolves during infection and that a similar pattern of evolution is observed in most patients (52, 53). Nevertheless, although some epidemic clones have been described, particularly in countries where patients are not segregated (54–58), the primary infective strain is frequently different for each patient, and its phenotype corresponds to a nonevolved strain. This may mean that the evolved strains are outcompeted when they are released from the chronically infected host. This possibility has been explained by means of a source/sink (51) behavior of generalist pathogens. The source/sink hypothesis states that when an organism is present in a large habitat (source) and colonizes a smaller habitat (sink), the adaptation to the sink produces deadaptation to the source, in which case the deadapted (evolved) bacteria will be outcompeted when returning to the source habitat (51). This may happen in the case of cystic fibrosis or chronic obstructive pulmonary disease, in which interpatient clonal transmission is not very a frequent event in most countries. The evolved strains adapted to the infected host (sink) return to their natural ecosystem (source), where they are most likely outcompeted by the wild-type strains. However, in the case of proficient interhost transmis-

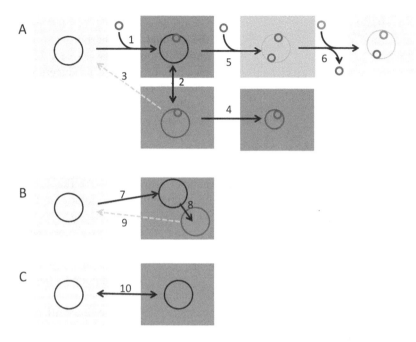

FIGURE 1 Evolutionary trajectories of bacterial pathogens. (A) The process of speciation of a pathogen (larger circles) such as *Y. pestis*. This process usually begins with the acquisition, by HGT, of a set of genes (red circle) that allow the shift of the pathogen's habitat from the environment to an infected host (1). If the rate of transmission is high enough, the newborn pathogen will disseminate among different individuals (2) and evolve by different mechanisms that include mutation and eventually genome reduction (4). These evolutionary processes might cause the deadaptation of the pathogen to its original habitat, in which case the chances of the microorganism recolonizing natural ecosystems will be low (3). Once the organism is a pathogen, it can change host specificity by acquiring novel genes (5) and eventually by losing of determinants unneeded in the novel host (6). In all cases, the integration of the acquired elements into the preformed bacterial metabolic and regulatory networks will be tuned by mutation. (B) The process of short-sighted evolution of opportunistic pathogens with an environmental origin, like *P. aeruginosa*. These microorganisms infect patients, presenting a basal disease, using virulence determinants already encoded in their genomes (7). During chronic infection, the infective strain evolves mainly by mutation and genome rearrangements (8). However, since it only infects people with a basal disease, transmission rates are usually low, which precludes clonal expansion and further diversification. Since adaptation to the new host is of no value for colonizing the environmental habitat (9), this is a dead-end evolutionary process. (C) The evolution of pathogens such as *V. cholerae* that present virulence determinants with a dual role in the environment and for infections, in which case the colonization of one of these two habitats does not severely compromise the colonization of the other (10). Reproduced with permission from reference 8.

sion, the evolved strains do not return to the source and further evolution, eventually leading to speciation may happens.

Although the term "short-sighted evolution" applies mainly to mutation-driven evolution, the same situation may arise in the case of HGT. Indeed, ecologically valuable genes (such as those for antibiotic resistance) can be transferred, but the acquisition of novel genes may impose a fitness cost, a fea-

ture that has been discussed in detail for antibiotic resistance genes and much less for virulence determinants, in which case they will disappear in the absence of selection (59, 60).

It has been suggested that HGT is rare in natural ecosystems (61). However, for detecting such transfer events, enrichment and eventually fixation are needed, and for fixation, positive selection is required. It is thus possible that HGT is more common than supposed in natural ecosystems, but we do not at the moment have the tools required to quantify transient transmission events that are not fixed in the population under selection pressure.

Evolution is frequently considered as a step-way nonreturn process. However, current information supports the idea that bacteria can explore evolutionary pathways without fixing the novel acquired traits. These "futile cycles" of evolution, which have been dubbed short-sighted evolution, likely play a fundamental role in the fast adaptation of bacterial populations to strong selective pressures such as the use of antibiotics.

ORIGIN AND FUNCTIONS OF ANTIBIOTIC RESISTANCE GENES

The most commonly used definition of antibiotic resistance, and consequently of antibiotic resistance genes, comes from the clinical world. An organism is resistant if the likelihood of treatment success is low. The genes contributing to this phenotype are antibiotic resistance genes and the mutations involved resistance mutations. The finding that some genes can be transferred and confer resistance to new hosts led to the hypothesis that these genes should also play the same role in their original hosts, where they evolved before being transferred to bacterial pathogens by HGT. When looking to the origin of resistance, it has been proposed that, since antibiotic producers need to protect themselves from the action of the antimicrobials they produce, they should be the source of resistance genes acquired by bacterial pathogens (62). Nevertheless, none of the resistance genes present in antibiotic producers has been found yet in a mobile element in a bacterial pathogen. It is true that both types of microorganisms present resistance genes belonging to the same functional families, but in the few cases in which the origin of HGT-acquired resistance genes has been tracked, the original hosts harboring them were not antibiotic producers (63–65). This does not mean that antibiotic producers cannot be a source of antibiotic resistance; rather, these results expand the potential origin of a mobile resistance gene to any bacteria present on Earth (66, 67).

While the function of resistance genes in producers as antibiotic decontaminant elements seems clear (62), the situation is not the same for non-antibiotic producers. Even in the case of antibiotic-inactivating enzymes present in antibiotic producers, a double function for them has been proposed: in addition to being involved in the degradation of the produced toxic compound, they can be involved in the modification of metabolic intermediates along the biosynthetic pathway (62). Concerning nonproducers, while resistance genes can serve on occasion to circumvent the activity of antibiotic inhibitors produced by competitors (68), in several cases current information does not support such a role. This is the situation for antibiotic resistance genes present in gut commensals, since producers of the antimicrobials currently in use for clinical practice have never been found in the gut microbiota. We can cite, among several others, the multidrug resistance (MDR) efflux pump AcrAB-TolC, a major determinant of antibiotic resistance in *Enterobacteriaceae*, whose actual function in these microorganisms is resisting the activity of bile salts (69, 70), a set of antibacterial detergents commonly found in the gut. Another widespread family of antibiotic resistance determinants is formed by the AmpC-type β-lactamases (71). Some of them have been found in plasmids, but on several occasions *ampC* genes are chromosomally encoded genes that belong to the bacterial core genome. It has been described that, besides contributing to antibiotic resistance, these enzymes can be involved in the building up and the recycling of the peptidoglycan layer (72–74). The same applies for other antibiotic resistance determinants, such as some aminoglycoside-inactivating enzymes that can recognize an antibiotic substrate because of its structural similarity to a peptidoglycan intermediate, which is the actual physiological substrate of the enzyme (75).

MDR efflux pumps are the group of clinically relevant antibiotic resistance determinants (76–79) for which the functions in natural ecosystems besides resistance have been better studied. In addition to helping to resist the activity of host-produced antibacterial compounds such as bile salts or antimicrobial peptides, it has been shown that such pumps can extrude quorum-sensing signal molecules, biocides, or plant-produced compounds, which indicates that their functions go beyond resisting the action of the antimicrobials currently in use in clinical practice (80–82).

We can thus conclude that what we have dubbed antibiotic resistance determinants might have a function in their environmental original host non-related with their capability of providing resistance to industrial antibiotics. However, their original, functional substrates are similar to antibiotics and hence are capable of modifying (antibiotic-inactivating enzymes) or extruding them (efflux pumps).

As stated above, this situation expands the number of potential donors of resistance to any bacteria on Earth. Any protein able to interact with the antibiotic or with its target in such a way that the action of the antimicrobial is impaired might also be a resistance determinant, irrespectively of whether or not its original function was impeding the action of antibiotics (9, 83, 84).

ECOLOGICAL VALUE OF VIRULENCE DETERMINANTS IN NONCLINICAL ECOSYSTEMS

The understanding of the ecology and evolution toward virulence of pathogens requires determining the needs and the benefits of the adaptation to a new habitat, the infected host.

As stated by Levin and Antia, "To pathogenic microparasites (viruses, bacteria, protozoa, or fungi), we and other mammals (living organisms at large) are little more than soft, thin-walled flasks of culture media" (85). In other words, the main reward of infection is gaining access to a new habitat that contains abundant and diversified nutrients (86) and where, at least in some cases (solid organ infection, prosthesis, bacteremia), the amounts of microbial competitors and of bacterial predators are low. For gaining access to the inside-host habitat, bacterial pathogens require two sets of elements. One of them is formed by those determinants required to resist the anti-infective host response. These elements include, among others, the innate immune response; the stomach's acidic pH; the production of antimicrobial compounds such as bile salts, antimicrobial peptides, or fatty acids; the host microbiota itself, which has anticolonization properties; and, more recently, the use of antibiotics, which can be considered as an anti-infective response product of the *cultural* human evolution (87). In addition to interfering with the host response, bacteria must present a metabolism capable of coping with the physicochemical characteristics of the *in-host* habitat. To produce an infection, a bacterium requires growing at 37°C as well as at the oxygen tension and at the osmolarity of host organs. In addition, it requires making use of the nutrients present in the human body, including harboring efficient iron-uptake systems, since iron availability is scarce inside the human body (88, 89). Some of the elements may deal with both aspects required for producing a proficient infection; this is the case for bacterial proteases that are used by microbial pathogens for degrading proteins involved in defense against infection and for disrupting the extracellular matrix, which are also useful for providing nutrients such as amino acids and peptides.

Even when a bacterial pathogen has evolved with the human ancestors (90) or when the only modification in the pathogen is the acquisition of elements allowing a host change from another organism to humans, what can be measured is the time frame since the acquisition of virulence determinants occurred. Indeed, the evolutionary history of HGT-acquired virulence genes differs from that of ancestral (core genome) genes (4). This indicates that the primary evolution of these determinants themselves occurred before their acquisition by the pathogen through HGT. Consequently, virulence determinants may have evolved outside the infective habitat, and hence they can have (as antibiotic resistance determinants) other functions beyond conferring on bacterial pathogens the capability of infecting the human host (8).

Some of the so-called virulence factors are involved in regular processes of bacterial physiology; these include iron-uptake systems, catabolic pathways, and structures involved in cell attachment (91–94). All these traits are relevant at the point of infection, but are relevant as well in other habitats presenting similar physiological requirements; for example, iron availability is low in most ecosystems and similar nutrients as those found in the human body can be found in other ecosystems. Cell attachment is needed as well for colonizing surfaces, in particular when detaching forces are acting (as with water bodies). For instance, *Vibrio cholerae* requires the colonization factor GbpA for attaching to epithelial surfaces and proficiently colonizing the intestinal tract. This colonization factor allows as well the bacterial attachment to chitin-containing shells of crustaceans present in coastal waters, the natural environmental habitat of *V. cholerae* (95).

A different situation may occur in the case of virulence factors playing more-specific roles in bacterial/host interactions. These include, among others, specific secretion systems capable of injecting a bacterial effector or a toxin straight inside the eukaryotic cell. In this case, an effect on novel bacterial metabolic capabilities is not expected.

Rather, they can be involved in general processes of interactions with multiple hosts. This is the case for *P. aeruginosa*, which produces a series of virulence determinants, such as siderophores, cyanide, proteases, or toxins, which are needed for infecting humans and also required for infecting plants, protozoans, worms, or insects (20–22, 96–99). If we take into consideration the evolutionary tree, it is conceivable that these virulence determinants evolved first for driving protozoan/bacterial interactions, likely before emergence of multicellularity, and have been coopted since for infecting other hosts, including humans. While prey/predator relationship might be in the basis of the evolution of these determinants, in other cases commensal interactions might play a role in their emergence. In favor of this possibility is the finding that several plant-associated bacteria present type III secretion systems, which function in mediating the plant/bacteria interactions (100). Coming back to the unicellular world, it is important to note that *Legionella pneumophila*, the causal agent of Legionnaires' disease, which is able to multiply into alveolar macrophages, is also capable of replicating inside amoebas and ciliated protozoa in its natural water habitat. Further, the mechanisms used by *L. pneumophila* for their intracellular growth are the same in macrophages and in its unicellular environmental hosts (101). Similarly, bacterial toxins that can harm the infected human host may have evolved to play a role in mediating predator/prey interactions. This may be the situation for the Shiga toxin, which, besides being a highly relevant virulence factor, allows bacteria to evade predation by the ciliate *Tetrahymena thermophila* (102, 103); or the *Listeria monocytogenes* listeriolysin O, which allows the intracellular survival of the pathogen during infection and induces lymphocytes' apoptosis. This major *L. monocytogenes* virulence determinant is needed for the survival of bacteria from predation by the bacterivorous ciliate *Tetrahymena pyriformis* (104).

To conclude, virulence determinants encoded in pathogenicity islands, which have been acquired by bacterial pathogens along their evolution, might be involved in intercellular interactions, including prey/predator and commensal interactions, as well as in regular aspects of bacterial metabolism in the nonclinical (environmental) ecosystems where the original hosts grow.

THE BUILDING UP OF A BACTERIAL PATHOGEN: *Y. PESTIS*, A RECENT CASE OF SPECIATION

As stated above, the acquisition by former nonvirulent organisms of novel traits into their genome allows for quantum leaps of evolution toward virulence (6, 48, 93). Since each pathogenic species (or clonal complex) shares the same or a very similar set of acquired virulence determinants, the evolution will be reflected in the clonal expansion of the strain that has acquired the virulence determinants (fitter in the new infective habitat than its ancestor), a situation that has been studied in the case of pathogens as *Bacillus anthracis*, *Y. pestis*, and *Francisella tularensis* (105).

With the description in 2011 of *Yersinia pekkanenii*, the genus *Yersinia* currently comprises 15 species (106); 3 of them, *Y. pestis*, *Y. pseudotuberculosis*, and *Y. enterocolitica*, are human pathogens (33, 36, 107). It has been shown that *Y. pestis* and *Y. pseudotuberculosis* diverged from *Y. enterocolitica* more than 40 million years ago, whereas *Y. pestis* is a clone that derived from *Y. pseudotuberculosis* less than 20,000 years ago (33, 36, 107). The successful expansion of the clone that is the origin of the *Y. pestis* species was caused by the incorporation into the genome of *Y. pseudotuberculosis* of a group of genes, the loss of others, and a final adaptation of the bacterial metabolism (Fig. 2). This novel set of determinants allowed the use by the emergent pathogen of a different transmission route through rodents and the bites of

infected fleas. In addition, the evolved microorganism produced a different kind of infection than its ancestor. Together, novel transmission routes and colonization of a different habitat within the human host allowed the expansion of a clone that is at the root of the *Y. pestis* speciation process. Indeed, *Y. pseudotuberculosis* is a foodborne pathogen that produces nonfatal gastrointestinal diseases, whereas *Y. pestis* has been the cause of septicemic, pneumonic, and bubonic plagues, which altogether have produced around 200 million deaths, and it is transmitted through inhalation or as the consequence of the bite by an infected flea (108). This recent process of speciation has required the acquisition of some genes and the loss of others as well. Among the latter, particularly relevant is the loss of insect toxins that will kill the insect host, impeding transmission of the pathogen. A higher capability of forming biofilms inside fleas has also improved the chances for interhost transmission to humans by bites of infected insects (32). It is important to note that, in addition to improving the transmissibility of *Y. pestis* to humans and consequently its epidemicity, another consequence of this evolutionary process is the adaptation of *Y. pestis* for acting as an insects' commensal. In addition to genome gain and loss, the evolution of *Y. pestis* involves the rewiring of the bacterial physiology to get a better adaptation for growing inside the host. This adaptation derives from the selection of mutants, mainly in regulatory elements (33), that are fitter for growing inside the infected host. A final step in the evolution of an organism might be the loss of those elements that are not required for colonizing the novel habitat. These processes of metabolic rewiring and genome reduction may impair the capabilities of the new virulent species for growing in the habitat of its ancestor, a situation that might further foster the speciation process.

Altogether, the studies on the reconstruction of the evolution of *Y. pestis* support the idea that, after a first HGT step, the acqui-

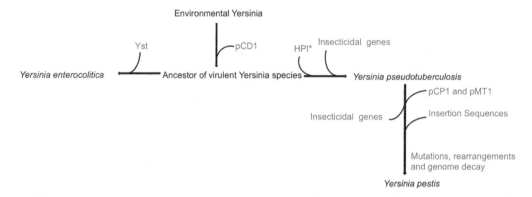

FIGURE 2 Evolution of *Y. pestis*. The process of *Y. pestis* speciation from an environmental, nonpathogenic ancestor is a good example of the evolutionary steps that are involved in the emergence of bacterial pathogens. This process began with the acquisition of the plasmid pCD1 by environmental *Yersinia*. This plasmid harbors genes encoding virulence determinants such as type III secretion systems and effector Yop proteins. From this ancestor of virulent *Yersinia* species, two branches have evolved. One diverged through the acquisition of the *Yersinia* stable toxin (Yst) and led to the speciation of *Y. enterocolitica*. This species has further evolved through acquisition and loss of genes (not shown in this figure). The other branch diverged through the acquisition of the high pathogenicity island (HPI*), which encodes an iron-uptake system and is present as well in different *Enterobacteriaceae*, and by the incorporation of insecticidal genes. *Y. pestis* is a successful clone that emerged recently from *Y. pseudotuberculosis* through the acquisition of the plasmids pCP1, which encodes the plasminogen activator gene, and pMT1, which allows colonization of the gut of fleas. The loss of insect toxins is an important event for the persistence of *Y. pestis* in its insect vectors. The acquisition of insertion sequences is the basis of the genome rearrangements and gene loss of *Y. pestis*. Finally, the entire process of adaptation to a new host is modulated by the mutation-driven optimization of the regulatory and metabolic networks of the pathogen. This evolutionary process is described in more detail in references 33, 37, and 105. Reproduced with permission from reference 8.

sition of other genes, together with genome reduction and selection of fitter mutants, foster the evolution of bacterial pathogens.

INSTANT EVOLUTION AND SPECIATION: TWO PATHWAYS IN THE EVOLUTION OF BACTERIAL PATHOGENS

The basic mechanisms of acquiring resistance genes and virulence factors are quite similar. It is true that virulence genes are more frequently present in large chromosomal arrangements (pathogenicity islands) and resistance genes are usually present in plasmids, but virulence plasmids and chromosomally encoded arrangements of resistance genes are also frequent, and combinations of virulence and antibiotic resistance genes in the same mobile element have been described (109–113). Despite these similarities in the genetic mechanisms of evolution, the consequences of acquiring virulence determinants or antibiotic resistance genes for the new host are completely different.

The acquisition of virulence determinants allows entry into a new habitat (the infected host). In the case that this also causes the deadaptation from the former ecosystem of the newly born pathogen, this situation is similar to geographic isolation (114, 115). This is the first step in a potential process of speciation, and hence the acquisition of virulence determinants by HGT is at the root of the speciation of bacterial pathogens (3–5).

The situation of antibiotic resistance is sharply different. From a human standpoint, resistance to antibiotics is a relevant process in the case of bacterial pathogens that have already gained access to the habitat that constitutes the human body. Resistance is needed for evasion of a deadly selective force, the presence of the antibiotic, and constitutes an instant evolutionary process (bacteria are resistant or they will die). Nevertheless, the reward is not the access to a new habitat, but just the possibility to keep multiplying in the old one, now polluted with antibiotics (87).

Although the acquisition of resistance can alter the bacterial metabolism and compensatory mutations can be selected after a first step in the evolution toward resistance (116–118), it is unsuitable that this situation should follow with a speciation process, as happens in the case of the acquisition of virulence determinants.

EXAPTATION AS A GENERAL PROCESS IN THE EVOLUTION OF BACTERIAL PATHOGENS

A common way of thinking is that evolution is a gradual process that operates through the sequential selection of minor genetic variants, each one rendering a fitter phenotype than the ancestor. Once the evolved variant is fixed, a novel genetic event occurs and the sequential selection of these improved variants is the basis of evolution. This gradual process, which explains well the selection of simple structures and traits, is more difficult to understand in the case of more complex systems that require being fully formed to be selected. One example of this is the feathers of birds. A bird can fly if it presents this complex structure. However, what are the selective forces behind the selection of intermediates between a regular hair and a feather if these evolutionary intermediates cannot be used for flying? For solving the problem of direct selection of complex systems, Gould introduced the concept of exaptation (119, 120). In the case of feathers, it is possible that their ancestors might have been gradually selected because of an improved capability (as compared with hair) for maintaining bird temperature homeostasis. This provides a potential selective force for this kind of structure. Only when the structure is complex enough will the bird will be able to fly, which constitutes an emerging property of feathers for which they were not previously selected during their evolution. The process of the acquisition of a new function is hence not driven by the selection of novel improved variants in a preexistent habitat but rather by a change of habitat where the novel selected properties can be used for a new function.

As we have seen before, antibiotic resistance genes and virulence determinants have evolved in their original hosts to play roles that are not necessarily resisting the presence of antibiotics or infecting a human host. Nevertheless, when confronted with the presence of antibiotics or when bacteria grow inside the new host, resistance and virulence are their more relevant functions. This situation fits well with the aforementioned type of adaptation in which evolution toward a new functionality happens as the consequence of a change of habitat more than because of the selection of a fitter variant.

While virulence determinants might have very similar roles in the natural environment and in the infected host, the situation is not the same in the case of antibiotic resistance genes. Indeed, a siderophore (88, 89) would produce the same effect for its bacterial host (getting iron) and a toxin may serve to kill a predator, which can be a unicellular protozoan or a macrophage, in which case the differences are more in the name of this element (virulence determinants) than in its actual function (getting nutrients and avoiding predators' activity in a given habitat). Nevertheless, in the case of antibiotic resistance genes, when they are transferred to a new host they are decoupled from the metabolic and regulatory networks of the host where they evolved. Further, the habitat colonized by the novel host does not necessarily contain the signals and cues for which the presence of these elements was needed. As an example, it has been shown that different *P. aeruginosa* efflux pumps can extrude quorum-sensing signals and their metabolic intermediates, suggesting that they can modulate the quorum-sensing response in this bacterial species (121–124). If these efflux pumps are acquired through HGT by a new host that does not produce the same quorum-sensing signals, they cannot play the role for which they were selected in nature. Under these circumstances of decontextualization, the unique function that HGT-acquired antibiotic resistance determinants may play is the one for which they have been selected after their transfer to a human pathogen: resistance to antimicrobials currently used for treating infectious diseases (Fig. 3).

The number of genes on Earth capable of conferring resistance to antibiotics is several orders of magnitude above those acquired by human pathogens. The introduction of antibiotics for therapeutic purposes has thus produced an enrichment of a specific subset of genes whose unique function is conferring resistance to antibiotics in an exaptation process that is a product of cultural human evolution (125–127).

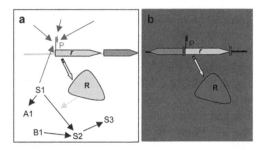

FIGURE 3 **Exaptation and gene decontextualization in the evolution of antibiotic resistance. Antibiotic resistance genes (*r*) have evolved for millions of years located in the chromosomes of their original hosts (a). During this evolution, the expression of these determinants (R) from their promoters (P) has been finely tuned to respond to several signals that might include the response to environmental and metabolic changes (blue arrows). Besides, the determinants encoded by these genes are integrated in physiological networks, where they can play a role as metabolic enzymes. S1 to S3 represent metabolites of the same pathway, and A1 and B1 metabolites of other interconnected pathways. When these genes are integrated in gene capture (for instance, an integron) and transfer units (for instance, a plasmid), they can be transferred to a new host and submitted to strong antibiotic selective pressure (b), and they can be constitutively expressed from a strong promoter (P) present in the capture unit and therefore lack the regulatory and physiological network encountered in the original host (gene decontextualization). Under these circumstances, the only function these determinants can play is antibiotic resistance, in such a way that this functional shift is not the consequence of adaptive changes in the determinants but rather of changes in their environment (exaptation). Reproduced with permission from reference 127.**

BOTTLENECKS IN THE ACQUISITION OF GENETIC ELEMENTS BY BACTERIAL PATHOGENS FROM ENVIRONMENTAL MICROORGANISMS

The increasing use of functional and sequence-based genomic and metagenomic approaches has demonstrated that genes capable of conferring resistance to antibiotics in a heterologous host are present in any ecosystem and in any bacteria. Although not studied in detail, a similar situation might also occur in the case of virulence determinants, which might eventually be present in nearly all metagenomes. In addition, similar virulence determinants are present in humans, animals, plants, and even protozoan pathogens. For the sake of simplicity and since information about virulence determinants in metage-

nomes has not been reviewed in depth, in this section I will mainly discuss the bottlenecks modulating the transfer of antibiotic resistance genes, although the conclusions are likely similar in the case of virulence determinants. In this context, it is worth mentioning that the variability of HGT-acquired antibiotic resistance genes is much lower than can be found in currently available metagenomes, which implies the existence of strong bottlenecks modulating the acquisition by bacterial pathogens of genetic elements from environmental microorganisms (11, 128).

The first one is ecological connectivity; the chances for the transfer of genetic material increase if the donor and the recipient bacteria are in the vicinity and belong to the same gene-exchange community. It is true that a chain of transfer events may allow the acquisition of an antibiotic resistance determinant by a bacterial pathogen even if the original host for this element is ecologically disconnected from this pathogen. Nevertheless, the success of this chain of transfer events would only be possible if selection operates along all steps. Because of this, although the first step in the acquisition of resistance determinants likely occurs in nonclinical, natural environments, where environmental and pathogenic microorganisms can encounter one another, the spread of these determinants occurs in places with high antibiotic loads such as hospitals and possibly other reservoirs like wastewater treatment plants, farms, and fisheries, in which selective pressure by antibiotics and other compounds, such as heavy metals or biocides, which are capable of select antibiotic resistance can be high on occasion (129–131).

The second bottleneck is the founder effect. Once a given bacterium has acquired a resistance gene, antibiotic selective pressure does not operate; bacteria are already resistant. Consequently, there is not any reward for incorporating a new gene conferring resistance to the antibiotic. If clonal expansion and HGT spread of the resistance determinant occur before such a second resistance gene is incorporated into the pathogens' population, the first one will spread among the population and the acquisition of novel resistance genes with the same antibiotic profile will be precluded. There are some situations in which the founder effect is a partial bottleneck (132). For instance, different elements conferring resistance to the same antibiotic can be selected at different geographic locations or in different clones if this happens

before the global spread of a single gene. Also, if the gene produces fitness costs (see below), extinction and reentrance episodes may occur, as well as the displacement of one resistance gene by a new, fitter one.

In the case of the acquisition of virulence determinants, the founder effect has a more drastic effect, since, as discussed above, the incorporation of traits that allow gaining access to the host may be the first step in a speciation process triggered through the clonal expansion of the clone that has acquired the novel traits. It is still possible that another clone from the same species incorporates a different subset of virulence determinants, but in this case the new evolved clone will be considered as belonging to a different clonal complex, as happens for intraintestinal and extraintestinal *E. coli* clones (133), which are not fully ecoequivalent. In the long term, this process can end in the speciation of the clones that have acquired different repertoires of virulence determinants.

The last bottleneck consists of fitness costs associated with the acquisition of novel genetic material (134–138). It has been suggested that these fitness costs should be the consequence of metabolic and energetic burden associated with the replication, transcription, and translation of the novel genes incorporated by the pathogen. If that is the case, the differences in fitness after incorporating one or another set of new genes will depend on the size of such genes as well as on the levels of their transcription and translation. Nevertheless, although some common trends can be found, different studies have shown that fitness costs associated with acquisition of antibiotic resistance and of foreign DNA depend on the type of gene, the environment, and even the microorganisms incorporating such genes (139–142). In addition, bacteria present mechanisms such as compensatory mutations or metabolic rewiring that ameliorate the costs of the acquisition of resistance (116, 118, 143–145). In this context, the fixation into the different members of the bacterial species of a new genetic element requires that it does not produce an unaffordable fitness cost or that fitness costs can be compensated (146). In the case of acquisition of antibiotic resistance, spread and fixation of the resistant strain requires low fitness costs in all habitats where these microorganisms can replicate, including natural, nonclinical ecosystems, where antibiotic selective pressure is low (147). However, in the case of virulence determinants, their incorporation may allow an increased fitness for colonizing the infected host at the cost of reducing the fitness for growing in their original environmental habitat. These differential fitness costs would be the basis of the speciation toward virulence of the new pathogen, which will be outcompeted by its ancestor in its original habitat while not having a competitor in the new one (infected host).

The number of genes capable of conferring antibiotic resistance present in available metagenomes is much larger than those currently acquired by human pathogens (83, 84, 129, 148, 149). This finding supports the premise that bottlenecks, such as the above-discussed ecological connectivity, founder effect, and fitness costs, modulate the acquisition, fixation, and spread of HGT-acquired genes in bacterial populations.

ACKNOWLEDGMENTS

My laboratory is supported by grants from the Spanish Ministry of Economy and Competitiveness (BIO2014-54507-R and JPI Water StARE JPIW2013-089-C02-01) and from the Instituto de Salud Carlos III (Spanish Network for Research on Infectious Diseases) (RD16/0016/0011).

CITATION

Martínez JL. 2017. Ecology and evolution of chromosomal gene transfer between environmental microorganisms and pathogens. Microbiol Spectrum 6(1):MTBP-0006-2016.

REFERENCES

1. **Ochman H, Groisman EA.** 1994. The origin and evolution of species differences in *Escherichia coli* and *Salmonella typhimurium*. *EXS* **69:**479–493.
2. **Maiden MC, Bygraves JA, Feil E, Morelli G, Russell JE, Urwin R, Zhang Q, Zhou J, Zurth K, Caugant DA, Feavers IM, Achtman M, Spratt BG.** 1998. Multilocus sequence typing: a portable approach to the identification of clones within populations of pathogenic microorganisms. *Proc Natl Acad Sci U S A* **95:**3140–3145.
3. **Achtman M, Wagner M.** 2008. Microbial diversity and the genetic nature of microbial species. *Nat Rev Microbiol* **6:**431–440.
4. **Ochman H, Lawrence JG, Groisman EA.** 2000. Lateral gene transfer and the nature of bacterial innovation. *Nature* **405:**299–304.
5. **Wiedenbeck J, Cohan FM.** 2011. Origins of bacterial diversity through horizontal genetic transfer and adaptation to new ecological niches. *FEMS Microbiol Rev* **35:**957–976.
6. **Groisman EA, Ochman H.** 1996. Pathogenicity islands: bacterial evolution in quantum leaps. *Cell* **87:**791–794.
7. **Rouli L, Merhej V, Fournier PE, Raoult D.** 2015. The bacterial pangenome as a new tool for analysing pathogenic bacteria. *New Microbes New Infect* **7:**72–85.
8. **Martínez JL.** 2013. Bacterial pathogens: from natural ecosystems to human hosts. *Environ Microbiol* **15:**325–333.
9. **Martínez JL.** 2008. Antibiotics and antibiotic resistance genes in natural environments. *Science* **321:**365–367.
10. **Martínez JL, Baquero F, Andersson DI.** 2007. Predicting antibiotic resistance. *Nat Rev Microbiol* **5:**958–965.
11. **Martinez JL, Fajardo A, Garmendia L, Hernandez A, Linares JF, Martínez-Solano L, Sánchez MB.** 2009. A global view of antibiotic resistance. *FEMS Microbiol Rev* **33:**44–65.
12. **Fajardo A, Linares JF, Martínez JL.** 2009. Towards an ecological approach to antibiotics and antibiotic resistance genes. *Clin Microbiol Infect* **15**(Suppl 1):14–16.
13. **Lukjancenko O, Wassenaar TM, Ussery DW.** 2010. Comparison of 61 sequenced *Escherichia coli* genomes. *Microb Ecol* **60:**708–720.
14. **Levin BR, Bergstrom CT.** 2000. Bacteria are different: observations, interpretations, speculations, and opinions about the mechanisms of adaptive evolution in prokaryotes. *Proc Natl Acad Sci U S A* **97:**6981–6985.
15. **Hacker J, Kaper JB.** 2000. Pathogenicity islands and the evolution of microbes. *Annu Rev Microbiol* **54:**641–679.

16. **Berg G, Martinez JL.** 2015. Friends or foes: can we make a distinction between beneficial and harmful strains of the *Stenotrophomonas malto-philia* complex? *Front Microbiol* **6:**241.

17. **Alonso A, Rojo F, Martínez JL.** 1999. Environmental and clinical isolates of *Pseudomonas aeruginosa* show pathogenic and biodegradative properties irrespective of their origin. *Environ Microbiol* **1:**421–430.

18. **Wiehlmann L, Wagner G, Cramer N, Siebert B, Gudowius P, Morales G, Köhler T, van Delden C, Weinel C, Slickers P, Tümmler B.** 2007. Population structure of *Pseudomonas aeruginosa*. *Proc Natl Acad Sci U S A* **104:**8101–8106.

19. **Morales G, Wiehlmann L, Gudowius P, van Delden C, Tümmler B, Martínez JL, Rojo F.** 2004. Structure of *Pseudomonas aeruginosa* populations analyzed by single nucleotide polymorphism and pulsed-field gel electrophoresis genotyping. *J Bacteriol* **186:**4228–4237.

20. **Rahme LG, Ausubel FM, Cao H, Drenkard E, Goumnerov BC, Lau GW, Mahajan-Miklos S, Plotnikova J, Tan MW, Tsongalis J, Walendziewicz CL, Tompkins RG.** 2000. Plants and animals share functionally common bacterial virulence factors. *Proc Natl Acad Sci U S A* **97:** 8815–8821.

21. **Mahajan-Miklos S, Rahme LG, Ausubel FM.** 2000. Elucidating the molecular mechanisms of bacterial virulence using non-mammalian hosts. *Mol Microbiol* **37:**981–988.

22. **Rahme LG, Stevens EJ, Wolfort SF, Shao J, Tompkins RG, Ausubel FM.** 1995. Common virulence factors for bacterial pathogenicity in plants and animals. *Science* **268:**1899–1902.

23. **Wolfgang MC, Kulasekara BR, Liang X, Boyd D, Wu K, Yang Q, Miyada CG, Lory S.** 2003. Conservation of genome content and virulence determinants among clinical and environmental isolates of *Pseudomonas aeruginosa. Proc Natl Acad Sci U S A* **100:**8484–8489.

24. **Libisch B, Gacs M, Csiszár K, Muzslay M, Rókusz L, Füzi M.** 2004. Isolation of an integron-borne bla_{VIM-4} type metallo-β-lactamase gene from a carbapenem-resistant *Pseudomonas aeruginosa* clinical isolate in Hungary. *Antimicrob Agents Chemother* **48:**3576–3578.

25. **Lee K, Lim JB, Yum JH, Yong D, Chong Y, Kim JM, Livermore DM.** 2002. bla_{VIM-2} cassette-containing novel integrons in metallo-β-lactamase-producing *Pseudomonas aeruginosa* and *Pseudomonas putida* isolates disseminated in a Korean hospital. *Antimicrob Agents Chemother* **46:**1053–1058.

26. **Yizhak K, Tuller T, Papp B, Ruppin E.** 2011. Metabolic modeling of endosymbiont genome

27. **Pérez-Brocal V, Gil R, Ramos S, Lamelas A, Postigo M, Michelena JM, Silva FJ, Moya A, Latorre A.** 2006. A small microbial genome: the end of a long symbiotic relationship? *Science* **314:**312–313.

28. **Gil R, Latorre A, Moya A.** 2004. Bacterial endosymbionts of insects: insights from comparative genomics. *Environ Microbiol* **6:**1109–1122.

29. **Tamas I, Klasson L, Canbäck B, Näslund AK, Eriksson AS, Wernegreen JJ, Sandström JP, Moran NA, Andersson SG.** 2002. 50 million years of genomic stasis in endosymbiotic bacteria. *Science* **296:**2376–2379.

30. **Brites D, Gagneux S.** 2015. Co-evolution of *Mycobacterium tuberculosis* and *Homo sapiens*. *Immunol Rev* **264:**6–24.

31. **Gagneux S.** 2012. Host-pathogen coevolution in human tuberculosis. *Philos Trans R Soc Lond B Biol Sci* **367:**850–859.

32. **Chouikha I, Hinnebusch BJ.** 2012. *Yersinia*—flea interactions and the evolution of the arthropod-borne transmission route of plague. *Curr Opin Microbiol* **15:**239–246.

33. **Zhou D, Yang R.** 2009. Molecular Darwinian evolution of virulence in *Yersinia pestis. Infect Immun* **77:**2242–2250.

34. **Lesic B, Carniel E.** 2005. Horizontal transfer of the high-pathogenicity island of *Yersinia pseudotuberculosis. J Bacteriol* **187:**3352–3358.

35. **Zhou D, Han Y, Song Y, Tong Z, Wang J, Guo Z, Pei D, Pang X, Zhai J, Li M, Cui B, Qi Z, Jin L, Dai R, Du Z, Bao J, Zhang X, Yu J, Wang J, Huang P, Yang R.** 2004. DNA microarray analysis of genome dynamics in *Yersinia pestis*: insights into bacterial genome microevolution and niche adaptation. *J Bacteriol* **186:**5138–5146.

36. **Achtman M, Morelli G, Zhu P, Wirth T, Diehl I, Kusecek B, Vogler AJ, Wagner DM, Allender CJ, Easterday WR, Chenal-Francisque V, Worsham P, Thomson NR, Parkhill J, Lindler LE, Carniel E, Keim P.** 2004. Microevolution and history of the plague bacillus, *Yersinia pestis*. *Proc Natl Acad Sci U S A* **101:**17837–17842.

37. **Wren BW.** 2003. The yersiniae—a model genus to study the rapid evolution of bacterial pathogens. *Nat Rev Microbiol* **1:**55–64.

38. **Achtman M, Zurth K, Morelli G, Torrea G, Guiyoule A, Carniel E.** 1999. *Yersinia pestis*, the cause of plague, is a recently emerged clone of *Yersinia pseudotuberculosis. Proc Natl Acad Sci U S A* **96:**14043–14048.

39. **Le Gall T, Clermont O, Gouriou S, Picard B, Nassif X, Denamur E, Tenaillon O.** 2007. Extraintestinal virulence is a coincidental by-product of commensalism in B2 phylogenetic group

Escherichia coli strains. *Mol Biol Evol* **24:**2373–2384.

40. **Smati M, Clermont O, Bleibtreu A, Fourreau F, David A, Daubié AS, Hignard C, Loison O, Picard B, Denamur E.** 2015. Quantitative analysis of commensal *Escherichia coli* populations reveals host-specific enterotypes at the intraspecies level. *MicrobiologyOpen* **4:**604–615.

41. **Zhang Y, Lin K.** 2012. A phylogenomic analysis of *Escherichia coli/Shigella* group: implications of genomic features associated with pathogenicity and ecological adaptation. *BMC Evol Biol* **12:**174.

42. **Alteri CJ, Mobley HL.** 2012. *Escherichia coli* physiology and metabolism dictates adaptation to diverse host microenvironments. *Curr Opin Microbiol* **15:**3–9.

43. **Carlos C, Pires MM, Stoppe NC, Hachich EM, Sato MI, Gomes TA, Amaral LA, Ottoboni LM.** 2010. *Escherichia coli* phylogenetic group determination and its application in the identification of the major animal source of fecal contamination. *BMC Microbiol* **10:**161.

44. **Luo C, Walk ST, Gordon DM, Feldgarden M, Tiedje JM, Konstantinidis KT.** 2011. Genome sequencing of environmental *Escherichia coli* expands understanding of the ecology and speciation of the model bacterial species. *Proc Natl Acad Sci U S A* **108:**7200–7205.

45. **Tenaillon O, Skurnik D, Picard B, Denamur E.** 2010. The population genetics of commensal *Escherichia coli*. *Nat Rev Microbiol* **8:**207–217.

46. **Milkman R.** 1997. Recombination and population structure in *Escherichia coli*. *Genetics* **146:**745–750.

47. **Wirth T, Falush D, Lan R, Colles F, Mensa P, Wieler LH, Karch H, Reeves PR, Maiden MC, Ochman H, Achtman M.** 2006. Sex and virulence in *Escherichia coli*: an evolutionary perspective. *Mol Microbiol* **60:**1136–1151.

48. **Heesemann J.** 2004. Darwin's principle of divergence revisited: small steps and quantum leaps set the path of microbial evolution. *Int J Med Microbiol* **294:**65–66.

49. **Ghosh AR.** 2013. Appraisal of microbial evolution to commensalism and pathogenicity in humans. *Clin Med Insights Gastroenterol* **6:**1–12.

50. **Levin BR, Bull JJ.** 1994. Short-sighted evolution and the virulence of pathogenic microorganisms. *Trends Microbiol* **2:**76–81.

51. **Sokurenko EV, Gomulkiewicz R, Dykhuizen DE.** 2006. Source-sink dynamics of virulence evolution. *Nat Rev Microbiol* **4:**548–555.

52. **Martínez-Solano L, Macia MD, Fajardo A, Oliver A, Martinez JL.** 2008. Chronic *Pseudomonas aeruginosa* infection in chronic obstructive pulmonary disease. *Clin Infect Dis* **47:**1526–1533.

53. **Oliver A, Cantón R, Campo P, Baquero F, Blázquez J.** 2000. High frequency of hypermutable *Pseudomonas aeruginosa* in cystic fibrosis lung infection. *Science* **288:**1251–1253.

54. **van Mansfeld R, de Vrankrijker A, Brimicombe R, Heijerman H, Teding van Berkhout F, Spitoni C, Grave S, van der Ent C, Wolfs T, Willems R, Bonten M.** 2016. The effect of strict segregation on *Pseudomonas aeruginosa* in cystic fibrosis patients. *PLoS One* **11:**e0157189.

55. **Wiehlmann L, Cramer N, Tümmler B.** 2015. Habitat-associated skew of clone abundance in the *Pseudomonas aeruginosa* population. *Environ Microbiol Rep* **7:**955–960.

56. **Oliver A, Mulet X, López-Causapé C, Juan C.** 2015. The increasing threat of *Pseudomonas aeruginosa* high-risk clones. *Drug Resist Updat* **21–22:**41–59.

57. **de Vrankrijker AM, Brimicombe RW, Wolfs TF, Heijerman HG, van Mansfeld R, van Berkhout FT, Willems RJ, Bonten MJ, van der Ent CK.** 2011. Clinical impact of a highly prevalent *Pseudomonas aeruginosa* clone in Dutch cystic fibrosis patients. *Clin Microbiol Infect* **17:**382–385.

58. **van Mansfeld R, Willems R, Brimicombe R, Heijerman H, van Berkhout FT, Wolfs T, van der Ent C, Bonten M.** 2009. *Pseudomonas aeruginosa* genotype prevalence in Dutch cystic fibrosis patients and age dependency of colonization by various *P. aeruginosa* sequence types. *J Clin Microbiol* **47:**4096–4101.

59. **San Millan A, Toll-Riera M, Qi Q, MacLean RC.** 2015. Interactions between horizontally acquired genes create a fitness cost in *Pseudomonas aeruginosa*. *Nat Commun* **6:**6845.

60. **Andersson DI, Hughes D.** 2010. Antibiotic resistance and its cost: is it possible to reverse resistance? *Nat Rev Microbiol* **8:**260–271.

61. **Forsberg KJ, Patel S, Gibson MK, Lauber CL, Knight R, Fierer N, Dantas G.** 2014. Bacterial phylogeny structures soil resistomes across habitats. *Nature* **509:**612–616.

62. **Benveniste R, Davies J.** 1973. Aminoglycoside antibiotic-inactivating enzymes in actinomycetes similar to those present in clinical isolates of antibiotic-resistant bacteria. *Proc Natl Acad Sci U S A* **70:**2276–2280.

63. **Poirel L, Rodriguez-Martinez JM, Mammeri H, Liard A, Nordmann P.** 2005. Origin of plasmid-mediated quinolone resistance determinant QnrA. *Antimicrob Agents Chemother* **49:**3523–3525.

64. **Humeniuk C, Arlet G, Gautier V, Grimont P, Labia R, Philippon A.** 2002. β-Lactamases of *Kluyvera ascorbata*, probable progenitors of some plasmid-encoded CTX-M types. *Antimicrob Agents Chemother* **46:**3045–3049.

65. **Yoon EJ, Goussard S, Touchon M, Krizova L, Cerqueira G, Murphy C, Lambert T, Grillot-Courvalin C, Nemec A, Courvalin P.** 2014. Origin in *Acinetobacter guillouiae* and dissemination of the aminoglycoside-modifying enzyme Aph(3′)-VI. *mBio* **5:**e01972-e14.

66. **Wright GD.** 2010. The antibiotic resistome. *Expert Opin Drug Discov* **5:**779–788.

67. **D'Costa VM, McGrann KM, Hughes DW, Wright GD.** 2006. Sampling the antibiotic resistome. *Science* **311:**374–377.

68. **Laskaris P, Tolba S, Calvo-Bado L, Wellington EM.** 2010. Coevolution of antibiotic production and counter-resistance in soil bacteria. *Environ Microbiol* **12:**783–796.

69. **Thanassi DG, Cheng LW, Nikaido H.** 1997. Active efflux of bile salts by *Escherichia coli*. *J Bacteriol* **179:**2512–2518.

70. **Ma D, Cook DN, Alberti M, Pon NG, Nikaido H, Hearst JE.** 1995. Genes *acrA* and *acrB* encode a stress-induced efflux system of *Escherichia coli*. *Mol Microbiol* **16:**45–55.

71. **Jacoby GA.** 2009. AmpC β-lactamases. *Clin Microbiol Rev* **22:**161–182.

72. **Morosini MI, Ayala JA, Baquero F, Martínez JL, Blázquez J.** 2000. Biological cost of AmpC production for *Salmonella enterica* serotype Typhimurium. *Antimicrob Agents Chemother* **44:**3137–3143.

73. **Wiedemann B, Pfeifle D, Wiegand I, Janas E.** 1998. β-Lactamase induction and cell wall recycling in gram-negative bacteria. *Drug Resist Updat* **1:**223–226.

74. **Henderson TA, Young KD, Denome SA, Elf PK.** 1997. AmpC and AmpH, proteins related to the class C β-lactamases, bind penicillin and contribute to the normal morphology of *Escherichia coli*. *J Bacteriol* **179:**6112–6121.

75. **Macinga DR, Rather PN.** 1999. The chromosomal 2′-*N*-acetyltransferase of *Providencia stuartii*: physiological functions and genetic regulation. *Front Biosci* **4:**D132–D140.

76. **Piddock LJ.** 2006. Clinically relevant chromosomally encoded multidrug resistance efflux pumps in bacteria. *Clin Microbiol Rev* **19:**382–402.

77. **Vila J, Martínez JL.** 2008. Clinical impact of the over-expression of efflux pump in nonfermentative Gram-negative bacilli, development of efflux pump inhibitors. *Curr Drug Targets* **9:**797–807.

78. **Li XZ, Plésiat P, Nikaido H.** 2015. The challenge of efflux-mediated antibiotic resistance in Gram-negative bacteria. *Clin Microbiol Rev* **28:**337–418.

79. **Hernando-Amado S, Blanco P, Alcalde-Rico M, Corona F, Reales-Calderón JA, Sánchez MB, Martínez JL.** 2016. Multidrug efflux pumps as main players in intrinsic and acquired resistance to antimicrobials. *Drug Resist Updat* **28:**13–27.

80. **Piddock LJ.** 2006. Multidrug-resistance efflux pumps—not just for resistance. *Nat Rev Microbiol* **4:**629–636.

81. **Alvarez-Ortega C, Olivares J, Martínez JL.** 2013. RND multidrug efflux pumps: what are they good for? *Front Microbiol* **4:**7.

82. **Martinez JL, Sánchez MB, Martínez-Solano L, Hernandez A, Garmendia L, Fajardo A, Alvarez-Ortega C.** 2009. Functional role of bacterial multidrug efflux pumps in microbial natural ecosystems. *FEMS Microbiol Rev* **33:**430–449.

83. **Martínez JL, Coque TM, Baquero F.** 2015. Prioritizing risks of antibiotic resistance genes in all metagenomes. *Nat Rev Microbiol* **13:**396.

84. **Martínez JL, Coque TM, Baquero F.** 2015. What is a resistance gene? Ranking risk in resistomes. *Nat Rev Microbiol* **13:**116–123.

85. **Levin BR, Antia R.** 2001. Why we don't get sick: the within-host population dynamics of bacterial infections. *Science* **292:**1112–1115.

86. **Eisenreich W, Dandekar T, Heesemann J, Goebel W.** 2010. Carbon metabolism of intracellular bacterial pathogens and possible links to virulence. *Nat Rev Microbiol* **8:**401–412.

87. **Martínez JL, Baquero F.** 2002. Interactions among strategies associated with bacterial infection: pathogenicity, epidemicity, and antibiotic resistance. *Clin Microbiol Rev* **15:**647–679.

88. **Martínez JL, Delgado-Iribarren A, Baquero F.** 1990. Mechanisms of iron acquisition and bacterial virulence. *FEMS Microbiol Rev* **6:**45–56.

89. **de Lorenzo V, Martinez JL.** 1988. Aerobactin production as a virulence factor: a reevaluation. *Eur J Clin Microbiol Infect Dis* **7:**621–629.

90. **Trueba G, Dunthorn M.** 2012. Many neglected tropical diseases may have originated in the Paleolithic or before: new insights from genetics. *PLoS Negl Trop Dis* **6:**e1393.

91. **Chouikha I, Germon P, Brée A, Gilot P, Moulin-Schouleur M, Schouler C.** 2006. A *selC*-associated genomic island of the extraintestinal avian pathogenic *Escherichia coli* strain BEN2908 is involved in carbohydrate uptake and virulence. *J Bacteriol* **188:**977–987.

92. **Luck SN, Turner SA, Rajakumar K, Sakellaris H, Adler B.** 2001. Ferric dicitrate transport system (Fec) of *Shigella flexneri* 2a YSH6000 is encoded on a novel pathogenicity island carrying multiple antibiotic resistance genes. *Infect Immun* **69:**6012–6021.

93. **Hacker J, Carniel E.** 2001. Ecological fitness, genomic islands and bacterial pathogenicity. A

Darwinian view of the evolution of microbes. *EMBO Rep* **2**:376–381.

94. **Schubert S, Rakin A, Karch H, Carniel E, Heesemann J.** 1998. Prevalence of the "high-pathogenicity island" of *Yersinia* species among *Escherichia coli* strains that are pathogenic to humans. *Infect Immun* **66**:480–485.

95. **Kirn TJ, Jude BA, Taylor RK.** 2005. A colonization factor links *Vibrio cholerae* environmental survival and human infection. *Nature* **438**:863–866.

96. **Miyata S, Casey M, Frank DW, Ausubel FM, Drenkard E.** 2003. Use of the *Galleria mellonella* caterpillar as a model host to study the role of the type III secretion system in *Pseudomonas aeruginosa* pathogenesis. *Infect Immun* **71**:2404–2413.

97. **Mahajan-Miklos S, Tan MW, Rahme LG, Ausubel FM.** 1999. Molecular mechanisms of bacterial virulence elucidated using a *Pseudomonas aeruginosa*-*Caenorhabditis elegans* pathogenesis model. *Cell* **96**:47–56.

98. **Carilla-Latorre S, Calvo-Garrido J, Bloomfield G, Skelton J, Kay RR, Ivens A, Martinez JL, Escalante R.** 2008. *Dictyostelium* transcriptional responses to *Pseudomonas aeruginosa*: common and specific effects from PAO1 and PA14 strains. *BMC Microbiol* **8**:109.

99. **Cosson P, Zulianello L, Join-Lambert O, Faurisson F, Gebbie L, Benghezal M, Van Delden C, Curty LK, Köhler T.** 2002. *Pseudomonas aeruginosa* virulence analyzed in a *Dictyostelium discoideum* host system. *J Bacteriol* **184**:3027–3033.

100. **Hueck CJ.** 1998. Type III protein secretion systems in bacterial pathogens of animals and plants. *Microbiol Mol Biol Rev* **62**:379–433.

101. **Gao LY, Harb OS, Abu Kwaik Y.** 1997. Utilization of similar mechanisms by *Legionella pneumophila* to parasitize two evolutionarily distant host cells, mammalian macrophages and protozoa. *Infect Immun* **65**:4738–4746.

102. **Lainhart W, Stolfa G, Koudelka GB.** 2009. Shiga toxin as a bacterial defense against a eukaryotic predator, *Tetrahymena thermophila*. *J Bacteriol* **191**:5116–5122.

103. **Steinberg KM, Levin BR.** 2007. Grazing protozoa and the evolution of the *Escherichia coli* O157:H7 Shiga toxin-encoding prophage. *Proc Biol Sci* **274**:1921–1929.

104. **Pushkareva VI, Ermolaeva SA.** 2010. *Listeria monocytogenes* virulence factor Listeriolysin O favors bacterial growth in co-culture with the ciliate *Tetrahymena pyriformis*, causes protozoan encystment and promotes bacterial survival inside cysts. *BMC Microbiol* **10**:26.

105. **Keim PS, Wagner DM.** 2009. Humans and evolutionary and ecological forces shaped the phylogeography of recently emerged diseases. *Nat Rev Microbiol* **7**:813–821.

106. **Murros-Kontiainen A, Johansson P, Niskanen T, Fredriksson-Ahomaa M, Korkeala H, Björkroth J.** 2011. *Yersinia pekkanenii* sp. nov. *Int J Syst Evol Microbiol* **61**:2363–2367.

107. **Morelli G, Song Y, Mazzoni CJ, Eppinger M, Roumagnac P, Wagner DM, Feldkamp M, Kusecek B, Vogler AJ, Li Y, Cui Y, Thomson NR, Jombart T, Leblois R, Lichtner P, Rahalison L, Petersen JM, Balloux F, Keim P, Wirth T, Ravel J, Yang R, Carniel E, Achtman M.** 2010. *Yersinia pestis* genome sequencing identifies patterns of global phylogenetic diversity. *Nat Genet* **42**:1140–1143.

108. **Perry RD, Fetherston JD.** 1997. *Yersinia pestis*—etiologic agent of plague. *Clin Microbiol Rev* **10**:35–66.

109. **Ramirez MS, Traglia GM, Lin DL, Tran T, Tolmasky ME.** 2014. Plasmid-mediated antibiotic resistance and virulence in Gram-negatives: the *Klebsiella pneumoniae* paradigm. *Microbiol Spectr* **2**:PLAS-0016-2013.

110. **Colonna B, Ranucci L, Fradiani PA, Casalino M, Calconi A, Nicoletti M.** 1992. Organization of aerobactin, hemolysin, and antibacterial resistance genes in lactose-negative *Escherichia coli* strains of serotype O4 isolated from children with diarrhea. *Infect Immun* **60**:5224–5231.

111. **Darfeuille-Michaud A, Jallat C, Aubel D, Sirot D, Rich C, Sirot J, Joly B.** 1992. R-plasmid-encoded adhesive factor in *Klebsiella pneumoniae* strains responsible for human nosocomial infections. *Infect Immun* **60**:44–55.

112. **Delgado-Iribarren A, Martinez-Suarez J, Baquero F, Perez-Diaz JC, Martinez JL.** 1987. Aerobactin-producing multi-resistance plasmids. *J Antimicrob Chemother* **19**:552–553.

113. **Martínez-Suárez JV, Martínez JL, López de Goicoechea MJ, Pérez-Díaz JC, Baquero F, Meseguer M, Liñares J.** 1987. Acquisition of antibiotic resistance plasmids in vivo by extraintestinal *Salmonella* spp. *J Antimicrob Chemother* **20**:452–453.

114. **Bentley SD, Parkhill J.** 2015. Genomic perspectives on the evolution and spread of bacterial pathogens. *Proc Biol Sci* **282**:20150488.

115. **de la Cruz F, Davies J.** 2000. Horizontal gene transfer and the origin of species: lessons from bacteria. *Trends Microbiol* **8**:128–133.

116. **Olivares J, Álvarez-Ortega C, Martínez JL.** 2014. Metabolic compensation of fitness costs associated with overexpression of the multidrug efflux pump MexEF-OprN in *Pseudomonas aeru-*

ginosa. Antimicrob Agents Chemother **58**:3904–3913.

117. **Schulz zur Wiesch P, Engelstädter J, Bonhoeffer S.** 2010. Compensation of fitness costs and reversibility of antibiotic resistance mutations. *Antimicrob Agents Chemother* **54**:2085–2095.

118. **Andersson DI.** 2006. The biological cost of mutational antibiotic resistance: any practical conclusions? *Curr Opin Microbiol* **9**:461–465.

119. **Gould SJ, Lloyd EA.** 1999. Individuality and adaptation across levels of selection: how shall we name and generalize the unit of Darwinism? *Proc Natl Acad Sci U S A* **96**:11904–11909.

120. **Gould SJ, Vrba S.** 1982. Exaptation: a missing term in the science of form. *Paleobiology* **8**:4–15.

121. **Olivares J, Alvarez-Ortega C, Linares JF, Rojo F, Köhler T, Martínez JL.** 2012. Overproduction of the multidrug efflux pump MexEF-OprN does not impair *Pseudomonas aeruginosa* fitness in competition tests, but produces specific changes in bacterial regulatory networks. *Environ Microbiol* **14**:1968–1981.

122. **Lamarche MG, Déziel E.** 2011. MexEF-OprN efflux pump exports the *Pseudomonas* quinolone signal (PQS) precursor HHQ (4-hydroxy-2-heptylquinoline). *PLoS One* **6**:e24310.

123. **Köhler T, van Delden C, Curty LK, Hamzehpour MM, Pechere JC.** 2001. Overexpression of the MexEF-OprN multidrug efflux system affects cell-to-cell signaling in *Pseudomonas aeruginosa. J Bacteriol* **183**:5213–5222.

124. **Evans K, Passador L, Srikumar R, Tsang E, Nezezon J, Poole K.** 1998. Influence of the MexAB-OprM multidrug efflux system on quorum sensing in *Pseudomonas aeruginosa. J Bacteriol* **180**:5443–5447.

125. **Martínez JL.** 2012. Natural antibiotic resistance and contamination by antibiotic resistance determinants: the two ages in the evolution of resistance to antimicrobials. *Front Microbiol* **3**:1.

126. **Martinez JL.** 2009. The role of natural environments in the evolution of resistance traits in pathogenic bacteria. *Proc Biol Sci* **276**:2521–2530.

127. **Baquero F, Alvarez-Ortega C, Martinez JL.** 2009. Ecology and evolution of antibiotic resistance. *Environ Microbiol Rep* **1**:469–476.

128. **Martínez JL.** 2012. Bottlenecks in the transferability of antibiotic resistance from natural ecosystems to human bacterial pathogens. *Front Microbiol* **2**:265.

129. **Berendonk TU, Manaia CM, Merlin C, Fatta-Kassinos D, Cytryn E, Walsh F, Bürgmann H, Sørum H, Norström M, Pons MN, Kreuzinger N, Huovinen P, Stefani S, Schwartz T, Kisand V, Baquero F, Martinez JL.** 2015. Tackling antibiotic resistance: the environmental framework. *Nat Rev Microbiol* **13**:310–317.

130. **Baquero F, Martínez JL, Cantón R.** 2008. Antibiotics and antibiotic resistance in water environments. *Curr Opin Biotechnol* **19**:260–265.

131. **Cabello FC, Godfrey HP, Tomova A, Ivanova L, Dölz H, Millanao A, Buschmann AH.** 2013. Antimicrobial use in aquaculture re-examined: its relevance to antimicrobial resistance and to animal and human health. *Environ Microbiol* **15**:1917–1942.

132. **Chen MY, Lira F, Liang HQ, Wu RT, Duan JH, Liao XP, Martínez JL, Liu YH, Sun J.** 2016. Multilevel selection of *bcrABDR*-mediated bacitracin resistance in *Enterococcus faecalis* from chicken farms. *Sci Rep* **6**:34895.

133. **Köhler CD, Dobrindt U.** 2011. What defines extraintestinal pathogenic *Escherichia coli*? *Int J Med Microbiol* **301**:642–647.

134. **San Millan A, Toll-Riera M, Qi Q, MacLean RC.** 2015. Interactions between horizontally acquired genes create a fitness cost in *Pseudomonas aeruginosa. Nat Commun* **6**:6845.

135. **Baltrus DA.** 2013. Exploring the costs of horizontal gene transfer. *Trends Ecol Evol* **28**:489–495.

136. **Starikova I, Harms K, Haugen P, Lunde TT, Primicerio R, Samuelsen Ø, Nielsen KM, Johnsen PJ.** 2012. A trade-off between the fitness cost of functional integrases and long-term stability of integrons. *PLoS Pathog* **8**:e1003043.

137. **Park C, Zhang J.** 2012. High expression hampers horizontal gene transfer. *Genome Biol Evol* **4**:523–532.

138. **Johnsen PJ, Levin BR.** 2010. Adjusting to alien genes. *Mol Microbiol* **75**:1061–1063.

139. **Knöppel A, Lind PA, Lustig U, Näsvall J, Andersson DI.** 2014. Minor fitness costs in an experimental model of horizontal gene transfer in bacteria. *Mol Biol Evol* **31**:1220–1227.

140. **Schaufler K, Semmler T, Pickard DJ, de Toro M, de la Cruz F, Wieler LH, Ewers C, Guenther S.** 2016. Carriage of extended-spectrum beta-lactamase-plasmids does not reduce fitness but enhances virulence in some strains of pandemic *E. coli* lineages. *Front Microbiol* **7**:336.

141. **Sánchez MB, Martínez JL.** 2012. Differential epigenetic compatibility of *qnr* antibiotic resistance determinants with the chromosome of *Escherichia coli. PLoS One* **7**:e35149.

142. **Björkman J, Nagaev I, Berg OG, Hughes D, Andersson DI.** 2000. Effects of environment on compensatory mutations to ameliorate costs of antibiotic resistance. *Science* **287**:1479–1482.

143. **Handel A, Regoes RR, Antia R.** 2006. The role of compensatory mutations in the emergence of drug resistance. *PLoS Comput Biol* **2**:e137.

144. **Maisnier-Patin S, Berg OG, Liljas L, Andersson DI.** 2002. Compensatory adaptation to the deleterious effect of antibiotic resistance in *Salmonella typhimurium. Mol Microbiol* **46:**355–366.

145. **Böttger EC, Springer B, Pletschette M, Sander P.** 1998. Fitness of antibiotic-resistant microorganisms and compensatory mutations. *Nat Med* **4:**1343–1344.

146. **Hernando-Amado S, Sanz-García F, Blanco P, Martínez JL.** 2017. Fitness costs associated with the acquisition of antibiotic resistance. *Essays Biochem* **61:**37–48.

147. **Martínez JL, Baquero F.** 2014. Emergence and spread of antibiotic resistance: setting a parameter space. *Ups J Med Sci* **119:**68–77.

148. **Fitzpatrick D, Walsh F.** 2016. Antibiotic resistance genes across a wide variety of metagenomes. *FEMS Microbiol Ecol* **92:**92.

149. **Hu Y, Yang X, Qin J, Lu N, Cheng G, Wu N, Pan Y, Li J, Zhu L, Wang X, Meng Z, Zhao F, Liu D, Ma J, Qin N, Xiang C, Xiao Y, Li L, Yang H, Wang J, Yang R, Gao GF, Wang J, Zhu B.** 2013. Metagenome-wide analysis of antibiotic resistance genes in a large cohort of human gut microbiota. *Nat Commun* **4:**2151.

Food-to-Humans Bacterial Transmission

PATRÍCIA ANTUNES,[1] CARLA NOVAIS,[2] and LUÍSA PEIXE[2]

INTRODUCTION

Food is considered one of the main environmental drivers shaping the human microbiota across the life span. Microorganisms vehiculated by food can be related to a variety of scenarios, including those benefiting health (e.g., stimulation of host antibodies, release of chemicals to stimulate the health of the overall system, or inhibition of pathogen development), those causing minimal change within the equilibrium of the host microbial community, and those that are pathogenic or have been associated with gut-host dysbiosis (1–3). Recently there has been an increase in knowledge on gut bacterial genera and species commonly affected by diet, as well as evidence suggesting that the intestinal microbiome plays an important role in modulating the risk of several chronic diseases (e.g., inflammatory bowel disease, obesity, type 2 diabetes, cardiovascular disease, and cancer) (1–3). Nevertheless, comprehensive information about the types of diet that transmit bacteria implicated in those diseases, as well as environmental and host factors favoring their colonization, remains scarce. Notwithstanding, food as a transmission mode for microorganisms reaching humans is extensively characterized for different pathogenic bacteria, the environment, animals, and humans being their main reservoirs

[1]Faculdade de Ciências da Nutrição e Alimentação, Universidade do Porto, Porto, Portugal; [2]Faculdade de Farmácia, Universidade do Porto, Porto, Portugal

Microbial Transmission in Biological Processes

Edited by Fernando Baquero, Emilio Bouza, J.A. Gutiérrez-Fuentes, and Teresa M. Coque

© 2018 American Society for Microbiology, Washington, DC

doi:10.1128/microbiolspec.MTBP-0019-2016

(Fig. 1) and the fecal-oral route their main transmission route (4–6). A triad including a contaminated food item, a susceptible human host, and bacterial pathogens able to survive and multiply in specific environmental conditions must be present for the occurrence of a foodborne disease. Nevertheless, transmission of typical foodborne pathogens can also occur more rarely by alternative transmission modes, as by direct contact of humans with infected animals or between humans (7).

In general, bacterial pathogens cause foodborne diseases by three mechanisms: ingestion of preformed toxins in foods (intoxication; e.g., *Staphylococcus aureus*), production of toxins within the gastrointestinal tract following ingestion of pathogens (food toxicoinfection; e.g., *Clostridium perfringens*), or invasion of the intestinal epithelial cells (infection; e.g., *Salmonella*) (6). Most foodborne bacterial pathogens are often associated with a self-limiting

gastroenteritis syndrome with nausea, vomiting, diarrhea, abdominal pain, and sometimes fever. Nevertheless, such bacteria might also cause severe illness with extraintestinal infections, postinfection sequelae, and even death, especially in individuals in high-risk groups (infants, young children, the elderly, and immunocompromised patients). Few bacterial pathogens (e.g., *Clostridium botulinum* and *Salmonella enterica* serovar Typhi) are associated with systemic clinical symptoms and more-severe clinical outcomes, even in individuals without risk factors (6).

In this review, we will focus on pathogenic bacteria for which food is conclusively demonstrated as their transmission mode to humans. The impact of foodborne diseases on public health, different scenarios evidencing relevant drivers for bacterial pathogen transmission, and the implication of the food chain in the widespread resistance to antibiotics that

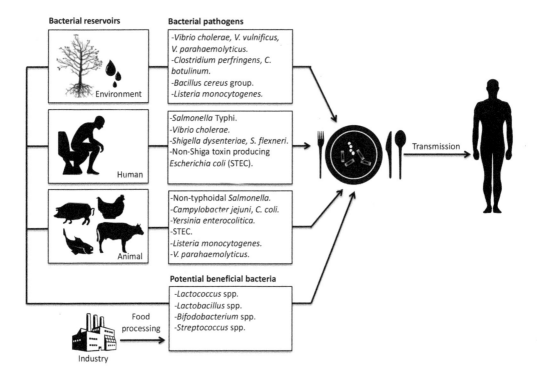

FIGURE 1 Reservoirs of the main pathogenic and potentially beneficial bacteria transmitted from food to humans.

is critical to the treatment of human infections will be presented.

FOODBORNE DISEASES
AND PUBLIC HEALTH

The first global estimates of foodborne diseases by the World Health Organization (WHO) indicate that about 1 in 10 people (600 million) around the world is sickened after eating contaminated food each year, with 420,000 deaths reported (8). The global burden of foodborne diseases has been measured in disability-adjusted life years (DALYs), which more fully capture disease symptoms and severity. In 2010, DALYs data showed the loss of 33 million healthy life years, most among children <5 years of age and in low-income countries (African and Southeast Asian regions) (8). The most frequent causes of foodborne disease worldwide are bacterial pathogens, the most important being the zoonotic *Campylobacter* and nontyphoidal *Salmonella* (NTS) (8). Certain diseases, such as those caused by NTS, are a public health concern across all regions of the world, in high- and low-income countries alike. Other diseases, such as typhoid fever, foodborne cholera, and those caused by pathogenic *Escherichia coli*, are much more common in low-income countries, while *Campylobacter* is an important pathogen in high-income countries (8). Besides the direct impact of foodborne diseases in human health, they also have health care, economic, and welfare costs, as in the case of the United Kingdom and the United States, where available data estimated a cost of £1.5 billion and of $14 billion, respectively (9, 10).

Currently, most human infections have a zoonotic origin, and ~75% of new and emerging pathogens originated from animals, including the foodborne ones (11). Transmission starts from the original habitat (the animal reservoir) to the food, along the complex farm-to-table pathway. Maintenance of a reservoir of zoonotic foodborne pathogens is favored by their transmission within the food animals and on-farm production environment, through diverse routes (e.g., contaminated feed and water, humans, rodents, and flies) (12).

Almost all type of foods (vehicles of transmission) can be contaminated by foodborne pathogens. Nevertheless, certain vehicles pose a greater threat than others, being classified as high-risk foods. They include raw or undercooked foods of animal origin (meat, poultry, eggs, fish, and milk) and, more recently, fresh produce (including leafy vegetables and sprouts) (13, 14). Also, food constituted with multiple ingredients and with a high level of handler manipulation has a greater potential to be associated with foodborne diseases (13). Some food types are considered unexpected vehicles of pathogens by the nature of the food matrices preventing microorganism multiplication, such as peanut butter, caramel apples, peppers, and chocolate. However, such food vehicles have been recently associated with large outbreaks, sometimes in wide geographic regions (15–19).

In recent decades, the epidemiology of foodborne outbreaks changed from acute and local to diffuse and widespread (e.g., geographically dispersed in many places at once), mostly due to production intensification and wide distribution of food (20–22). This challenge spurred the development of rapid and more sensitive molecular methods for foodborne pathogen surveillance, such as whole-genome sequencing (WGS). It became crucial not only to rapidly identify the responsible pathogen (classical and newly emergent ones) and source of origin (including the contexts that led to food contamination) but also to identify new or unsuspected transmission routes and to support public health interventions in global food markets (23, 24). For example, WGS has been applied to source attribution of campylobacteriosis (25, 26), outbreak investigations of salmonellosis (10, 18, 21, 27) and listeriosis (19, 28), as well as to differentiating persistent contamination by *Listeria monocytogenes* from reintroduction in food-associated environments (29). Beyond high-resolution subtyping, WGS could also allow characterization of foodborne pathogen virulence markers (linked to greater pathogenicity) and stress tolerance as well as antimicrobial resistance prediction, both features important to microbial risk assessment (23, 24). For example, in 2011, Shiga toxin-producing *E. coli* (STEC) O104:H4 caused one of the largest foodborne outbreaks of recent history, with >3,000 cases of infection and >40 deaths reported, in multiple European countries and North America. Within a week, WGS revealed that the unusually virulent outbreak strain belonged to a distinct group of enteroaggregative *E. coli* that had acquired the combination of genes coding for Shiga toxin 2, antimicrobial resistance, and other virulence factors (30). Despite the promising application of WGS to improve foodborne pathogen surveillance, the use of standardized methods that can be practiced among routine laboratories remains a challenge, namely, the selection of standardized analytical tools as well as epidemiologic interpretation of WGS data (23, 24).

DRIVERS OF FOOD-TO-HUMAN BACTERIAL PATHOGENIC TRANSMISSION

Several drivers have been identified to promote the increase of food-to-human bacterial pathogenic transmission and foodborne diseases worldwide by leading to the introduction and amplification of pathogens along the complex farm-to-human pathway (31–37). This section will address the driving factors promoting such events associated with the features of bacterial pathogens, the food chain, and the human host (Fig. 2). Diverse examples of transmission scenarios involving those drivers will be given.

Drivers Related to the Food Chain

Changes in the food chain, involving intensive and large-scale production and distribution, climate change, and globalization of food and live animal suppliers, are considered particu-

larly significant drivers for the emergence of foodborne diseases (34, 36).

Transmission Scenarios Related to Intensive and Large-Scale Food Production and Distribution

Shifts in food production, processing, and distribution during the last several decades have contributed to the increased risk and complexity of foodborne diseases, resulting in new opportunities for pathogen transmission to humans, particularly of zoonotic agents (e.g., *Salmonella* and *Campylobacter*). The increased demand for food due to worldwide population growth contributed to the growth of industrial-scale production systems, including intensification of animal production plus agriculture and large-scale food processing and distribution (31, 33).

Intensive livestock practices with high animal densities promote persistence and dissemination of zoonotic pathogens in food animals and farm production environments, leading to the maintenance of a reservoir of foodborne pathogens directly transmitted to foods of animal origin and indirectly to fresh produce (12). This is illustrated by pandemic *S. enterica* serovar Enteritidis in the 1980s and '90s, mostly attributed to intensive production of eggs/broilers, which was later overcome with successful control programs, including adequate biosecurity measures (38). More recently, in the European Union, contamination in the large turkey production chain was associated with a large outbreak of *S. enterica* serovar Stanley (39). Also, in the case of *Campylobacter* it was shown that the major contamination source of chicken meat was at the large production rearing farm (40). More recently, changing farming practices for free-range and organic animal production (allowing outdoor access for farm animals) have raised new questions about food safety, as this type of production is also associated with several hazards, including *Campylobacter* and *Salmonella* (41).

The intensification of vegetable and fruit production has been also associated with sev-

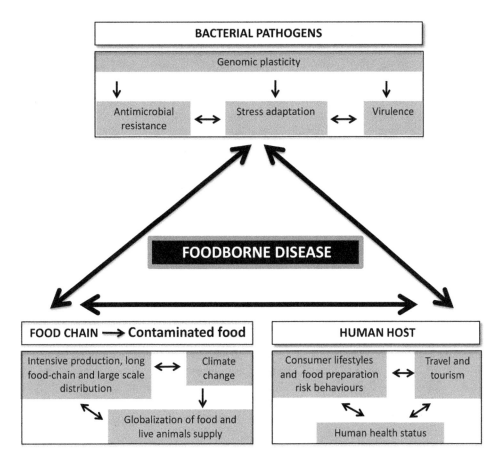

FIGURE 2 **Factors that drive transmission of pathogenic bacteria from food to humans.**

eral risks related to the use of unsafe irrigation water and manure, poor worker hygiene, inadequate pest control, and improper cleaning of sanitizing or harvest equipment and utensils, among others (42). It has been shown that organic agriculture practices related to seed production (e.g., contaminated irrigation water and/or manure) have contributed to identification of sprouted seeds as a high-risk food for STEC and *Salmonella* (43). In the United States, unsanitary conditions identified in one farm and processing operations environment (failure in sanitizing and fruit precooling; ineffective cleaning due to inadequate facilities and equipment design) resulted in contamination of cantaloupes with diverse *L. monocytogenes* strains, leading to a large and fatal outbreak (147 cases, 33 deaths, and 1 miscar-

riage) (22, 44). Other foodborne outbreaks associated with fruits and vegetables through contact with surface or irrigation water have been reported and recently revised (45).

Besides production practices, climate change also can impact crops, food animals, and the growth and survival of pathogens, as well as exposure and transmission pathways of foodborne diseases (46, 47). Climate changes potentially enhance the ability of pathogens to survive and persist in soil, crops, and water, increasing the probability of their transmission thorough water, seafood, or vegetables (46, 48–50).

The complexity of the food chain due to industrial-scale production systems can also increase the risk of foodborne outbreaks, with some occurring during long periods of time

(51–54). A simple failure in a single industrial-scale production resulting from contamination with pathogens during food processing (e.g., from the environment, surface, or food ingredients) can result in distribution of contaminated food batches to millions of consumers, affecting their health in different locations at the same time. In 2000, a massive outbreak of food intoxication from milk products in Japan resulted in >10,000 cases, the contamination point being a production line valve of a major dairy-products processing plant in Osaka that became contaminated with staphylococcal enterotoxin type A (51). Recently, a 2017–2018 outbreak in the European Union due to contaminated infant formula from a French dairy company with *S. enterica* serovar Agona led to the recall of >10 million boxes from multiple countries (52). A 2-year (2015–2016) contaminated food-processing environment resulted in a deadly *L. monocytogenes* outbreak linked to bagged salads (33 cases and 4 deaths in the United States and Canada) (53). One example of a contaminated food ingredient affecting multiple products was the large outbreak (714 cases and 9 deaths in 46 states in the United States) of *S. enterica* serovar Typhimurium linked to peanut products from a plant evidencing diverse possibilities of pathogen transmission (e.g., rodent-accessible entryways, an unsealed air-handling system, and rain leakage into peanut storage areas) to food (17). There are also comprehensive published examples of food safety failures (e.g., ignored positive tests of microbiological hazards, falsification of food safety documents, inadequate controls to prevent contamination and kill bacteria, and insufficient cleaning and sanitation) that led to large outbreaks and deaths from foodborne diseases, demonstrating that maintaining a food safety culture within the entire organization is crucial (55).

Transmission Scenarios Related to Globalization of the Food Supply

A growing international food trade resulting in the export and import of contaminated farm animals, food products (e.g., vegetables, fruit, seeds, meat and poultry, and ethnic foods), and single meals containing ingredients from multiple regions is contributing to changing trends in foodborne diseases. Most of the food products consumed in developed countries are produced on industrial scale, being also increasingly imported (not grown or produced locally) due to changing consumer demand for a wide diversity of foods and fresh produce year-round (33, 56). However, import from other countries includes those with lower food safety standards (e.g., lacking meat processing plant inspections) or without appropriate food production and processing safety practices (e.g., untreated human/animal manure, contaminated water, or untreated wastewater sewage) (33, 42). In the European Union, the most-imported food categories in 2016 were fruits and nuts among vegetable products and fish, crustaceans, and aquatic invertebrates among animal products (57), as occurs in the United States, where most seafood and a moiety of fruits are imported (56). Both types of foodstuffs have been reported in developed regions as presenting an increased association with foodborne disease outbreaks in recent years (13, 14, 27, 56, 58).

In addition, the trade of live animals and food-animal products has also been implicated in the transmission of foodborne pathogens to humans. In Europe, this is exemplified by contaminated products resulting in multicountry foodborne outbreaks, as the 2017–2018 *S.* Enteritidis outbreak linked to eggs (table eggs and consumed raw in some recipes) from Poland, with its origin in egg-packing centers and laying-hen farms (59). Recently, poultry products imported from Brazil, one of the biggest exporters, have been linked to the spread of epidemic clones of an uncommon and multidrug-resistant (MDR) *S. enterica* serotype, *S.* Heidelberg, into European countries (60, 61). Aquaculture practices applied in seafood and fish production in many exporting countries, mostly in Asia (e.g., integrated fish-pig farms in Southeast Asia), are also related to food contamination by pathogens (33, 62). For example, using a novel combination of

WGS analysis and geographic metadata to create a transmission network, it was possible to trace the origin of a U.S. outbreak of *S. enterica* serovar Bareilly to scraped tuna imported from a fishery facility in India (10).

Recent studies showed that illegal importation of food-animal products (including bush meat and livestock meat) from Africa to Europe through airport passengers' luggage was commonly verified, some of those illegal food items being contaminated with foodborne pathogens such as NTS, suggesting a potential public health risk by a neglected route of transmission (63, 64). Also, uncontrolled entry of foodstuffs into the European Union (including from the black market at the EU border) have been recently reported as a neglected route of potential methicillin-resistant *S. aureus* (MRSA) transmission (65).

Drivers Related to the Host

Changes in consumer demands for foods, lifestyles, and behaviors related to food safety as well as the increasing proportion of vulnerable human host groups can also increase exposure to bacterial pathogens and susceptibility to infectious diseases (33, 34, 36).

Transmission Scenarios Related to Changes in Consumer Lifestyles and Risk Behaviors

In recent decades, consumer demand for more-diverse (e.g., tropical products, fruits and vegetables year-round), convenient ready-to-eat (RTE) (e.g., pre-prepared meals, ready-washed fruit and vegetables, and quick-cook sauces), and healthy foods (e.g., those with less salt), known to be associated with higher foodborne pathogen contamination, constitutes a driving factor in the emergence of foodborne diseases. One of the major examples is the increasing consumption of fresh produce due to health concerns, which have been frequently associated with foodborne outbreaks linked to leafy green vegetables (e.g., spinach and lettuce), sprouts, and fruits (e.g., melons and papayas) in developed countries (56, 66).

The increasing trend of consumption of uncooked or undercooked food of animal origin (e.g., meat and poultry, fish, seafood-and-meat recipes, and raw milk) and convenience foods like RTE also potentiate transmission of foodborne pathogenic bacteria (34). For example, consumption of raw milk, in which interest is growing in the European Union, was identified as clearly associated with transmission of human disease caused by *Campylobacter*, *Salmonella*, and STEC (67). Moreover, the increasing consumption of minimally processed foods with extended shelf lives, such as refrigerated or frozen RTE products, was proposed as a possible factor in the promotion of human listeriosis in Europe (68). Also, several cases and outbreaks of *Vibrio parahaemolyticus* infections have been reported in European countries, associated with higher consumption of raw and undercooked fish and shellfish (including imported) in recent years coupled with an increase in the number of susceptible individuals consuming seafood products and with warming of marine waters as a result of global climatic change (50, 69, 70).

Besides consumer demand for specific food products, the new generation of active consumers frequently eat out of the home, being more exposed to transmission of foodborne pathogens by contaminated food prepared in public places. According to the European Food Safety Authority (EFSA), in the European Union almost half of foodborne outbreaks occurred in food service establishments (13). Eating out exposes consumers to food-handler behaviors, whose food safety practices (e.g., personal hygiene to avoid microbial spread, proper food handling to avoid cross-contamination, and efficient cooking and storage temperatures to avoid microbial growth) are crucial to prevent transmission of foodborne pathogenic bacteria to humans. A recent report studying EU salmonellosis cases associated with catering facilities over a 15-year period identified food-handler behaviors (e.g., cross-contamination between heat-treated foods and raw materials or improperly cleaned food-contact surfaces) as potential risk factors (71). Also, it was shown that food risk behaviors (e.g., serving chicken at barbecues when unsure it was fully cooked—a *Campylobacter* risk factor) in U.K. kitchens were widely prevalent among chefs and catering students and the public (72).

Consumers have more opportunities to travel today, positioning travel and tourism as driving forces contributing to exposure to contaminated food (73, 74). For example, an international outbreak of *S.* Heidelberg associated with in-flight catering meals affected 25 people of 5 nationalities (74). In addition, food tourism creates more opportunities for consumers to be exposed to pathogenic bacteria by consumption of traditional food recipes or exotic cuisine (75). This was illustrated by the association of Peruvian goat cheese (often made with unpasteurized milk) with brucellosis (11) and reptile meal with salmonellosis (75). Migration may also change food preparation behaviors and consumption habits (34). This was the case with an outbreak of listeriosis among Mexican immigrants (mostly affecting pregnant women) in the United States as the result of consumption of illicit, noncommercial, homemade, Mexican-style cheese produced from contaminated raw milk sold to unlicensed cheese makers by a local dairy (76).

However, it is of note that a large number of foodborne outbreaks occur in the home/domestic kitchen (13). Such events are mostly associated with poor food-handling behaviors, such as inadequate time-temperature control, cross-contamination, poor personal hygiene, insufficient cleaning, and using food from unsafe sources (6, 77). It was noted that unsafe practices (including those related to storage time and temperatures) are not uncommon with elderly people (>10% of the persons studied), one of the risk group consumers, having a potential impact on the human listeriosis risk (68). In addition, it was recently reported that the temperatures in EU domestic refrigerators are high (ranging from −8 to −4 to 11 to 21°C), which could

potentiate *L. monocytogenes* growth (68). Also, questionable is the proper use of home cooking or reheating methods like microwave and other emerging cooking machines ("cooking robots"). For example, the use of ready-to-cook products for microwave preparation before consumption could be a risk if the temperatures are not sufficient to kill pathogens like *Salmonella* (33, 34). This is illustrated by an outbreak of *Salmonella* possibly related to failures in the microwave cooking of frozen, not-ready-to-eat, microwaveable foods due to misinterpretation of the product's cooking label instructions and/or unfamiliarity with the oven's wattage (78). Also, during summer activities (picnics, barbecues, and summer festivals), the increased risk of cross-contamination and lack of personal hygiene together with the difficulty of keeping food at safe temperatures coincides with peaks of some foodborne infections (47).

Transmission Scenarios Related to Host Risk Population

In recent decades, the worldwide increase of vulnerable people, particularly the elderly and the immunocompromised (e.g., due to cancer, transplant interventions, AIDS, diabetes, liver or kidney disease, and malnutrition), contributed to more-effective transmission of particular pathogens to a wide number of susceptible hosts. Around 15 to 20% of people of developed countries, such as the United Kingdom and United States, belong to this group, with increased vulnerability resulting in development of foodborne disease by a lower infectious dose than typically expected or in diseases with increased severity (79). *L. monocytogenes* is recognized as one of the main foodborne pathogens with great impact in vulnerable groups. In a recent EFSA report, the only clearly identified risk factor for the increasing trend in cases of listeriosis in the European Union was the increase in the elderly population (68). In France, patients with chronic lymphocytic leukemia had a listeriosis incidence >1,000 times greater than that of the population with no risk factors

(80), and low infectious doses of *Listeria* associated with milkshakes affected only hospitalized patients in the United States (81). The elderly was the group most likely to die after infection with STEC, and children <5 years old develop more-severe infections (82). Infant botulism is associated with honey consumption and with the growth of *Clostridium botulinum* and neurotoxin production in the gut of infants <1 year old (83). It was also demonstrated that in patients with chronic liver diseases (cirrhosis), elevated serum iron levels, or immunodeficiency, *Vibrio vulnificus* causes frequently rapid fatal septicemia, mostly associated with previous consumption of raw oysters (84, 85). The wide use of antacids (particularly proton pump inhibitors) or constipating drugs (e.g., antipsychotics) by people whether or not they are in the vulnerable groups might also increase susceptibility to foodborne diseases, at least during a transitional period (79, 86). There is evidence that patients with hypochlorhydria or achlorhydria or who have been treated with proton pump inhibitors or H_2 receptor antagonists are more susceptible to *Campylobacter*, *E. coli* O157:H7, *L. monocytogenes*, *Salmonella*, *Shigella*, and *Vibrio cholerae* than healthy persons (79, 87–89). The increasing numbers of vulnerable populations and their risk of easily acquiring a foodborne disease impose the need for food safety management systems among food suppliers of hospitals, nursing homes, elderly-care homes, schools, and day care centers for children (79).

Drivers Related to Foodborne Bacterial Pathogens

Foodborne bacterial pathogens face a variety of adverse effects or stresses during transmission events from their reservoirs to the human host. Stressful conditions occur from the agriculture level to food processing, storage, distribution, cooking, and within the human host (12, 90–93). Such stresses often co- and/or sequentially occur in the same ecosystem (e.g., application of hurdle technology

in food preservation), during ecosystem transition (e.g., from acid food to acid pH in stomach and bile salts in animal and human gut), or during infection (e.g., high temperature or acidic pH within macrophages), imposing on bacteria the necessity for ceaseless adaptation (90, 91, 93–97).

Bacteria stress responses can be stable or transient. Stable phenotypes, for example, associated with genetic mutation, can be positively selected and fixed in the bacterial population under stressful conditions. A transient stress response can be associated with differential expression of particular genes and generally occurring while the stress is present. These types of responses contribute to protect vital processes, to restore cellular homeostasis, to repair the damage, to counteract or eliminate the stress agent, and/or to increase the cellular resistance against subsequent stress challenges (96). The ability to overcome sublethal or normally lethal stressful conditions was described for such diverse foodborne pathogens as *Campylobacter jejuni* (e.g., to oxidative stress, osmotic stress, or antibiotics) (98–100), *Salmonella* (e.g., to acid, low water activity, thermal treatment, high hydrostatic pressure, metals, or antibiotics) (101–106), STEC (e.g., to acid, osmotic stress, oxidative stress, or heat) (99, 107, 108), *L. monocytogenes* (e.g., to acid, osmotic stress, or disinfectants) (99, 109–111), *V. parahaemolyticus* (e.g. to salt, acid, or cold) (112), *Bacillus cereus* (e.g. to acid, cold, or reducing atmospheres) (96, 113), and *Cronobacter sakazakii* (e.g., to heat, osmotic stress, or desiccation) (99, 114), among others, stress responses being strain dependent, i.e., variable among members of the same species (90). Moreover, the presence of a particular stress can modulate bacterial response to that stress as well as to other ones, the latter phenomenon denominated stress cross-protection (90, 91). In fact, preexposure to sublethal levels of a given stress protects bacteria during subsequent exposure to normally lethal conditions, as was described for *Salmonella* adaptation to bile or to acid (115, 116). Diverse *Salmonella* serotypes (*S.* Typhimurium, *S.* Enteritidis, *S.* Newport, and *S.* Infantis) were cross-protected against UV irradiation, various sanitizing agents, dry heat, and bile salts when under desiccation stress (117). Induced response after contact with sublethal stress or cross-protection events can be found in the literature for other foodborne pathogens, including *V. parahaemolyticus*, *L. monocytogenes*, and STEC (112, 118, 119).

Against all the above, it is evident that bacterial stress response can be a complex scenario, dependent on the interplay of microbial-specific features and intrinsic (e.g., food matrix), extrinsic (e.g., temperature), or food-processing factors (e.g., hurdle technology). According to the nature of such interactions (e.g., bacterial species, strain type, stress concentrations, one or multiple stresses, food components, and competing microbiota in the host), different outcomes in bacterial survival, multiplication, and persistence in the food chain and human host can occur, with potential implications for foodborne pathogen transmission dynamics. In fact, the ability of bacteria to survive and multiply under the stressful conditions occurring in the food chain might increase human exposure to a greater number of pathogenic bacterial cells in food (e.g., through higher pathogen shedding from animal reservoirs, survival of food processing, or persistence in food-processing facilities) as well as to induced stress strains producing greater amounts of toxins responsible for food poisoning symptoms or requiring lower infectious doses than typically expected (120–125).

Bacterial Strain Diversity Favoring Pathogen-Food-Human Transmission Scenarios

It is well known that bacteria adapt to environmental conditions by the acquisition of specific genetic clusters through horizontal transfer, genetic recombination, or mutations as well as by differential expression of regulatory pathways (126). With the advances of genomic, transcriptomic, and single-cell studies applied to foodborne pathogens, it is be-

coming evident that the dynamic response of microorganisms to changing environmental conditions depends on the behavior of individual cells within the bacterial population (127, 128). Thus, it is critical to understand the genetic context, epigenetic mechanisms, and occurrence of heterogeneous behaviors of individual bacteria, as they could have an impact on the success of food-processing and -preservation strategies, on bacterial persistence within food facilities, and on the food-to-human transmission of particular strains (e.g., serotypes or clonal lineages). Some examples illustrate variable features among bacteria that potentially contribute to pathogen-food-human transmission scenarios.

At the farm level, emergent clinically relevant *S. enterica* serotype Rissen/ST469 and the European clone of *S.* Typhimurium/ST34 or *S. enterica* serotype 4,[5],12:i:-/ST34 of pig origin are more tolerant to toxic concentrations of copper under anaerobiosis, due to the genetic horizontal acquisition of the *sil* gene cluster, than other *Salmonella* serotypes from the same origin that are less associated with human infections (102). Such data suggest that the widespread use of copper as a feed additive in pigs might contribute to the selection of these fitter clones, and consequently to pig meat contamination and their transmission to humans.

At food-processing facilities, *L. monocytogenes* acquiring the *qacH* and *bcrABC* genes had a survival advantage when sublethal concentrations of quaternary ammonium compounds (QACs) often used in disinfection remained on surfaces due to insufficient rinsing methods (110). QAC tolerance genes were often found in isolates belonging to clonal lineage II-serotype 1/2a-ST121, the dominant persistent ST type worldwide associated with food-processing plants and occasionally isolated from human infections (129–132), as well as in lineage I-serotype IVb-ST6 isolates associated with human meningitis (111). Using a WGS approach combined with assays evaluating the ability of *L. monocytogenes* to grow in cold (4°C), salt (6% NaCl, 25°C), and acid (pH 5, 25°C), it was found that the bacterial stress response seems to be related to serotype and clonal complex, among other factors (133).

At the food cooking level, it was shown that *E. coli* AW1.7 isolated from commercial beef slaughter plants had a D60°C of 71 min, with cell counts reducing by only <5 log_{10} CFU g^{-1} in ground-beef patties cooked to an internal 71°C, the temperature considered effective for bacterial elimination in beef (134). This thermal resistance was linked to the acquisition of an island termed locus of heat resistance (LHR) present in only 2% of *E. coli* genomes, including clinical ones (107, 135). These data suggest the potential inefficacy of standard thermal conditions applied in food safety when particular strains are present.

Uncommon bacterial genotypes occurring through DNA acquisition and recombination events allied to transmission-favorable contexts might also contribute to the emergence of unusual problems. In 2011 in the European Union, thousands of people were infected by MDR and highly virulent STEC O104:H4, linked to sprout consumption, a serotype that rarely caused human infection in the past. WGS revealed an unexpected genetic context of a hybrid enteroaggregative (EAEC)/ enterohemorrhagic (EHEC) *E. coli* strain, potentially supporting the high pathogenicity. The evolution analysis of STEC O104:H4 strains, by the description of the genome and population structure of the outbreak and non-outbreak isolates obtained from sporadic infections, suggested that outbreak STEC O104:H4 might have evolved to public health importance from EAEC by exploiting a specific cocktail of mobile genetic elements (e.g., prophage with *stx2*, plasmids carrying CTX-M15 or aggregative adherence fimbriae, high-pathogenicity island [HPI], among others), underlining the possibility of further outbreaks if strains achieve novel combinations of mobile genetic elements (136–139).

Finally, the heterogeneous behavior of individual cells within the bacterial population can differentially evolve to cope with the same stress at different levels, or with changing stresses (104, 115, 140). For example, a heterogeneous and multifactorial response to high pressure in *S. enterica* was described with respect to both degree of inactivation and mechanisms (related to the cell membrane and RpoS regulon) used to overcome it. Parker et al. (140) showed that outbreak *E. coli* O157:H7 strains isolated from patients and the spinach production environment (all indistinguishable by pulsed-field gel electrophoresis [PFGE]) differ in their stress responses, and that marketed spinach bags carried a mix of both subpopulations. Clinical strains carrying the mutated *rpoS* gene were more susceptible to acid, osmotic shock, or oxidation than environmental ones with wild-type *rpoS*. However, clinical strains had a greater nutrient-scavenging ability, potentially favoring survival and rapid adaptation of *E. coli* O157:H7 at critical points of its transmission cycle from "field to fork."

Interplay between Bacterial Strains and Food Matrix Favoring Pathogen-Food-Human Transmission Scenarios

Despite the fact that bacterial strain variability could determine its transmission success to the human host, the interplay of strains with supporting food matrices seems to be critical for such an event. Food composition might determine the natural colonization of food with particular strains (e.g., due to specificities of nutrient availability), protect foodborne pathogens from being eliminated during food processing or during their passage into the host gastrointestinal tract (e.g., bacteria can use food molecules to overcome stress), and can induce the expression of virulence features or of cross-protection regulatory pathways dealing with multiple stresses in particular strains (96). Thus, bacterial stress response stimulated by the food matrix could have multiple food safety implications, namely, in the efficacy of hurdle technology used in bacterial growth control (e.g., combination and sequence of stresses applied) (90). Moreover, more opportunities for pathogen-food-human transmission might arise through the consumption of new food vehicles associated with market availability of a variety of food products with specific intrinsic (e.g., different types of lettuce species) or processing factors (e.g., sublethal salt concentrations or low acid content), possibly allowing survival and multiplication of specific strains. Some examples illustrate the interplay between bacterial strains and food matrices that potentially contribute to pathogen-food-human transmission scenarios.

Vegetables constitute variable challenges (based, e.g., on nutrient availability, solar irradiation, and microbiota competition) to foodborne pathogens, which could fit better or worse accordingly with the interplay of strain type, plant species, or even plant age (141). For example, with the use of whole-transcriptome analysis, Crozier et al. (124) observed plant species-specific metabolic responses (e.g., to acid and nutrient stress) when *E. coli* O157:H7 (Sakai strain associated with a sprout outbreak in Japan) was exposed to lettuce or spinach extracts as well as to different parts of the same plant (leafs or roots). Brandl et al. (142) demonstrated that population sizes of *E. coli* O157:H7 (lettuce-associated outbreak H1827 clinical strain) and *S. enterica* serovar Thompson (cilantro-associated outbreak RM1987 clinical strain) were higher in young romaine lettuce leaves (enriched in total nitrogen and carbon) than in middle leaves harvested from mature lettuce heads, positioning younger leaves as vehicles of greater risk to transmit human pathogens. Moreover, several studies found that some foodborne pathogens (e.g., *Salmonella*, *E. coli*, and *L. monocytogenes*) have the ability to internalize in vegetables' edible parts (e.g., tomatoes and lettuce), impairing their removal by standard disinfection methods before human consumption (143–146). Thus, knowing the interaction of specific strains with particular vegetables might contribute to predictive modeling or risk-based analysis of the potential for microbial contamination, colonization, and persistence in different horticultural crops (each day

more often associated with outbreaks) (147) and to better understanding of the transmission routes and vehicles of particular strains.

Food matrices could have an impact on the global stress response of particular strains due to the expression of stress cross-protection mechanisms, often described in foodborne pathogens (91, 103, 117, 148). Poimenidou et al. (149) found that tomato-habituated *L. monocytogenes* under cold temperatures was more tolerant to acid or osmotic stress than that habituated on lettuce, and lettuce-habituated *L. monocytogenes* was more tolerant during heat challenge at 60°C compared to tomato-habituated cells. Also, *Salmonella* resistant to low water activity found in some food types (e.g. flour, chocolate, cocoa and hazelnut shells, and dried milk) was more thermotolerant (99).

It has been suggested that food molecules (e.g., specific amino acids, carbohydrates, urea, and fatty acids) could protect bacteria from stressful conditions (96). Using a simulated gastric passage model (pH 2.5; pepsin; bile salt and enzymes), Aviles et al. (150) showed that a peanut butter outbreak-associated *S. enterica* serovar Tennessee strain was better able to survive the acid environment when vehiculated in peanut butter matrix with low water activity and high fat content than in low-fat formulations. Also, Birk et al. (151) showed that *S. enterica* serovar Dublin was better protected when some types of proteins (pepsin, ovalbumin, and turkey meat) were included in a simulated gastric digestion compared with bovine serum albumin, indicating that protection could be protein specific. In a different context, Liu et al. (152) showed that *E. coli* LTH5807 differed in thermal resistance when heated to 60°C on mung bean, radish, or alfalfa seeds (153).

Bacterial stress protection by the food matrix seems to be also related to low infectious doses, as in the case of salmonellosis epidemiological linked to values of the order of 10 to 100 CFU vehiculated by food with low water activity, compared to >10^5 CFU in other food types (103). Another explanation for such low infectious doses is that bacteria could be missed by standard microbiological food methods, as dehydration could induce the bacterial filament form (underestimate the true number of cells) or the viable but nonculturable (VBNC) state (impairing bacterial growth). Filamentous bacteria seem to be more acid or bile resistant and retained their virulence *in vitro* and *in vivo* in a mouse model (154), and cells in the VBNC state were described in some cases to maintain their pathogenic capacity after resuscitation (103, 155). For example, it was demonstrated that VBNC cells of *C. jejuni* maintained the ability to adhere to intestinal cells (156) and VBNC cells of *E. coli* O157:H7 expressed *stx1* and *stx2* toxin-coding genes and produced the toxin (157, 158). The VBNC state was also described for other foodborne pathogens such as *Shigella* spp., *Yersinia enterocolitica*, *Aeromonas* spp., *Brucella* spp., and *Vibrio* spp. (155), being induced by several stresses occurring in the food matrices and during food processing or storage (155, 159). Considering the large number of foodborne outbreaks described without the identification of the etiological agent, implicated food vehicle, or reservoir (13), more knowledge is needed to clarify how often VBNC bacteria could be involved in undetected pathogen-food-human transmission events. For example, the STEC O104:H4 of the sprout-associated European outbreak in 2011 was never isolated from the suspected origin (fenugreek seeds), and it was shown to be able to enter the VNBC state and resuscitate (160).

Finally, the components of food matrices or the processing factors applied to them might have an impact on the expression of foodborne pathogen virulence factors. This is the case for enterotoxins produced by *Staphylococcus* spp., *B. cereus*, or STEC, in which toxin expression seem to be dependent on the interplay between toxin type, strain, thermal treatment, and food matrix, although different studies reported disparate data (95, 121, 123,161–167). Thus, the certainty of as-sessing *Staphylococcus* or *B. cereus* food poisoning risk through colony-forming units present in food products has been disproven, with the scientific community and food business operators aware of the threat arising from unforeseeable enterotoxin production under stress conditions.

Interplay between Bacterial Strains and Host Favoring Pathogen-Food-Human Transmission Scenarios

A successful host colonization occurs by the ability of a pathogen to outcompete and out-grow native host microbiota, mostly in the intestinal tract (97, 168). For that, foodborne pathogens must survive specific stressful conditions (e.g., stomach acid, macrophages, and oxidative stress) as well as modulate host microbiota (e.g., changing the equilibrium of particular species), the immune system (e.g., inducing inflammatory reactions), and, indirectly, the gut physicochemical environment (e.g., available nutrients and oxygen tension) (95, 97, 168, 169). A previous contact with stressful conditions in the food chain might allow a preadaptation of the pathogen to those similarly occurring in the host, or even increase its virulence due to coregulation of stress and virulence genes (90, 105, 109). After the colonization step, foodborne pathogens shedding from their hosts vary in the amount of bacteria expelled and in the duration that shedding occurs, resulting in diverse levels of environmental, animal carcass, or vegetable contamination, with impact on pathogen transmission dynamics (168, 170). On the other hand, the interplay between bacterial genetic evolution and environmental challenges imposed by the specific physiology of each host (e.g., related to the variable gut environment in different animal reservoirs, changing diets, or antimicrobials used in intensive animal production) might increase bacterial shedding from particular individuals and drive strains' evolution pathways toward specialist (e.g., one host) or generalist (multiple hosts) lifestyles (5, 168, 171). A selection of generalist strains conducts to greater transmission opportunities among a variety of reservoirs and hosts (172). In contrast, specialist strains have fewer opportunities to be transmitted but usually cause more severe, chronic and asymptomatic infections, with the possibility of long periods of host shedding, sometimes undetected (5). Some examples illustrate the interplay of strain-host scenarios potentially contributing to foodborne pathogen-food-human transmission.

C. jejuni is a major foodborne human pathogen vehiculated mainly by contaminated poultry (13, 173). *C. jejuni* can highly colonize poultry (up to 10^{10} CFU/g feces), and it is suggested that the high body temperatures (41 to 45°C) of poultry species, the poultry gut environment, and the inefficiency of poultry immune system activation contribute to the persistent colonization of the avian gut with thermotolerant and microaerophilic *C. jejuni* and, consequently, to its continuous shedding and transmission to the environment and other poultry hosts (173, 174). Also, for STEC O157:H7, individual host features allied to strain and environmental factors could determine the level of host colonization and shedding. Cattle are pointed to as the main reservoir of STEC O157:H7, with some animals classified as "super-shedders" when they release $\geq 10^4$ CFU/g of feces (175). Strain specificities (e.g., ability to colonize the rectal-anal junction of cattle), animal features (e.g., composition of the cattle native microbiome), and animal age and diet seem to determine whether *E. coli* O157:H7 can proliferate sufficiently for the host to obtain super-shedder status (168, 175–177). The supper-shedding state or a prolonged release period of bacteria in the feces has also been associated with consumption of antibiotics with impact on the host microbiota. This was detected for *S.* Typhimurium in mouse infection models, releasing bacteria on the order of $>10^8$ CFU/g, or in outbreaks of *S.* Typhimurium from roast pork, in which antibiotic consumption by patients increased the carrier state period (125, 178). Prolonged

human symptomatic infections (from weeks to several years) with other NTS serotypes (*S. enterica* serovars Mbandaka, Bredeney, Infantis, and Virchow) have also been described, with antibiotic consumption also cited as one of the factors contributing to their persistence (170).

High host shedding of foodborne pathogen strains allied to favorable transmission patterns might increase opportunities to colonize multiple available hosts (e.g., several animal species), which depend on bacteria making rapid adjustments to each new host ecosystem. However, the high prevalence and wide distribution of the so-called "generalist clonal lineages" complicates source attribution, as in the case of *C. jejuni* ST21/ST45 clonal complexes isolated from poultry, cattle, and infected humans (172). In spite of this, Sheppard et al. (179) showed that within ST21/ST45 clonal complexes exist sublineages with host association, determined by the occurrence of the *panBCD* genes encoding the vitamin B5 biosynthesis pathway, more prevalent in cattle (diet composed of grass with low vitamin B5) isolates than in chicken (diet composed of cereal and grains abundant in vitamin B5) ones. The discovery by WGS of gene loci gained or lost makes genetic elements possible targets for source tracking, with the genetic makeup of a human isolate theoretically helping in the potential identification of the isolate source and of transmission food vehicles (180). Generalist and specialist lifestyles could also be related to *Salmonella* serotypes, with *S.* Typhi (specialist serotype) associated with human reservoirs and infections, and the main emerging *S.* Typhimurium and *S.* Enteritidis (generalist serotypes) associated with human infections and colonization of diverse animals (13, 181). It remains to clarify whether generalism is a stable strategy taking advantage of the large number of transmission opportunities in agriculture or whether it reflects insufficient time for well-adapted host specialist lineages to have evolved in the recent man-made environment. For example, studies on *S.* Typhimurium ST313, causing invasive infections in immunocompromised populations in Africa, point to the presence of degraded genome capacity in the form of pseudogenes and deletions, suggesting evolution from a generalist to a specialist lifestyle, with transmission among humans potentially exerting genomic selection pressure (181). Understanding the differences of foodborne pathogen lifestyles is important to establish effective control measures adapted to the context of specific hosts as well as to preview future transmission scenarios of specific foodborne strains through particular reservoirs and food types.

ANTIMICROBIAL-RESISTANT FOODBORNE BACTERIA TRANSMISSION ALONG THE FOOD CHAIN

Antimicrobial resistance is considered a major global public health issue for humans and animals, and a major priority in food safety by a number of entities (the European Commission, WHO, and Food and Agriculture Organization of the United Nations) (182–186). According to Centers for Diseases Control and Prevention (CDC) estimates, antibiotic-resistant infections caused 23,000 deaths per year in the United States, and about one of five resistant infections were caused by microorganisms from food and animals (185, 187–189). Nevertheless, the contribution of food to the transmission to humans of bacteria carrying clinically relevant resistance genes is still poorly established, including the real enrichment of the human microbiota with such bacteria and genes.

Although in recent years great effort has been made by different organizations (e.g., the WHO, EFSA, and CDC) to understand the magnitude and burden of antimicrobial resistance transmission through the food chain, it remains uncertain at the global level (190). It is particularly underestimated in low- and middle-income countries where drivers of antimicrobial resistance (e.g., unregulated farming and food-production practices con-

cerning food safety and antibiotic use; poor hygienic conditions, namely, related to water and sewage; and human travel and migration) are significant, eventually affecting the spread of antimicrobial resistance by the food chain in a wide geographic area (189, 191). The regular use of antimicrobials in livestock (therapeutic, metaphylactic, prophylactic, or growth-promoting use) associated with modern intensive food-animal production has been considered the main driver of the selection of both antibiotic-resistant bacteria and genetic elements worldwide, with food products (e.g., meat, poultry, eggs, vegetables, and farmed fish) the most relevant transmission mode to humans (186, 188, 189, 192). In fact, new WHO guidelines on the use of medically important antimicrobials in food-producing animals stressed that antibiotic-resistant bacteria in this sector were reduced by up to 39% after interventions restricting ntibiotic use at the farm level (186). However, other nonantibiotic compounds with antimicrobial activity and widely used in food-animal production (e.g., copper) may also contribute to the selection of antibiotic-resistant zoonotic bacteria and to less successful intervention scenarios related to reduction of antibiotic use (101, 102, 188, 193).

Antimicrobial-resistant bacteria with human relevance include pathogenic zoonotic organisms (e.g., *Salmonella* and *Campylobacter*) as well as likely commensal zoonotic bacteria (e.g., *E. coli* and *Enterococcus*). Both groups have been recognized as important or major contributors to the burden of antimicrobial resistance (188, 192, 194). Antimicrobial-resistant zoonotic pathogenic bacteria may be associated with more-prolonged infections; treatment failures as a result of invasive infections; or the use of last-line antimicrobials for therapy, which are more expensive and/or toxic. Commensal zoonotic bacteria could be reservoirs of clinically relevant antibiotic resistance genes mobilizable to pathogens and be potentially involved in extraintestinal opportunistic infections (e.g., urinary tract or bloodstream infections) after transmission by food and colonization of humans (Fig. 3) (190, 194). In general, these commensal strains with likely animal origin are widespread in multiple hosts and often participate in genetic exchange events with other microorganisms sharing the same ecosystems, making direction of transmission (e.g., food-human, environment-human, or human-human) hard to assess (189, 190).

For several decades, the contribution of food-animal reservoirs and food vehicles in the transmission of antimicrobial-resistant bacteria relevant to human health has been controversial. However, accumulating evidence linking livestock production with antimicrobial resistance burden in humans has been reported (188–190, 192, 195), which we classify in three categories.

Association between the Use of Antimicrobial Agents and the Occurrence of Antimicrobial-Resistant Bacteria in Food-Producing Animals and/or Humans

The correlation between antibiotic use and the occurrence of antimicrobial resistance in bacteria isolated from the food chain and humans is evident in studies from the last 25 years, including those of zoonotic pathogens or commensal bacteria. Among the more illustrative cases was the consequences of licensing the fluoroquinolone enrofloxacin for animal use in the 1990s, especially in poultry. It led to increased rates of ciprofloxacin resistance in *S.* Typhimurium DT104 recovered from animals/food and humans in the United

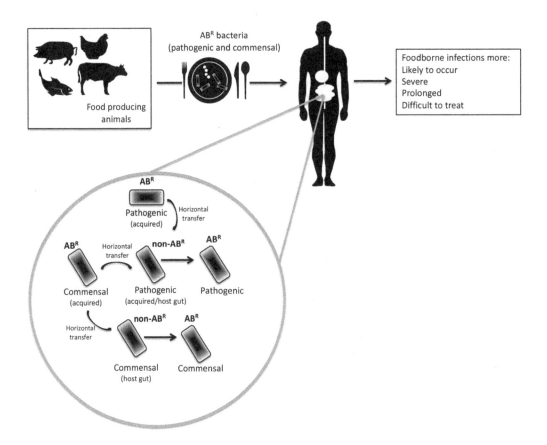

FIGURE 3 Implications of antibiotic-resistant bacteria transmitted from food to humans. AB^R, antibiotic resistance.

Kingdom (196) and of *C. jejuni* from humans in the United States (197) and from chickens and humans in The Netherlands (198). More recently, a voluntary withdrawal of ceftiofur by poultry producers in Canada was correlated with decreasing occurrence of ceftiofur-resistant *S.* Heidelberg (one of the most common serotypes associated with salmonellosis in this country) from both human infections and retail poultry. After reintroduction of ceftiofur 2 years later in poultry production, an increase in resistance levels in poultry and humans was once more observed (199). Another example was the ban of the glycopeptide avoparcin as a growth promoter in Europe in the 1990s, which led to the reduction of vancomycin-resistant *Enterococcus* in community settings (producing animals and healthy humans) (200–203). Evidence on the correlation between antibiotic consumption and resistance among foodborne pathogens from humans and food-producing animals was also corroborated by the last European Centre for Disease Prevention and Control (ECDC)/EFSA/European Medicines Agency (EMA) joint report involving univariate/multivariate analysis in almost 30 European countries. It demonstrated that resistance to fluoroquinolones in *Salmonella* and *Campylobacter* and resistance to macrolides in *Campylobacter coli* from humans were related to the consumption of fluoroquinolones or macrolides, respectively, in animals (204). Previous findings have also suggested a link between *S.* Enteritidis resistance to nitrofurans and their illegal use in food-producing poultry in Portugal (205).

Correlation between Rates of Antibiotic Resistance among Bacteria from Food-Producing Animals, Food, and Humans Obtained from Systematic Surveillance Data

The 2016 EFSA reported that resistance to widely used antimicrobials (including critical ones important for the treatment of severe human infections) was commonly detected in *Campylobacter* and *Salmonella* from humans

and poultry. This is illustrated by the high level of resistance to ciprofloxacin in *C. jejuni* isolated from broilers (69.8%), broiler meat (65.7%), and humans (60.2%). In the case of *Salmonella*, it was reported that resistance to ciprofloxacin was markedly higher in some serotypes commonly associated with poultry (*S.* Enteritidis, *S.* Infantis, and *S. enterica* serovar Kentucky), suggesting a greater contribution of the poultry production chain to the human burden (183). Moreover, a high prevalence of MDR *Salmonella* in humans (26%) and poultry meat (broiler, 24,8%; turkey, 30.5%) (including the ampicillin/streptomycin/sulfonamides and tetracycline resistance [ASSuT] profile) was also described (183). Data from the National Antimicrobial Resistance Monitoring System (NARMS) reported an increase of *S.* 4,[5],12:i:- with the ASSuT-MDR phenotype in humans, from 43 to 60% between 2014 and 2015, and of 65% in swine from 2015 (206).

In low- and middle-income countries (e.g., in Asia, African, and Latin America), the rates of antibiotic resistance, including to clinically relevant antibiotics (ciprofloxacin, extended-spectrum cephalosporins, colistin, and carbapenems), are undoubtedly higher than in high-income countries, with food products presenting a potential role in its emergence (189). For example, high levels of *Salmonella* nonsusceptible to ciprofloxacin (15 to 48%) and cephalosporins (38% to ceftriaxone) were observed in humans from Asian countries (207, 208). These data are in agreement with several studies documenting a high prevalence of resistance to fluoroquinolones (>22.5% to ciprofloxacin) and cephalosporins (12.5 to >23.4% to ceftriaxone and 26.6% to ceftazidime) in *Salmonella* from poultry meat obtained in South Korea and China (209, 210), as well as in *E. coli* from farmed fish (36.7% reduced susceptibility to ciprofloxacin) in China (211). Also, a recent Chinese surveillance study revealed high rates of the new plasmid-mediated colistin resistance gene *mcr-1* in diverse foodborne bacteria recovered from water (71% of samples), animal feces

(51%), food products (36%, mostly meat), and humans (28% of human subjects surveyed), further supporting the role of the food chain in the transmission of colistin-resistant bacteria and the *mcr-1* gene to humans (212). However, direct zoonotic transmission of *mcr-1* could not be excluded, as stated by the association of colonization of farmers with *mcr-1*-carrying bacteria with exposure to *mcr-1*-positive chickens from small-scale poultry farms in Vietnam (213).

The role of low- and middle-income countries as largely exporters of food to different geographic regions of the world, their changing from extensive farming systems to large-scale ones with a higher use of antibiotics due to consumer demand for protein, and the largely unregulated use of antibiotics in animal production suggest that international trade of contaminated breeding animals (e.g., poultry production depends on a pyramid-like breeding system), feed, and meat products with antibiotic-resistant foodborne pathogens may contribute to the rapid worldwide spread of these bacteria, with impact on human health (214). The last DANMAP (Danish Integrated Antimicrobial Resistance Monitoring and Research Programme) report described higher levels of extended-spectrum β-lactamase (ESBL)/ AmpC-producing *E. coli* (56% of samples, including ST131 clone) and ciprofloxacin resistance in *C. jejuni* (71% of isolates) from imported broiler meat compared with domestically produced broiler meat (23% of the samples with ESBL/AmpC-producing *E. coli* and 22% of *C. jejuni* isolates with ciprofloxacin resistance) (215). Recently, Brazilian imported poultry meat contaminated with extended-spectrum cephalosporin-resistant bla_{CMY-2}-producing *S.* Heidelberg (a poultry-related serotype uncommon in Europe) was reported in Europe and included strains with indistinguishable PFGE profiles from epidemic clones with invasive potential that caused outbreaks in the United States, alerting for potential risk to human health (60, 61). The spread of *E. coli* carrying bla_{CMY-2} from flocks of imported broiler parents to broiler meat (including potentially human-pathogenic types), even in a country with no cephalosporin use (216), suggests that the globalization of trade of food animals and food products is an important driver of antibiotic resistance spread through the food chain.

Transmission of Clinically Relevant Antibiotic Resistance Genes on Mobile Genetic Elements and/or Antibiotic-Resistant Clones of Zoonotic Pathogens and Commensal Bacteria from Producing Animals and Food to Humans

Transmission of antibiotic-resistant clones and genetic elements between bacteria (pathogens and commensal) from the food chain to humans has been described in recent decades (189, 191, 195, 217, 218). With the evolution of molecular methods (WGS versus multilocus sequence typing [MLST] and PFGE), the accuracy of such linkages may be clearer in the near future as data accumulate, by facilitating the identification of new cases as well as confirming or contesting older ones. Table 1 shows examples illustrating linkage and transmission of *Salmonella*, *E. coli*, and *Enterococcus* spp. clones from the food chain to humans. It includes studies developed in diverse time frames that established such linkages. Other examples including only mobilization of genetic elements are discussed in the paragraphs below.

In several European countries, multiple clones of pathogenic *Salmonella* serotypes ESBL producers (e.g., CTX-M-2, CTX-M-9, and TEM-52) shared between poultry and human cases have been reported (Table 1). A recent example describes an MDR and ESBL-producing (CTX-M-1) clone of *S.* Infantis causing human infections and isolated from poultry (including meat) in Italy during 2001 and 2014 (Table 1) (219). In Canada, the transmission of *S.* Heidelberg (one of the top MDR poultry-related serotypes in North America) between abattoir, retail poultry, and humans as well as the transmission of a common

TABLE 1 Antibiotic-resistant pathogens and commensal zoonotic bacteria recovered from food products and humans[a]

Bacteria	Clonality approach	Clinically relevant antibiotic resistance gene(s)	Genetic element PL – Inc group	Food source (human source)	Country(ies)/year(s)	Reference(s)
Salmonella						
S. 1,4,[5],12:i:-	PFGE	MCR-1	PL-X4, HI2	Pork products (clinical cases)	Portugal/2011–2015	222
S. Enteritidis	PFGE, phage typing	ESBL-CTX-M-15	PL – FII	Chicken meat, chicken feces, or diseased chicken (clinical cases)	Korea/2009	245
S. Heidelberg	WGS-based hqSNV	AmpC-CMY-2	PL – I1	Retail poultry, abattoir poultry (clinical cases)	Canada/2012	220
S. Heidelberg	PFGE, MLST	AmpC-CMY-2	PL – I1, A/C	Imported poultry meat (clinical cases)	Portugal/2014–2015; The Netherlands/1999–2013	60, 61
S. Heidelberg	PFGE	AmpC-CMY-2	PL – I1	Chicken abattoir, chicken retail, bovine and porcine (clinical cases)	Canada/2002–2004	246
S. Indiana	PFGE	ESBL-CTX-M-65, CTX-M-14; PMQR-AAC (6')-IB-CR+OQXAB	PL-NR	Chicken (clinical cases)	China/2009–2013	224
S. Infantis	PFGE, MLST, WGS-based SNP	ESBL-CTX-M-1, CTX-M-65	PL-I1+P	Broiler meat, broiler chickens (clinical cases)	Italy/2011–2014	219
S. Infantis	PFGE	ESBL-TEM-52	PL – I1	Poultry (clinical cases)	Belgium/2001–2005	247
S. Kentucky (ST198-X1-SGI1)	PFGE, MLST	CipR-	PL – I1	Poultry and turkey meat, seafood, broilers (clinical cases)	Europe, Asia/2000–2013	221
S. Typhimurium	PFGE	ESBL-CTX-M-2	PL – NR	Poultry (clinical cases)	Brazil/2003–2004	248
S. Typhimurium	PFGE	ESBL-CTX-M-1	PL – N	Swine meat (human)	Germany/2007	249
S. Virchow	PFGE, MLST	ESBL-CTX-M-15	PL-HI2	Poultry meat, pig farms (clinical cases)	Korea/2012	98
S. Virchow	PFGE	ESBL-CTX-M-2	PL – NR	Poultry (clinical cases)	Belgium-France/2000–2003	250
S. Virchow	PFGE	ESBL-CTX-M-9	NR	Broilers (clinical cases)	Spain/2000–2004	251
Escherichia coli						
A-ST-10, ST-117	MLST	ESBL-diverse		Chicken meat, other meats (healthy humans-fecal, and human blood)	The Netherlands	228
O25sH4-B2-ST131	MLST, PFGE	ESBL-CTX-M-9		Chicken meat and avian (human infections)	Spain/1993–2010	252
A-ST-10, ST-117	MLST	ESBL-CTX-M-1, TEM-52	PL-I1 (ST3, ST7, ST10)	Poultry (blood and urine isolates)	The Netherlands/2006–2010	230
A, B1, D	MLST, AFLP, PFGE	ESBL	PL	Chicken meat (human carrier or blood isolates)	The Netherlands/2008–2009	227
ST38	WGS-based SNP; MLST	AmpC-CMY-2	PL-K	Chicken meat (clinical isolates-urinary tract infections)	Norway/2012–2014	232
Enterococcus						
Enterococcus faecium	PFGE	aac(6')-le-aph(2'')-la	NR	Poultry carcasses (healthy human feces)	Portugal/2001	233
Enterococcus faecalis	PFGE	aac(6')-le-aph(2'')-la	NR	Poultry carcasses (healthy human feces)	Portugal/2001	233
	PFGE	aac(6')-le-aph(2'')-la	NR	Poultry carcasses (outpatients' feces)	United States/1998–2000	234
	PFGE	aac(6')-le-aph(2'')-la	NR	Ground pork (healthy human feces)	United States/1998–2000	234

[a]Abbreviations: AFLP, amplified fragment length polymorphism; hqSNV, high-quality core genome single-nucleotide variant; NR, not reported; NT, plasmids that were not typeable with the scheme used; PL, plasmid.

CMY-2 plasmid among those strains was suggested (220). Also of concern is the dissemination of the ciprofloxacin-resistant *S.* Kentucky ST198 strain (with a reservoir in northern Africa [Egypt]) in Europe and elsewhere since 2010, including that associated with an increasing number of contaminated sources, mainly poultry but also seafood (221). A possible transmission from pork products to humans of *mcr-1* colistin resistance observed in an MDR and copper-tolerant clinically relevant *S.* 1,4,[5],12:i:- clonal lineage was suggested in a Portuguese study (222). Other studies also point to the food chain as an important reservoir of *mcr-1*-bearing plasmids transmitted among different bacterial clones and species (213, 223) and suggest that *mcr-1* first arose in animals before being transmitted to humans, due to colistin use in food-animal production (152). Other descriptions of shared genetic elements include identical *oqxAB*-carrying plasmids carried by *Salmonella* and *E. coli* and identified in food products and humans, particularly in China (177), with a few reports of shared clones (224).

In relation to commensal zoonotic bacteria, evidence of antibiotic resistance transmission between animals/food and humans is harder to establish, with some studies reaching different conclusions (195, 225, 226). Those suggesting such transmission through the food chain were based on the detection of common clinically relevant genes, mobile genetic elements (e.g., plasmids), and/or clones between food and humans (including those associated with infections). For example, transmission from livestock and/or retail meat to humans of ESBL and AmpC β-lactamase genes on plasmids (including plasmids shared with pathogenic bacteria like *Salmonella*) and/or of *E. coli* clones has been suggested (195, 218, 226–232). The last DANMAP also reported the observation of phylogenetically related (WGS-based single-nucleotide polymorphism [SNP]) ST131 bla_{CMY-2}-producing *E. coli* from imported meat and human bloodstream infections in Denmark during 2015-2016, thus suggesting a potential zoonotic link between imported

broiler meat and severe human infections (215). Among *Enterococcus* spp. the same clones of a gentamicin-resistant *E. faecalis* or *E. faecium* were found in the feces of healthy humans and in poultry carcasses for human consumption in Portugal (233). Clonal linkage between poultry or ground pork for human consumption and humans was also detected in the United States (234). Freitas et al. (235) detected the same MDR, vancomycin-resistant *E. faecium* clone (CC5-PFGE A) in a piggery environment, feces from live and slaughtered swine, healthy human feces, and hospitalized patients, strongly suggesting its transmission across the food chain in Europe and the United States between 1995 and 2008. Tn*1546-vanA* with the same structure and shared by humans and food animals was also described (236, 237).

More recently, new alerts of public health threats, but those with indefinable risks for human health, linked to food animals and food products have been observed. This is the case for carbapenem-resistant pathogenic or commensal MDR bacteria (e.g., VIM-1-producing *Enterobacteriaceae* and NDM-1- or OXA-23-producing *Acinetobacter* spp.) isolated from food-animal farms and food products of animal origin (217, 231, 238, 239) and from other potential new food vehicles like seafood and produce (239–242). Also, the potential risk of transmission of MRSA carrying different antimicrobial resistance and virulence genes through the food chain cannot be ignored (238). Evidence of food-to-human transmission of livestock-associated MRSA was recently described, with broiler chicken and turkey meat implicated as probable vehicles of the hybrid CC9/CC398 lineage (243, 244). However, more data will be critical to clarify the contribution of the food chain to the transmission of carbapenem-resistant bacteria and MRSA to humans.

CONCLUSIONS

Transmission of bacterial pathogens from food to humans has a relevant impact on public health, aggravated by the acquisition of antimicrobial resistance. Despite the improvements in food safety measures in different parts of the world, the modern era imposed a plethora of drivers for transmission of bacteria to humans through food consumption. The multiplicity and interplay of drivers related to the intensification, diversification, and globalization of food production; consumer health status, lifestyles, and behaviors; and bacterial adaptation to different challenges from farm to human make the prevention of bacteria-food-human transmission a modern and continuous challenge. To minimize the selection and spread of foodborne zoonotic pathogens and commensals, including MDR, it is critical to improve biosecurity measures from the farm (e.g., high hygiene standards and vaccination) and throughout the food chain (e.g., slaughtering and food processing, food handling, and education of consumers); to control antibiotic use, and the live-animal and food trade; as well as to explore bacterial adaptation mechanisms to food production ecosystems. A global One Health approach is mandatory to better understand and minimize the transmission pathways of human pathogens through the food chain (8, 189).

ACKNOWLEDGMENTS

We thank the European Society of Clinical Microbiology and Infectious Diseases (ESCMID) Food- and Water-borne Infections Study Group (EFWISG).

CITATION

Antunes P, Novais C, Peixe L. 2018. Food-to-humans bacterial transmission. Microbiol Spectrum 5(3):MTBP-0019-2016.

REFERENCES

1. **Josephs-Spaulding J, Beeler E, Singh OV.** 2016. Human microbiome versus food-borne pathogens: friend or foe. *Appl Microbiol Biotechnol* **100:** 4845–4863.

2. **Kamada N, Chen GY, Inohara N, Núñez G.** 2013. Control of pathogens and pathobionts by the gut microbiota. *Nat Immunol* **14:**685–690.

3. **Voreades N, Kozil A, Weir TL.** 2014. Diet and the development of the human intestinal microbiome. *Front Microbiol* **5:**494.

4. **Antonovics J, Wilson AJ, Forbes MR, Hauffe HC, Kallio ER, Leggett HC, Longdon B, Okamura B, Sait SM, Webster JP.** 2017. The evolution of transmission mode. *Philos Trans R Soc Lond B Biol Sci* **372:**20160083.

5. **Bäumler A, Fang FC.** 2013. Host specificity of bacterial pathogens. *Cold Spring Harb Perspect Med* **3:**a010041.

6. **Acheson DK.** 2009. Food and waterborne illnesses, p 480–506. *In* Schaechter M (ed), *The Desk Encyclopedia of Microbiology,* 2nd ed. Elsevier, San Diego, CA.

7. **Scallan E, Hoekstra RM, Angulo FJ, Tauxe RV, Widdowson MA, Roy SL, Jones JL, Griffin PM.** 2011. Foodborne illness acquired in the United States—major pathogens. *Emerg Infect Dis* **17:** 7–15.

8. **World Health Organization.** 2015. *WHO Estimates of the Global Burden of Foodborne Diseases: Foodborne Disease Burden Epidemiology Reference Group 2007–2015.* World Health Organization, Geneva, Switzerland. http://apps.who.int/iris/bitstream/10665/199350/1/9789241565165_eng.pdf.

9. **Food Standards Agency.** 2011. *Foodborne Disease Strategy 2010–15: An FSA Programme for the Reduction of Foodborne Diseases in the UK.* Food Standards Agency, London, United Kingdom. https://acss.food.gov.uk/sites/default/files/multimedia/pdfs/fds2015.pdf.

10. **Hoffmann M, Luo Y, Monday SR, Gonzalez-Escalona N, Ottesen AR, Muruvanda T, Wang C, Kastanis G, Keys C, Janies D, Senturk IF, Catalyurek UV, Wang H, Hammack TS, Wolfgang WJ, Schoonmaker-Bopp D, Chu A, Myers R, Haendiges J, Evans PS, Meng J, Strain EA, Allard MW, Brown EW.** 2016. Tracing origins of the *Salmonella* Bareilly strain causing a food-borne outbreak in the United States. *J Infect Dis* **213:**502–508.

11. **Cutler SJ.** 2014. Bacterial zoonoses: an overview, p 1771–1780. *In* Sussman M, Liu D, Poxton I, Schwartzman J (ed), *Molecular Medical Microbiology,* 2nd ed, **vol 1.** Elsevier, San Diego, CA.

12. **Berry ED, Wells JE.** 2016. Reducing foodborne pathogen persistence and transmission in animal production environments: challenges and opportunities. *Microbiol Spectr* **4:**PFS-0006-2014.

13. **European Food Safety Authority.** 2017. The European Union summary report on trends and

sources of zoonoses, zoonotic agents and foodborne outbreaks in 2016. *EFSA J* **15**:e05077.

14. **Painter JA, Hoekstra RM, Ayers T, Tauxe RV, Braden CR, Angulo FJ, Griffin PM.** 2013. Attribution of foodborne illnesses, hospitalizations, and deaths to food commodities by using outbreak data, United States, 1998–2008. *Emerg Infect Dis* **19**:407–415.

15. **Werber D, Dreesman J, Feil F, van Treeck U, Fell G, Ethelberg S, Hauri AM, Roggentin P, Prager R, Fisher IS, Behnke SC, Bartelt E, Weise E, Ellis A, Siitonen A, Andersson Y, Tschäpe H, Kramer MH, Ammon A.** 2005. International outbreak of *Salmonella* Oranienburg due to German chocolate. *BMC Infect Dis* **5**:7.

16. **Sheth AN, Hoekstra M, Patel N, Ewald G, Lord C, Clarke C, Villamil E, Niksich K, Bopp C, Nguyen TA, Zink D, Lynch M.** 2011. A national outbreak of *Salmonella* serotype Tennessee infections from contaminated peanut butter: a new food vehicle for salmonellosis in the United States. *Clin Infect Dis* **53**:356–362.

17. **Cavallaro E, Date K, Medus C, Meyer S, Miller B, Kim C, Nowicki S, Cosgrove S, Sweat D, Phan Q, Flint J, Daly ER, Adams J, Hyytia-Trees E, Gerner-Smidt P, Hoekstra RM, Schwensohn C, Langer A, Sodha SV, Rogers MC, Angulo FJ, Tauxe RV, Williams IT, Behravesh CB, Salmonella Typhimurium Outbreak Investigation Team.** 2011. *Salmonella* Typhimurium infections associated with peanut products. *N Engl J Med* **365**:601–610.

18. **Lienau EK, Strain E, Wang C, Zheng J, Ottesen AR, Keys CE, Hammack TS, Musser SM, Brown EW, Allard MW, Cao G, Meng J, Stones R.** 2011. Identification of a salmonellosis outbreak by means of molecular sequencing. *N Engl J Med* **364**:981–982.

19. **Angelo KM, Conrad AR, Saupe A, Dragoo H, West N, Sorenson A, Barnes A, Doyle M, Beal J, Jackson KA, Stroika S, Tarr C, Kucerova Z, Lance S, Gould LH, Wise M, Jackson BR.** 2017. Multistate outbreak of *Listeria monocytogenes* infections linked to whole apples used in commercially produced, prepackaged caramel apples: United States, 2014–2015. *Epidemiol Infect* **145**: 848–856.

20. **Navarro-Garcia F.** 2014. *Escherichia coli* O104: H4 pathogenesis: an enteroaggregative *E. coli*/ Shiga Toxin-Producing *E. coli* explosive cocktail of high virulence. *Microbiol Spectr* **2**:EHEC-0008-2013.

21. **Inns T, Ashton PM, Herrera-Leon S, Lighthill J, Foulkes S, Jombart T, Rehman Y, Fox A, Dallman T, DE Pinna E, Browning L, Coia JE, Edeghere O, Vivancos R.** 2017. Prospective use of whole genome sequencing (WGS) detected a multi-country outbreak of *Salmonella* Enteritidis. *Epidemiol Infect* **145**:289–298.

22. **McCollum JT, Cronquist AB, Silk BJ, Jackson KA, O'Connor KA, Cosgrove S, Gossack JP, Parachini SS, Jain NS, Ettestad P, Ibraheem M, Cantu V, Joshi M, DuVernoy T, Fogg NW Jr, Gorny JR, Mogen KM, Spires C, Teitell P, Joseph LA, Tarr CL, Imanishi M, Neil KP, Tauxe RV, Mahon BE.** 2013. Multistate outbreak of listeriosis associated with cantaloupe. *N Engl J Med* **369**:944–953.

23. **Deng X, den Bakker HC, Hendriksen RS.** 2016. Genomic epidemiology: whole-genome-sequencing-powered surveillance and outbreak investigation of foodborne bacterial pathogens. *Annu Rev Food Sci Technol* **7**:353–374.

24. **Ronholm J, Nasheri N, Petronella N, Pagotto F.** 2016. Navigating microbiological food safety in the era of whole-genome sequencing. *Clin Microbiol Rev* **29**:837–857.

25. **Ravel A, Hurst M, Petrica N, David J, Mutschall SK, Pintar K, Taboada EN, Pollari F.** 2017. Source attribution of human campylobacteriosis at the point of exposure by combining comparative exposure assessment and subtype comparison based on comparative genomic fingerprinting. *PLoS One* **12**:e0183790.

26. **Kovanen S, Kivistö R, Llarena AK, Zhang J, Kärkkäinen UM, Tuuminen T, Uksila J, Hakkinen M, Rossi M, Hänninen ML.** 2016. Tracing isolates from domestic human *Campylobacter jejuni* infections to chicken slaughter batches and swimming water using whole-genome multilocus sequence typing. *Int J Food Microbiol* **226**:53–60.

27. **Byrne L, Fisher I, Peters T, Mather A, Thomson N, Rosner B, Bernard H, McKeown P, Cormican M, Cowden J, Aiyedun V, Lane C, on behalf of the International Outbreak Control Team.** 2014. A multi-country outbreak of *Salmonella* Newport gastroenteritis in Europe associated with watermelon from Brazil, confirmed by whole genome sequencing: October 2011 to January 2012. *Euro Surveill* **19**:6–13.

28. **European Centre for Disease Control and Prevention.** 2017. *Rapid Risk Assessment: Multi-country outbreak of* Listeria monocytogenes *PCR serogroup IVb, MLST ST6.* European Centre for Disease Prevention and Control, Stockholm, Sweden. https://ecdc.europa.eu/sites/portal/files/documents/RRA-Listeria-monocytogenes-2017_0.pdf.

29. **Stasiewicz MJ, Oliver HF, Wiedmann M, den Bakker HC.** 2015. Whole-genome sequencing allows for improved identification of persistent *Listeria monocytogenes* in food-associated environments. *Appl Environ Microbiol* **81**:6024–6037.

30. **Mellmann A, Harmsen D, Cummings CA, Zentz EB, Leopold SR, Rico A, Prior K, Szczepanowski R, Ji Y, Zhang W, McLaughlin SF, Henkhaus JK, Leopold B, Bielaszewska M, Prager R, Brzoska PM, Moore RL, Guenther S, Rothberg JM, Karch H.** 2011. Prospective genomic characterization of the German enterohemorrhagic *Escherichia coli* O104:H4 outbreak by rapid next generation sequencing technology. *PLoS One* **6:**e22751.

31. **Nyachuba DG.** 2010. Foodborne illness: is it on the rise? *Nutr Rev* **68:**257–269.

32. **Newell DG, Koopmans M, Verhoef L, Duizer E, Aidara-Kane A, Sprong H, Opsteegh M, Langelaar M, Threfall J, Scheutz F, van der Giessen J, Kruse H.** 2010. Food-borne diseases— the challenges of 20 years ago still persist while new ones continue to emerge. *Int J Food Microbiol* **139**(Suppl 1):S3–S15.

33. **Tauxe RV, Doyle MP, Kuchenmüller T, Schlundt J, Stein CE.** 2010. Evolving public health approaches to the global challenge of foodborne infections. *Int J Food Microbiol* **139**(Suppl 1): S16–S28.

34. **Quested TE, Cook PE, Gorris LG, Cole MB.** 2010. Trends in technology, trade and consumption likely to impact on microbial food safety. *Int J Food Microbiol* **139**(Suppl 1):S29–S42.

35. **Boqvist S, Söderqvist K, Vågsholm I.** 2018. Food safety challenges and One Health within Europe. *Acta Vet Scand* **60:**1.

36. **Semenza JC, Lindgren E, Balkanyi L, Espinosa L, Almqvist MS, Penttinen P, Rocklöv J.** 2016. Determinants and drivers of infectious disease threat events in Europe. *Emerg Infect Dis* **22:**581–589.

37. **Engering A, Hogerwerf L, Slingenbergh J.** 2013. Pathogen-host-environment interplay and disease emergence. *Emerg Microbes Infect* **2:**e5.

38. **Rodrigue DC, Tauxe RV, Rowe B.** 1990. International increase in *Salmonella enteritidis*: a new pandemic? *Epidemiol Infect* **105:**21–27.

39. **Kinross P, van Alphen L, Martinez Urtaza J, Struelens M, Takkinen J, Coulombier D, Makela P, Bertrand S, Mattheus W, Schmid D, Kanitz E, Rucker V, Krisztalovics K, Paszti J, Szogyenyi Z, Lancz Z, Rabsch W, Pfefferkorn B, Hiller P, Mooijman K, Gossner C.** 2014. Multidisciplinary investigation of a multicountry outbreak of *Salmonella* Stanley infections associated with turkey meat in the European Union, August 2011 to January 2013. *Euro Surveill* **19:**20801.

40. **Skarp CP, Hänninen ML, Rautelin HI.** 2016. Campylobacteriosis: the role of poultry meat. *Clin Microbiol Infect* **22:**103–109.

41. **Kijlstra A, Meerburg BG, Bos AP.** 2009. Food safety in free-range and organic livestock systems: risk management and responsibility. *J Food Prot* **72:**2629–2637.

42. **Jung Y, Jang H, Matthews KR.** 2014. Effect of the food production chain from farm practices to vegetable processing on outbreak incidence. *Microb Biotechnol* **7:**517–527.

43. **European Food Safety Authority.** 2011. STEC and other pathogenic bacteria in seeds and sprouted seeds. *EFSA J* **9:**2424.

44. **Lomonaco S, Verghese B, Gerner-Smidt P, Tarr C, Gladney L, Joseph L, Katz L, Turnsek M, Frace M, Chen Y, Brown E, Meinersmann R, Berrang M, Knabel S.** 2013. Novel epidemic clones of *Listeria monocytogenes*, United States, 2011. *Emerg Infect Dis* **19:**147–150.

45. **Markland SM, Ingram D, Kniel KE, Sharma M.** 2017. Water for agriculture: the convergence of sustainability and safety. *Microbiol Spectr* **5:**PFS-0014-2016.

46. **Kniel KE, Spanninger P.** 2017. Preharvest food safety under the influence of a changing climate. *Microbiol Spectr* **5:**PFS-0015-2016.

47. **Schijven J, Bouwknegt M, de Roda Husman AM, Rutjes S, Sudre B, Suk JE, Semenza JC.** 2013. A decision support tool to compare waterborne and foodborne infection and/or illness risks associated with climate change. *Risk Anal* **33:**2154–2167.

48. **Hellberg RS, Chu E.** 2016. Effects of climate change on the persistence and dispersal of foodborne bacterial pathogens in the outdoor environment: a review. *Crit Rev Microbiol* **42:**548–572.

49. **Effler E, Isaäcson M, Arntzen L, Heenan R, Canter P, Barrett T, Lee L, Mambo C, Levine W, Zaidi A, Griffin PM.** 2001. Factors contributing to the emergence of *Escherichia coli* O157 in Africa. *Emerg Infect Dis* **7:**812–819.

50. **Vezzulli L, Grande C, Reid PC, Hélaouët P, Edwards M, Höfle MG, Brettar I, Colwell RR, Pruzzo C.** 2016. Climate influence on *Vibrio* and associated human diseases during the past half-century in the coastal North Atlantic. *Proc Natl Acad Sci U S A* **113:**E5062–E5071.

51. **Asao T, Kumeda Y, Kawai T, Shibata T, Oda H, Haruki K, Nakazawa H, Kozaki S.** 2003. An extensive outbreak of staphylococcal food poisoning due to low-fat milk in Japan: estimation of enterotoxin A in the incriminated milk and powdered skim milk. *Epidemiol Infect* **130:**33–40.

52. **European Centre for Disease Prevention and Control.** 2018. Salmonella *Agona outbreak associated with infant formula milk.* European Centre for Disease Prevention and Control, Stockholm, Sweden. https://ecdc.europa.eu/en/news-events/salmonella-agona-outbreak-associated-infant-formula-milk.

53. **Centers for Disease Control and Prevention.** 2016. *Multistate outbreak of listeriosis linked to packaged salads produced at Springfield, Ohio Dole processing facility (final update).* Centers for Disease Control and Prevention, Atlanta, GA. https://www.cdc.gov/listeria/outbreaks/bagged-salads-01-16/index.html.

54. **Centers for Disease Control and Prevention.** 2015. *Multistate outbreak of listeriosis linked to Blue Bell Creameries products (final update).* Centers for Disease Control and Prevention, Atlanta, GA. https://www.cdc.gov/listeria/outbreaks/ice-cream-03-15/index.html.

55. **Powell DA, Jacob CJ, Chapman BJ.** 2011. Enhancing food safety culture to reduce rates of foodborne illness. *Food Control* **22:**817–822.

56. **Gould LH, Kline J, Monahan C, Vierk K.** 2017. Outbreaks of disease associated with food imported into the United States, 1996–2014.[1] *Emerg Infect Dis* **23:**525–528.

57. **Eurostat—Statistics Explained.** 2017. *Extra-EU trade in agricultural goods.* http://ec.europa.eu/eurostat/statistics-explained/index.php/Extra-EU_trade_in_agricultural_goods.

58. **Centers for Disease Control and Prevention.** 2017. *Reports of* Salmonella *outbreak investigations from 2017.* Centers for Disease Control and Prevention, Atlanta, GA. https://www.cdc.gov/salmonella/outbreaks-2017.html.

59. **European Food Safety Authority, European Centre for Disease Prevention and Control.** 2017. *Multi-country outbreak of* Salmonella *Enteritidis infections linked to Polish eggs.* European Food Safety Authority, Parma, Italy. http://onlinelibrary.wiley.com/doi/10.2903/sp.efsa.2017.EN-1353/epdf.

60. **Campos J, Mourão J, Silveira L, Saraiva M, Correia CB, Maçãs AP, Peixe L, Antunes P.** 2018. Imported poultry meat as a source of extended-spectrum cephalosporin-resistant CMY-2-producing *Salmonella* Heidelberg and *Salmonella* Minnesota in the European Union, 2014–2015. *Int J Antimicrob Agents* **51:**151–154.

61. **Liakopoulos A, Geurts Y, Dierikx CM, Brouwer MS, Kant A, Wit B, Heymans R, van Pelt W, Mevius DJ.** 2016. Extended-spectrum cephalosporin-resistant *Salmonella enterica* serovar Heidelberg strains, the Netherlands.[1] *Emerg Infect Dis* **22:**1257–1261.

62. **Li K, Petersen G, Barco L, Hvidtfeldt K, Liu L, Dalsgaard A.** 2017. *Salmonella* Weltevreden in integrated and non-integrated tilapia aquaculture systems in Guangdong, China. *Food Microbiol* **65:**19–24.

63. **Rodríguez-Lázaro D, Ariza-Miguel J, Diez-Valcarce M, Stessl B, Beutlich J, Fernández-Natal I, Hernández M, Wagner M, Rovira J.** 2015. Identification and molecular characterization of pathogenic bacteria in foods confiscated from non-EU flights passengers at one Spanish airport. *Int J Food Microbiol* **209:**20–25.

64. **Beutlich J, Hammerl JA, Appel B, Nöckler K, Helmuth R, Jöst K, Ludwig ML, Hanke C, Bechtold D, Mayer-Scholl A.** 2015. Characterization of illegal food items and identification of foodborne pathogens brought into the European Union via two major German airports. *Int J Food Microbiol* **209:**13–19.

65. **Rodríguez-Lázaro D, Oniciuc EA, García PG, Gallego D, Fernández-Natal I, Dominguez-Gil M, Eiros-Bouza JM, Wagner M, Nicolau AI, Hernández M.** 2017. Detection and characterization of *Staphylococcus aureus* and methicillin-resistant *S. aureus* in foods confiscated in EU borders. *Front Microbiol* **8:**1344.

66. **Callejón RM, Rodríguez-Naranjo MI, Ubeda C, Hornedo-Ortega R, Garcia-Parrilla MC, Troncoso AM.** 2015. Reported foodborne outbreaks due to fresh produce in the United States and European Union: trends and causes. *Foodborne Pathog Dis* **12:**32–38.

67. **EFSA Panel on Biological Hazards (BIOHAZ).** 2015. Scientific opinion on the public health risks related to the consumption of raw drinking milk. *EFSA J* **13:**3940.

68. **EFSA Panel on Biological Hazards (BIOHAZ), Ricci A, Allende A, Bolton D, Chemaly M, Davies R, Escámez PS, Girones R, Herman L, Koutsoumanis K, Nørrung B, Robertson L, Ru G, Sanaa M, Simmons M, Skandamis P, Snary E, Speybroeck N, Ter Kuile B, Threlfall J, Wahlström H, Takkinen J, Wagner M, Arcella D, Da Silva Felicio MT, Georgiadis M, Messens W, Lindqvist R.** 2018. *Listeria monocytogenes* contamination of ready-to-eat foods and the risk for human health in the EU. *EFSA J* **16:**5134.

69. **Baker-Austin C, Stockley L, Rangdale R, Martinez-Urtaza J.** 2010. Environmental occurrence and clinical impact of *Vibrio vulnificus* and *Vibrio parahaemolyticus*: a European perspective. *Environ Microbiol Rep* **2:**7–18.

70. **Le Roux F, Wegner KM, Baker-Austin C, Vezzulli L, Osorio CR, Amaro C, Ritchie JM, Defoirdt T, Destoumieux-Garzón D, Blokesch M, Mazel D, Jacq A, Cava F, Gram L, Wendling CC, Strauch E, Kirschner A, Huehn S.** 2015. The emergence of *Vibrio* pathogens in Europe: ecology, evolution, and pathogenesis (Paris, 11–12th March 2015). *Front Microbiol* **6:**830.

71. **Osimani A, Aquilanti L, Clementi F.** 2016. Salmonellosis associated with mass catering: a survey of European Union cases over a 15-year period. *Epidemiol Infect* **144:**3000–3012.

72. Jones AK, Cross P, Burton M, Millman C, O'Brien SJ, Rigby D. 2017. Estimating the prevalence of food risk increasing behaviours in UK kitchens. *PLoS One* **12:**e0175816.

73. El Omeiri N, Puell-Gomez L, Camps N, Bartolome-Comas R, Simon-Soria F, Soler-Crespo P, Martin-Granado A, Echeita-Sarrionandia A, Herrera-Guibert D. 2007. International outbreak of salmonellosis in a hotel in Lloret de Mar, Spain, August 2007. *Euro Surveill* **12:**E071018.3.

74. Rebolledo J, Garvey P, Ryan A, O'Donnell J, Cormican M, Jackson S, Cloak F, Cullen L, Swaan CM, Schimmer B, Appels RW, Nygard K, Finley R, Sreenivasan N, Lenglet A, Gossner C, McKeown P. 2014. International outbreak investigation of *Salmonella* Heidelberg associated with in-flight catering. *Epidemiol Infect* **142:**833–842.

75. Hochberg NS, Bhadelia N. 2015. Infections associated with exotic cuisine: the dangers of delicacies. *Microbiol Spectr* **3:**IOL5-0010-2015.

76. MacDonald PD, Whitwam RE, Boggs JD, MacCormack JN, Anderson KL, Reardon JW, Saah JR, Graves LM, Hunter SB, Sobel J. 2005. Outbreak of listeriosis among Mexican immigrants as a result of consumption of illicitly produced Mexican-style cheese. *Clin Infect Dis* **40:**677–682.

77. World Health Organization. 2006. *Five Keys to Safer Food Manual.* World Health Organization, Geneva, Switzerland. http://apps.who.int/iris/bitstream/10665/43546/1/9789241594639_eng.pdf?ua=1.

78. Mody RK, Meyer S, Trees E, White PL, Nguyen T, Sowadsky R, Henao OL, Lafon PC, Austin J, Azzam I, Griffin PM, Tauxe RV, Smith K, Williams IT. 2014. Outbreak of *Salmonella enterica* serotype I 4,5,12:i:- infections: the challenges of hypothesis generation and microwave cooking. *Epidemiol Infect* **142:**1050–1060.

79. Lund BM, O'Brien SJ. 2011. The occurrence and prevention of foodborne disease in vulnerable people. *Foodborne Pathog Dis* **8:**961–973.

80. Goulet V, Hebert M, Hedberg C, Laurent E, Vaillant V, De Valk H, Desenclos JC. 2012. Incidence of listeriosis and related mortality among groups at risk of acquiring listeriosis. *Clin Infect Dis* **54:**652–660.

81. Pouillot R, Klontz KC, Chen Y, Burall LS, Macarisin D, Doyle M, Bally KM, Strain E, Datta AR, Hammack TS, Van Doren JM. 2016. Infectious dose of *Listeria monocytogenes* in outbreak linked to ice cream, United States, 2015. *Emerg Infect Dis* **22:**2113–2119.

82. Gould LH, Demma L, Jones TF, Hurd S, Vugia DJ, Smith K, Shiferaw B, Segler S, Palmer A, Zansky S, Griffin PM. 2009. Hemolytic uremic syndrome and death in persons with *Escherichia coli* O157:H7 infection, foodborne diseases active surveillance network sites, 2000–2006. *Clin Infect Dis* **49:**1480–1485.

83. Rosow LK, Strober JB. 2015. Infant botulism: review and clinical update. *Pediatr Neurol* **52:**487–492.

84. Daniels NA. 2011. *Vibrio vulnificus* oysters: pearls and perils. *Clin Infect Dis* **52:**788–792.

85. Baker-Austin C, Oliver JD. 2018. *Vibrio vulnificus*: new insights into a deadly opportunistic pathogen. *Environ Microbiol* **20:**423–430.

86. Bos J, Smithee L, McClane B, Distefano RF, Uzal F, Songer JG, Mallonee S, Crutcher JM. 2005. Fatal necrotizing colitis following a foodborne outbreak of enterotoxigenic *Clostridium perfringens* type A infection. *Clin Infect Dis* **40:**e78–e83.

87. Bowen A, Newman A, Estivariz C, Gilbertson N, Archer J, Srinivasan A, Lynch M, Painter J. 2007. Role of acid-suppressing medications during a sustained outbreak of *Salmonella enteritidis* infection in a long-term care facility. *Infect Control Hosp Epidemiol* **28:**1202–1205.

88. Gillespie IA, McLauchlin J, Little CL, Penman C, Mook P, Grant K, O'Brien SJ. 2009. Disease presentation in relation to infection foci for non-pregnancy-associated human listeriosis in England and Wales, 2001 to 2007. *J Clin Microbiol* **47:**3301–3307.

89. Tam CC, Higgins CD, Neal KR, Rodrigues LC, Millership SE, O'Brien SJ, Campylobacter Case-Control Study Group. 2009. Chicken consumption and use of acid-suppressing medications as risk factors for *Campylobacter* enteritis, England. *Emerg Infect Dis* **15:**1402–1408.

90. Begley M, Hill C. 2015. Stress adaptation in foodborne pathogens. *Annu Rev Food Sci Technol* **6:**191–210.

91. Wesche AM, Gurtler JB, Marks BP, Ryser ET. 2009. Stress, sublethal injury, resuscitation, and virulence of bacterial foodborne pathogens. *J Food Prot* **72:**1121–1138.

92. Yousef AE, Courtney PD. 2003. Basics of stress adaptation and implications in new-generation foods, p 1–30. *In* Yousef AE, Juneja VK (ed), *Microbial Stress Adaptation and Food Safety.* CRC Press, Boca Raton, FL.

93. Browne HP, Neville BA, Forster SC, Lawley TD. 2017. Transmission of the gut microbiota: spreading of health. *Nat Rev Microbiol* **15:**531–543.

94. Singh S, Shalini R. 2016. Effect of hurdle technology in food preservation: a review. *Crit Rev Food Sci Nutr* **56:**641–649.

95. Fang FC, Frawley ER, Tapscott T, Vázquez-Torres A. 2016. Bacterial stress responses during host infection. *Cell Host Microbe* **20:**133–143.

96. **Alvarez-Ordóñez A, Broussolle V, Colin P, Nguyen-The C, Prieto M.** 2015. The adaptive response of bacterial food-borne pathogens in the environment, host and food: implications for food safety. *Int J Food Microbiol* **213:**99–109.

97. **Anderson CJ, Kendall MM.** 2017. *Salmonella enterica* serovar Typhimurium strategies for host adaptation. *Front Microbiol* **8:**1983.

98. **Kim JC, Oh E, Kim J, Jeon B.** 2015. Regulation of oxidative stress resistance in *Campylobacter jejuni*, a microaerophilic foodborne pathogen. *Front Microbiol* **6:**751.

99. **Burgess CM, Gianotti A, Gruzdev N, Holah J, Knøchel S, Lehner A, Margas E, Esser SS, Sela Saldinger S, Tresse O.** 2016. The response of foodborne pathogens to osmotic and desiccation stresses in the food chain. *Int J Food Microbiol* **221:**37–53.

100. **Wieczorek K, Osek J.** 2013. Antimicrobial resistance mechanisms among *Campylobacter. BioMed Res Int* **2013:**340605.

101. **Mourão J, Novais C, Machado J, Peixe L, Antunes P.** 2015. Metal tolerance in emerging clinically relevant multidrug-resistant *Salmonella enterica* serotype 4,[5],12:i:- clones circulating in Europe. *Int J Antimicrob Agents* **45:**610–616.

102. **Mourão J, Marçal S, Ramos P, Campos J, Machado J, Peixe L, Novais C, Antunes P.** 2016. Tolerance to multiple metal stressors in emerging non-typhoidal MDR *Salmonella* serotypes: a relevant role for copper in anaerobic conditions. *J Antimicrob Chemother* **71:**2147–2157.

103. **Finn S, Condell O, McClure P, Amézquita A, Fanning S.** 2013. Mechanisms of survival, responses and sources of *Salmonella* in low-moisture environments. *Front Microbiol* **4:**331.

104. **Tamber S.** 2018. Population-wide survey of *Salmonella enterica* response to high-pressure processing reveals a diversity of responses and tolerance mechanisms. *Appl Environ Microbiol* **84:**e01673-17.

105. **Dawoud TM, Davis ML, Park SH, Kim SA, Kwon YM, Jarvis N, O'Bryan CA, Shi Z, Crandall PG, Ricke SC.** 2017. The potential link between thermal resistance and virulence in *Salmonella*: a review. *Front Vet Sci* **4:**93.

106. **Álvarez-Ordóñez A, Prieto M, Bernardo A, Hill C, López M.** 2012. The acid tolerance response of *Salmonella* spp.: an adaptive strategy to survive in stressful environments prevailing in foods and the host. *Food Res Int* **45:**482–492.

107. **Mercer RG, Zheng J, Garcia-Hernandez R, Ruan L, Gänzle MG, McMullen LM.** 2015. Genetic determinants of heat resistance in *Escherichia coli. Front Microbiol* **6:**932.

108. **Vidovic S, Korber DR.** 2016. *Escherichia coli* O157: insights into the adaptive stress physiology and the influence of stressors on epidemiology and ecology of this human pathogen. *Crit Rev Microbiol* **42:**83–93.

109. **NicAogáin K, O'Byrne CP.** 2016. The role of stress and stress adaptations in determining the fate of the bacterial pathogen *Listeria monocytogenes* in the food chain. *Front Microbiol* **7:**1865.

110. **Møretrø T, Schirmer BC, Heir E, Fagerlund A, Hjemli P, Langsrud S.** 2017. Tolerance to quaternary ammonium compound disinfectants may enhance growth of *Listeria monocytogenes* in the food industry. *Int J Food Microbiol* **241:**215–224.

111. **Kremer PH, Lees JA, Koopmans MM, Ferwerda B, Arends AW, Feller MM, Schipper K, Valls Seron M, van der Ende A, Brouwer MC, van de Beek D, Bentley SD.** 2017. Benzalkonium tolerance genes and outcome in *Listeria monocytogenes* meningitis. *Clin Microbiol Infect* **23:**265.e1–265.e7.

112. **Kalburge SS, Whitaker WB, Boyd EF.** 2014. High-salt preadaptation of *Vibrio parahaemolyticus* enhances survival in response to lethal environmental stresses. *J Food Prot* **77:**246–253.

113. **Duport C, Jobin M, Schmitt P.** 2016. Adaptation in *Bacillus cereus*: from stress to disease. *Front Microbiol* **7:**1550.

114. **Orieskova M, Kajsik M, Szemes T, Holy O, Forsythe S, Turna J, Drahovska H.** 2016. Contribution of the thermotolerance genomic island to increased thermal tolerance in *Cronobacter* strains. *Antonie Van Leeuwenhoek* **109:**405–414.

115. **Hernández SB, Cota I, Ducret A, Aussel L, Casadesús J.** 2012. Adaptation and preadaptation of *Salmonella enterica* to bile. *PLoS Genet* **8:**e1002459.

116. **Lianou A, Nychas GE, Koutsoumanis KP.** 2017. Variability in the adaptive acid tolerance response phenotype of *Salmonella enterica* strains. *Food Microbiol* **62:**99–105.

117. **Gruzdev N, Pinto R, Sela S.** 2011. Effect of desiccation on tolerance of *Salmonella enterica* to multiple stresses. *Appl Environ Microbiol* **77:**1667–1673.

118. **Begley M, Gahan CG, Hill C.** 2002. Bile stress response in *Listeria monocytogenes* LO28: adaptation, cross-protection, and identification of genetic loci involved in bile resistance. *Appl Environ Microbiol* **68:**6005–6012.

119. **Chung HJ, Bang W, Drake MA.** 2006. Stress response of *Escherichia coli. Compr Rev Food Sci Food Saf* **5:**52–64.

120. **Schelin J, Wallin-Carlquist N, Cohn MT, Lindqvist R, Barker GC, Rådström P.** 2011. The formation of *Staphylococcus aureus* enterotoxin in food environments and advances in risk assessment. *Virulence* **2:**580–592.

121. Ehling-Schulz M, Frenzel E, Gohar M. 2015. Food-bacteria interplay: pathometabolism of emetic *Bacillus cereus*. *Front Microbiol* **6:**704.

122. Kapperud G, Gustavsen S, Hellesnes I, Hansen AH, Lassen J, Hirn J, Jahkola M, Montenegro MA, Helmuth R. 1990. Outbreak of *Salmonella typhimurium* infection traced to contaminated chocolate and caused by a strain lacking the 60-megadalton virulence plasmid. *J Clin Microbiol* **28:**2597–2601.

123. Lenzi LJ, Lucchesi PM, Medico L, Burgán J, Krüger A. 2016. Effect of the food additives sodium citrate and disodium phosphate on Shiga toxin-producing *Escherichia coli* and production of *stx*-phages and Shiga toxin. *Front Microbiol* **7:**992.

124. Crozier L, Hedley PE, Morris J, Wagstaff C, Andrews SC, Toth I, Jackson RW, Holden NJ. 2016. Whole-transcriptome analysis of verocytotoxigenic *Escherichia coli* O157:H7 (Sakai) suggests plant-species-specific metabolic responses on exposure to spinach and lettuce extracts. *Front Microbiol* **7:**1088.

125. Lawley TD, Bouley DM, Hoy YE, Gerke C, Relman DA, Monack DM. 2008. Host transmission of *Salmonella enterica* serovar Typhimurium is controlled by virulence factors and indigenous intestinal microbiota. *Infect Immun* **76:**403–416.

126. Brooks AN, Turkarslan S, Beer KD, Lo FY, Baliga NS. 2011. Adaptation of cells to new environments. *Wiley Interdiscip Rev Syst Biol Med* **3:**544–561.

127. Abee T, Koomen J, Metselaar KI, Zwietering MH, den Besten HM. 2016. Impact of pathogen population heterogeneity and stress-resistant variants on food safety. *Annu Rev Food Sci Technol* **7:**439–456.

128. Guldimann C, Guariglia-Oropeza V, Harrand S, Kent D, Boor KJ, Wiedmann M. 2017. Stochastic and differential activation of σ^B and PrfA in *Listeria monocytogenes* at the single cell level under different environmental stress conditions. *Front Microbiol* **8:**348.

129. Ortiz S, López V, Martínez-Suárez JV. 2014. Control of *Listeria monocytogenes* contamination in an Iberian pork processing plant and selection of benzalkonium chloride-resistant strains. *Food Microbiol* **39:**81–88.

130. Moura A, Criscuolo A, Pouseele H, Maury MM, Leclercq A, Tarr C, Björkman JT, Dallman T, Reimer A, Enouf V, Larsonneur E, Carleton H, Bracq-Dieye H, Katz LS, Jones L, Touchon M, Tourdjman M, Walker M, Stroika S, Cantinelli T, Chenal-Francisque V, Kucerova Z, Rocha EP, Nadon C, Grant K, Nielsen EM, Pot B, Gerner-Smidt P, Lecuit M, Brisse S. 2016. Whole genome-based population biology and epidemiological surveillance of *Listeria monocytogenes*. *Nat Microbiol* **2:**16185.

131. Schmitz-Esser S, Müller A, Stessl B, Wagner M. 2015. Genomes of sequence type 121 *Listeria monocytogenes* strains harbor highly conserved plasmids and prophages. *Front Microbiol* **6:**380.

132. Ferreira V, Wiedmann M, Teixeira P, Stasiewicz MJ. 2014. *Listeria monocytogenes* persistence in food-associated environments: epidemiology, strain characteristics, and implications for public health. *J Food Prot* **77:**150–170.

133. Hingston P, Chen J, Dhillon BK, Laing C, Bertelli C, Gannon V, Tasara T, Allen K, Brinkman FS, Truelstrup Hansen L, Wang S. 2017. Genotypes associated with *Listeria monocytogenes* isolates displaying impaired or enhanced tolerances to cold, salt, acid, or desiccation stress. *Front Microbiol* **8:**369.

134. Dlusskaya EA, McMullen LM, Gänzle MG. 2011. Characterization of an extremely heat-resistant *Escherichia coli* obtained from a beef processing facility. *J Appl Microbiol* **110:**840–849.

135. Mercer RG, Walker BD, Yang X, McMullen LM, Gänzle MG. 2017. The locus of heat resistance (LHR) mediates heat resistance in *Salmonella enterica*, *Escherichia coli* and *Enterobacter cloacae*. *Food Microbiol* **64:**96–103.

136. Zhou K, Ferdous M, de Boer RF, Kooistra-Smid AM, Grundmann H, Friedrich AW, Rossen JW. 2015. The mosaic genome structure and phylogeny of Shiga toxin-producing *Escherichia coli* O104:H4 is driven by short-term adaptation. *Clin Microbiol Infect* **21:**468.e7–468.e18.

137. Grad YH, Godfrey P, Cerquiera GC, Mariani-Kurkdjian P, Gouali M, Bingen E, Shea TP, Haas BJ, Griggs A, Young S, Zeng Q, Lipsitch M, Waldor MK, Weill FX, Wortman JR, Hanage WP. 2013. Comparative genomics of recent Shiga toxin-producing *Escherichia coli* O104:H4: short-term evolution of an emerging pathogen. *mBio* **4:**e00452-12.

138. Baquero F, Tobes R. 2013. Bloody *coli*: a gene cocktail in *Escherichia coli* O104:H4. *mBio* **4:**e00066-13.

139. Karch H, Denamur E, Dobrindt U, Finlay BB, Hengge R, Johannes L, Ron EZ, Tønjum T, Sansonetti PJ, Vicente M. 2012. The enemy within us: lessons from the 2011 European *Escherichia coli* O104:H4 outbreak. *EMBO Mol Med* **4:**841–848.

140. Parker CT, Kyle JL, Huynh S, Carter MQ, Brandl MT, Mandrell RE. 2012. Distinct transcriptional profiles and phenotypes exhibited by *Escherichia coli* O157:H7 isolates related to the 2006 spinach-associated outbreak. *Appl Environ Microbiol* **78:**455–463.

141. Martínez-Vaz BM, Fink RC, Diez-Gonzalez F, Sadowsky MJ. 2014. Enteric pathogen-plant

interactions: molecular connections leading to colonization and growth and implications for food safety. *Microbes Environ* **29**:123–135.

142. **Brandl MT, Amundson R.** 2008. Leaf age as a risk factor in contamination of lettuce with *Escherichia coli* O157:H7 and *Salmonella enterica. Appl Environ Microbiol* **74**:2298–2306.

143. **Gu G, Hu J, Cevallos-Cevallos JM, Richardson SM, Bartz JA, van Bruggen AH.** 2011. Internal colonization of *Salmonella enterica* serovar Typhimurium in tomato plants. *PLoS One* **6**: e27340.

144. **Kroupitski Y, Golberg D, Belausov E, Pinto R, Swartzberg D, Granot D, Sela S.** 2009. Internalization of *Salmonella enterica* in leaves is induced by light and involves chemotaxis and penetration through open stomata. *Appl Environ Microbiol* **75**: 6076–6086.

145. **Shenoy AG, Oliver HF, Deering AJ.** 2017. *Listeria monocytogenes* internalizes in romaine lettuce grown in greenhouse conditions. *J Food Prot* **80**: 573–581.

146. **Erickson MC, Webb CC, Davey LE, Payton AS, Flitcroft ID, Doyle MP.** 2014. Biotic and abiotic variables affecting internalization and fate of *Escherichia coli* O157:H7 isolates in leafy green roots. *J Food Prot* **77**:872–879.

147. **Wadamori Y, Gooneratne R, Hussain MA.** 2017. Outbreaks and factors influencing microbiological contamination of fresh produce. *J Sci Food Agric* **97**:1396–1403.

148. **Leenanon B, Drake MA.** 2001. Acid stress, starvation, and cold stress affect poststress behavior of *Escherichia coli* O157:H7 and nonpathogenic *Escherichia coli. J Food Prot* **64**:970–974.

149. **Poimenidou SV, Chatzithoma DN, Nychas GJ, Skandamis PN.** 2016. Adaptive response of *Listeria monocytogenes* to heats Salinity and low pH, after habituation on cherry tomatoes and lettuce leaves. *PLoS One* **11**:e0165746.

150. **Aviles B, Klotz C, Smith T, Williams R, Ponder M.** 2013. Survival of *Salmonella enterica* serotype Tennessee during simulated gastric passage is improved by low water activity and high fat content. *J Food Prot* **76**:333–337.

151. **Birk T, Kristensen K, Harboe A, Hansen TB, Ingmer H, De Jonge R, Takumi K, Aabo S.** 2012. Dietary proteins extend the survival of *Salmonella* Dublin in a gastric acid environment. *J Food Prot* **75**:353–358.

152. **Liu Y, Gill A, McMullen L, Gänzle MG.** 2015. Variation in heat and pressure resistance of verotoxigenic and nontoxigenic *Escherichia coli. J Food Prot* **78**:111–120.

153. **Li H, Gänzle M.** 2016. Some like it hot: heat resistance of *Escherichia coli* in food. *Front Microbiol* **7**:1763.

154. **Stackhouse RR, Faith NG, Kaspar CW, Czuprynski CJ, Wong AC.** 2012. Survival and virulence of *Salmonella enterica* serovar Enteritidis filaments induced by reduced water activity. *Appl Environ Microbiol* **78**:2213–2220.

155. **Zhao X, Zhong J, Wei C, Lin CW, Ding T.** 2017. Current perspectives on viable but non-culturable state in foodborne pathogens. *Front Microbiol* **8**:580.

156. **Patrone V, Campana R, Vallorani L, Dominici S, Federici S, Casadei L, Gioacchini AM, Stocchi V, Baffone W.** 2013. CadF expression in *Campylobacter jejuni* strains incubated under low-temperature water microcosm conditions which induce the viable but non-culturable (VBNC) state. *Antonie Van Leeuwenhoek* **103**:979–988.

157. **Yaron S, Matthews KR.** 2002. A reverse transcriptase-polymerase chain reaction assay for detection of viable *Escherichia coli* O157:H7: investigation of specific target genes. *J Appl Microbiol* **92**:633–640.

158. **Dinu LD, Bach S.** 2011. Induction of viable but nonculturable *Escherichia coli* O157:H7 in the phyllosphere of lettuce: a food safety risk factor. *Appl Environ Microbiol* **77**:8295–8302.

159. **Orruño M, Kaberdin VR, Arana I.** 2017. Survival strategies of *Escherichia coli* and *Vibrio* spp.: contribution of the viable but nonculturable phenotype to their stress-resistance and persistence in adverse environments. *World J Microbiol Biotechnol* **33**:45.

160. **Aurass P, Prager R, Flieger A.** 2011. EHEC/EAEC O104:H4 strain linked with the 2011 German outbreak of haemolytic uremic syndrome enters into the viable but non-culturable state in response to various stresses and resuscitates upon stress relief. *Environ Microbiol* **13**:3139–3148.

161. **Schelin J, Susilo YB, Johler S.** 2017. Expression of staphylococcal enterotoxins under stress encountered during food production and preservation. *Toxins (Basel)* **9**:E401.

162. **Walker-York-Moore L, Moore SC, Fox EM.** 2017. Characterization of enterotoxigenic *Bacillus cereus sensu lato* and *Staphylococcus aureus* isolates and associated enterotoxin production dynamics in milk or meat-based broth. *Toxins (Basel)* **9**:E225.

163. **Wallin-Carlquist N, Cao R, Márta D, da Silva AS, Schelin J, Rådström P.** 2010. Acetic acid increases the phage-encoded enterotoxin A expression in *Staphylococcus aureus. BMC Microbiol* **10**:147.

164. **Zeaki N, Rådström P, Schelin J.** 2015. Evaluation of potential effects of NaCl and sorbic acid on staphylococcal enterotoxin A formation. *Microorganisms* **3**:551–566.

165. **Regenthal P, Hansen JS, André I, Lindkvist-Petersson K.** 2017. Thermal stability and struc-

tural changes in bacterial toxins responsible for food poisoning. *PLoS One* **12**:e0172445.

166. **Ikeda T, Tamate N, Yamaguchi K, Makino S.** 2005. Mass outbreak of food poisoning disease caused by small amounts of staphylococcal enterotoxins A and H. *Appl Environ Microbiol* **71:** 2793–2795.

167. **Jørgensen HJ, Mathisen T, Løvseth A, Omoe K, Qvale KS, Loncarevic S.** 2005. An outbreak of staphylococcal food poisoning caused by enterotoxin H in mashed potato made with raw milk. *FEMS Microbiol Lett* **252**:267–272.

168. **Munns KD, Selinger LB, Stanford K, Guan L, Callaway TR, McAllister TA.** 2015. Perspectives on super-shedding of *Escherichia coli* O157:H7 by cattle. *Foodborne Pathog Dis* **12:**89–103.

169. **Bäumler AJ, Sperandio V.** 2016. Interactions between the microbiota and pathogenic bacteria in the gut. *Nature* **535:**85–93.

170. **Marzel A, Desai PT, Goren A, Schorr YI, Nissan I, Porwollik S, Valinsky L, McClelland M, Rahav G, Gal-Mor O.** 2016. Persistent Infections by nontyphoidal *Salmonella* in humans: epidemiology and genetics. *Clin Infect Dis* **62:**879–886.

171. **Feasey NA, Dougan G, Kingsley RA, Heyderman RS, Gordon MA.** 2012. Invasive non-typhoidal *Salmonella* disease: an emerging and neglected tropical disease in Africa. *Lancet* **379:**2489–2499.

172. **Dearlove BL, Cody AJ, Pascoe B, Méric G, Wilson DJ, Sheppard SK.** 2016. Rapid host switching in generalist *Campylobacter* strains erodes the signal for tracing human infections. *ISME J* **10:** 721–729.

173. **Alemka A, Corcionivoschi N, Bourke B.** 2012. Defense and adaptation: the complex interrelationship between *Campylobacter jejuni* and mucus. *Front Cell Infect Microbiol* **2:**15.

174. **Robyn J, Rasschaert G, Pasmans F, Heyndrickx M.** 2015. Thermotolerant *Campylobacter* during broiler rearing: risk factors and intervention. *Compr Rev Food Sci Food Saf* **14:**81–105.

175. **Stein RA, Katz DE.** 2017. *Escherichia coli*, cattle and the propagation of disease. *FEMS Microbiol Lett* **364:**fnx050.

176. **Xu Y, Dugat-Bony E, Zaheer R, Selinger L, Barbieri R, Munns K, McAllister TA, Selinger LB.** 2014. *Escherichia coli* O157:H7 super-shedder and non-shedder feedlot steers harbour distinct fecal bacterial communities. *PLoS One* **9:**e98115.

177. **Wang O, Liang G, McAllister TA, Plastow G, Stanford K, Selinger B, Guan L.** 2016. Comparative transcriptomic analysis of rectal tissue from beef steers revealed reduced host immunity in *Escherichia coli* O157:H7 super-shedders. *PLoS One* **11:**e0151284.

178. **Murase T, Yamada M, Muto T, Matsushima A, Yamai S.** 2000. Fecal excretion of *Salmonella enterica* serovar Typhimurium following a foodborne outbreak. *J Clin Microbiol* **38:**3495–3497.

179. **Sheppard SK, Didelot X, Meric G, Torralbo A, Jolley KA, Kelly DJ, Bentley SD, Maiden MC, Parkhill J, Falush D.** 2013. Genome-wide association study identifies vitamin B5 biosynthesis as a host specificity factor in *Campylobacter*. *Proc Natl Acad Sci U S A* **110:**11923–11927.

180. **Llarena AK, Taboada E, Rossi M.** 2017. Whole-genome sequencing in epidemiology of *Campylobacter jejuni* infections. *J Clin Microbiol* **55:** 1269–1275.

181. **Crump JA, Sjölund-Karlsson M, Gordon MA, Parry CM.** 2015. Epidemiology, clinical presentation, laboratory diagnosis, antimicrobial resistance, and antimicrobial management of invasive *Salmonella* infections. *Clin Microbiol Rev* **28:**901–937.

182. **European Commission.** 2017. *A European One Health Action Plan against Antimicrobial Resistance (AMR)*. European Commission, Brussels, Belgium https://ec.europa.eu/health/amr/sites/amr/files/amr_action_plan_2017_en.pdf.

183. **European Food Safety Authority, European Centre for Disease Prevention and Control.** 2016. The European Union summary report on antimicrobial resistance in zoonotic and indicator bacteria from humans, animals and food in 2014. *EFSA J* **14:**4380. http://onlinelibrary.wiley.com/doi/10.2903/j.efsa.2016.4380/epdf.

184. **World Health Organization.** 2015. *Global Action Plan on Antimicrobial Resistance*. World Health Organization, Geneva, Switzerland. http://apps.who.int/iris/bitstream/10665/193736/1/9789241509763_eng.pdf?ua=1.

185. **Food and Agriculture Organization of the United Nations.** 2016. *The FAO Action Plan on Antimicrobial Resistance 2016–2020*. Food and Agriculture Organization of the United Nations, Rome, Italy. http://www.fao.org/3/a-i5996e.pdf.

186. **World Health Organization.** 2017. *WHO Guidelines on Use of Medically Important Antimicrobials in Food-Producing Animals*. World Health Organization, Geneva, Switzerland. http://apps.who.int/iris/bitstream/10665/258970/1/9789241550130-eng.pdf?ua=1.

187. **Centers for Disease Control and Prevention.** 2013. *Antibiotic Resistance Threats in the United States, 2013*. Centers for Disease Control and Prevention, Atlanta, GA. https://www.cdc.gov/drugresistance/threat-report-2013/pdf/ar-threats-2013-508.pdf.

188. **European Food Safety Authority.** 2009. Joint opinion on antimicrobial resistance (AMR) focused on zoonotic infections. *EFSA J* **7:**1372.

189. **Founou LL, Founou RC, Essack SY.** 2016. Antibiotic resistance in the food chain: a developing country-perspective. *Front Microbiol* **7:**1881.

190. **Chang Q, Wang W, Regev-Yochay G, Lipsitch M, Hanage WP.** 2015. Antibiotics in agriculture and the risk to human health: how worried should we be? *Evol Appl* **8:**240–247.

191. **Holmes AH, Moore LS, Sundsfjord A, Steinbakk M, Regmi S, Karkey A, Guerin PJ, Piddock LJ.** 2016. Understanding the mechanisms and drivers of antimicrobial resistance. *Lancet* **387:**176–187.

192. **Aarestrup FM.** 2015. The livestock reservoir for antimicrobial resistance: a personal view on changing patterns of risks, effects of interventions and the way forward. *Philos Trans R Soc Lond B Biol Sci* **370:**20140085.

193. **Silveira E, Freitas AR, Antunes P, Barros M, Campos J, Coque TM, Peixe L, Novais C.** 2014. Co-transfer of resistance to high concentrations of copper and first-line antibiotics among *Enterococcus* from different origins (humans, animals, the environment and foods) and clonal lineages. *J Antimicrob Chemother* **69:**899–906.

194. **Toutain PL, Ferran AA, Bousquet-Melou A, Pelligand L, Lees P.** 2016. Veterinary medicine needs new green antimicrobial drugs. *Front Microbiol* **7:**1196.

195. **EFSA Panel on Biological Hazards (BIOHAZ).** 2011. Scientific opinion on the public health risks of bacterial strains producing extended-spectrum β-lactamases and/or AmpC β-lactamases in food and food-producing animals. *EFSA J* **9:**2322.

196. **Threlfall EJ, Ward LR, Frost JA, Cheasty T, Willshaw GA.** The emergence and spread of antibiotic resistance in food-borne bacteria in the United Kingdom. *AUPA Newsletter* **17:**1–7.

197. **Nachamkin I, Ung H, Li M.** 2002. Increasing fluoroquinolone resistance in *Campylobacter jejuni*, Pennsylvania, USA,1982–2001. *Emerg Infect Dis* **8:**1501–1503.

198. **Endtz HP, Ruijs GJ, van Klingeren B, Jansen WH, van der Reyden T, Mouton RP.** 1991. Quinolone esistance in *Campylobacter* isolated from man and poultry following the introduction of fluoroquinolones in veterinary medicine. *J Antimicrob Chemother* **27:**199–208.

199. **Dutil L, Irwin R, Finley R, Ng LK, Avery B, Boerlin P, Bourgault AM, Cole L, Daignault D, Desruisseau A, Demczuk W, Hoang L, Horsman GB, Ismail J, Jamieson F, Maki A, Pacagnella A, Pillai DR.** 2010. Ceftiofur resistance in *Salmonella enterica* serovar Heidelberg from chicken meat and humans, Canada. *Emerg Infect Dis* **16:**48–54.

200. **van den Bogaard AE, Bruinsma N, Stobberingh EE.** 2000. The effect of banning avoparcin on VRE carriage in The Netherlands. *J Antimicrob Chemother* **46:**146–148.

201. **Klare I, Badstübner D, Konstabel C, Böhme G, Claus H, Witte W.** 1999. Decreased incidence of VanA-type vancomycin-resistant enterococci isolated from poultry meat and from fecal samples of humans in the community after discontinuation of avoparcin usage in animal husbandry. *Microb Drug Resist* **5:**45–52.

202. **Bager F, Aarestrup FM, Madsen M, Wegener HC.** 1999. Glycopeptide resistance in *Enterococcus faecium* from broilers and pigs following discontinued use of avoparcin. *Microb Drug Resist* **5:**53–56.

203. **Pantosti A, Del Grosso M, Tagliabue S, Macrì A, Caprioli A.** 1999. Decrease of vancomycin-resistant enterococci in poultry meat after avoparcin ban. *Lancet* **354:**741–742.

204. **European Centre for Disease Prevention and Control (ECDC), European Food Safety Authority (EFSA), European Medicines Agency (EMA).** 2017. ECDC/EFSA/EMA second joint report on the integrated analysis of the consumption of antimicrobial agents and occurrence of antimicrobial resistance in bacteria from humans and food producing animals. Joint Interagency Antimicrobial Consumption and Resistance Analysis (JIACRA) report. *EFSA J* **15:**4872.

205. **Antunes P, Machado J, Peixe L.** 2006. Illegal use of nitrofurans in food animals: contribution to human salmonellosis? *Clin Microbiol Infect* **12:**1047–1049.

206. **National Antimicrobial Resistance Monitoring System.** 2017. *NARMS 2015 Integrated Report.* Food and Drug Administration, Laurel, MD. https://www.fda.gov/downloads/AnimalVeterinary/Safety Health/AntimicrobialResistance/NationalAnti microbialResistanceMonitoringSystem/UCM 581468.pdf.

207. **Lee HY, Su LH, Tsai MH, Kim SW, Chang HH, Jung SI, Park KH, Perera J, Carlos C, Tan BH, Kumarasinghe G, So T, Chongthaleong A, Hsueh PR, Liu JW, Song JH, Chiu CH.** 2009. High rate of reduced susceptibility to ciprofloxacin and ceftriaxone among nontyphoid *Salmonella* clinical isolates in Asia. *Antimicrob Agents Chemother* **53:**2696–2699.

208. **Van TT, Nguyen HN, Smooker PM, Coloe PJ.** 2012. The antibiotic resistance characteristics of non-typhoidal *Salmonella enterica* isolated from food-producing animals, retail meat and humans in South East Asia. *Int J Food Microbiol* **154:**98–106.

209. **Yang B, Cui Y, Shi C, Wang J, Xia X, Xi M, Wang X, Meng J, Alali WQ, Walls I, Doyle MP.** 2014. Counts, serotypes, and antimicrobial resistance of *Salmonella* isolates on retail raw poultry in the People's Republic of China. *J Food Prot* **77:**894–902.

210. **Yoon RH, Cha SY, Wei B, Roh JH, Seo HS, Oh JY, Jang HK.** 2014. Prevalence of *Salmonella* isolates and antimicrobial resistance in poultry

meat from South Korea. *J Food Prot* **77:**1579–1582.

211. **Jiang HX, Tang D, Liu YH, Zhang XH, Zeng ZL, Xu L, Hawkey PM.** 2012. Prevalence and characteristics of β-lactamase and plasmid-mediated quinolone resistance genes in *Escherichia coli* isolated from farmed fish in China. *J Antimicrob Chemother* **67:**2350–2353.

212. **Chen K, Chan EW, Xie M, Ye L, Dong N, Chen S.** 2017. Widespread distribution of *mcr-1*-bearing bacteria in the ecosystem, 2015 to 2016. *Euro Surveill* **22:**17-00206.

213. **Trung NV, Matamoros S, Carrique-Mas JJ, Nghia NH, Nhung NT, Chieu TTB, Mai HH, van Rooijen W, Campbell J, Wagenaar JA, Hardon A, Mai NT, Hieu TQ, Thwaites G, de Jong MD, Schultsz C, Hoa NT.** 2017. Zoonotic transmission of *mcr-1* colistin resistance gene from small-scale poultry farms, Vietnam. *Emerg Infect Dis* **23:**529–532.

214. **Van Boeckel TP, Brower C, Gilbert M, Grenfell BT, Levin SA, Robinson TP, Teillant A, Laxminarayan R.** 2015. Global trends in antimicrobial use in food animals. *Proc Natl Acad Sci U S A* **112:**5649–5654.

215. **Statens Serum Institut; National Veterinary Institute, Technical University of Denmark; National Food Institute, Technical University of Denmark.** 2017. *DANMAP 2016—Use of Antimicrobial Agents and Occurrence of Antimicrobial Resistance in Bacteria from Food Animals, Food and Humans in Denmark.* https://www.danmap.org/~/media/Projektsites/Danmap/DANMAPReports/DANMAP2016/DANMAP_2016_web.ashx.

216. **Agersø Y, Jensen JD, Hasman H, Pedersen K.** 2014. Spread of extended spectrum cephalosporinase-producing *Escherichia coli* clones and plasmids from parent animals to broilers and to broiler meat in a production without use of cephalosporins. *Foodborne Pathog Dis* **11:**740–746.

217. **Seiffert SN, Hilty M, Perreten V, Endimiani A.** 2013. Extended-spectrum cephalosporin-resistant Gram-negative organisms in livestock: an emerging problem for human health? *Drug Resist Updat* **16:**22–45.

218. **Manges AR, Johnson JR.** 2015. Reservoirs of extraintestinal pathogenic *Escherichia coli. Microbiol Spectr* **3:**UTI-0006-2012.

219. **Franco A, Leekitcharoenphon P, Feltrin F, Alba P, Cordaro G, Iurescia M, Tolli R, D'Incau M, Staffolani M, Di Giannatale E, Hendriksen RS, Battisti A.** 2015. Emergence of a clonal lineage of multidrug-resistant ESBL-producing *Salmonella infantis* transmitted from broilers and broiler meat to humans in Italy between 2011 and 2014. *PLoS One* **10:**e0144802.

220. **Edirmanasinghe R, Finley R, Parmley EJ, Avery BP, Carson C, Bekal S, Golding G, Mulvey MR.** 2017. A whole-genome sequencing approach to study cefoxitin-resistant *Salmonella enterica* serovar Heidelberg isolates from various sources. *Antimicrob Agents Chemother* **61:**e01919-16.

221. **Le Hello S, Bekhit A, Granier SA, Barua H, Beutlich J, Zając M, Münch S, Sintchenko V, Bouchrif B, Fashae K, Pinsard JL, Sontag L, Fabre L, Garnier M, Guibert V, Howard P, Hendriksen RS, Christensen JP, Biswas PK, Cloeckaert A, Rabsch W, Wasyl D, Doublet B, Weill FX.** 2013. The global establishment of a highly-fluoroquinolone resistant *Salmonella enterica* serotype Kentucky ST198 strain. *Front Microbiol* **4:**395.

222. **Campos J, Cristino L, Peixe L, Antunes P.** 2016. MCR-1 in multidrug-resistant and copper-tolerant clinically relevant *Salmonella* 1,4,[5],12:i:- and *S.* Rissen clones in Portugal, 2011 to 2015. *Euro Surveill* **21:**30270.

223. **Zurfluh K, Nüesch-Inderbinen M, Klumpp J, Poirel L, Nordmann P, Stephan R.** 2017. Key features of *mcr-1*-bearing plasmids from *Escherichia coli* isolated from humans and food. *Antimicrob Resist Infect Control* **6:**91.

224. **Bai L, Zhao J, Gan X, Wang J, Zhang X, Cui S, Xia S, Hu Y, Yan S, Wang J, Li F, Fanning S, Xu J.** 2016. Emergence and diversity of *Salmonella enterica* serovar Indiana isolates with concurrent resistance to ciprofloxacin and cefotaxime from patients and food-producing animals in China. *Antimicrob Agents Chemother* **60:**3365–3371.

225. **Dorado-García A, Smid JH, van Pelt W, Bonten MJ, Fluit AC, van den Bunt G, Wagenaar JA, Hordijk J, Dierikx CM, Veldman KT, de Koeijer A, Dohmen W, Schmitt H, Liakopoulos A, Pacholewicz E, Lam TJ, Velthuis AG, Heuvelink A, Gonggrijp MA, van Duijkeren E, van Hoek AH, de Roda Husman AM, Blaak H, Havelaar AH, Mevius DJ, Heederik DJ.** 2018. Molecular relatedness of ESBL/AmpC-producing *Escherichia coli* from humans, animals, food and the environment: a pooled analysis. *J Antimicrob Chemother* **73:**339–347.

226. **de Been M, Lanza VF, de Toro M, Scharringa J, Dohmen W, Du Y, Hu J, Lei Y, Li N, Tooming-Klunderud A, Heederik DJ, Fluit AC, Bonten MJ, Willems RJ, de la Cruz F, van Schaik W.** 2014. Dissemination of cephalosporin resistance genes between *Escherichia coli* strains from farm animals and humans by specific plasmid lineages. *PLoS Genet* **10:**e1004776.

227. **Kluytmans JA, Overdevest IT, Willemsen I, Kluytmans-van den Bergh MF, van der Zwaluw K, Heck M, Rijnsburger M, Vandenbroucke-**

Grauls CM, Savelkoul PH, Johnston BD, Gordon D, Johnson JR. 2013. Extended-spectrum β-lactamase-producing *Escherichia coli* from retail chicken meat and humans: comparison of strains, plasmids, resistance genes, and virulence factors. *Clin Infect Dis* **56**:478–487.

228. Overdevest I, Willemsen I, Rijnsburger M, Eustace A, Xu L, Hawkey P, Heck M, Savelkoul P, Vandenbroucke-Grauls C, van der Zwaluw K, Huijsdens X, Kluytmans J. 2011. Extended-spectrum β-lactamase genes of *Escherichia coli* in chicken meat and humans, The Netherlands. *Emerg Infect Dis* **17**:1216–1222.

229. Vincent C, Boerlin P, Daignault D, Dozois CM, Dutil L, Galanakis C, Reid-Smith RJ, Tellier PP, Tellis PA, Ziebell K, Manges AR. 2010. Food reservoir for *Escherichia coli* causing urinary tract infections. *Emerg Infect Dis* **16**:88–95.

230. Leverstein-van Hall MA, Dierikx CM, Cohen Stuart J, Voets GM, van den Munckhof MP, van Essen-Zandbergen A, Platteel T, Fluit AC, van de Sande-Bruinsma N, Scharinga J, Bonten MJ, Mevius DJ, National ESBL surveillance group. 2011. Dutch patients, retail chicken meat and poultry share the same ESBL genes, plasmids and strains. *Clin Microbiol Infect* **17**:873–880.

231. Madec JY, Haenni M, Nordmann P, Poirel L. 2017. Extended-spectrum β-lactamase/AmpC- and carbapenemase-producing *Enterobacteriaceae* in animals: a threat for humans? *Clin Microbiol Infect* **23**:826–833.

232. Berg ES, Wester AL, Ahrenfeldt J, Mo SS, Slettemeas JS, Steinbakk M, Samuelsen Ø, Grude N, Simonsen GS, Løhr IH, Jørgensen SB, Tofteland S, Lund O, Dahle UR, Sunde M. 2017. Norwegian patients and retail chicken meat share cephalosporin-resistant *Escherichia coli* and IncK/*bla*$_{CMY-2}$ resistance plasmids. *Clin Microbiol Infect* **23**:407.e9–407.e15.

233. Novais C, Coque TM, Sousa JC, Peixe LV. 2006. Antimicrobial resistance among faecal enterococci from healthy individuals in Portugal. *Clin Microbiol Infect* **12**:1131–1134.

234. Donabedian SM, Thal LA, Hershberger E, Perri MB, Chow JW, Bartlett P, Jones R, Joyce K, Rossiter S, Gay K, Johnson J, Mackinson C, Debess E, Madden J, Angulo F, Zervos MJ. 2003. Molecular characterization of gentamicin-resistant enterococci in the United States: evidence of spread from animals to humans through food. *J Clin Microbiol* **41**:1109–1113.

235. Freitas AR, Coque TM, Novais C, Hammerum AM, Lester CH, Zervos MJ, Donabedian S, Jensen LB, Francia MV, Baquero F, Peixe L. 2011. Human and swine hosts share vancomycin-resistant *Enterococcus faecium* CC17 and CC5 and *Enterococcus faecalis* CC2 clonal clusters harboring Tn*1546* on indistinguishable plasmids. *J Clin Microbiol* **49**:925–931.

236. Willems RJ, Top J, van den Braak N, van Belkum A, Mevius DJ, Hendriks G, van Santen-Verheuvel M, van Embden JD. 1999. Molecular diversity and evolutionary relationships of Tn*1546*-like elements in enterococci from humans and animals. *Antimicrob Agents Chemother* **43**: 483–491.

237. Novais C, Freitas AR, Sousa JC, Baquero F, Coque TM, Peixe LV. 2008. Diversity of Tn*1546* and its role in the dissemination of vancomycin-resistant enterococci in Portugal. *Antimicrob Agents Chemother* **52**:1001–1008.

238. Michael GB, Freitag C, Wendlandt S, Eidam C, Feßler AT, Lopes GV, Kadlec K, Schwarz S. 2015. Emerging issues in antimicrobial resistance of bacteria from food-producing animals. *Future Microbiol* **10**:427–443.

239. Köck R, Daniels-Haardt I, Becker K, Mellmann A, Friedrich AW, Mevius D, Schwarz S, Jurke A. 2018. Carbapenem-resistant *Enterobacteriaceae* in wildlife, food-producing, and companion animals: a systematic review. *Clin Microbiol Infect*.

240. Roschanski N, Guenther S, Vu TT, Fischer J, Semmler T, Huehn S, Alter T, Roesler U. 2017. VIM-1 carbapenemase-producing *Escherichia coli* isolated from retail seafood, Germany 2016. *Euro Surveill* **22**:17-00032.

241. Janecko N, Martz SL, Avery BP, Daignault D, Desruisseau A, Boyd D, Irwin RJ, Mulvey MR, Reid-Smith RJ. 2016. Carbapenem-resistant *Enterobacter* spp. in retail seafood imported from Southeast Asia to Canada. *Emerg Infect Dis* **22**: 1675–1677.

242. Pletz MW, Wollny A, Dobermann UH, Rödel J, Neubauer S, Stein C, Brandt C, Hartung A, Mellmann A, Trommer S, Edel B, Patchev V, Makarewicz O, Maschmann J. 2018. A nosocomial foodborne outbreak of a VIM carbapenemase-expressing *Citrobacter freundii*. *Clin Infect Dis* **67**:58–64.

243. Larsen J, Stegger M, Andersen PS, Petersen A, Larsen AR, Westh H, Agersø Y, Fetsch A, Kraushaar B, Käsbohrer A, Feßler AT, Schwarz S, Cuny C, Witte W, Butaye P, Denis O, Haenni M, Madec JY, Jouy E, Laurent F, Battisti A, Franco A, Alba P, Mammina C, Pantosti A, Monaco M, Wagenaar JA, de Boer E, van Duijkeren E, Heck M, Domínguez L, Torres C, Zarazaga M, Price LB, Skov RL. 2016. Evidence for human adaptation and foodborne transmission of livestock-associated methicillin-resistant *Staphylococcus aureus*. *Clin Infect Dis* **63**:1349–1352.

244. **Fetsch A, Kraushaar B, Käsbohrer A, Hammerl JA.** 2017. Turkey meat as source of CC9/CC398 methicillin-resistant *Staphylococcus aureus* in humans? *Clin Infect Dis* **64:**102–103.
245. **Tamang MD, Nam HM, Kim TS, Jang GC, Jung SC, Lim SK.** 2011. Emergence of extended-spectrum β-lactamase (CTX-M-15 and CTX-M-14)-producing nontyphoid *Salmonella* with reduced susceptibility to ciprofloxacin among food animals and humans in Korea. *J Clin Microbiol* **49:**2671–2675.
246. **Andrysiak AK, Olson AB, Tracz DM, Dore K, Irwin R, Ng LK, Gilmour MW, Canadian Integrated Program for Antimicrobial Resistance Surveillance Collaborative.** 2008. Genetic characterization of clinical and agri-food isolates of multi drug resistant *Salmonella enterica* serovar Heidelberg from Canada. *BMC Microbiol* **8:**89.
247. **Cloeckaert A, Praud K, Doublet B, Bertini A, Carattoli A, Butaye P, Imberechts H, Bertrand S, Collard JM, Arlet G, Weill FX.** 2007. Dissemination of an extended-spectrum-β-lactamase *bla*$_{TEM-52}$ gene-carrying IncI1 plasmid in various *Salmonella enterica* serovars isolated from poultry and humans in Belgium and France between 2001 and 2005. *Antimicrob Agents Chemother* **51:**1872–1875.
248. **Fernandes SA, Paterson DL, Ghilardi-Rodrigues AC, Adams-Haduch JM, Tavechio AT, Doi Y.** 2009. CTX-M-2-producing *Salmonella* Typhimurium isolated from pediatric patients and poultry in Brazil. *Microb Drug Resist* **15:**317–321.
249. **Rodríguez I, Barownick W, Helmuth R, Mendoza MC, Rodicio MR, Schroeter A, Guerra B.** 2009. Extended-spectrum β-lactamases and AmpC β-lactamases in ceftiofur-resistant *Salmonella enterica* isolates from food and livestock obtained in Germany during 2003–07. *J Antimicrob Chemother* **64:**301–309.
250. **Bertrand S, Weill FX, Cloeckaert A, Vrints M, Mairiaux E, Praud K, Dierick K, Wildemauve C, Godard C, Butaye P, Imberechts H, Grimont PA, Collard JM.** 2006. Clonal emergence of extended-spectrum β-lactamase (CTX-M-2)-producing *Salmonella enterica* serovar Virchow isolates with reduced susceptibilities to ciprofloxacin among poultry and humans in Belgium and France (2000 to 2003). *J Clin Microbiol* **44:**2897–2903.
251. **Riaño I, García-Campello M, Sáenz Y, Alvarez P, Vinué L, Lantero M, Moreno MA, Zarazaga M, Torres C.** 2009. Occurrence of extended-spectrum beta-lactamase-producing *Salmonella enterica* in northern Spain with evidence of CTX-M-9 clonal spread among animals and humans. *Clin Microbiol Infect* **15:**292–295.
252. **Mora A, Herrera A, Mamani R, López C, Alonso MP, Blanco JE, Blanco M, Dahbi G, García-Garrote F, Pita JM, Coira A, Bernárdez MI, Blanco J.** 2010. Recent emergence of clonal group O25b:K1:H4-B2-ST131 *ibeA* strains among *Escherichia coli* poultry isolates, including CTX-M-9-producing strains, and comparison with clinical human isolates. *Appl Environ Microbiol* **76:**6991–6997.

Insects and the Transmission of Bacterial Agents

10

MAUREEN LAROCHE,[1] DIDIER RAOULT,[2] and PHILIPPE PAROLA[1]

INTRODUCTION

Arthropods are a phylum of invertebrate animals with an exoskeleton, including >1 million species and accounting for >80% of all known living animal species (1).

Some hematophagous arthropods known as vectors possess the capacity to transmit infectious agents to human and other vertebrate animals (2). To date, the majority of arthropod vector species belong to the classes of insects and arachnids, which include mosquitoes and ticks, respectively (3).

Mosquitoes are the primary vectors of human infectious diseases, including malaria, dengue, and filariasis (4). Moreover, the recent epidemics of Chikungunya and Zika throughout the world are some examples of the expansion of mosquito-borne diseases (5). Dissemination is now seen as a global problem. Most of the vector-borne diseases that have been brought to the attention of the public in recent years are arboviral diseases. Arthropod-borne bacterial diseases are considered neglected, with the exception of tick-borne diseases, thanks to the identification and emergence of Lyme disease and many rickettsial diseases in recent years (6, 7). However, knowledge of the transmission of bacterial disease agents by insects, and how some agents might disseminate, is poor.

[1]Aix Marseille Univ, IRD, AP-HM, SSA, VITROME, IHU-Méditerranée Infection, Marseille, France; [2]Aix Marseille Univ, IRD, AP-HM, MEPHI, IHU-Méditerranée Infection, Marseille, France.
Microbial Transmission in Biological Processes
Edited by Fernando Baquero, Emilio Bouza, J.A. Gutiérrez-Fuentes, and Teresa M. Coque
© 2018 American Society for Microbiology, Washington, DC
doi:10.1128/microbiolspec.MTBP-0017-2016

As a matter of fact, the potential for dissemination is linked to the so-called vectorial capacity of the insect. This term includes several factors linked to the role of an arthropod in microorganism transmission, including arthropod abundance and longevity, host specificity, the time for the microorganism to develop and/or multiply within the vector, the route of transmission, but also environmental, ecological, behavioral, cellular, biochemical, and molecular factors. The vector competence of an arthropod is a subcomponent of vectorial capacity. It corresponds to the intrinsic ability of the arthropod to acquire a microorganism, allow its replication, and subsequently transmit it to a susceptible host.

Although microorganisms enter their arthropod vector during the blood meal, their transmission to an animal is more varied. Furthermore, a pathogen often needs to overcome several physical barriers in the arthropod before finding an exit and a pathway to be transmitted. Furthermore, the immune response of the arthropod can limit the development of microorganisms and thus the success of the transmission.

Salivation is the most common way for vectors to transmit infectious agents. As an illustration, all arthropod-borne viruses are transmitted this way, and the virus is directly injected into the host during probing or blood feeding. A key step in the transmission of most vector-borne diseases is therefore the entry of the microorganism into the salivary glands of the arthropod (8). For the success of their blood feeding, the salivary glands of arthropods produce a variety of substances, including enzymes and vasodilators, as well as anti-inflammatory, antihemostatic, and immunosuppressive substances (9). However, salivation cannot be employed for the transmission of microorganisms that remain in the gut or the hemocoel of an arthropod, as this would require their entry into the salivary glands. The two major alternate mechanisms of horizontal transmission that can be used include exit with arthropod feces (stercoration) and regurgitation.

Here we focus on bacterial disease agents that are or at least can be transmitted by insects (mosquitoes, sand flies, lice, fleas, and bugs), with illustrative examples of pathways of transmission and the potential for dissemination.

MOSQUITOES

The ability of mosquitoes to transmit bacterial diseases to humans is poorly understood and has not been a topic of research or even of interest until recently. Particularly *Wolbachia* spp., bacteria known as endosymbionts in many arthropods, have been associated with mosquitoes (10). Mosquitoes have also been presented as the mechanical vectors of *Francisella tularensis*, the agent of tularemia in humans, and possible transmission through adult mosquitoes that have acquired the pathogen from their aquatic larval habitats has been suggested (11).

In opposition to mechanical transmission, biological transmission is the way in which mosquitoes transmit arboviruses such as dengue, Chikungunya, and yellow fever viruses through their bite. The competence of mosquitoes in transmitting arboviruses has long been well known; however, nothing was known about their potential competence in transmitting bacterial agents until attempts to decipher *Rickettsia felis'* epidemiology. *Rickettsia felis* is an obligate intracellular bacterium that differs from other officially recognized rickettsial species. Many aspects of the ecology and epidemiology of *R. felis* are not completely understood and remain to be uncovered. Our team definitively described this organism in 2002 (12). A growing number of recent reports have implicated *R. felis* as a human pathogen, paralleling the increasing detection of *R. felis* in arthropod hosts across the globe (13). In Sub-Saharan Africa, epidemiological studies revealed that *R. felis* was detected in up to 15% of patients with fever of unknown origin (14). Various arthropods, but primarily fleas, have been associated with *R. felis*, and more specifically, the cat flea *Ctenocephalides felis* is the arthropod in which *R. felis* has been most frequently detected (15). For a long time, it was the sole confirmed biological vector of *R. felis*. Interestingly, *Aedes albopictus* and *Anopheles gambiae* mosquito cells support *R. felis* growth. In 2012, we found that *A. albopictus* (a major vector of Chikungunya, dengue, and Zika virus) from Gabon and *An. gambiae* (the primary African malarial vector) from Ivory Coast both tested positive for *R. felis* by species-specific real-time quantitative PCR (15). Also, we found several mosquito species from Senegal that harbor *R. felis*. These data raised new issues with respect to the epidemiology of *R. felis* in Africa, including the degree of vector competence of mosquitoes. Recently, we demonstrated that *An. gambiae* mosquitoes, the primary malarial vectors in Sub-Saharan Africa, have the potential to be vectors of *R. felis* infection (16). *An. gambiae* mosquitoes were fed with either *R. felis*-infected blood meal or infected cellular media administered through an artificial membrane feeding system. In an *in vivo* model, mosquitoes were fed on *R. felis*-infected mice. The acquisition and persistence of *R. felis* in *An. gambiae* were demonstrated by quantitative PCR detection of the bacteria up to day 15 postinfection. Furthermore, *R. felis* was visualized by immunofluorescence in the salivary glands and in the ovaries, although no vertical transmission was observed. *Rickettsia felis* was also found in the cotton used for mosquito sucrose feeding, which implies potential transmission through the mosquito's bite. Bites from *R. felis*-infected *An. gambiae* were able to cause transient rickettsemia in mice, indicating that this mosquito species has the potential to be a vector of *R. felis* infection (16).

LICE

Three louse ecotypes are known to parasitize humans: pubic lice, which are a sexually transmitted disease but not known vectors of infectious diseases; as well as head lice and body lice. The latter are two very close ecotypes on both the genetic and morphological levels (17). Infectious diseases transmission mainly involve body lice. Until the 19th century, the presence of body lice in the general population was extremely common. Today, these arthropods are only found in poor populations such as homeless populations or in critical situations such as war zones. Lice were involved in the most explosive outbreaks known, such as louse-borne relapsing fever, epidemic typhus, and trench fever, which were caused by *Borrelia recurrentis*, *Rickettsia prowazekii*, and *Bartonella quintana*, respectively (18). Although one might presume that these diseases belong to the past, very peculiar situations have allowed them now to resurge. Rwanda and Burundi had civil wars that allowed the proliferation of body louse populations, along with an epidemic typhus resurgence, causing 10,000 deaths toward the end of the 20th century (19). At the same time, it was identified that *B. quintana* was cocirculating with *R. prowazekii* in the same population (19). *Rickettsia prowazekii* is thought to have been introduced in Europe from Mexico, where it has been detected in ticks. The first human cases of epidemic typhus were detected by paleomicrobiology and reported from the War of the Spanish Succession of the early 18th century. Moreover, paleomicrobiology allowed the detection of *B. quintana* DNA in a 4,000-year-old human tooth (20), and also in Napoleon's soldiers buried in Vilnius, causing an outbreak of trench fever that might have impacted the French retreat from Russia (21).

More recently, two major questions emerged regarding the role of lice in the transmission of infectious diseases. The first is the ability of the louse to transmit *Yersinia pestis*, the causative agent of plague. Indeed, paleomicrobiology demonstrated that both plagues (of Justinian and the Middle Ages) were caused by *Y. pestis* (22, 23). However, the admitted biological cycle of transmission of the pathogen is not able to explain the dynamics of the outbreak in Europe, which involved 90% of the population at phenomenal speed. For these reasons, the validity of *Y. pestis* as the etiological agent of the Middle Ages plague was challenged. Rats and fleas alone can't explain the violence of the outbreak. However, this type of explosive outbreak is common for louse-borne infectious diseases. Ancient studies reported that lice could be infected by *Y. pestis*, and we demonstrated in an experimental model that the louse is competent for the transmission of *Y. pestis* in laboratory conditions. Finally, more recently, we reported *Y. pestis* in body lice collected in areas where plague is endemic in Democratic Republic of the Congo (DRC) (24). Here it appears highly plausible that lice were the origin of the infection. The data suggest that rural plague is probably followed by urban plague cases that are further amplified by body lice.

The second question regarding lice and infectious diseases concerns the inability of head lice to transmit pathogenic microorganisms. *Bartonella quintana*'s DNA was detected in head lice, and its presence in human cases in Dielmo, Senegal, has been reported. It appears that head lice may be vectors of *B. quintana*, which was considered impossible until now. Finally, we recently identified *Y. pestis* in head lice collected in DRC, which raises the question of the potential role of head lice in the transmission of this pathogenic bacterium.

Lice probably played a major role in the outbreaks of the last centuries. The potential role of head lice in the transmission of infectious disease is of far greater concern in the 21st century because of its wide distribution, and how outbreaks could spread. Lice are not very specific, since the microorganisms are transmitted through their feces, not directly by the bite. The itching induced by the louse's saliva allow the pathogen to penetrate the skin through scratching lesions. Therefore, it appears that the transmission of infectious disease by the louse is more likely guided by the opportunism of the ingested microorganism than true host-bacterium specificity.

FLEAS

There are currently ~2,500 species and subspecies of fleas (25). These insects are small, wingless, bilaterally flat parasites, principally of mammals and sometimes of birds (26). Fleas are holometabolous arthropods, which means that their development from the egg to the hematophagous adult includes a larval, then a pupal stage. Like many other blood-sucking insects, fleas are involved in the transmission of vector-borne pathogens. However, current data suggest that fleas transmit pathogens through their feces and not through their bite. The microorganisms later enter the vertebrate skin through scratch lesions.

Despite the large number of known flea species, only a few tend to bite humans (27). Even *Pulex irritans*, which is known as the human flea, is more frequently associated with swine and dogs in some parts of the world (26). Yet because of their high affinity for domestic animals, *C. felis* fleas are very frequently found associated with human dwellings.

We still have much to decipher about flea-borne diseases. However, much is already known regarding the competence of these arthropods in transmitting human pathogens, and many microorganisms have been molecularly detected in fleas (28). Indeed, fleas have been and still are involved in the transmission of *Y. pestis*, the causative agent of plague (29). *Yersinia pestis* multiplies in the flea's proventriculus, a structure between the esophagus and the midgut, and therefore obstructs the passage of ingested blood. Infected fleas then regurgitate infected blood during their attempts to feed (30). Around 30 flea species, particularly of the *Xenopsylla* genus, are demonstrated vectors of *Y. pestis* (31). Fleas are also recognized as vectors of *Rickettsia typhi*, an agent of murine typhus and of endemic typhus. Transmitted through flea feces, the bacteria then infect the mammalian host's endothelial cells (32). The disease then manifests with fever, headache, myalgia, and nausea (33).

If the role of mosquitoes in the transmission of *R. felis* is now in the spotlight, this bacterium was initially detected and isolated from the cat flea (15). *Rickettsia felis* transmission was shown both vertically and horizontally in fleas, making them a probable reservoir of the bacterium (34, 35). Since *R. felis* was detected in the salivary glands of fleas, transmission through the bite is highly suspected (36).

Fleas have recently been implicated in the transmission of bartonelloses. Cat scratch disease, caused by *Bartonella henselae*, is transmitted through cat scratch, but likely also by cat bite and by *C. felis* (37). Although most cat cases resolve spontaneously (37), immunocompromised patients may develop a potentially fatal bacillary angiomatosis (38). Moreover, infections with *B. henselae* in patients with valvulopathies may lead to fatal endocarditis, since the mortality can reach 25% (39). *Bartonella quintana* infections were quite frequently reported during previous centuries and are now resurging among disadvantaged populations, among which the louse, its primary vector, is thriving (18). This bacterium has been detected in cat fleas (40), and an experimental model was designed to assess the ability of *C. felis* to transmit *B. quintana* in laboratory conditions. The pathogen was excreted alive in the flea's feces, allowing further contamination of the vertebrate host through scratching (41).

Because of their high affinity for their animal hosts and low attraction to humans, it appears unlikely that fleas could be the origin of explosive outbreaks.

TRUE BUGS

The true bugs order is the largest insect order, composed of ~90,000 species distributed worldwide. These insects are generally characterized by two pairs of wings and a wing morphology dividing the order in two suborders: homopterans, which possess two highly similar pairs of wings; and heteropterans, for which the wing is composed of two thickened and two membranous parts. They are also characterized by piercing mouthparts that enable them to feed on different biological fluids such as plant juice, hemolymph, or vertebrate blood. Although homopterans are mostly phytophagous, heteropterans include hematophagous insects of medical and veterinary importance (26).

Kissing bugs (*Triatominae*) and bed bugs (*Cimicidae*) are the *Hemiptera* subfamily and family, respectively, involved in human health issues. All developmental stages of these flattened insects are hematophagous, and while bed bugs are wingless and relatively small, around 6 mm, kissing bugs are winged insects reaching up to 5 cm long. The ability of these insects to naturally transmit bacteria to humans is still unknown.

Triatomines (*Reduviidae; Triatominae*) are among the largest blood-sucking arthropods and live in diverse ecotopes. They can be totally sylvatic and feed on small mammals or they can be invasive, even domiciliated, and then feed principally on humans (42). When they are infected, they can transmit the flagellate protozoan *Trypanosoma cruzi* through their feces, which is the causative agent of Chagas disease. A major parasitic disease in the Americas, it is responsible for heart failure in up to 30% of individuals 10 to 30 years postinfection (43). Around 10,000 people died in 2014 from the manifestations of Chagas disease in 2014, and more than 25 million people are at risk of acquiring the disease. For a long time, the vectors and parasites were restricted to the New World. However, due to the intensification of human exchanges, arthropods are now disseminated all over the world, and triatomines are no exception. *Triatoma rubrofaciata* is now fully implanted in Vietnam (44), and the parasite itself is also present outside America in emigrant communities such as the Latin

American migrant community of Italy (45). Because of the public health impact and the rising threat of Chagas disease worldwide, almost no investigations have been conducted to assess the presence of other arthropod-borne pathogens in triatomines. Recent studies reported the molecular detection of a new *Bartonella* species, closely related to *B. bacilliformis*, the etiological agent of Carrion's disease, in invasive triatomines (42). The pathogenicity of this bacterium, however, remains to be demonstrated.

Bed bugs (*Cimex* species) are strict parasites of humans. They feed on human blood and are therefore a major pest when they infest human dwellings, hotels, trains, etc. (46). The host reaction following the bite is variable, but bed bugs are responsible for severe allergic reactions and dermatitis (47). Their implication in vector-borne pathogen transmission in the wild is still poorly known. Recent studies pointed out their vector competence in transmitting bacteria. The molecular detection of *B. quintana* in bed bugs collected from a prison in Rwanda raised the question of their role in the transmission of this louse-borne pathogen (48). Trench fever, caused by *B. quintana*, was broadly reported during World War I and II and is now resurging among homeless populations. In experimental models of infection, bed bugs were able to eliminate living bacteria through their feces, which allowed further cultivation of the microorganisms (49). To date, *B. quintana* is the only bacterial pathogen detected in bed bugs with demonstration of transmission in laboratory conditions.

CONCLUSION

Arthropod-borne bacteria will constitute an important reservoir of emerging infectious diseases in the future. Regarding the behavior and pathway of transmission, mosquito-borne diseases have the best potential for global transmission and causing large outbreaks. For example, the vectorial competence of *A. albopictus*, the Asian tiger mosquito, remains unknown but requires investigation. *Rickettsia felis* has already been detected in these highly anthropophilic mosquitoes, which played a major role in the spread of the Chikungunya and Zika outbreaks, and *R. felis* might be the next *A. albopictus*-borne outbreak agent (50).

CITATION

Laroche M, Raoult D, Parola P. 2018. Insects and the Transmission of Bacterial Agents, Microbiol Spectrum 6(5):MTBP-0017-2016.

REFERENCES

1. **Giribet G, Ribera C.** 2000. A review of arthropod phylogeny: new data based on ribosomal DNA sequences and direct character optimization. *Cladistics* 16:204–231.
2. **Pérez-Eid C.** 2007. *Les tiques: identification, biologie, importance médicale et vétérinaire.* Tec & Doc Lavoisier.
3. **Mathison BA, Pritt BS.** 2014. Laboratory identification of arthropod ectoparasites. *Clin Microbiol Rev* 27:48–67.
4. **Zeller H, Marrama L, Sudre B, Van Bortel W, Warns-Petit E.** 2013. Mosquito-borne disease surveillance by the European Centre for Disease Prevention and Control. *Clin Microbiol Infect* 19:693–698.
5. **Musso D, Gubler DJ.** 2016. Zika virus. *Clin Microbiol Rev* 29:487–524.
6. **Stanek G, Wormser GP, Gray J, Strle F.** 2012. Lyme borreliosis. *Lancet* 379:461–473.
7. **Parola P, Paddock CD, Socolovschi C, Labruna MB, Mediannikov O, Kernif T, Abdad MY, Stenos J, Bitam I, Fournier PE, Raoult D.** 2013. Update on tick-borne rickettsioses around the world: a geographic approach. *Clin Microbiol Rev* 26:657–702.
8. **Mueller AK, Kohlhepp F, Hammerschmidt C, Michel K.** 2010. Invasion of mosquito salivary glands by malaria parasites: prerequisites and defense strategies. *Int J Parasitol* 40:1229–1235.
9. **Andersen JF.** 2010. Structure and mechanism in salivary proteins from blood-feeding arthropods. *Toxicon* 56:1120–1129.
10. **Benelli G, Jeffries CL, Walker T.** 2016. Biological control of mosquito vectors: past, present, and future. *Insects* 7:E52.
11. **Bäckman S, Näslund J, Forsman M, Thelaus J.** 2015. Transmission of tularemia from a water

source by transstadial maintenance in a mosquito vector. *Sci Rep* **5:**7793.

12. **La Scola B, Meconi S, Fenollar F, Rolain JM, Roux V, Raoult D.** 2002. Emended description of *Rickettsia felis* (Bouyer et al. 2001), a temperature-dependent cultured bacterium. *Int J Syst Evol Microbiol* **52:**2035–2041.

13. **Parola P.** 2011. *Rickettsia felis*: from a rare disease in the USA to a common cause of fever in sub-Saharan Africa. *Clin Microbiol Infect* **17:**996–1000.

14. **Mediannikov O, Socolovschi C, Edouard S, Fenollar F, Mouffok N, Bassene H, Diatta G, Tall A, Niangaly H, Doumbo O, Lekana-Douki JB, Znazen A, Sarih M, Ratmanov P, Richet H, Ndiath MO, Sokhna C, Parola P, Raoult D.** 2013. Common epidemiology of *Rickettsia felis* infection and malaria, Africa. *Emerg Infect Dis* **19:**1775–1783.

15. **Angelakis E, Mediannikov O, Parola P, Raoult D.** 2016. *Rickettsia felis*: the complex journey of an emergent human pathogen. *Trends Parasitol* **32:**554–564.

16. **Dieme C, Bechah Y, Socolovschi C, Audoly G, Berenger JM, Faye O, Raoult D, Parola P.** 2015. Transmission potential of *Rickettsia felis* infection by *Anopheles gambiae* mosquitoes. *Proc Natl Acad Sci U S A* **112:**8088–8093.

17. **Boutellis A, Abi-Rached L, Raoult D.** 2014. The origin and distribution of human lice in the world. *Infect Genet Evol* **23:**209–217.

18. **Raoult D, Roux V.** 1999. The body louse as a vector of reemerging human diseases. *Clin Infect Dis* **29:**888–911.

19. **Raoult D, Ndihokubwayo JB, Tissot-Dupont H, Roux V, Faugere B, Abegbinni R, Birtles RJ.** 1998. Outbreak of epidemic typhus associated with trench fever in Burundi. *Lancet* **352:**353–358.

20. **Drancourt M, Tran-Hung L, Courtin J, Lumley H, Raoult D.** 2005. *Bartonella quintana* in a 4000-year-old human tooth. *J Infect Dis* **191:**607–611.

21. **Raoult D, Dutour O, Houhamdi L, Jankauskas R, Fournier PE, Ardagna Y, Drancourt M, Signoli M, La VD, Macia Y, Aboudharam G.** 2006. Evidence for louse-transmitted diseases in soldiers of Napoleon's Grand Army in Vilnius. *J Infect Dis* **193:**112–120.

22. **Drancourt M, Aboudharam G, Signoli M, Dutour O, Raoult D.** 1998. Detection of 400-year-old *Yersinia pestis* DNA in human dental pulp: an approach to the diagnosis of ancient septicemia. *Proc Natl Acad Sci U S A* **95:**12637–12640.

23. **Raoult D, Aboudharam G, Crubézy E, Larrouy G, Ludes B, Drancourt M.** 2000. Molecular identification by "suicide PCR" of *Yersinia pestis* as the agent of medieval black death. *Proc Natl Acad Sci U S A* **97:**12800–12803.

24. **Piarroux R, Abedi AA, Shako JC, Kebela B, Karhemere S, Diatta G, Davoust B, Raoult D, Drancourt M.** 2013. Plague epidemics and lice, Democratic Republic of the Congo. *Emerg Infect Dis* **19:**505–506.

25. **Lewis RE.** 1993. Checklist of the valid genus-group names in the Siphonaptera, 1758–1991. *J Med Entomol* **30:**64–79.

26. **Mullen GR, Durden LA.** 2009. *Medical and Veterinary Entomology*, 2nd ed. Academic Press, Burlington, MA.

27. **Bitam I, Dittmar K, Parola P, Whiting MF, Raoult D.** 2010. Fleas and flea-borne diseases. *Int J Infect Dis* **14:**e667–e676.

28. **Leulmi H, Socolovschi C, Laudisoit A, Houemenou G, Davoust B, Bitam I, Raoult D, Parola P.** 2014. Detection of *Rickettsia felis*, *Rickettsia typhi*, *Bartonella* species and *Yersinia pestis* in fleas (Siphonaptera) from Africa. *PLoS Negl Trop Dis* **8:**e3152.

29. **Stenseth NC, Atshabar BB, Begon M, Belmain SR, Bertherat E, Carniel E, Gage KL, Leirs H, Rahalison L.** 2008. Plague: past, present, and future. *PLoS Med* **5:**e3.

30. **Prentice MB, Rahalison L.** 2007. Plague. *Lancet* **369:**1196–1207.

31. **Perry RD, Fetherston JD.** 1997. *Yersinia pestis*—etiologic agent of plague. *Clin Microbiol Rev* **10:**35–66.

32. **Azad AF, Radulovic S, Higgins JA, Noden BH, Troyer JM.** 1997. Flea-borne rickettsioses: ecologic considerations. *Emerg Infect Dis* **3:**319–327.

33. **Dumler JS, Taylor JP, Walker DH.** 1991. Clinical and laboratory features of murine typhus in south Texas, 1980 through 1987. *JAMA* **266:**1365–1370.

34. **Hirunkanokpun S, Thepparit C, Foil LD, Macaluso KR.** 2011. Horizontal transmission of *Rickettsia felis* between cat fleas, *Ctenocephalides felis*. *Mol Ecol* **20:**4577–4586.

35. **Thepparit C, Hirunkanokpun S, Popov VL, Foil LD, Macaluso KR.** 2013. Dissemination of blood-meal acquired *Rickettsia felis* in cat fleas, *Ctenocephalides felis*. *Parasit Vectors* **6:**149.

36. **Macaluso KR, Pornwiroon W, Popov VL, Foil LD.** 2008. Identification of *Rickettsia felis* in the salivary glands of cat fleas. *Vector Borne Zoonotic Dis* **8:**391–396.

37. **Moriarty RA, Margileth AM.** 1987. Cat scratch disease. *Infect Dis Clin North Am* **1:**575–590.

38. **Fournier PE, Lelievre H, Eykyn SJ, Mainardi JL, Marrie TJ, Bruneel F, Roure C, Nash J, Clave D, James E, Benoit-Lemercier C, Deforges L,**

Tissot-Dupont H, Raoult D. 2001. Epidemiologic and clinical characteristics of *Bartonella quintana* and *Bartonella henselae* endocarditis: a study of 48 patients. *Medicine (Baltimore)* **80:** 245–251.

39. Ives TJ, Marston EL, Regnery RL, Butts JD. 2001. In vitro susceptibilities of *Bartonella* and *Rickettsia* spp. to fluoroquinolone antibiotics as determined by immunofluorescent antibody analysis of infected Vero cell monolayers. *Int J Antimicrob Agents* **18:**217–222.

40. Rolain JM, Franc M, Davoust B, Raoult D. 2003. Molecular detection of *Bartonella quintana, B. koehlerae, B. henselae, B. clarridgeiae, Rickettsia felis,* and *Wolbachia pipientis* in cat fleas, France. *Emerg Infect Dis* **9:**338–342.

41. Kernif T, Leulmi H, Socolovschi C, Berenger JM, Lepidi H, Bitam I, Rolain JM, Raoult D, Parola P. 2014. Acquisition and excretion of *Bartonella quintana* by the cat flea, *Ctenocephalides felis felis. Mol Ecol* **23:**1204–1212.

42. Laroche M, Berenger JM, Mediannikov O, Raoult D, Parola P. 2017. Detection of a potential new *Bartonella* species "Candidatus *Bartonella rondoniensis*" in human biting kissing bugs (Reduviidae; Triatominae). *PLoS Negl Trop Dis* **11:**e0005297.

43. Bern C. 2015. Chagas' disease. *N Engl J Med* **373:**456–466.

44. Dujardin JP, Lam TX, Khoa PT, Schofield CJ. 2015. The rising importance of *Triatoma rubrofasciata. Mem Inst Oswaldo Cruz* **110:**319–323.

45. Guerri-Guttenberg RA, Ciannameo A, Di Girolamo C, Milei JJ. 2009. Chagas disease: an emerging public health problem in Italy? *Infez Med* **17:**5–13. (In Italian.)

46. Delaunay P. 2012. Human travel and traveling bedbugs. *J Travel Med* **19:**373–379.

47. Delaunay P, Blanc V, Dandine M, Del Giudice P, Franc M, Pomares-Estran C, Marty P, Chosidow O. 2009. Bedbugs and healthcare-associated dermatitis, France. *Emerg Infect Dis* **15:**989–990.

48. Angelakis E, Socolovschi C, Raoult D. 2013. *Bartonella quintana* in *Cimex hemipterus,* Rwanda. *Am J Trop Med Hyg* **89:**986–987.

49. Leulmi H, Bitam I, Berenger JM, Lepidi H, Rolain JM, Almeras L, Raoult D, Parola P. 2015. Competence of *Cimex lectularius* bed bugs for the transmission of *Bartonella quintana,* the agent of trench fever. *PLoS Negl Trop Dis* **9:** e0003789.

50. Parola P, Musso D, Raoult D. 2016. *Rickettsia felis*: the next mosquito-borne outbreak? *Lancet Infect Dis* **16:**1112–1113.

PATIENT-TO-PATIENT TRANSMISSION

11

Biology of Hand-to-Hand
Bacterial Transmission

ROSA DEL CAMPO,[1,2] LAURA MARTÍNEZ-GARCÍA,[1,2]
ANA MARÍA SÁNCHEZ-DÍAZ,[1,2] and FERNANDO BAQUERO[1,3]

INTRODUCTION

Oliver Wendell Hol-mes was the first to describe the direct transmission of possible infective ("pestilent") agents to puerperal women through the physician's contaminated hands (1). In 1855, he published a book entitled *Puerperal Fever, as a Private Pestilence* in the United States (2). Nevertheless, the worldwide recognition of this relevant observation was classically attributed to Ignaz Philipp Semmelweis, who published a scientifically based demonstration of the role of hand disinfection in his thesis titled "The Etiology, the Concept and the Prophylaxis of Childbed Fever," developing seminal observations carried out in the year 1847 (3). Both authors implicated, for first time, the role of human hands contaminated with "cadaverous particles" in the deadly transmission process. Their legacy persists today, with considerable influence on current medicine, in which hand hygiene remains a liturgy in surgical procedures and is also a general measure with a pivotal role in the prevention and control of communicable diseases (4, 5).

[1]Servicio de Microbiología, Hospital Universitario Ramón y Cajal and Instituto Ramón y Cajal de Investigación Sanitaria (IRYCIS), Madrid, Spain; [2]Red Española de Investigación en Patología Infecciosa (REIPI), Madrid, Spain; [3]CIBER Epidemiología y Salud Pública (CIBERESP), Madrid, Spain.
Microbial Transmission in Biological Processes
Edited by Fernando Baquero, Emilio Bouza, J.A. Gutiérrez-Fuentes, and Teresa M. Coque
© 2018 American Society for Microbiology, Washington, DC
doi:10.1128/microbiolspec.MTBP-0011-2016

An interesting epistemological thought is that the overwhelming clarity, prestige, and influence of widely accepted and applied practices might repress fundamental research in this particular field—the idea that because it works beyond any reasonable doubt, there is no need to look for explanations. Semmelweis himself discarded as "irrelevant" the use of the microscope to explain his own results (6–10). These classical observations fostered the development of microbiology (11), but were not seminal for research on the biological bases of transmission of bacteria by hands, which remains largely unexplored.

HANDWASHING PREVENTS BACTERIAL TRANSMISSION

It is now accepted worldwide that adequate hand hygiene among hospital staff is the best measure to prevent nosocomial infections and outbreaks (12). To standardize the handwashing process by health care workers, in 2009, the World Health Organization published universal guidelines (13). Although numerous scientific studies have confirmed the clear relationship between proper hand hygiene on the part of the hospital staff and lower nosocomial infection rates, overall compliance is only ~40% (14).

Alcoholic solutions have recently been incorporated for hand hygiene. These solutions eliminate 99.99% of resident hand microbiota, whereas water washing only reaches 95% of the total decontamination (15, 16). It should be noted that these are indicative numbers, which are probably variable and dependent on the methodology of sampling and enumerating bacterial organisms (17, 18). Most importantly, we have minimal data from which to elucidate whether deeper hand microbiota decontamination is the recommended option to prevent bacterial transmission. As occurs in other microbiota localizations, the commensal native hand microbiota might play a crucial role in preventing the colonization and growth of external pathogens. In that sense, controlled reduction of hand microbiota density might be more recommendable than complete disinfection (19). The "mechanism" of bacterial killing with various procedures and the microecology of decontamination are also critical aspects that remain to be investigated.

MICROECOLOGY OF HAND SURFACES

In classical water washing, the majority of the bacterial reduction is due to the dragging effect, whereas alcohol solutions have an additional bactericidal effect by removing membrane lipids in both bacterial and human cells (15, 20). The real usefulness of these alcoholic solutions for hand hygiene has recently been noted (21). Lipids are important components of the epidermis-binding corneocytes that form the skin barrier and that prevent water loss. Moreover, some antimicrobial properties have been attributed to some of these skin lipids (22, 23). The compromise of the skin barrier after lipid removal via alcoholic solutions has not been sufficiently studied; more importantly, the role of these human lipids in the bacterial transmission process has not been explored. In fact, scientific evidence on skin moisture as a relevant factor for bacterial hand transmission can be found (24–26), and this transmission is more efficient when the skin is wet.

Skin microbiota density and composition is strongly conditioned by physical interaction with the environment, where the intensity of the friction of the skin with objects influences its final bacterial density. Friction effects are particularly relevant in specific areas, such as the fingers and palms, which are the most environment-interactive parts of our body. Our epidermis is completely renovated every 4 weeks, and the numerous squamous particles containing dead human cells but also viable bacteria are discharged daily. However, the dynamics of shedding and how it is influenced by the nature of biotic (including other persons) or abiotic contact objects remain poorly studied, as well as the number and type of microorganisms preferentially detached with squamous particles.

Physiological characteristics such as pH, humidity, and temperature influence the microecology and final microbial composition of our skin microbiota (18). Their structure varies by skin localization and depends on the distribution and density of hair follicles; sebaceous, eccrine, and apocrine glands; and scars and anatomic imperfections (27). Differences in the microbiota depending on the skin stratum have been observed, with indigenous bacteria corresponding to deeper skin layers, whereas transient bacteria are located only in the most superficial layers (28).

Significant differences among individuals have been detected in the skin microbiome composition. The intraindividual composition, however, remains relatively stable across time, although it undergoes important daily fluctuations in density, most of them after handwashing or external friction (29, 30). Furthermore, gender differences have also been confirmed; women have significantly higher bacterial diversity in their hands as well as differences in the bacterial composition of the dominant and nondominant hands (29). Age and race effects have not been sufficiently evaluated, although skin microbiota particularities of the Chinese population (31) and differences related to altitude have recently been reported (32).

THE HAND'S MICROBIOME

As occurs in other human microbial-associated ecosystems, new molecular tools based on 16S rRNA massive sequencing have revealed a more diverse skin microbiota than those found by traditional microbiological cultures (33). Most of the microorganisms inhabiting human skin belong to the *Corynebacterium*, *Propionibacterium*, and *Staphylococcus* genera, with a median bacterial load (population size) of ~1 ×

10^7 bacteria per cm^2 (34). More than 150 bacterial species have been found in the palms, most belonging to the *Actinobacteria*, *Firmicutes*, and *Proteobacteria* phyla (29).

It is of relevance to differentiate between autochthonous resident microbiota and transitory microbiota that we can acquire after physical interactions with contaminated surfaces (35). Furthermore, transitory microbiota might have a commensal or a pathogenic behavior, depending on their interaction with the immune system. As occurs in other parts of our body, the skin microbiota have a continuous dialogue with the immune system, which recognizes and destroys the external (alien) pathogens. In a healthy state, the resident microbiota do not represent an insult to the innate immune system, although they could occasionally activate it, particularly when reaching a high population density. In this sense, the immune system could be implicated in the regulation of the microbial skin ecosystem, which also maintains resilience properties that allow it to recover its composition and structure after attacks (36). In general, the skin constitutes a defensive barrier against the external microbial world. Not only shedding, but physical (pH, low humidity), chemical (skin antimicrobial fatty acids), biological (local enzymes, such as serine proteases, and constitutively produced cationic antimicrobial peptides, such as β-defensins and cathelicidins), and innate immunity effectors (inflammatory cytokines, such as interleukin-1, interleukin-17, and epidermal Toll-like receptors) contribute in an inducible, coordinated, and overlapping way to maintain a limitation on the density of microbial skin populations, and thus the interhuman transmission ability (37–41). Some skin structural features are critical to maintaining skin microbial homeostasis; in particular, the role of filaggrin (filament aggregating protein) ensures binding to keratin fibers in epithelial cells, which results in lipid barrier integrity and water retention and finally skin hydration (42).

HAND CONTAMINATION
BY NONRESIDENT ORGANISMS

Alien bacterial organisms are those not represented in the normal skin microbiome, and consequently include those that are incorporated into the hand's surface by occasional environmental contamination. The acquisition of external bacteria by hand exposure to contaminated fomites or surfaces is a critical source of nosocomial infection, particularly for health workers (43). However, bacterial interchange events between the environment and hands occur daily on countless occasions during routine actions such as eating (44), paying with cash (45, 46), or touching mobile phones (47). Undoubtedly, a major source of external bacterial contamination is the microbiota from other places on our own body (for instance, nostril-to-finger transmission), and also from family or friends. External bacteria rarely reach high populations, however, and often do not trigger a response from the innate immune system (e.g., by antimicrobial peptides), which reveals the inoffensiveness of these quotidian contaminations (40).

In the hand transmission process, environmentally tolerant microorganisms have more opportunities to be successfully transmitted to the hand. In fact, each type of bacterial organism, including pathogens, has a particular transmission efficiency rate that is influenced by its initial inoculum at the source as well as its capability to adhere to new surfaces. *Staphylococcus saprophyticus*, *Pseudomonas aeruginosa*, and *Serratia* spp. were transferred in greater numbers than was *Escherichia coli* from a contaminated to a clean piece of fabric after hand contact (48).

Curiously, in the bacterial hand transmission process, the transmission efficiency of human-to-human exchanges has scarcely been evaluated (49), and intrapersonal particularities have not yet been explored. In the next sections, we share recent data obtained by our group on the human role in hand-to-hand bacterial transmission, particularly in terms of interindividual differences.

DESIGN OF A MODEL FOR TESTING
INTRAINDIVIDUAL FINGER-TO-FINGER
TRANSMISSION EFFICIENCY

In a recent publication by our group, experimental results regarding intraindividual bacterial hand transmission efficiency of 30 healthy volunteers (20 women and 10 men) with four different *Enterococcus faecium* clones were presented (50). We designed a new test to explore the finger-to-finger bacterial transmission of the volunteers, as shown in Fig. 1. Each finger was put in close static contact (ensuring full surface contact, but with minimal pressure and without twists or wipes) for ~10 sec. Interestingly, this simple experiment provided consistently significant differences in host finger-to-finger transmission among individuals and bacterial isolates. The 30 individuals were classified into three transmission efficiency categories: poor, medium, and high finger-to-finger bacterial transmitters. An interesting result not previously described is that the 10 male volunteers were classified as poor or high transmitters, whereas almost all 20 of the women were grouped in the medium category. As was mentioned earlier, men and women have significant differences in their skin composition. Men usually have lower pH values in their skin, but there are also differences in sweat and sebum production, skin moisture, skin thickness, and hormone levels (51). Possible interindividual differences in the lipid composition of the human skin might also be considered. Chemical and physical interactions between bacterial and human lipids might determine the final adherence of the bacteria to the superficial skin layer. However, for a microorganism to colonize a new environment, such as a receptor hand, the lipid interactions of the invasive bacteria with the human lipids or the external lipids of the resident skin microbiota can be decisive. In addition, the physical attraction or repulsion forces between lipids can determine the permanence of a microorganism. Although the bacterial hand transmission process has considerable clinical repercussions

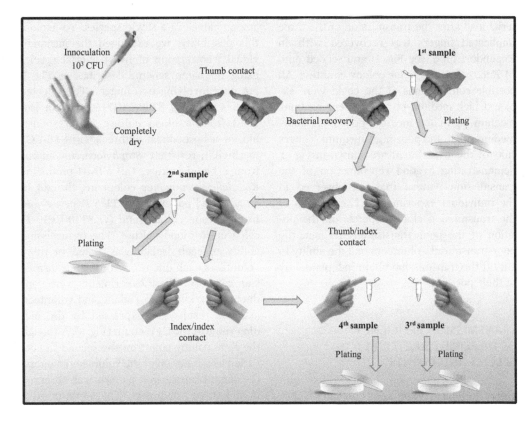

FIGURE 1 Schematic representation of the intraindividual finger-to-finger transmission efficiency test, which employs a total of four fingers of the same individual. The remaining bacteria on the finger surface are recovered after the contact between fingers and immediately plated on M-*Enterococcus* agar plates, which are counted after 24 to 48 h.

in terms of human infections, particularly those associated with health care centers, the microecological determination of transmission has not been sufficiently explored.

TESTING THE FINGER-TO-FINGER INTERINDIVIDUAL TRANSMISSION CHAIN

In the last section, we discussed the possibility of differences between individuals in their own finger-to-finger transmission potential. The best transmitters are typically those who more effectively release the bacterial population and/or those who more completely bind to the released bacteria from the donor finger. In any case, we can hypothesize that the best

transmitters from their own fingers are also good transmitters for other individuals. We evaluated this hypothesis by constructing a finger-to-finger transmission chain with various individuals. For this purpose, we selected three volunteers to represent each category (high, medium, and poor transmitters), and we chose the foodborne *E. faecium* L50 strain as the most transmissible. The scheme used for this purpose was similar to that described previously, but with finger contact among the three volunteers: the first individual received a bacterial load of 10^7 CFU of *E. faecium* L50 on the thumb, which was put in contact for 10 sec with the thumb of the second volunteer, when it was completely dry, and this thumb was put in contact with the thumb of the third volunteer. The remaining bacterial load after the transmission of the three implicated fingers was recovered with an Eppendorf tube (see Fig. 1) and seeded onto M-*Enterococcus* agar for colony counting. All possible combinations of the chain were explored: high-medium-poor, high-poor-medium, medium-high-poor, medium-poor-high, poor-medium-high, and poor-high-medium. The results of this experiment are shown in Fig. 2, demonstrating a good reproduction of the transmission pattern that we observed in the individual experiments. The success of the transmission chain depends on the position of the poor transmitter. In fact, the poor-transmitter volunteers had the ability to cut off the transmission chain independently of their position.

TRANSMISSION EFFICIENCY OF DIFFERENT BACTERIAL SPECIES AND CLONES

Finger-to-finger transmission efficiency is conditioned by the particular characteristics of both the human and the bacterial organisms. In fact, there appears to be differences even among clones in a single species. To explore this possibility, we examined the intraindividual transmission of five bacterial species using the same scheme described in Fig. 1, but only involving two fingers. The selected species were (i) ST18-CC17 *E. faecium* isolated from a blood culture and responsible for a nosocomial outbreak, (ii) ST5-CC5 methicillin-resistant *Staphylococcus aureus* from a blood culture, (iii) VIM-1-producing *Klebsiella pneumoniae* colonizing the gut of an admitted patient, (iv) ST175 *P. aeruginosa* from a blood culture, and (v) ST10-CC10 *E. coli* from a blood culture. The transmission ability of each isolate was tested in three volunteers each one representing a transmission category. These experiments were conducted in triplicate per clone and volunteer, and the results are expressed by the median value of the CFU count (Fig. 3). Although the final colony count on the second fingers varied as a function of the volunteer category, the same transmission pattern was observed in the three volunteers. The Gram-positive organisms, *E. faecium* and *S. aureus*, exhibited the highest transmission efficiency, whereas the Gram-negative organisms were less effi-

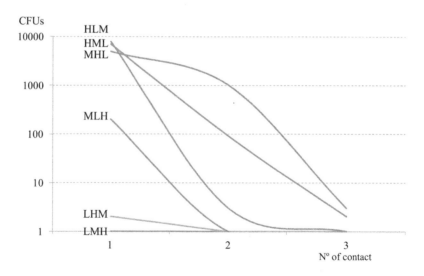

FIGURE 2 **The transmission chain process was explored using three volunteers—high, medium, and poor transmitters—and the foodborne *E. faecium* L50 clone. All six possible combinations of the three volunteers were assayed.**

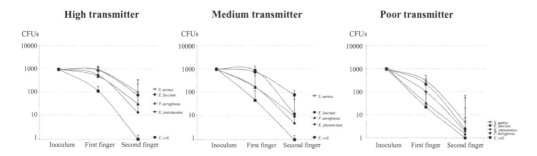

FIGURE 3 Differences in the transmission efficiency of five bacterial species using one volunteer per transmission category. The transmission pattern was repeated for the three individuals.

cient. Unexpectedly, *E. coli*, which is one of the most universal and ubiquitous bacteria, had the lowest transmission rate. The nosocomial character of the species was the selection criterion employed for our experiment, but these data could be completed with other species/clones and volunteers to better understand the transmission differences between bacteria and humans (38, 39).

FUTURE PROSPECTS IN BASIC BIOLOGY OF HAND TRANSMISSION: DIGGING INTO SKIN MICROENVIRONMENTS

The biology of hand transmission requires a much more detailed characterization of hand surface microenvironments, their variability among humans, and possibly circadian changes within each host. We need to know the hands' skin microecological conditions, including basic physicochemical traits such as temperature, water content, osmolality, pH, ions, iron, proteins (including enzymes), peptides, sugars, short-chain fatty acids, and bacterial microbiota profile—and ultimately antibody screening arrays, molecule-oriented antibodies or full-sample mass spectrometry (matrix-assisted laser desorption ionization–time of flight mass spectrometry) profiles—to obtain a full-environment fingerprint. Compact telemetry devices could be developed to obtain all these data. The final aim of such an

approach is the bioinformatic (phylogenetic-like) construction of "microenvironment trees," thus closing the circle of the microbe-environment evolutionary unit (52). Whether the structure of particular "individual-specific skin microenvironments" favoring bacterial survival and transmission correlates with particular human genotypes (as suggested by studies in atopic dermatitis) remains an interesting topic of research. These studies might indeed reveal whether some individuals (or human populations) are genetically prone to be better at human-to-human transmission of organisms causing infectious diseases (53), certainly a hot topic for preventive measures and targeted interventions.

ACKNOWLEDGMENTS

This work was supported by the PI13-00205 project (Instituto de Salud Carlos III-FIS), from the Ministry of Economy and Competitiveness (MINECO, Spain), and cofinanced by the European Development Regional Fund "A way to achieve Europe", Spanish Network for the Research in Infectious Diseases (REIPI RD12/0015/0004).

CITATION

del Campo R, Martínez-García L, Sánchez-Díaz AM, Baquero F. 2018. Biology of hand-to-hand bacterial transmission, Microbiol Spectrum 5(3):MTBP-0011-2016.

REFERENCES

1. **Lane HJ, Blum N, Fee E.** 2010. Oliver Wendell Holmes (1809–1894) and Ignaz Philipp Semmelweis (1818–1865): preventing the transmission of puerperal fever. *Am J Public Health* **100:**1008–1009.
2. **Holmes OW.** 1855. *Puerperal Fever as a Private Pestilence.* Ticknor and Fields, Boston, MA.
3. **Loudon I.** 2005. Semmelweis and his thesis. *J R Soc Med* **98:**555.
4. **Stewardson A, Allegranzi B, Sax H, Kilpatrick C, Pittet D.** 2011. Back to the future: rising to the Semmelweis challenge in hand hygiene. *Future Microbiol* **6:**855–876.
5. **Monnet DL, Sprenger M.** 2012. Hand hygiene practices in healthcare: measure and improve. *Euro Surveill* **17:**20166.
6. **Miranda CM, Navarrete TL.** 2008. Semmelweis and his outstanding contribution to medicine: washing hands saves lives. *Rev Chilena Infectol* **25:**54–57. (In Spanish.)
7. **Bauer J.** 1963. The tragic fate of Ignaz Philipp Semmelweis. *Calif Med* **98:**264–266.
8. **Dunn PM.** 2005. Ignaz Semmelweis of Budapest and the prevention of puerperal fever. *Arch Dis Child Fetal Neonatal* **90:**345–348.
9. **Raju TN.** 1999. Ignác Semmelweis and the etiology of fetal and neonatal sepsis. *J Perinatol* **19:** 307–310.
10. **Tan SY, Brown J.** 2006. Ignac Philipp Semmelweis (1818–1865): handwashing saves lives. *Singapore Med J* **47:**6–7.
11. **Wyklicky H, Skopec M.** 1983. Ignaz Philipp Semmelweis, the prophet of bacteriology. *Infect Control* **4:**367–370.
12. **Pittet D, Allegranzi B, Sax H, Dharan S, Pessoa-Silva CL, Donaldson L, Boyce JM, WHO Global Patient Safety Challenge, World Alliance for Patient Safety.** 2006. Evidence-based model for hand transmission during patient care and the role of improved practices. *Lancet Infect Dis* **6:**641–652.
13. **World Health Organization.** 2009. *WHO Guidelines on Hand Hygiene in Health Care.* World Health Organization, Geneva, Switzerland. http://apps.who.int/iris/bitstream/10665/44102/1/9789241597906_eng.pdf.
14. **Erasmus V, Daha TJ, Brug H, Richardus JH, Behrendt MD, Vos MC, van Beeck EF.** 2010. Systematic review of studies on compliance with hand hygiene guidelines in hospital care. *Infect Control Hosp Epidemiol* **31:**283–294.
15. **Girou E, Loyeau S, Legrand P, Oppein F, Brun-Buisson C.** 2002. Efficacy of handrubbing with alcohol based solution versus standard handwashing with antiseptic soap: randomised clinical trial. *BMJ* **325:**362.

16. **Edmonds SL, Macinga DR, Mays-Suko P, Duley C, Rutter J, Jarvis WR, Arbogast JW.** 2012. Comparative efficacy of commercially available alcohol-based hand rubs and World Health Organization-recommended hand rubs: formulation matters. *Am J Infect Control* **40:**521–525.
17. **Baquero F, Patrón C, Cantón R, Martínez Ferrer M.** 1991. Laboratory and *in-vitro* testing of skin antiseptics: a prediction for *in-vivo* activity? *J Hosp Infect* **18**(Suppl B):5–11.
18. **Zapka C, Leff J, Henley J, Tittl J, De Nardo E, Butler M, Griggs R, Fierer N, Edmonds-Wilson S.** 2017. Comparison of standard culture-based method to culture-independent method for evaluation of hygiene effects on the hand microbiome. *mBio* **8:**e00093-17.
19. **Vandegrift R, Bateman AC, Siemens KN, Nguyen M, Wilson HE, Green JL, Van Den Wymelenberg KG, Hickey RJ.** 2017. Cleanliness in context: reconciling hygiene with a modern microbial perspective. *Microbiome* **5:**76.
20. **Trick WE, Vernon MO, Hayes RA, Nathan C, Rice TW, Peterson BJ, Segreti J, Welbel SF, Solomon SL, Weinstein RA.** 2003. Impact of ring wearing on hand contamination and comparison of hand hygiene agents in a hospital. *Clin Infect Dis* **36:**1383–1390.
21. **Foddai AC, Grant IR, Dean M.** 2016. Efficacy of instant hand sanitizers against foodborne pathogens compared with hand washing with soap and water in food preparation settings: a systematic review. *J Food Prot* **79:**1040–1054.
22. **Drake DR, Brogden KA, Dawson DV, Wertz PW.** 2008. Thematic review series: skin lipids. Antimicrobial lipids at the skin surface. *J Lipid Res* **49:**4–11.
23. **Plichta JK, Droho S, Curtis BJ, Patel P, Gamelli RL, Radek KA.** 2014. Local burn injury impairs epithelial permeability and antimicrobial peptide barrier function in distal unburned skin. *Crit Care Med* **42:**e420–e431.
24. **Marples RR, Towers AG.** 1979. A laboratory model for the investigation of contact transfer of micro-organisms. *J Hyg (Lond)* **82:**237–248.
25. **Patrick DR, Findon G, Miller TE.** 1997. Residual moisture determines the level of touch-contact-associated bacterial transfer following hand washing. *Epidemiol Infect* **119:**319–325.
26. **Sattar SA, Springthorpe S, Mani S, Gallant M, Nair RC, Scott E, Kain J.** 2001. Transfer of bacteria from fabrics to hands and other fabrics: development and application of a quantitative method using *Staphylococcus aureus* as a model. *J Appl Microbiol* **90:**962–970.
27. **Grice EA, Segre JA.** 2011. The skin microbiome. *Nat Rev Microbiol* **9:**244–253.

28. **Zeeuwen PL, Boekhorst J, van den Bogaard EH, de Koning HD, van de Kerkhof PM, Saulnier DM, van Swam II, van Hijum SA, Kleerebezem M, Schalkwijk J, Timmerman HM.** 2012. Microbiome dynamics of human epidermis following skin barrier disruption. *Genome Biol* **13:** R101.

29. **Fierer N, Hamady M, Lauber CL, Knight R.** 2008. The influence of sex, handedness, and washing on the diversity of hand surface bacteria. *Proc Natl Acad Sci U S A* **105:**17994–17999.

30. **Schommer NN, Gallo RL.** 2013. Structure and function of the human skin microbiome. *Trends Microbiol* **21:**660–668.

31. **Leung MH, Wilkins D, Lee PK.** 2015. Insights into the pan-microbiome: skin microbial communities of Chinese individuals differ from other racial groups. *Sci Rep* **5:**11845.

32. **Lee M, Jung Y, Kim E, Lee HK.** 2017. Comparison of skin properties in individuals living in cities at two different altitudes: an investigation of the environmental effect on skin. *J Cosmet Dermatol* **16:**26–34.

33. **Kong HH, Segre JA.** 2012. Skin microbiome: looking back to move forward. *J Invest Dermatol* **132:**933–939.

34. **Edmonds-Wilson SL, Nurinova NI, Zapka CA, Fierer N, Wilson M.** 2015. Review of human hand microbiome research. *J Dermatol Sci* **80:**3–12.

35. **Jumaa PA.** 2005. Hand hygiene: simple and complex. *Int J Infect Dis* **9:**3–14.

36. **Cogen AL, Nizet V, Gallo RL.** 2008. Skin microbiota: a source of disease or defence? *Br J Dermatol* **158:**442–455.

37. **Gunathilake R.** 2015. The human epidermal antimicrobial barrier: current knowledge, clinical relevance and therapeutic implications. *Recent Pat Antiinfect Drug Discov* **10:**84–97.

38. **Elias PM.** 2007. The skin barrier as an innate immune element. *Semin Immunopathol* **29:**3–14.

39. **Feingold KR.** 2007. Thematic review series: skin lipids. The role of epidermal lipids in cutaneous permeability barrier homeostasis. *J Lipid Res* **48:** 2531–2546.

40. **Feng Z, Jia X, Adams MD, Ghosh SK, Bonomo RA, Weinberg A.** 2014. Epithelial innate immune response to *Acinetobacter baumannii* challenge. *Infect Immun* **82:**4458–4465.

41. **Ryu S, Song PI, Seo CH, Cheong H, Park Y.** 2014. Colonization and infection of the skin by *S. aureus*: immune system evasion and the response to cationic antimicrobial peptides. *Int J Mol Sci* **15:**8753–8772.

42. **Ovaere P, Lippens S, Vandenabeele P, Declercq W.** 2009. The emerging roles of serine protease cascades in the epidermis. *Trends Biochem Sci* **34:** 453–463.

43. **Larocque M, Carver S, Bertrand A, McGeer A, McLeod S, Borgundvaag B.** 2016. Acquisition of bacteria on health care workers' hands after contact with patient privacy curtains. *Am J Infect Control* **44:**1385–1386.

44. **Baker KA, Han IY, Bailey J, Johnson L, Jones E, Knight A, MacNaughton M, Marvin P, Nolan K, Martinez-Dawson R, Dawson PL.** 2015. Bacterial transfer from hands while eating popcorn. *Food Nutr Sci* **6:**1333–1338.

45. **Gedik H, Voss TA, Voss A.** 2013. Money and transmission of bacteria. *Antimicrob Resist Infect Control* **2:**22.

46. **Angelakis E, Azhar EI, Bibi F, Yasir M, Al-Ghamdi AK, Ashshi AM, Elshemi AG, Raoult D.** 2014. Paper money and coins as potential vectors of transmissible disease. *Future Microbiol* **9:**249–261.

47. **Pal S, Juyal D, Adekhandi S, Sharma M, Prakash R, Sharma N, Rana A, Parihar A.** 2015. Mobile phones: reservoirs for the transmission of nosocomial pathogens. *Adv Biomed Res* **4:**144.

48. **Mackintosh CA, Hoffman PN.** 1984. An extended model for transfer of micro-organisms via the hands: differences between organisms and the effect of alcohol disinfection. *J Hyg (Lond)* **92:** 345–355.

49. **Bellissimo-Rodrigues F, Pires D, Soule H, Gayet-Ageron A, Pittet D.** 2017. Assessing the likelihood of hand-to-hand cross-transmission of bacteria: an experimental study. *Infect Control Hosp Epidemiol* **38:**553–558.

50. **del Campo R, Sánchez-Díaz AM, Zamora J, Torres C, Cintas LM, Franco E, Cantón R, Baquero F.** 2014. Individual variability in finger-to-finger transmission efficiency of *Enterococcus faecium* clones. *MicrobiologyOpen* **3:**128–132.

51. **Ying S, Zeng DN, Chi L, Tan Y, Galzote C, Cardona C, Lax S, Gilbert J, Quan ZX.** 2015. The influence of age and gender on skin-associated microbial communities in urban and rural human populations. *PLoS One* **10:**e0141842.

52. **Baquero F.** 2015. Causes and interventions: need of a multiparametric analysis of microbial ecobiology. *Environ Microbiol Rep* **7:**13–14.

53. **Rupec RA, Boneberger S, Ruzicka T.** 2010. What is really in control of skin immunity: lymphocytes, dendritic cells, or keratinocytes? facts and controversies. *Clin Dermatol* **28:**62–66.

Transmission Surveillance for Antimicrobial-Resistant Organisms in the Health System

12

JOHANN D. D. PITOUT[1]

INTRODUCTION

The use of antimicrobial agents has resulted in the subsequent development of resistance by bacteria to such agents, with increased transmission of several significant antimicrobial-resistant pathogenic microorganisms within the health care system (1; see also https://www.cdc.gov/drugresistance/pdf/ar-threats-2013-508.pdf and http://www.jpiamr.eu/document-library/strategicresearch agenda). These bacteria include methicillin-resistant *Staphylococcus aureus* (MRSA), vancomycin-resistant *Enterococcus* (VRE), extended-spectrum β-lactamase (ESBL)-producing Gram-negative bacteria, and carbapenemase-producing Gram-negative enteric bacteria (CPE). The transmission of these antimicrobial-resistant organisms (AROs) has the potential to negatively impact patient morbidity and mortality (2).

The global spread of antimicrobial resistance was recently identified by the World Health Organization (WHO) as one of the three greatest threats to human health and is considered to be a public health threat (3; see also http://www.wpro.who.int/entity/drug_resistance/resources/global_action_plan_eng.

[1]Departments of Pathology & Laboratory Medicine, Microbiology, Immunology and Infectious Diseases, Cumming School of Medicine, University of Calgary, Calgary, Alberta, Canada; Division of Microbiology, Calgary Laboratory Services, Calgary, Alberta, Canada; and Department of Medical Microbiology, University of Pretoria, Pretoria, South Africa.

Microbial Transmission in Biological Processes
Edited by Fernando Baquero, Emilio Bouza, J.A. Gutiérrez-Fuentes, and Teresa M. Coque
© 2018 American Society for Microbiology, Washington, DC
doi:10.1128/microbiolspec.MTBP-0010-2016

pdf). The emergence of bacteria resistant to all or most existing antibiotics, especially in the realm of Gram-negative bacteria, constitutes a crisis: a return to the pre-antimicrobial era is a real possibility in the 21st century (4).

The spread of AROs is problematic for the medical community at large since it undermines empirical treatment regimens by delaying the administration of appropriate antibiotic therapy and by reducing the options for appropriate treatment. This contributes to increased patient mortality and morbidity (5). The problem is so serious that it threatens the achievements of modern medicine. Many aspects of modern medical care rely on the therapeutic or prophylactic use of antibiotics to minimize the morbidity and mortality associated with infections due to immunosuppression (e.g., chemotherapy) or breaching of the body's natural barriers (e.g., surgery). The emergence and widespread occurrence of bacteria that are resistant to antibiotics thus threatens not only the treatment of common bacterial infectious diseases but also the management of patients in diverse clinical settings.

There is evidence that the transmission rate of AROs is directly related to effective infection prevention and control practices within health care settings (6, 7). The early effective interventions that focus on the prevention of cross-transmission of AROs between patients have a greater relative impact in controlling and preventing endemicity of AROs in a facility (8). An infection prevention and control program for AROs that emphasizes the early identification of colonized patients through using active surveillance cultures and the use of contact precautions for the prevention of transmission of AROs reduces the overall prevalence and incidence of both colonization and infection, improves patient outcomes, and reduces health care costs (9). With the rise in the global prevalence of MRSA, VRE, ESBL-producing bacteria, and CPB, there is a need for effective measures to prevent and control the spread of these AROs. Since the usual method of acquisition of MRSA and VRE infection is via direct or indirect contact, it is possible to prevent infections caused by these microorganisms by instituting a set of practices and procedures that will prevent transmission of MRSA and VRE to patients. Such prevention and control efforts are necessary to protect the health and improve outcomes of clients/patients/residents but also to lessen the burden of MRSA and VRE on health care systems (10).

The increased risk for acquiring AROs is related both to the patient's own host risk factors as well as to the amount of time that the patient spent in a health care setting and was exposed to these microorganisms (2). Host risk factors include those conditions that put an individual at higher risk of acquiring an infection due to a compromised immune system. They include clinical conditions such as HIV and burn injury, being the recipient of a transplant, as well as treatments that bypass the immune system, such as the use of indwelling medical devices. Exposure to certain classes of antibiotics also puts individuals at increased risk for infection. Some environments have been shown to be more conducive than others to acquisition of AROs (2). These include in-hospital areas such as critical care units, intensive care units, burn units, and units that have had recent outbreaks of AROs.

Successful treatment of serious infections requires timely administration of effective chemotherapeutic agents. Clinical decisions about the empirical treatment require knowledge of the likely pathogen(s) and the likely susceptibility of these pathogens to antibiotics. Such knowledge is gained in part by clinical experience over time, but more objectively and robustly through surveillance. The U.S. Centers for Disease Control and Prevention (CDC) defines surveillance as "the ongoing systematic collection, analysis and interpretation of health data essential to the planning, implementation and evaluation of public health practice, closely integrated with the timely dissemination of these data to those who need to know" (1). Surveillance is the generation and timely provision of information to inform decision making and using such information to empirically treat a wide range of infections. For surveillance to directly influence decision making at the bedside, it requires a readily available source of data. For surveillance of AROs, the essential core data are generated by clinical microbiology laboratories that routinely identify and determine the susceptibility or resistance patterns of bacteria isolated from clinical specimens. These results are stored in the laboratory computer system and, if accessed, collected, and analyzed, can be used to predict the degree of antibiotic resistance seen in different bacterial isolates responsible for different types of infection. Changes or variations in antibiotic resistance either geographically or over time should also be monitored. This review will focus primarily on examples of existing global surveillance systems (Table 1) and provide a brief overview on the molecular typing of AROs.

SURVEILLANCE PROGRAMS FOR ANTIBIOTIC RESISTANCE

To impede the pending antibiotic resistance crisis, a worldwide response is urgently needed to find and develop new antimicrobial agents that will meet therapeutic needs for infections due to AROs. The Infectious Diseases Society of America recently launched a sustainable global antibacterial drug research and development enterprise referred to as the "10 × '20" initiative, with the power

TABLE 1 Summary of surveillance networks discussed herein

Network	Brief description
Tigecycline Evaluation and Surveillance Trial (TEST)	TEST is an ongoing global antimicrobial susceptibility surveillance study that examines the *in vitro* activity of tigecycline and comparators against clinically important pathogens.
EuCORE (European Cubicin Outcome Registry and Experience)	EuCORE is noncomparative database of daptomycin use in patients who have received at least one daptomycin dose. The primary objective is to evaluate the clinical outcomes of patients treated with this drug.
WHO Antimicrobial Resistance Monitoring program	WHONET (http://www.whonet.org) is freely accessible software that is widely used as a common platform for antibiotic resistance data collection, management, and sharing and serves as a strategy to facilitate global surveillance of antimicrobial resistance, including in low- and middle-income countries.
European Antimicrobial Resistance Surveillance Network (EARS-Net)	The main function of EARS-Net is to document the emergence and dissemination of AROs within European countries and to increase awareness among the citizenry, scientists, and public health authorities.
U.S. CDC National Healthcare Safety Network (NHSN)	The NHSN provides facilities, states, and regions with data needed to identify problem areas, measure progress of prevention efforts, and ultimately eliminate health care-associated infections.
U.S. Department of Defense's Antimicrobial Resistance Monitoring and Research Program (ARMoR)	ARMoR consists of a network of epidemiologists, bioinformaticists, microbiology researchers, policymakers, hospital-based infection preventionists, and health care providers who collaborate to collect relevant antimicrobial resistance data, conduct centralized molecular characterization, and use antimicrobial resistance characterization feedback to implement appropriate infection prevention and control measures and influence policy.
SMART (Study for Monitoring Antimicrobial Resistance Trends) and AstraZeneca global surveillance program	Both programs provide important information about changes in the spectrum of microbial pathogens and trends in the antimicrobial resistance patterns in nosocomial and community-acquired intra-abdominal infections and provide important surveillance data on AROs from resource-limited countries.

in the short term to develop 10 new, safe, and effective antibiotics by 2020 (3). The medical community at large also needs to improve the use of currently available antibiotics and to prevent and control the transmission of bacteria resistant to antibiotics, especially within the health care system (11). Such actions can only be guided by reliable epidemiological information about the prevalence and impact of resistant bacteria in different settings. Although antibiotic resistance is a universal public health concern, great gaps remain in our current understanding of the magnitude of the problem. Improved surveillance of antibiotic resistance in bacteria is essential to fill those gaps (12). The ultimate goal of strengthening surveillance is to formulate strategies and interventions to address the challenge of antibiotic resistance and improve the outcome of individual patients.

Surveillance also plays an essential role in detecting the emergence and spread of previously uncommon or completely novel types of antimicrobial resistance (13). Such types of surveillance systems should include international, national, and local alert systems for notifying clinical microbiologists of the emergence of new types of antibiotic resistance. Alerts typically describe the nature of the resistance, the extent of its known spread (if any), and how the resistance can be detected in diagnostic laboratories.

Essential and interrelated roles of surveillance systems are to enhance the understanding of the epidemiology of AROs and the factors that influence their emergence and spread, with a view to devising interventions aimed at reducing their burden, and then to assess the effectiveness of interventions by monitoring rates of resistance following their implementation.

Surveillance programs funded by industry to monitor the emergence and selection of resistance to new antibiotics have recently been established and include the Tigecycline Evaluation and Surveillance Trial (TEST) (i.e., tigecycline and linezolid) and EuCORE (European Cubicin Outcome Registry and Experience). TEST is an ongoing global antimicrobial susceptibility surveillance study that examines the *in vitro* activity of tigecycline and comparators against clinically important pathogens. Data are available at the ATLAS (Antimicrobial Testing Leadership and Surveillance) website (https://atlas-surveillance.com/#/login). EuCORE is an ongoing retrospective, European, postmarketing, noncomparative database of daptomycin use in patients who have received at least one daptomycin dose. The primary objective is to evaluate the clinical outcomes of patients treated with this drug. These industry-funded types of surveillance programs are important for monitoring and detecting resistance against newer antibiotics.

WHO: Antibiotic Resistance Surveillance on a Global Scale

The WHO issued a comprehensive report in 2014 on global antimicrobial resistance surveillance (14). Data from 129 member countries were sought for a selected set of nine bacteria-antibacterial drug combinations. Overall, 114 countries provided information regarding at least one of nine bacteria-antibacterial drug combinations; only 22 countries contributed data for all nine combinations. The most important findings of the WHO report were: "a) Very high rates of resistance have been observed in all WHO regions in common bacteria (for example, *Escherichia coli*, *Klebsiella pneumoniae* and *S. aureus*) that cause common health-care associated and community-acquired infections (i.e. urinary tract infections, wound infections, bloodstream infections and pneumonia). b) Many gaps exist in information on pathogens of major public health importance." The WHO report identified significant gaps in surveillance and a lack of standards for methodology, data sharing, and coordination. Overall, the report also stated that the global surveillance of antibiotic resistance is neither coordinated nor harmonized. The paucity and inconsistency in the availability of data reveals the lack of surveillance infrastructure at the national level that can be drawn upon to collect information from individual member countries. Most of the country-level data originated from the European region and the region of the Americas, where regional surveillance efforts have been more successful, and less so from Asia and Africa. Furthermore, data sources were biased toward bacterial infections associated with health care, at the expense of community-acquired infections. Overall, the lack of a global consensus on the methodology and data collection was acknowledged as a major obstacle for effective surveillance of antibiotic-resistant bacteria.

Using the findings of the 2014 report, the WHO is currently developing a global action plan for antimicrobial resistance that will include following: "a) the development of tools and standards for harmonized surveillance of antimicrobial resistance in humans, as well as integrated surveillance in food-producing animals and the food chain; b) the elaboration of strategies for population-based surveillance of antimicrobial resistance and its health and economic impact; c) the collaboration between antimicrobial surveillance networks and centres to create or strengthen coordinated regional and global surveillance."

The WHO also established a program in 1997 to tackle the problem of global antimicrobial resistance (15). It is known as the Antimicrobial Resistance Monitoring program. It required accurate and easily accessible data on antimicrobial resistance to support the decision making and to take action from the local to the global level. To achieve all this, the WHO has devised an electronic format named WHONET (http://www.whonet.org), freely accessible software (created and maintained by J. Stelling and T. F. O'Brien, Boston, MA) that is widely used as a common platform for antibiotic resistance data collection, management, and sharing and serves as a strategy to facilitate global surveillance of antimicrobial resistance, including

in low- and middle-income countries (16). The WHONET system has been successfully introduced in countries such as Nepal to monitor, analyze, and share the antimicrobial susceptibility data at various levels within that country (17).

Europe: Example of Successful Integrated Surveillance

The European Antimicrobial Resistance Surveillance Network (EARS-Net) is a multi-country surveillance network that collects routine clinical antibiotic susceptibility data from national surveillance systems within Europe (18). The European Centre for Disease Prevention and Control (ECDC) has hosted EARS-Net since 2010. The main function of EARS-Net is to document the emergence and dissemination of AROs within European countries and to increase awareness among the citizenry, scientists, and public health authorities. EARS-Net is the largest publicly funded surveillance system for antimicrobial resistance in the European region. At present it includes 900 public health laboratories serving more than 1,400 hospitals in Europe and providing services to an estimated population of 100 million European citizens. Several focused scientific papers and maps, graphs, and tables from annual reports are available through a Web-based data query tool (https://ecdc.europa.eu/en/surveillance-and-disease-data). There are two other ECDC surveillance networks that operate in close association with EARS-Net: the European Surveillance of Antimicrobial Consumption Network (ESAC-Net) and the Healthcare-Associated Infections Surveillance Network (HAI-Net). HAI-Net is responsible for coordinating a yearly point prevalence survey of health care-associated infections in acute care hospitals throughout Europe. EARS-Net also cooperates with the European Committee on Antimicrobial Susceptibility Testing (EUCAST) to establish guidelines and quality assurance activities among member countries. The ECDC has also developed a communication platform tool dedicated to antimicrobial resistance in health care-associated infections, which is referred to as the Epidemic Intelligence Information System (EPIS) AMR-HAI. EPIS AMR-HAI allows experts of national risk assessment bodies within the European Union to rapidly and securely exchange information related to microorganisms with emerging antimicrobial resistance that have a potential impact in Europe. EPIS AMR-HAI is a very useful tool for information exchange and subsequent rapid interventions.

The most recent reports from EARS-Net reveal a continuous increase between 2010 and 2014 in resistance to third-generation cephalosporins in *K. pneumoniae* and *E. coli* mediated by ESBLs, with coresistance to fluoroquinolones and aminoglycosides especially in Southern and Eastern European countries. Carbapenem-resistant and multi-drug-resistant *Pseudomonas aeruginosa* and *Acinetobacter* spp. are also on the increase. Carbapenem-resistant *K. pneumoniae* occurred in high proportions in Greece, Italy, and Romania but remained infrequent in the rest of European countries (19).

The surveillance systems described above contain limited data regarding antibiotic-resistant bacteria and antibiotic consumption among children. The Antibiotic Resistance and Prescribing in European Children (ARPEC) project, created to fill that void, revealed that the profiles of antibiotic resistance in bloodstream isolates from children differ from those reported by EARS-Net. This finding indicates that caution should be used when generalizing data from surveillance to special populations (20).

United States: National and Regional Surveillance Becomes a Presidential Priority

In 2005, the U.S. CDC established the National Healthcare Safety Network (NHSN) as a system to track health care-associated infections. The NHSN is the United States'

most widely used health care-associated infection tracking system and provides facilities, states, and regions with data needed to identify problem areas, measure progress of prevention efforts, and ultimately eliminate health care-associated infections. The NHSN now encompasses more than 17,000 medical facilities that include acute care hospitals, long-term acute care hospitals (LTACHs), psychiatric hospitals, rehabilitation hospitals, outpatient dialysis centers, ambulatory surgery centers, and nursing homes, with hospitals and dialysis facilities representing the majority of facilities reporting data. The NHSN annual reports include the Antimicrobial Resistance Reports, National and State Healthcare Associated Infections Progress Reports, and additional NHSN reports and resources. The most recent report from 2008–2014 describes significant reductions in central line-associated bloodstream infections and surgical-site infections, progress in MRSA bloodstream infections, and increases in catheter-associated urinary tract infections (https://www.cdc.gov/HAI/pdfs/progress-report/hai-progress-report.pdf).

Surveillance of antibiotic resistance among bacteria causing health care-associated infections through the NHSN describes increasing multidrug resistance and carbapenem resistance in Gram-negative bacteria from a large proportion of facilities (21). A more detailed assessment of the status of carbapenem-resistant *Enterobacteriaceae* infections in the United States as of 2012 was made possible by supplementing information derived from the NSHN with data collected through the Multi-site Gram-negative Surveillance Initiative (MuGSI), a population-based surveillance project conducted by the CDC's Emerging Infections Program (EIP), and from the Surveillance Network, an electronic surveillance database of antibiotic resistance encompassing several hundred microbiology laboratories across the country (22). Approximately 4% of hospitals reported infections due to carbapenem-resistant *Enterobacteriaceae*, as did as many as 18% of LTACHs. The proportion of *Klebsiella* spp. resistant to carbapenems averaged 10%, occurring mostly in patients with substantial health care exposures (23). These findings served to increase awareness and have motivated public health action to counter the dissemination of CRE in U.S. health care facilities. Specifically, the EIP MuGSI surveillance project determines the extent of CRE and multidrug-resistant *Acinetobacter* disease in the United States, identifies people most at risk for illness from these organisms, and measures trends of disease over time (https://www.cdc.gov/hai/eip/mugsi.html).

Important efforts to advance surveillance of CRE and other antibiotic-resistant bacteria in the United States have occurred at the regional level. Statewide networks for the detection of CRE have been established in certain states (24, 25). In northeast Ohio, a regional network examined the microbiological and genetic determinants of clinical outcomes in hospitalized patients with carbapenem-resistant *K. pneumoniae*; two subtypes were identified within the predominant ST258, which correspond to clades I and II, as determined by genomic analyses (26). In the region around Chicago, a multidrug-resistant organism surveillance network involving 25 short-stay acute care hospitals and seven LTACHs served to carry out a single-day prevalence survey demonstrating CRE in 30% of patients from LTACHs, and in only 3% of patients from acute care hospitals (27).

The impact of the CRE epidemic in U.S. community hospitals is revealed by data from 25 hospitals in North Carolina, South Carolina, Virginia, and Georgia that are members of the Duke Infection Control Outreach Network (DICON). The rate of CRE detection, albeit low, increased >5-fold from 2008 (0.26 cases per 100,000 patient-days) to 2012 (1.4 cases per 100,000 patient-days) (28).

Responding to escalating antimicrobial resistance, the U.S. Department of Defense implemented an enterprise-wide collaboration in 2009, the Antimicrobial Resistance Monitoring and Research Program (ARMoR), to aid in infection prevention and control. It consisted of a network of epidemiologists, bioinformaticists, microbiology researchers, policymakers, hospital- based infection preventionists, and health care providers who collaborate to collect relevant antimicrobial resistance data, conduct centralized molecular characterization, and use antimicrobial resistance characterization feedback to implement appropriate infection prevention and control measures and influence policy. A fundamental aspect of the ARMoR program is the transmission of laboratory and surveillance data back to participating hospitals through periodic reports on target bacteria. Similarly, these reports are communicated to leaders and policymakers within the health care facilities and the organization. Although it is challenging to establish a causal effect, there has been a significant decrease in the prevalence of CRE after the implementation of the ARMoR program. Indeed, this program serves as a model for comprehensive programs to combat antimicrobial resistance to be adopted by other health care organizations in the United States (29).

The U.S. White House recently released the National Action Plan for Combating Antibiotic-Resistant Bacteria, which outlines steps for implementing a national strategy and addressing policy recommendations of the President's Council of Advisors on Science and Technology report on combating antibiotic resistance. It was developed in response to Executive Order 13676: Combating Antibiotic-Resistant Bacteria, which was issued by President Barack Obama on September 18, 2014. The goals of the National Action Plan include the following: (i) slow the emergence of AROs and prevent the spread of resistant infections; (ii) strengthen national One-Health surveillance efforts to combat resistance; (iii) advance development and use of rapid and innovative diagnostic tests for identification and characterization of AROs; (iv) accelerate basic and applied research and development for new antibiotics, other therapeutics, and vaccines; and (v) improve international collaboration and capacities for antibiotic resistance prevention, surveillance, control, and antibiotic research and development (http://www.cdc.gov/drugresistance/federal-engagement-in-ar/).

United Kingdom: Voluntary Reporting Combined with Centralized Sentinel Sites

The voluntary reporting of microbiological diagnoses by hospital laboratories to Public Health England and its predecessors, the Health Protection Agency and the Public Health Laboratory Service, has been a mainstay of infectious disease surveillance in England for many decades. Since 1989, clinical microbiologists working in laboratories in England have been encouraged to report both the identification and antibiotic susceptibility of blood culture isolates to a national database called LabBase2. Initially, reporting was on paper forms, but it moved to electronic transmission of results in the 1990s. The outputs from this surveillance system have tended to focus on national trends in resistance in common pathogens (30).

In addition to the collection of routinely generated laboratory results, surveillance systems have also been established that involve the collection of bacterial isolates from sentinel laboratories for testing in a centralized facility, typically a national reference laboratory. In the United Kingdom, two such schemes, one for respiratory isolates and the other for bacteremia isolates, are sponsored by the British Society for Antimicrobial Chemotherapy and have been running continuously since 1999 and 2001, respectively (31).

Limited-Resource Countries: Gaps in Surveillance

Important gaps in the surveillance of antibiotic-resistant bacteria are evident in developing countries, as highlighted by the WHO 2014 report (14). Ironically, it is often in these countries where the challenge posed by resistant bacteria is the greatest, threatening to erode the important contribution of antibiotics to the health of the population.

The SMART (Study for Monitoring Antimicrobial Resistance Trends) surveillance program is managed by IHMA, Inc. for Merck & Co., Inc. It started in 2002 to monitor antimicrobial resistance trends among bacterial isolates from intra-abdominal infection obtained from 213 sites in 54 countries in Africa, Asia, Latin America, Europe, North America, the South Pacific, and the Middle East and was expanded to include urinary tract isolates in 2009. SMART surveillance includes a wide representation of microbiology laboratories among resource-limited countries (32). All isolates from SMART were from intra-abdominal infections or urinary tract infections, and only one isolate per species per patient per year was accepted. The molecular characterization of the SMART isolates started in 2008. Up to 100 consecutive nonselected Gram-negative aerobic and facultative bacilli per year from each of the participating hospitals were included. All organisms were deemed clinically significant based upon the criteria of the local investigators. The SMART program provides important information about changes in the spectrum of microbial pathogens and trends in the antimicrobial resistance patterns in nosocomial and community-acquired intra-abdominal infections and provides important surveillance data on AROs from resource-limited countries (33). The program supports measures for the prevention of infection along with conservation and appropriate use of all antibiotics, including the implementation of the WHO's Global Action Plan, calling for comprehensive stewardship programs and activities that enhance health system capability to use antibiotics appropriately.

The AstraZeneca global surveillance program is another global surveillance program managed by IHMA, Inc. This program is conducted in 202 sites from 40 countries (from Africa, Asia, Latin America, Europe, North

America, the South Pacific, and the Middle East), was initiated in 2012, and also includes a wide representation of microbiology laboratories among resource-limited countries (34). Up to 100 consecutive nonselected Gram-negative aerobic and facultative bacilli from each participating hospital were included. All organisms were deemed clinically significant based upon the criteria of the local investigators and were obtained from urinary tract, skin-structure, intra-abdominal, and lower respiratory tract specimens. Molecular characterization of AROs is a characteristic of the AstraZeneca global surveillance program, and this program has provided important molecular information about AROs among resource-limited countries (33).

Vietnam has demonstrated the need and potential impact of surveillance systems in combating antibiotic resistance among resource-limited countries. In this Southeast Asian country with >90 million inhabitants, Gram-negative bacteria reach high levels of resistance (i.e., >40% of ESBL-producing *Enterobacteriaceae* among hospitalized patients), likely due to limited infection control, diagnostic capabilities, and widespread overuse and misuse of antibiotics (35). To respond to this challenge, an ambitious program is underway in Vietnam that aims to implement infection control and antimicrobial stewardship programs. The Vietnamese Ministry of Health has committed to build a surveillance program to monitor hospital antibiotic use and resistance, community antibiotic use and resistance, and antibiotic use and resistance in animals, and to provide a reference laboratory and quality assurance mechanisms for local microbiology laboratories. Additionally, Viet Nam Resistance (VINARES) is being implemented as a capacity-building initiative designed to equip 16 hospitals with the tools to perform self-sufficient antibiotic surveillance and carry out antimicrobial stewardship. The VINARES project was started in the autumn of 2012 led by researchers from Sweden, the United Kingdom, and Vietnam. Hospitals submit monthly data on antibiotic consumption, infection control surveillance, and susceptibility of bacterial pathogens (using WHONET); hospitals receive regular reports, which compare their performance to that of other hospitals (36). These objectives and framework are eminently transferable to other developing countries and compatible with Resolution 67.25 from the World Health Assembly, which urged countries, especially low- and middle-income countries, to develop capacity to combat antimicrobial resistance through strengthened surveillance and laboratory capacity (37).

Indeed, they resonate with a surveillance initiative undertaken in Colombia, a middle-income country in South America. Since 2003, the Centro Internacional de Entrenamiento e Investigaciones Médicas (CIDEIM) has developed a surveillance project that now comprises 23 hospitals in 10 cities, with the objective of tracking antibiotic resistance among Gram-negative bacteria. Research in CIDEIM is developed along three broad lines—prevention and control, host-pathogen interaction, and chemotherapy and resistance—which together constitute an integrated approach to infectious diseases. The three lines are directed toward the same goal: defining solutions to health problems from the perspective of diverse disciplines in the basic and applied sciences. In the most recent 4-year period, analysis using WHONET, demonstrated increasing trends in the proportion of multidrug-resistant bacteria. Detailed molecular characterization of resistance determinants and strain typing of carbapenem-resistant organisms was carried out in a central laboratory. Feedback on their respective data on antibiotic resistance, molecular mechanisms, and strain typing is transmitted to participating hospitals. These reports, in turn, help inform infection control and antimicrobial stewardship actions at the local level. Additionally, they provide insight into the molecular epidemiology of antibiotic-resistant Gram-negative bacteria in Colombia and permit comparisons to be drawn at the continental and global levels (38).

SUMMARY: CHALLENGES AND OPPORTUNITIES IN SURVEILLANCE

This review highlighted some aspects of global surveillance systems for tracking the emergence and transmission of AROs. These surveillance programs play a crucial role in enhanced diagnostics, development of potential vaccines, and development of novel antibiotics with activity against AROs, notwithstanding their current limitations. Furthermore, the molecular analysis of bacterial isolates through surveillance projects yields important insights into the transmission dynamics and mechanisms responsible for such resistance. The threat posed by the emergence and dissemination of AROs dictates the bolstering and development of current regional, national, and global surveillance systems. We urgently need to use surveillance and surveillance programs to identify areas for further research. This was highlighted in the last workshop on surveillance supported by the European Union throughout the Joint Programming Initiative on Antimicrobial Resistance (https://www.jpiamr.eu/jpiamr-workshop-the-interplay-between-amr-surveillance-and-science/).

The impact of surveillance can be improved by incorporating data on antimicrobial usage and antibiotic resistance, as well as data from different components of health care. A "One-Health" approach, integrating multiple disciplines working locally, nationally, and globally to improve the health of people, animals, and the environment, is a template very well suited to expand surveillance schemes. Unfortunately, surveillance systems as such are very restricted in this regard. Another crucial shortcoming of antimicrobial resistance surveillance is that data are consigned in one-time or annual reports and do not reflect a real-time assessment of antibiotic consumption and resistance. ARTEMIS (Antimicrobial Resistance Trend Monitoring System), a pilot network of seven European health care institutions introduced in 2012 sharing data about drug resistance and consumption using a Semantic Web-based model, provides an example of how this problem can be overcome. Queries obtained within a few seconds provide real-time information about antimicrobial resistance that is accurate, comparable to data from EARS-Net. ARTEMIS involved the introduction of monitoring architecture that can be used to build transnational antimicrobial resistance surveillance networks. Results indicated that the Semantic Web-based approach provided an efficient and reliable solution for development of eHealth architectures that enable online antimicrobial resistance monitoring from heterogeneous data sources. ARTEMIS can be used to detect emerging bacterial resistance in a multinational context and support public health actions. This or similar platforms can serve as the backbone of future multisite and multinational surveillance networks that allow rapid detection of emerging resistance to antibiotics and guide immediate infection control and public health actions (39).

Another example of an antimicrobial resistance monitoring system is one from Portugal called HAITool (http://haitool.ihmt.unl.pt/). HAITool is a hospital infections management and antibiotic prescribing decision-making information system that has been implemented in several Portuguese hospitals. The main objectives of this project are to identify and evaluate the existing health care-associated infections management processes in the participating hospitals; collect data about antimicrobial resistance among health care-associated infections; and use these data to design, implement, and evaluate a new toolkit for assisting health professionals dealing with antimicrobial-resistant health care-associated infections. Ultimately, this program aims to enable Internet access to the toolkit for other European and Portuguese-speaking countries.

An alternative approach is to monitor trends in antibiotic resistance using automated semantic and scientometric analysis of PubMed entries. When the relationship between the introduction of novel antibiotic classes into the market and emergence of bacterial resistance was investigated and compared with data from EARS-Net, only a partial correlation was observed between scientometric analysis and development of resistance (40).

The application of genomic tools to the characterization of antibiotic resistance determinants (such as mobile genetic elements) and isolates will provide insights into transmission and ultimately enhance surveillance. A U.S. study used long-read genome sequencing (PacBio) with full end-to-end assembly and illustrated that carbapenem resistance genes are located on a wide array of plasmid platforms, with evidence of horizontal gene transfer between clinical and environmental bacteria (41).

Local, national, and global integrated ARO surveillance programs with sufficient data linkage with enhanced genomics accompanied by user-friendly bioinformatics systems promise to overcome some of the stumbling blocks encountered in understanding the emergence and spread of AROs. Hopefully surveillance programs will be able to benefit society at large (16).

Global surveillance programs have shown that antibiotic resistance is a major threat to the public. Surveillance systems must also be utilized to assess the effectiveness and impacts of initiatives and interventions to reduce the development and spread of AROs. Timely and targeted dissemination of surveillance data will continue to be an essential component of efforts to combat the threat of AROs. The dissemination of surveillance data should not be restricted to the scientific and medical community but must include all major stakeholders, including the public as well as policymakers and governments.

CITATION

Pitout JDD. 2018. Transmission surveillance for antimicrobial-resistant organisms in the health system. *Microbiol Spectrum* 6(5):MTBP-0010-2016.

REFERENCES

1. **Medina E, Pieper DH.** 2016. Tackling threats and future problems of multidrug-resistant bacteria. *Curr Top Microbiol Immunol* **398:**3–33.
2. **Huskins WC.** 2007. Interventions to prevent transmission of antimicrobial-resistant bacteria in the intensive care unit. *Curr Opin Crit Care* **13:** 572–577.
3. **Infectious Diseases Society of America.** 2010. The 10 × '20 Initiative: pursuing a global commitment to develop 10 new antibacterial drugs by 2020. *Clin Infect Dis* **50:**1081–1083.
4. **Baker S.** 2015. Infectious disease. A return to the pre-antimicrobial era? *Science* **347:**1064–1066.
5. **Schwaber MJ, Navon-Venezia S, Kaye KS, Ben-Ami R, Schwartz D, Carmeli Y.** 2006. Clinical and economic impact of bacteremia with extended-spectrum-β-lactamase-producing *Enterobacteriaceae. Antimicrob Agents Chemother* **50:**1257–1262.
6. **Grayson ML, Jarvie LJ, Martin R, Johnson PD, Jodoin ME, McMullan C, Gregory RH, Bellis K, Cunnington K, Wilson FL, Quin D, Kelly AM, Hand Hygiene Study Group and Hand Hygiene Statewide Roll-out Group, Victorian Quality Council.** 2008. Significant reductions in methicillin-resistant *Staphylococcus aureus* bacteraemia and clinical isolates associated with a multisite, hand hygiene culture-change program and subsequent successful statewide roll-out. *Med J Aust* **188:**633–640.
7. **Nolan SM, Gerber JS, Zaoutis T, Prasad P, Rettig S, Gross K, McGowan KL, Reilly AF, Coffin SE.** 2009. Outbreak of vancomycin-resistant enterococcus colonization among pediatric oncology patients. *Infect Control Hosp Epidemiol* **30:**338–345.
8. **Calfee DP, Farr BM.** 2002. Infection control and cost control in the era of managed care. *Infect Control Hosp Epidemiol* **23:**407–410.
9. **Muto CA, Jernigan JA, Ostrowsky BE, Richet HM, Jarvis WR, Boyce JM, Farr BM, SHEA.** 2003. SHEA guideline for preventing nosocomial transmission of multidrug-resistant strains of *Staphylococcus aureus* and *Enterococcus. Infect Control Hosp Epidemiol* **24:**362–386.
10. **Farr BM.** 2004. Prevention and control of methicillin-resistant *Staphylococcus aureus* infections. *Curr Opin Infect Dis* **17:**317–322.
11. **Spellberg B, Bartlett JG, Gilbert DN.** 2013. The future of antibiotics and resistance. *N Engl J Med* **368:**299–302.
12. **Grundmann H, Klugman KP, Walsh T, Ramon-Pardo P, Sigauque B, Khan W, Laxminarayan R, Heddini A, Stelling J.** 2011. A framework for global surveillance of antibiotic resistance. *Drug Resist Updat* **14:**79–87.

13. **Johnson AP.** 2015. Surveillance of antibiotic resistance. *Philos Trans R Soc Lond B Biol Sci* **370:** 20140080.

14. **World Health Organization (WHO).** 2014. *Antimicrobial Resistance: Global Report on Surveillance 2014.* WHO, Geneva, Switzerland.

15. **Stelling JM, O'Brien TF.** 1997. Surveillance of antimicrobial resistance: the WHONET program. *Clin Infect Dis* **24**(Suppl 1):S157–S168.

16. **O'Brien TF, Stelling J.** 2011. Integrated multilevel surveillance of the world's infecting microbes and their resistance to antimicrobial agents. *Clin Microbiol Rev* **24:**281–295.

17. **Ghosh AN, Bhatta DR, Ansari MT, Tiwari HK, Mathuria JP, Gaur A, Supram HS, Gokhale S.** 2013. Application of WHONET in the antimicrobial resistance surveillance of uropathogens: a first user experience from Nepal. *J Clin Diagn Res* **7:**845–848.

18. **Weist K, Diaz Högberg L.** 2014. ECDC publishes 2013 surveillance data on antimicrobial resistance and antimicrobial consumption in Europe. *Euro Surveill* **19:**20962.

19. **European Centre for Disease Prevention and Control (ECDC).** 2015. *Antimicrobial Resistance Surveillance in Europe 2014.* Annual Report of the European Antimicrobial Resistance Surveillance Network (EARS-Net). ECDC, Stockholm, Sweden.

20. **Bielicki JA, Lundin R, Sharland M, Project A, ARPEC Project.** 2015. Antibiotic resistance prevalence in routine bloodstream isolates from children's hospitals varies substantially from adult surveillance data in Europe. *Pediatr Infect Dis J* **34:**734–741.

21. **Sievert DM, Ricks P, Edwards JR, Schneider A, Patel J, Srinivasan A, Kallen A, Limbago B, Fridkin S, National Healthcare Safety Network (NHSN) Team and Participating NHSN Facilities.** 2013. Antimicrobial-resistant pathogens associated with healthcare-associated infections: summary of data reported to the National Healthcare Safety Network at the Centers for Disease Control and Prevention, 2009–2010. *Infect Control Hosp Epidemiol* **34:**1–14.

22. **Karlowsky JA, Kelly LJ, Thornsberry C, Jones ME, Evangelista AT, Critchley IA, Sahm DF.** 2002. Susceptibility to fluoroquinolones among commonly isolated Gram-negative bacilli in 2000: TRUST and TSN data for the United States. *Int J Antimicrob Agents* **19:**21–31.

23. **Centers for Disease Control and Prevention (CDC).** 2013. Vital signs: carbapenem-resistant Enterobacteriaceae. *MMWR Morb Mortal Wkly Rep* **62:**165–170.

24. **Brennan BM, Coyle JR, Marchaim D, Pogue JM, Boehme M, Finks J, Malani AN, VerLee KE, Buckley BO, Mollon N, Sundin DR, Washer LL, Kaye KS.** 2014. Statewide surveillance of carbapenem-resistant Enterobacteriaceae in Michigan. *Infect Control Hosp Epidemiol* **35:**342–349.

25. **Johnson JK, Wilson LE, Zhao L, Richards K, Thom KA, Harris AD, Maryland Multidrug-Resistant Organism Prevention Collaborative.** 2014. Point prevalence of *Klebsiella pneumoniae* carbapenemase-producing *Enterobacteriaceae* in Maryland. *Infect Control Hosp Epidemiol* **35:** 443–445.

26. **Wright MS, Perez F, Brinkac L, Jacobs MR, Kaye K, Cober E, van Duin D, Marshall SH, Hujer AM, Rudin SD, Hujer KM, Bonomo RA, Adams MD.** 2014. Population structure of KPC-producing *Klebsiella pneumoniae* isolates from midwestern U.S. hospitals. *Antimicrob Agents Chemother* **58:**4961–4965.

27. **Lin MY, Lyles-Banks RD, Lolans K, Hines DW, Spear JB, Petrak R, Trick WE, Weinstein RA, Hayden MK, Centers for Disease Control and Prevention Epicenters Program.** 2013. The importance of long-term acute care hospitals in the regional epidemiology of *Klebsiella pneumoniae* carbapenemase-producing Enterobacteriaceae. *Clin Infect Dis* **57:**1246–1252.

28. **Thaden JT, Lewis SS, Hazen KC, Huslage K, Fowler VG Jr, Moehring RW, Chen LF, Jones CD, Moore ZS, Sexton DJ, Anderson DJ.** 2014. Rising rates of carbapenem-resistant Enterobacteriaceae in community hospitals: a mixed-methods review of epidemiology and microbiology practices in a network of community hospitals in the southeastern United States. *Infect Control Hosp Epidemiol* **35:**978–983.

29. **Lesho EP, Waterman PE, Chukwuma U, McAuliffe K, Neumann C, Julius MD, Crouch H, Chandrasekera R, English JF, Clifford RJ, Kester KE.** 2014. The Antimicrobial Resistance Monitoring and Research (ARMoR) Program: the US Department of Defense response to escalating antimicrobial resistance. *Clin Infect Dis* **59:**390–397.

30. **Livermore DM, Hope R, Reynolds R, Blackburn R, Johnson AP, Woodford N.** 2013. Declining cephalosporin and fluoroquinolone non-susceptibility among bloodstream Enterobacteriaceae from the UK: links to prescribing change? *J Antimicrob Chemother* **68:**2667–2674.

31. **White AR, BSAC Working Parties on Resistance Surveillance.** 2008. The British Society for Antimicrobial Chemotherapy Resistance Surveillance Project: a successful collaborative model. *J Antimicrob Chemother* **62**(Suppl 2):ii3–ii14.

32. **Lascols C, Peirano G, Hackel M, Laupland KB, Pitout JD.** 2013. Surveillance and molecular epi-

demiology of *Klebsiella pneumoniae* isolates that produce carbapenemases: first report of OXA-48-like enzymes in North America. *Antimicrob Agents Chemother* **57**:130–136.

33. **Peirano G, Bradford PA, Kazmierczak KM, Badal RE, Hackel M, Hoban DJ, Pitout JD.** 2014. Global incidence of carbapenemase-producing *Escherichia coli* ST131. *Emerg Infect Dis* **20**:1928–1931.

34. **Kazmierczak KM, Biedenbach DJ, Hackel M, Rabine S, de Jonge BL, Bouchillon SK, Sahm DF, Bradford PA.** 2016. Global dissemination of bla_{KPC} into bacterial species beyond *Klebsiella pneumoniae* and *in vitro* susceptibility to ceftazidime-avibactam and aztreonam-avibactam. *Antimicrob Agents Chemother* **60**:4490–4500.

35. **Nguyen KV, Thi Do NT, Chandna A, Nguyen TV, Pham CV, Doan PM, Nguyen AQ, Thi Nguyen CK, Larsson M, Escalante S, Olowokure B, Laxminarayan R, Gelband H, Horby P, Thi Ngo HB, Hoang MT, Farrar J, Hien TT, Wertheim HF.** 2013. Antibiotic use and resistance in emerging economies: a situation analysis for Viet Nam. *BMC Public Health* **13**:1158.

36. **Wertheim HF, Chandna A, Vu PD, Pham CV, Nguyen PD, Lam YM, Nguyen CV, Larsson M, Rydell U, Nilsson LE, Farrar J, Nguyen KV, Hanberger H.** 2013. Providing impetus, tools, and guidance to strengthen national capacity for antimicrobial stewardship in Viet Nam. *PLoS Med* **10**:e1001429.

37. **Shallcross LJ, Davies SC.** 2014. The World Health Assembly resolution on antimicrobial resistance. *J Antimicrob Chemother* **69**:2883–2885.

38. **Hernández-Gómez C, Blanco VM, Motoa G, Correa A, Vallejo M, Villegas MV, Grupo de Resistencia Bacteriana Nosocomial en Colombia.** 2014. Evolution of antimicrobial resistance in Gram negative bacilli from intensive care units in Colombia. *Biomedica* **34**(Suppl 1): 91–100. (In Spanish.)

39. **Teodoro D, Pasche E, Gobeill J, Emonet S, Ruch P, Lovis C.** 2012. Building a transnational biosurveillance network using semantic web technologies: requirements, design, and preliminary evaluation. *J Med Internet Res* **14**:e73.

40. **Brandt C, Makarewicz O, Fischer T, Stein C, Pfeifer Y, Werner G, Pletz MW.** 2014. The bigger picture: the history of antibiotics and antimicrobial resistance displayed by scientometric data. *Int J Antimicrob Agents* **44**:424–430.

41. **Conlan S, Thomas PJ, Deming C, Park M, Lau AF, Dekker JP, Snitkin ES, Clark TA, Luong K, Song Y, Tsai YC, Boitano M, Dayal J, Brooks SY, Schmidt B, Young AC, Thomas JW, Bouffard GG, Blakesley RW, NISC Comparative Sequencing Program, Mullikin JC, Korlach J, Henderson DK, Frank KM, Palmore TN, Segre JA, Segre JA.** 2014. Single-molecule sequencing to track plasmid diversity of hospital-associated carbapenemase-producing Enterobacteriaceae. *Sci Transl Med* **6**:254ra126.

The Evolution of Genotyping Strategies to Detect, Analyze, and Control Transmission of Tuberculosis

13

DARÍO GARCÍA DE VIEDMA[1,2,3] and LAURA PÉREZ-LAGO[1,2]

INTRODUCTION

The introduction of DNA fingerprinting tools for the analysis of *Mycobacterium tuberculosis* (MTB) isolates has transformed the way we control the transmission of this pathogen. As with any other infection transmitted via aerosolized particles harboring infective bacteria, obtaining accurate data on the index case and subsequent contacts involved in a transmission chain is challenging.

The traditional approach to identifying tuberculosis (TB) transmission events was based on contact tracing (1–3), in which it was necessary to interview every TB patient in order to identify other potential active TB cases and secondary cases that could also have been exposed to the index case. Research is based on a concentric circles approach; i.e., it moves in an outward direction, starting from a context in which closer contacts are more frequent and prolonged and moving on to contexts in which the frequency and duration of exposure are lower. This strategy has proven to be useful (2–4) when the exposure/transmission events occur in the domestic or work environment, although it

[1]Department of Microbiology and Infectious Diseases, Gregorio Marañón General University Hospital, Madrid, Spain; [2]Instituto Investigación Sanitaria Gregorio Marañón (IiSGM), Madrid, Spain; [3]CIBER Enfermedades respiratorias CIBERES, Spain.

Microbial Transmission in Biological Processes
Edited by Fernando Baquero, Emilio Bouza, J.A. Gutiérrez-Fuentes, and Teresa M. Coque
© 2018 American Society for Microbiology, Washington, DC
doi:10.1128/microbiolspec.MTBP-0002-2016

has severe limitations for tracking transmission events linked to leisure activities or resulting from more sporadic contacts.

New molecular epidemiology-based approaches emerged to overcome the limitations of standard epidemiology. The rationale of these approaches was to use the DNA fingerprint of the MTB isolates to identify cases that were likely involved in the same transmission chain, i.e., infected by isolates sharing an identical pattern, namely, clustered isolates.

Therefore, the identification of TB cases involved in clusters constituted an alternative approach to identifying and analyzing TB transmission events. The methods applied to characterize MTB isolates for the study of molecular epidemiology have evolved since the first genotyping tools were introduced as support elements in the surveillance of transmission. However, and more importantly, these methodological developments have been accompanied by considerable changes in our approach to analyzing and tracking the transmission of MTB.

In this chapter, we analyze the parallel evolution of two lines: (i) the development of laboratory methods, initially genotypic and finally genomic, that have been applied to analyze the genetic features of MTB isolates; and (ii) how we apply these tools to optimize the way we track transmission of TB.

Á LA CARTE GENOTYPING

MTB genotyping was initially applied only when the epidemiologist needed support to confirm or clarify a suspected outbreak or microepidemic. MTB genotyping was no more than a confirmatory tool to either prove that the cases suspected of being part of the outbreak were truly linked, once genotyping confirmed an identical fingerprint for all the isolates, or to rule out the involvement of cases when the corresponding isolate was genotypically different. The first unexpected finding in the application of genotyping tools

in this "á la carte" approach was that some microepidemics that were highly suspected owing to the high possibility of exposure between the cases were not later confirmed by molecular analysis. Consequently, different genotypes were detected for some or all of the cases involved. In a study performed on 33 microepidemics involving 44 epidemiologically linked case pairs (5), 7 microepidemics were finally not confirmed because they showed genotypic differences, and 5 of these microepidemics were highly suspected because the patients lived in the same house. Furthermore, some theoretically linked cases have been shown to not share a genotype with the index case (e.g., 30% of the cases in a study in San Francisco [6] and 29% in a study in seven sentinel areas in the United States [7]). In high-incidence settings, such as the suburbs of Cape Town in South Africa, the figures recorded were even higher, and only 46% of the cases shared a fingerprint pattern with another member of the same household (8).

The message of these early studies was that transmission did not occur exclusively as the result of close and prolonged contacts but, on the contrary, that cases occasionally resulted from unexpected links outside the scenarios envisaged by the standard concentric circle-based approach. This observation led to the first major transformation in molecular epidemiology, in which genotyping restricted to the analysis of cases suspected of being part of transmission events by the epidemiologist shifted toward a universal genotyping format. The rationale behind this decision was that only the systematic analysis of each and every case of TB in a whole population would enable us to identify all the links in the transmission chains active in that population.

UNIVERSAL GENOTYPING

If we analyze all the cases of TB in a population, we can identify all the transmission chains. However, in TB, exposure to the pathogen is not always sequential; i.e., TB may or may not develop after exposure. However, if it does, it could happen some time after the exposure, depending on host factors. The possible lack of sequence in TB, from exposure to disease, complicates the analysis of transmission and obliges us to apply systematic genotyping for a minimum time period (>3 years) (9) before we can be confident that we have successfully identified the links involved in ongoing transmission chains.

Universal genotyping proved extremely useful for detailed examination of the transmission dynamics of TB in a complete population, especially in settings where socioepidemiological transformations were occurring. These developments coincided with dramatic epidemiological transformations in many cities in Europe and the United States arising from the arrival of immigrants, usually from countries with higher rates of TB than the host country. It was therefore possible to compare the percentage of TB cases due to recent transmission (those included in clusters) with those corresponding to reactivation of imported infections (nonclustered orphan cases), compare recent transmission rates between autochthonous and immigrant cases, and even identify cross-transmission between both populations. These relevant features went far beyond the possibilities of standard epidemiology.

Several major studies that applied universal genotyping (10–14) drew similar conclusions. Most immigrant TB cases were unclustered, indicating that they were the result of reactivations of exposures in the country of origin. The percentage of immigrant cases that were clustered owing to recent transmission after arrival in the host country was low for clusters including other immigrant cases and clusters also including autochthonous cases.

In Spain, findings differed from those reported elsewhere. Here, immigration is a much more recent phenomenon than in other countries, and the profile of nationalities differed markedly depending on the area of the country where the immigrants settled. Universal genotyping enabled us to observe trans-mission dynamics in two different observation nodes: Madrid, a large city with immigrants mainly from Latin America (15); and Almería, a small province in southeast Spain receiving immigrants mainly from North and Sub-Saharan Africa (16). In both settings, we observed that even among immigrants from countries with high rates of TB, not all cases of TB corresponded to reactivations of imported infections, which had been assumed before the availability of molecular epidemiology techniques. In some patients (29% in Madrid and 36.8% in Almería), the MTB isolates clustered with other cases in the population, likely owing to recent transmissions. Different nationalities were involved in 50% of the clusters in Madrid and 28.9% of those in Almería, and >50% of these clusters involved both immigrant and autochthonous cases in the same cluster. These data revealed a singular finding in Spain that we termed "transmission permeability," which differed from observations in other countries, and suggested the existence of complex socioepidemiological transmission dynamics that were revealed thanks to universal genotyping strategies.

Therefore, universal genotyping has huge potential for unraveling the complexity and singularities of TB transmission dynamics in different populations. However, studies were carried out retrospectively, and while they made it possible to analyze transmission dynamics in detail, they were of no practical use for control of transmission, since transmission was studied at a point in time when intervention was not possible. This situation was due in part to the genotyping method used, which in most cases was IS6110 restriction fragment length polymorphism (RFLP) analysis. Of the methods used in the early stages of the study of the molecular epidemiology of TB, IS6110-RFLP (17) (Fig. 1) had good discriminatory power, and its development and validation were supported by international consensus (18). The technique is based on the purification of DNA, digestion by restriction enzymes, separation of the digested fragments by electrophoresis, and

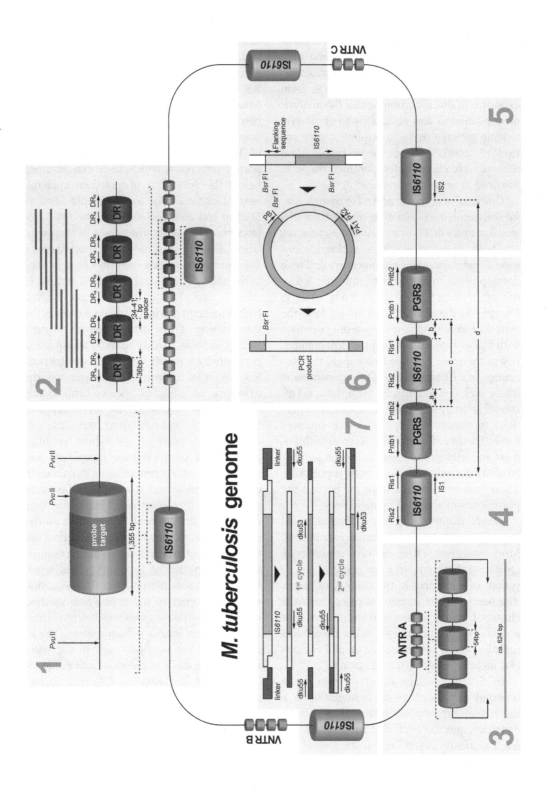

M. tuberculosis genome

hybridization with a DNA probe complementary to the IS*6110* transposon sequence. As the number of IS*6110* copies and their distribution along the MTB chromosome differed between isolates, the technique generated a band pattern that differed in the number and size of bands for each strain. Comparison of RFLP types for different isolates enabled us to identify cases infected by the same strain and thus define transmission clusters.

Since IS*6110*-RFLP requires a large amount of purified DNA, long incubation times are necessary (up to 6 to 8 weeks owing to the slow-growing nature of MTB). In addition, the technique itself is cumbersome and time-consuming, and the proven epidemiological value of genotyping data highlighted the need for faster results.

REAL-TIME MOLECULAR EPIDEMIOLOGY

The next step in studying the molecular epidemiology of TB required a shift from retrospective studies, which had proven extremely useful for precisely defining the transmission dynamics of TB in complex transformations, to prospective application of genotyping strategies for identification of transmission clusters and application of timely interventions. This shift could only come about with a faster genotyping tool, thus necessitating a switch to PCR-based methods, which were faster and did not require well-grown MTB cultures.

Several attempts have been made to establish new techniques to replace RFLP-based genotyping as the gold standard for MTB fingerprinting. One of the most widely applied was spoligotyping (19), which is a PCR-based method followed by reverse hybridization that analyzes a clustered regularly interspaced short palindromic repeat (CRISPR) region comprising 43 spacers distributed between DNA repetitions in the direct repeat (DR) locus of MTB. Depending on the variability in the number of spacers between strains, we obtain different patterns, or spoligotypes. Although spoligotyping is fast and inexpensive, its discriminatory power is lower than that of RFLP. Consequently, spoligotyping is now frequently used as a tool for evolutionary/phylogenetic studies and for assigning lineages, families, and subfamilies for global surveillance (20). However, its discriminatory power is not sufficient to enable it to identify recent transmission events at the population level, since it must be used in combination

FIGURE 1 Schematic representation of the chromosome of a hypothetical *M. tuberculosis* complex isolate with marked repetitive elements as targets for different typing methods. The principle of those methods is pictorially outlined. (1) In IS*6110*-RFLP typing, mycobacterial DNA is cleaved with the restriction endonuclease PvuII, and the resulting fragments are separated electrophoretically on an agarose gel, transferred onto a nylon membrane by Southern blotting, and hybridized to a probe complementary to the 3' end of the IS*6110* (probe target), yielding a characteristic banding pattern in which every band represents a single IS*6110* element. (2) Spoligotyping relies upon PCR amplification of a single DR locus that harbors 36-bp DRs interspersed with unique 34- to 41-bp spacer sequences. The PCR products (red horizontal lines) are hybridized to a membrane containing 43 oligonucleotides corresponding to the spacers from *M. tuberculosis* H37Rv and *Mycobacterium bovis* BCG. The presence or absence of each of those 43 spacers in the DR region of the analyzed isolate will be represented as the pattern of positive or negative hybridization signals. (3) The VNTR loci or MIRUs are PCR-amplified, and the obtained products (yellow horizontal line) are sized on agarose gels to deduce the number of repeats in each individual locus. (4, 5) Two PCR-based typing methods, that is, DRE-PCR and amplityping, are designed to amplify DNA between clusters of IS*6110* and polymorphic GC-rich sequences (PGRS) or between clusters of IS*6110* elements, respectively. Different distances between the repetitive elements and their different copy numbers result in variability of banding patterns, composed of DNA fragments amplified (a to d) and produced for individual isolates. Other typing methods (less frequently used) are also shown: heminested inverse PCR (6) and ligation-mediated PCR (7). Figure reprinted and legend adapted from reference 83, CC BY 3.0.

with another genotyping method. New efforts made to improve the approach are based on the following: (i) enhancement of the discriminatory power of spoligotyping by increasing the number of spacers analyzed (20); (ii) extending the informative value of the technique by including resistance mutations; and (iii) streamlining performance by modifying the analysis format from solid to liquid hybridization, thus taking advantage of high-throughput analysis in Luminex platforms (21, 22).

Amplified fragment length polymorphism (AFLP) analysis was yet another alternative to RFLP, whether in its standard format, which is based on radiolabeled primers (AFLP) (23), or in its improved fluorescent version (fAFLP) (24). The method is laborious because it is based on DNA restriction, ligation to adaptors, and subsequent PCR primed with these adaptors. Its discriminatory power is no higher than that of RFLP, and it is mostly restricted to typing of nontuberculous mycobacteria (25, 26). Other methods have been developed and evaluated as alternatives for MTB fingerprinting, although they have proven either to be cumbersome (pulsed-field gel electrophoresis [PFGE] [27]) or to lack reproducibility (double-repetitive-element PCR [DRE-PCR] [28] and randomly amplified polymorphic DNA [RAPD] [29]).

These inconclusive efforts were followed by a novel, promising development, namely, mycobacterial interspersed repetitive-unit–variable-number tandem-repeat (MIRU-VNTR) analysis, which is based on the analysis of the number of tandem repeats in a selection of targets in the MTB chromosome. The first design of the method involved 12 loci (30, 31), which was soon increased to 15 loci (only 6 of the previous loci were retained owing to the poor discriminatory power of the first format) (32). The number of loci analyzed was increased to 24 in a subsequent version, which is considered to offer the highest discriminatory power (32, 33).

After the release of this new, fast genotyping technique, various studies compared its efficiency with the previous gold standard, RFLP, and found the concordance between them to be ~78 to 85%. However, the remaining discrepancies between the techniques (either RFLP clusters split by MIRU-VNTR or vice versa) were difficult to resolve. Some authors suggested that MIRU-VNTR should be accompanied by spoligotyping to improve its discriminatory power (33, 34). However, most studies agreed that MIRU-VNTR was not inferior to RFLP and highlighted its marked superiority in terms of speed, ease of performance, and interlaboratory sharing of data based on a numerical code (33, 35, 36). In a study carried out in Spain, the discriminatory power of MIRU-VNTR made it possible to clarify major RFLP-defined clusters that were not epidemiologically supported. MIRU-VNTR split the clusters into smaller subclusters with more consistent geographical and epidemiological significance (37). With respect to the times of response to obtain data, a prospective study applying RFLP and VNTR-MIRU in parallel demonstrated that the clusters were defined by MIRU-VNTR in a much shorter time range (2 to 3 weeks versus >5 weeks for RFLP) (38). Similar to the international consensus achieved before proposing IS6110-RFLP as the reference method for genotyping of MTB, an international quality control scheme aimed to ensure proper application of MIRU-VNTR in different settings (39, 40).

The latest versions of MIRU-VNTR involve adaptation of the technique to a multiplex PCR format in which the amplified products from triplex PCRs, which use fluorescent primers, are sized using capillary electrophoresis and read in independent channels to assign the alleles. This format enabled semiautomated high-throughput and highly precise analysis of isolates (41). Unfortunately, it requires capillary electrophoresis and a certain degree of expertise. A version of the 24-loci multiplex MIRU-VNTR has also been adapted for settings that do not have access to capillary electrophoresis but need an easy genotyping format to resolve simple issues. MIRU-VNTR length polymorphism triplex (MLP3) (42) is based on comparison of the mobility of the triplex-PCR products in standard gel electrophoresis. It enables only a qualitative comparison between patterns for rapid identification of similarities or differences between the isolates, although it does not make it possible to assign alleles. In any case, the technique provides a straightforward approach to outbreaks, microepidemic alarms, and laboratory cross-contamination alerts and differentiates between reactivations and reinfections in recurrences.

Nevertheless, despite the availability of a new fast, discriminative, and high-throughput genotyping tool, the time needed to obtain the MTB cultures continues to be a limitation. The only way to ensure availability of genotyping data sufficiently early for intervention would be to ensure that clusters are identified close to the diagnosis of each new case, once the TB bacilli have been identified by microscopy but before cultures are available. Consequently, MIRU-VNTR must be applied directly on positive respiratory specimens. The application of multiplex MIRU-VNTR directly on respiratory specimens was evaluated in a selection of 61 sputa from independent patients: a complete MIRU-VNTR pattern was identified in all but 1 sputum, which failed in a single locus of the 24 (43). A subsequent study showed similar applicability, although incomplete patterns were obtained for specimens below a specific bacterial load (44).

OPTIMIZING PRECISION IN ASSIGNING CLUSTERS

Once the issue of speed had been resolved, the move to real-time molecular epidemiology seemed possible. However, it was still necessary to address the precision needed to define clusters. The remaining areas of uncertainty included the identification of isolates with genotypes that were similar but not identical to other isolates in a cluster, the possible misassignment of genotypic patterns owing to

mixed infections by >1 strain, and the detection of clustered cases in which an epidemiological link could not be found among some or all of the clustered cases. In the following sections, we examine the advances made to address these uncertainties.

Highlighting the Value of Clonal Variants and Mixed Infections

Misassignment of clustered isolates as orphans is a cause for concern. It can result from not being aware of the two types of TB that are considered examples of "clonally complex" infections (45–50), namely, those involving clonal variants emerging from a parental strain and mixed infections involving >1 MTB strain.

The possible impact of the clonal complexity of MTB on the interpretation of molecular epidemiology data must be taken into account. As for clonal variants, the standard approach was not to consider clustered those isolates showing subtle differences in the genotypic pattern shared by the cases included in a specific cluster. However, the plasticity of the MTB genome means that subtle differences between fingerprinting patterns can result from microevolution phenomena, which lead to the emergence of clonal variants from the same parental strain (46, 48). These clonal variants have been described both in independent isolates from a single patient and in different patients in the same transmission chain (46, 48, 51, 52). If clonal variants are systematically interpreted as unrelated, we might underestimate the true percentage of recent transmission in a population and miss the epidemiological links that could fully describe the cluster. Second-line complementary genotyping techniques would help us to decide whether to include the variants in the clusters under study. In this sense, the importation of isolates with patterns similar to those of a cluster has been shown to increase the number of significant epidemiological links (53).

In the case of coinfection by two strains, it is important to rule out the inclusion of a false genotype in the analysis. When the tool used is RFLP or spoligotyping, the genotype obtained would take the form of a mixed pattern comprising the patterns corresponding to each of the coinfecting strains, in other words, a false pattern that cannot be part of the clusters under study and that will always be assigned as an orphan cluster. Fortunately, MIRU-VNTR analysis identifies mixed infections through identification of double alleles in some of the loci analyzed that take the form of double bands in gel electrophoresis or double peaks in capillary electrophoresis (54–56). After identification of a case of mixed infection, the MIRU-VNTR pattern for each coinfecting strain can be assigned by subculturing the primary culture and analyzing single colonies (56).

Optimizing the Epidemiological Support of Clusters

The fact that a certain percentage of the clusters in a population were not supported based on available epidemiological data leads us to consider that these epidemiological data could be limited and do not reveal the true relationships between the clustered cases.

Various efforts have been made to improve the quality and quantity of the epidemiological data obtained from patients. Standardized questionnaires were designed to extend data compilation far beyond interviews and now include data on leisure activities, social aspects, use of public transport, and presence in shopping areas. The introduction of such meticulous questionnaires increased to 86% the number of RFLP-clustered cases in which an epidemiological link was revealed (57). Another innovative approach applied in Texas was based on pursuing visual recognition between TB cases. The authors observed that patients in clusters clearly recognized the patients sharing their cluster but not patients from different clusters (58).

Both advances were combined in a complex socioepidemiological scenario in Almería, southeast Spain, where the high proportion of immigrants, many of whom are undocumented, increased the difficulties in obtaining precise epidemiological data. The study was piloted on the 12 clusters identified in the sector with the highest proportion of immigrants, Poniente. Epidemiological links were found in only 2 of the 12 clusters; these corresponded to 2 clusters that did not include immigrants but did involve exposure within the same family. When the refined strategy combining standardized questionnaires in interviews and photographic recognition was applied, the number of clusters where epidemiological links were finally revealed increased to 10 out of 12. These newly detected epidemiological links were related to leisure activities, drug consumption at the same location, and sporadic sharing of substandard housing, none of which are easily detected in standard epidemiological surveys. Consequently, refined epidemiological research seems to enhance the correlation between molecular data and epidemiological data.

Finally, geographic information systems have also been applied as an advanced system for localization of transmission hot spots by integrating GPS coordinates and genotypic clustering data. This approach was used in Texas and showed that the areas with the highest incidence of TB coincided with those with the highest proportion of recent transmission, as indicated by the percentage of cases involved in clusters (59).

Improving Discriminatory Power in Genotyping

The fact that identification of some clusters was not supported by epidemiological links between the cases, even after refining the epidemiological survey, could reflect the lack of sufficient discriminatory power in the fingerprinting tools applied, which could in turn lead to unrelated cases being considered clustered.

The discriminatory power of the 24-loci MIRU-VNTR technique is better than that of the previous reference method, IS*6110*-RFLP.

Adaptations of this method have even been developed to ensure suitable discrimination where the standard format fails, for example, when the population being analyzed is rich in isolates from the Beijing lineage (60). For these contexts, adapted versions that ensure correct discrimination between isolates have been designed (61).

However, even with the most discriminatory versions of the MIRU-VNTR formats, we can still interrogate only 24 specific targets along the chromosome. In other words, we are defining the transmission clusters in our populations based on comparisons of ~0.03% of the 4.4 Mb of total MTB genomic content.

If we aim to achieve true discrimination to ensure the highest possible precision in the definition of transmission clusters, we must access all the information in the chromosome. Consequently, the fingerprinting tool must be whole-genome sequencing (WGS). The reduction in the cost of WGS and the development of more-accessible platforms have led to it being used in the analysis of TB transmission and thus facilitated the transition to genomic epidemiology.

As occurred when RFLP was replaced by MIRU-VNTR, the first analysis focused on comparing discriminatory power and, therefore, the assignment of cases as clusters or orphans when WGS was applied. As expected, the discriminatory power of WGS surpassed that of MIRU-VNTR, with the result that some MIRU-defined clusters were split into subclusters when WGS was applied. The fact that these subclusters were more consistent with the geographical distribution of the cases and with the epidemiological links between them (62–64) paved the way for genomic epidemiology.

When a new approach is implemented for comparing isolates, the first step is to establish the similarity thresholds that will be used to determine when two MTB isolates are to be considered as belonging to the same strain (clustered) or to different strains (orphan). These similarity cutoffs were established in a solid study (63) of isolates that were representative of different categories: serial isolates from single patients, clustered isolates with strong epidemiological support, clustered isolates with weaker links, and unrelated isolates. Based on their data, the authors proposed as reference values that two isolates would be considered to be clustered if they showed ≤5 single nucleotide polymorphisms (SNPs) between them and to be orphan if they accumulated >12 SNPs. Subsequent studies have shown the appropriateness of these (65, 66). However, caution has been advised against establishing strict universal thresholds (67), mainly because in some transmission events, the microevolution rate can be higher than expected, thus potentially leading to an accumulation of SNPs between truly related isolates and to isolates being misclassified as orphan.

Apart from the informative high discriminatory power offered by WGS analysis, it must be highlighted that based on these data, we gain access to extremely valuable information about the chronology of the transmission clusters that was previously unavailable. Before WGS, the identification of a cluster informed us only about the involvement of cases in the same transmission chain. However, the precise chronology of the transmission chain could not be determined because of the lack of a constant interval between the time a patient is exposed and the time he or she becomes ill. Now, for the first time, if the epidemiological data allow us to determine the index case, the chronology of a transmission within a cluster can be defined, since in MTB, once a SNP is acquired, it does not reverse. We can therefore position clustered cases chronologically according to the dynamics of accumulation of the SNPs in that cluster (Fig. 2). This same analysis also allows us to depict the topology of the transmission, through which we now see a chain more as a network than as a series of longitudinal links (Fig. 2). The topology of transmission networks can be extremely complex (Fig. 3). Some networks are highly informative, such as those with a star-like shape,

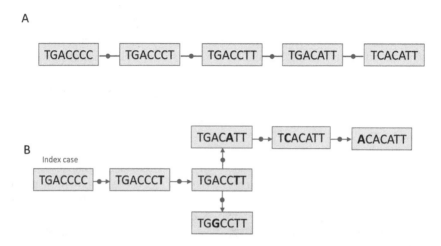

FIGURE 2 Schematic representation of how the chronologies of transmission can be inferred from the analysis of SNPs from clustered isolates. Each dot represents a SNP. Each box represents a patient. (A) Hypothetical transmission involving five patients, each differing in one SNP with the closest isolate. Neither the directionality of the transmission nor the index case can be inferred. (B) Hypothetical transmission involving seven patients. If the epidemiological data allow us to determine the index case, the direction of transmission (indicated by arrows) can be deduced.

which indicate the existence of many secondary cases caused directly by a single index case. A network with this topology alerts to the presence of a superspreader, who must be specifically targeted to ensure effective control of transmission.

NOVEL INTEGRATIVE SCHEMES

Our review of MTB genotyping applied to optimize the detection and analysis of TB transmission has identified two milestones: (i) MIRU-VNTR-enabled real-time molecular epidemiology when applied directly on respiratory specimens and (ii) the excellent discriminatory power of WGS. However, each of these milestones has a major pitfall: (i) the limited discriminatory power of MIRU-VNTR compared with WGS and (ii) the delay in identifying clusters based on SNPs because WGS analysis depends on MTB cultures. Therefore, it is essential to find a novel integrative scheme that reconciles the speed of PCR with the discriminatory power of WGS in order to pave the way for a new,

highly discriminatory, real-time epidemiological approach.

Efforts have been made in this direction. We published a proposal (68) to change the paradigm in which we supported the molecular epidemiology of TB. Our proposal involves modifying the current system, which is based exclusively on universal systematic genotyping of all the MTB isolates in a population to identify all clusters in it. The application of these programs has enabled us to identify clusters that are especially relevant because of their magnitude, difficult control, speed of producing secondary cases, and involvement of high-risk strains (imported, resistant, and virulent). The new proposal is aimed at developing new strategies for targeted surveillance of specific clusters/strains and redirecting the generally limited resources dedicated to TB control toward the clusters/strains that are responsible for most of the secondary cases in a population.

Our proposal comprises four steps: (i) identification of the most actively transmitted strains in a population or those that warrant special attention owing to their high-risk

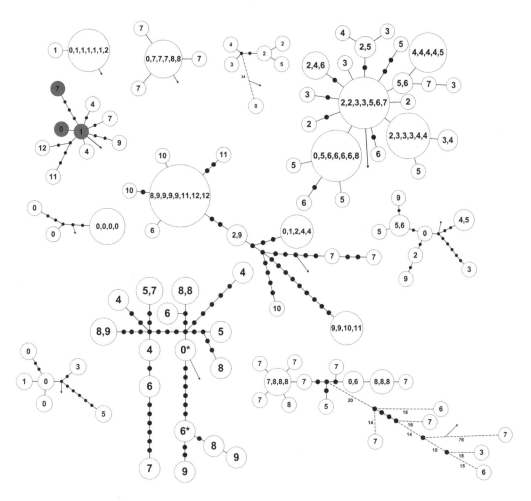

FIGURE 3 Different networks of clusters based on the analysis of SNPs obtained from WGS. Each black dot represents a SNP. All the isolates sharing identical SNP composition are included in the same circle. The size of the circle is proportional to the number of isolates included. An example of star-like topology, expected for networks including superspreader case, can be found in the cluster with the central node highlighted in red (second line, leftside). Reprinted from reference 63 with permission from Elsevier CC-BY-4.0.

phenotype, (ii) analysis of the strains selected by WGS to identify SNPs that are specific to them, (iii) design of allele-specific PCRs to identify strains, and (iv) prospective application of the strain-specific PCRs to track new cases infected by the surveyed strains.

This new strategy has been evaluated in various scenarios, for example, when tracking widely transmitted strains that are part of uncontrolled transmission clusters and in the rapid analysis of the presence of outbreak-related strains in a population.

Surveillance of Prevalent Strains

Strain-specific PCRs to track transmission of strains considered to be highly transmissible owing to their involvement in outbreaks are not a new development. Various PCRs targeting strain-specific genetic features were developed to identify cases infected by specific Beijing strains of MTB, all of which were involved in outbreaks or highly prevalent in their populations of origin. These PCRs include the multiplex assay that is specific for the multiresistant W-Beijing strain that caused a severe outbreak in New York. The assay was evaluated in 193 *M. tuberculosis* isolates and correctly identified all 48 W-Beijing isolates (69). Another strategy based on real-time PCR targeting highly prevalent Beijing strains in Russia also proved to be efficient (70).

All of these assays require an in-depth knowledge of the genetic composition of strains in order to be able to identify a genetic rearrangement or singular feature that can be targeted by PCR primers. Thanks to WGS, these singular features, namely, SNPs, are more accessible in the strains of interest. WGS extends the possibility of designing specific PCRs for each strain and simplifies the format of the specific PCR assay to be applied, namely, allele-specific oligonucleotide PCR (ASO-PCR).

We used WGS to design a duplex ASO-PCR to track the two most actively transmitted strains in Almería (68). The assay was known as targeted regional allele-specific PCR (TRAP). First, we took advantage of geographic information systems technology to identify geographic hot spots with a high concentration of clustered cases. This approach enabled us to identify the two strains responsible for the two clusters that were the most difficult to control in the eastern area of Almería province. We analyzed the strains using WGS and compared the sequence data with those of the reference strain to obtain the list of SNPs from our strains that were not found in the reference strain. We then compared these SNPs with those in global databases, including several hundred MTB strains circulating worldwide, to filter out the SNPs from our two strains that were also found in other strains. This process refined the list of potentially strain-specific SNPs. A duplex allele-specific PCR was designed to offer different amplification patterns depending on whether a new TB case is infected by each of the surveyed strains or by another strain.

With respect to the reconciliation between high discrimination and speed, TRAP was able to investigate the involvement of the surveyed strains in a new case at the time of diagnosis and was sufficiently sensitive to offer an interpretable result when applied directly on respiratory specimens (68).

As a final step in our strategy, we sought to transfer the TRAP tool to the clinical microbiology laboratory at the hospital in Almería, which was the local node responsible for managing the prevalent strains in the area. The technique was sufficiently robust to be easily adapted to the new experimental conditions and provided results even when applied directly on clinical specimens. It enabled staff to identify new cases infected by both strains and to retrospectively identify other strains involved in the same clusters that had not been previously suspected (68).

The approach we describe will make it possible to activate a new model for surveillance of TB transmission (Fig. 4). This new model will involve a shift from the current system, which is generally based on centralized reference centers that receive the isolates and perform standard genotyping analysis to return the final clustering data to the local nodes, normally after prolonged delays, to a system based on a delocalized network of laboratories applying simple tools for rapid *in situ* tracking of transmission problems at each local node.

Surveillance of Outbreak Strains

Strain-specific PCRs designed from WGS data have proven successful in the prospective surveillance of active transmission. However, they have also provided robust support for the analysis of strains that have been involved in outbreaks.

A good example of this approach was seen in the need for rapid tracking in Madrid of a Beijing strain that had caused a severe outbreak in Gran Canaria in the 1990s (GC strain) (71). Rapid tracking was necessary as a result of the identification of a patient who had had active TB for 8 years, with prolonged periods of infectivity owing to intermittent adherence to therapy. The alarm was raised

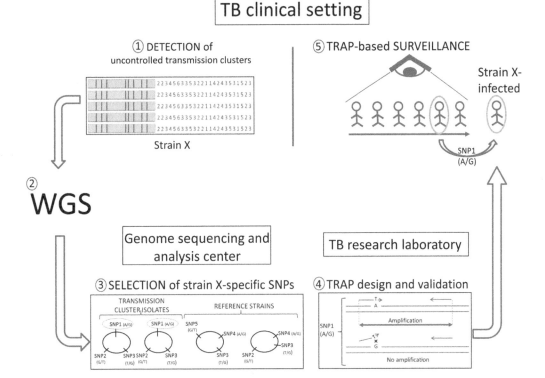

FIGURE 4 Chart illustrating work flow between the clinical setting, the genome and analysis center, and the TB research laboratory. (1) Strain X is identified as belonging to an uncontrolled transmission cluster. Strains are analyzed from raw sequencing data (2) to detect polymorphisms at the genome sequencing center. (3) SNPs are detected after comparison of the strain X sequence with those of the reference strains. SNP1 is shared by the strains belonging to the cluster and is not present in the global strain collection. (4) The TB research laboratory will use the transmission cluster-specific SNP to design specific assays. An allele-specific-oligonucleotide PCR assay, TRAP, was chosen to distinguish between strains belonging to the cluster. Once the assay is validated, it is easily transferred to a local clinical setting (5) for screening of ongoing surveillance (both from culture and from direct samples) of the spread of the targeted highly transmissible strains and as support to the local TB control program. Reprinted from reference 68 with permission.

when the patient was shown to be infected by the GC outbreak strain. It was therefore urgent to determine the potential presence of secondary cases infected by this patient. Two collections of isolates at two large hospitals in Madrid (~26% of all TB cases) were analyzed by applying a GC strain-specific PCR to target four strain-specific SNPs that were identified after WGS of the strain. The ASO-PCR was applied directly on a crude inactivated extract of frozen stored aliquots without the need for subculture or purification of DNA. This approach made it possible to analyze

868 isolates in 7 working days and finally identified 2 cases infected by the GC strain. The cases corresponded to persons who had recently arrived from Guinea Conakry, a neighbor of Liberia and the country of origin of the index patient who caused the GC outbreak. Surprisingly, the data recorded ruled out secondary cases arising from the persistently infected case, despite the enormous opportunities the strain had to be transmitted. Several months would have been needed to resolve this issue if the analysis had been based on standard genotyping.

Another relevant study where strain-specific PCR was applied to refine the analysis of an outbreak was performed in Bern, Switzerland. An outbreak had been reported in the city (22 cases in 1993) before the study was started. A strain-specific real-time PCR was designed based on TaqMan probes to specifically identify the outbreak strain. The systematic application of the assay to 1,642 isolates revealed 68 new cases infected with the outbreak strain, thus making it possible to redefine the true magnitude of the outbreak (72).

FUTURE CONSIDERATIONS

In this chapter, we have reviewed the development of fingerprinting tools for genotyping MTB in epidemiological studies. We also performed a parallel analysis of how our approach to tracking transmission of TB has changed.

We conclude that our objective in the coming years must be to reconcile both speed and precision to ensure high-quality surveillance of the transmission of TB. Speed and precision will ultimately be ensured when we are able to perform the analysis based on WGS directly from respiratory specimens and develop analytical tools and pipelines capable of recording MTB data while eliminating potential interference from other human or bacterial DNA.

The MTB bacilli present in clinical specimens have yet to be analyzed directly. The only trial to accelerate the time in which WGS can be applied to analyze MTB was based on optimizing procedures to enrich MTB DNA purified directly from the primary liquid culture instead of requiring a new subculture to eliminate accompanying material. In this study, the quality of the WGS sequences was good, yet the design still required additional days of incubation after diagnosis (73).

The recent development of platforms for the capture of specific DNA in complex samples makes it possible to perform WGS directly on clinical specimens. These platforms have been used for the study of the human exome in various types of cancer and also for the study of the viroma (74, 75). Trials performed with *Mycobacterium lepromatosis* and *Mycobacterium leprae* have yielded positive results (76, 77). One group used biotinylated RNA baits designed specifically for *M. tuberculosis* DNA that captured full *M. tuberculosis* genomes directly from infected sputum samples, thus enabling WGS without the need for culture (78).

In addition to the efforts made to gain access to WGS data directly from clinical specimens, it is important to remember the need to develop optimized fast, user-friendly pipelines to ensure that once WGS data have been obtained, major efforts in analysis will be unnecessary, thus minimizing the time until the final identification of clusters. In the same sense, we must standardize the data obtained in order to facilitate comparison and transfer between different laboratories. One proposal has attempted to imitate the approach of multilocus sequence typing (MLST). Core genome MLST (cgMLST) transforms the information obtained from the WGS analysis into a standardized allele-numbering system. As in other pathogens, such as *Streptococcus pneumoniae*, *Escherichia coli*, and *Neisseria meningitidis* (79–81), a standard set of 3,041 genes has been proposed for the cgMLST of MTB (82). A pilot study performed on 26 MTB strains showed that the cgMLST-based strategy offered a discriminatory power equivalent to that obtained when the complete WGS data set was used for standard SNP-based typing.

Finally, all forthcoming efforts must always be accompanied by the parallel development of alternative strategies to obtain simple, inexpensive, and easily implementable tools to ensure that advanced analysis of transmission will not be restricted to those nodes with access to complex devices and expertise. We must make a concerted effort to reduce the gap between the wealthy nodes and the many areas of the world that lack resources in order to truly optimize surveillance worldwide.

CITATION

García De Viedma D, Pérez-Lago L. 2018. The evolution of genotyping strategies to detect, analyze, and control transmission of tuberculosis. Microbiol Spectrum 6(5):MTBP-0002-2016.

REFERENCES

1. **Grupo de trabajo del area TIR de SEPAR.** 2002. SEPAR guidelines. Guidelines for tuberculosis prevention. *Arch Bronconeumol* **38:**441–451. (In Spanish.)

2. **Fox GJ, Barry SE, Britton WJ, Marks GB.** 2013. Contact investigation for tuberculosis: a systematic review and meta-analysis. *Eur Respir J* **41:**140–156.

3. **National Tuberculosis Controllers Association, Centers for Disease Control and Prevention (CDC).** 2005. Guidelines for the investigation of contacts of persons with infectious tuberculosis. Recommendations from the National Tuberculosis Controllers Association and CDC. *MMWR Recomm Rep* **54**(RR-15):1–47.

4. **Thind D, Charalambous S, Tongman A, Churchyard G, Grant AD.** 2012. An evaluation of 'Ribolola': a household tuberculosis contact tracing programme in North West Province, South Africa. *Int J Tuberc Lung Dis* **16:**1643–1648.

5. **Martín A, Iñigo J, Chaves F, Herranz M, Ruiz-Serrano MJ, Palenque E, Bouza E, García de Viedma D.** 2009. Re-analysis of epidemiologically linked tuberculosis cases not supported by IS6110-RFLP-based genotyping. *Clin Microbiol Infect* **15:**763–769.

6. **Behr MA, Hopewell PC, Paz EA, Kawamura LM, Schecter GF, Small PM.** 1998. Predictive value of contact investigation for identifying recent transmission of *Mycobacterium tuberculosis*. *Am J Respir Crit Care Med* **158:**465–469.

7. **Bennett DE, Onorato IM, Ellis BA, Crawford JT, Schable B, Byers R, Kammerer JS, Braden CR.** 2002. DNA fingerprinting of *Mycobacterium tuberculosis* isolates from epidemiologically linked case pairs. *Emerg Infect Dis* **8:**1224–1229.

8. **Verver S, Warren RM, Munch Z, Richardson M, van der Spuy GD, Borgdorff MW, Behr MA, Beyers N, van Helden PD.** 2004. Proportion of tuberculosis transmission that takes place in households in a high-incidence area. *Lancet* **363:**212–214.

9. **Vynnycky E, Nagelkerke N, Borgdorff MW, van Soolingen D, van Embden JD, Fine PE.** 2001. The effect of age and study duration on the relationship between 'clustering' of DNA fingerprint patterns and the proportion of tuberculosis disease attributable to recent transmission. *Epidemiol Infect* **126:**43–62.

10. **Chin DP, DeRiemer K, Small PM, de Leon AP, Steinhart R, Schecter GF, Daley CL, Moss AR, Paz EA, Jasmer RM, Agasino CB, Hopewell PC.** 1998. Differences in contributing factors to tuberculosis incidence in U.S.-born and foreign-born persons. *Am J Respir Crit Care Med* **158:**1797–1803.

11. **Dahle UR, Sandven P, Heldal E, Caugant DA.** 2003. Continued low rates of transmission of *Mycobacterium tuberculosis* in Norway. *J Clin Microbiol* **41:**2968–2973.

12. **Kunimoto D, Sutherland K, Wooldrage K, Fanning A, Chui L, Manfreda J, Long R.** 2004. Transmission characteristics of tuberculosis in the foreign-born and the Canadian-born populations of Alberta, Canada. *Int J Tuberc Lung Dis* **8:**1213–1220.

13. **Diel R, Rüsch-Gerdes S, Niemann S.** 2004. Molecular epidemiology of tuberculosis among immigrants in Hamburg, Germany. *J Clin Microbiol* **42:**2952–2960.

14. **Kamper-Jørgensen Z, Andersen AB, Kok-Jensen A, Kamper-Jørgensen M, Bygbjerg IC, Andersen PH, Thomsen VO, Lillebaek T.** 2012. Migrant tuberculosis: the extent of transmission in a low burden country. *BMC Infect Dis* **12:**60.

15. **Alonso Rodríguez N, Chaves F, Iñigo J, Bouza E, García de Viedma D, Andrés S, Cías R, Daza R, Domingo D, Esteban J, García J, Gómez Mampaso E, Herranz M, Palenque E, Ruiz Serrano MJ, TB Molecular Epidemiology Study Group of Madrid.** 2009. Transmission permeability of tuberculosis involving immigrants, revealed by a multicentre analysis of clusters. *Clin Microbiol Infect* **15:**435–442.

16. **Martínez-Lirola M, Alonso-Rodriguez N, Sánchez ML, Herranz M, Andrés S, Peñafiel T, Rogado MC, Cabezas T, Martínez J, Lucerna MA, Rodríguez M, Bonillo MC, Bouza E, García de Viedma D.** 2008. Advanced survey of tuberculosis transmission in a complex socioepidemiologic scenario with a high proportion of cases in immigrants. *Clin Infect Dis* **47:**8–14.

17. **van Embden JD, Cave MD, Crawford JT, Dale JW, Eisenach KD, Gicquel B, Hermans P, Martin C, McAdam R, Shinnick TM, Small PM.** 1993. Strain identification of *Mycobacterium tuberculosis* by DNA fingerprinting: recommen-

dations for a standardized methodology. *J Clin Microbiol* **31**:406–409.

18. van Soolingen D, de Haas PE, Kremer K. 2001. Restriction fragment length polymorphism typing of mycobacteria. *Methods Mol Med* **54**:165–203.

19. Kamerbeek J, Schouls L, Kolk A, van Agterveld M, van Soolingen D, Kuijper S, Bunschoten A, Molhuizen H, Shaw R, Goyal M, van Embden J. 1997. Simultaneous detection and strain differentiation of *Mycobacterium tuberculosis* for diagnosis and epidemiology. *J Clin Microbiol* **35**:907–914.

20. Brudey K, Driscoll JR, Rigouts L, Prodinger WM, Gori A, Al-Hajoj SA, Allix C, Aristimuño L, Arora J, Baumanis V, Binder L, Cafrune P, Cataldi A, Cheong S, Diel R, Ellermeier C, Evans JT, Fauville-Dufaux M, Ferdinand S, Garcia de Viedma D, Garzelli C, Gazzola L, Gomes HM, Guttierez MC, Hawkey PM, van Helden PD, Kadival GV, Kreiswirth BN, Kremer K, Kubin M, Kulkarni SP, Liens B, Lillebaek T, Ho ML, Martin C, Martin C, Mokrousov I, Narvskaïa O, Ngeow YF, Naumann L, Niemann S, Parwati I, Rahim Z, Rasolofo-Razanamparany V, Rasolonavalona T, Rossetti ML, Rüsch-Gerdes S, Sajduda A, Samper S, Shemyakin IG, Singh UB, Somoskovi A, Skuce RA, van Soolingen D, Streicher EM, Suffys PN, Tortoli E, Tracevska T, Vincent V, Victor TC, Warren RM, Yap SF, Zaman K, Portaels F, Rastogi N, Sola C. 2006. *Mycobacterium tuberculosis* complex genetic diversity: mining the fourth international spoligotyping database (SpolDB4) for classification, population genetics and epidemiology. *BMC Microbiol* **6**:23.

21. Zhang J, Abadia E, Refregier G, Tafaj S, Boschiroli ML, Guillard B, Andremont A, Ruimy R, Sola C. 2010. *Mycobacterium tuberculosis* complex CRISPR genotyping: improving efficiency, throughput and discriminative power of 'spoligotyping' with new spacers and a microbead-based hybridization assay. *J Med Microbiol* **59**:285–294.

22. Gomgnimbou MK, Hernández-Neuta I, Panaiotov S, Bachiyska E, Palomino JC, Martin A, del Portillo P, Refregier G, Sola C. 2013. Tuberculosis-spoligo-rifampin-isoniazid typing: an all-in-one assay technique for surveillance and control of multidrug-resistant tuberculosis on Luminex devices. *J Clin Microbiol* **51**:3527–3534.

23. Janssen P, Coopman R, Huys G, Swings J, Bleeker M, Vos P, Zabeau M, Kersters K. 1996. Evaluation of the DNA fingerprinting method AFLP as a new tool in bacterial taxonomy. *Microbiology* **142**:1881–1893.

24. Goulding JN, Stanley J, Saunders N, Arnold C. 2000. Genome-sequence-based fluorescent amplified-fragment length polymorphism analysis of *Mycobacterium tuberculosis*. *J Clin Microbiol* **38**:1121–1126.

25. Pfaller SL, Aronson TW, Holtzman AE, Covert TC. 2007. Amplified fragment length polymorphism analysis of *Mycobacterium avium* complex isolates recovered from southern California. *J Med Microbiol* **56**:1152–1160.

26. Chemlal K, Huys G, Laval F, Vincent V, Savage C, Gutierrez C, Laneelle MA, Swings J, Meyers WM, Daffe M, Portaels F. 2002. Characterization of an unusual *Mycobacterium*: a possible missing link between *Mycobacterium marinum* and *Mycobacterium ulcerans*. *J Clin Microbiol* **40**:2370–2380.

27. Tenover FC, Arbeit RD, Goering RV, Mickelsen PA, Murray BE, Persing DH, Swaminathan B. 1995. Interpreting chromosomal DNA restriction patterns produced by pulsed-field gel electrophoresis: criteria for bacterial strain typing. *J Clin Microbiol* **33**:2233–2239.

28. Friedman CR, Stoeckle MY, Johnson WD Jr, Riley LW. 1995. Double-repetitive-element PCR method for subtyping *Mycobacterium tuberculosis* clinical isolates. *J Clin Microbiol* **33**:1383–1384.

29. Linton CJ, Jalal H, Leeming JP, Millar MR. 1994. Rapid discrimination of *Mycobacterium tuberculosis* strains by random amplified polymorphic DNA analysis. *J Clin Microbiol* **32**:2169–2174.

30. Frothingham R, Meeker-O'Connell WA. 1998. Genetic diversity in the *Mycobacterium tuberculosis* complex based on variable numbers of tandem DNA repeats. *Microbiology* **144**:1189–1196.

31. Supply P, Mazars E, Lesjean S, Vincent V, Gicquel B, Locht C. 2000. Variable human minisatellite-like regions in the *Mycobacterium tuberculosis* genome. *Mol Microbiol* **36**:762–771.

32. Supply P, Allix C, Lesjean S, Cardoso-Oelemann M, Rüsch-Gerdes S, Willery E, Savine E, de Haas P, van Deutekom H, Roring S, Bifani P, Kurepina N, Kreiswirth B, Sola C, Rastogi N, Vatin V, Gutierrez MC, Fauville M, Niemann S, Skuce R, Kremer K, Locht C, van Soolingen D. 2006. Proposal for standardization of optimized mycobacterial interspersed repetitive unit-variable-number tandem repeat typing of *Mycobacterium tuberculosis*. *J Clin Microbiol* **44**:4498–4510.

33. Oelemann MC, Diel R, Vatin V, Haas W, Rüsch-Gerdes S, Locht C, Niemann S, Supply P. 2007. Assessment of an optimized mycobacterial interspersed repetitive-unit-variable-number tandem-repeat typing system combined with spoligotyping for population-based molecular epidemiology studies of tuberculosis. *J Clin Microbiol* **45**:691–697.

34. **Cowan LS, Diem L, Monson T, Wand P, Temporado D, Oemig TV, Crawford JT.** 2005. Evaluation of a two-step approach for large-scale, prospective genotyping of *Mycobacterium tuberculosis* isolates in the United States. *J Clin Microbiol* **43:**688–695.

35. **van Deutekom H, Supply P, de Haas PE, Willery E, Hoijng SP, Locht C, Coutinho RA, van Soolingen D.** 2005. Molecular typing of *Mycobacterium tuberculosis* by mycobacterial interspersed repetitive unit-variable-number tandem repeat analysis, a more accurate method for identifying epidemiological links between patients with tuberculosis. *J Clin Microbiol* **43:**4473–4479.

36. **de Beer JL, van Ingen J, de Vries G, Erkens C, Sebek M, Mulder A, Sloot R, van den Brandt AM, Enaimi M, Kremer K, Supply P, van Soolingen D.** 2013. Comparative study of IS*6110* restriction fragment length polymorphism and variable-number tandem-repeat typing of *Mycobacterium tuberculosis* isolates in the Netherlands, based on a 5-year nationwide survey. *J Clin Microbiol* **51:**1193–1198.

37. **Rodríguez NA, Lirola MM, Chaves F, Iñigo J, Herranz M, Ritacco V, EpiMOLTB Madrid, INDAL-TB group, Bouza E, García de Viedma D.** 2010. Differences in the robustness of clusters involving the *Mycobacterium tuberculosis* strains most frequently isolated from immigrant cases in Madrid. *Clin Microbiol Infect* **16:**1544–1554.

38. **Alonso-Rodriguez N, Martínez-Lirola M, Sánchez ML, Herranz M, Peñafiel T, Bonillo MC, Gonzalez-Rivera M, Martínez J, Cabezas T, Diez-García LF, Bouza E, García de Viedma D.** 2009. Prospective universal application of mycobacterial interspersed repetitive-unit-variable-number tandem-repeat genotyping to characterize *Mycobacterium tuberculosis* isolates for fast identification of clustered and orphan cases. *J Clin Microbiol* **47:**2026–2032.

39. **de Beer JL, Kremer K, Ködmön C, Supply P, van Soolingen D, Global Network for the Molecular Surveillance of Tuberculosis 2009.** 2012. First worldwide proficiency study on variable-number tandem-repeat typing of *Mycobacterium tuberculosis* complex strains. *J Clin Microbiol* **50:**662–669.

40. **de Beer JL, Ködmön C, van Ingen J, Supply P, van Soolingen D, Global Network for Molecular Surveillance of Tuberculosis 2010.** 2014. Second worldwide proficiency study on variable number of tandem repeats typing of *Mycobacterium tuberculosis* complex. *Int J Tuberc Lung Dis* **18:**594–600.

41. **Supply P, Lesjean S, Savine E, Kremer K, van Soolingen D, Locht C.** 2001. Automated high-throughput genotyping for study of global epidemiology of *Mycobacterium tuberculosis* based on mycobacterial interspersed repetitive units. *J Clin Microbiol* **39:**3563–3571.

42. **Sislema-Egas F, Ruiz-Serrano MJ, Bouza E, García-de-Viedma D.** 2013. Qualitative analysis to ascertain genotypic identity of or differences between *Mycobacterium tuberculosis* isolates in laboratories with limited resources. *J Clin Microbiol* **51:**4230–4233.

43. **Alonso M, Herranz M, Martínez Lirola M, González-Rivera M, Bouza E, García de Viedma D, INDAL-TB Group.** 2012. Real-time molecular epidemiology of tuberculosis by direct genotyping of smear-positive clinical specimens. *J Clin Microbiol* **50:**1755–1757.

44. **Bidovec-Stojkovič U, Seme K, Žolnir-Dovč M, Supply P.** 2014. Prospective genotyping of *Mycobacterium tuberculosis* from fresh clinical samples. *PLoS One* **9:**e109547.

45. **Stavrum R, Mphahlele M, Ovreås K, Muthivhi T, Fourie PB, Weyer K, Grewal HM.** 2009. High diversity of *Mycobacterium tuberculosis* genotypes in South Africa and preponderance of mixed infections among ST53 isolates. *J Clin Microbiol* **47:**1848–1856.

46. **Al-Hajoj SA, Akkerman O, Parwati I, al-Gamdi S, Rahim Z, van Soolingen D, van Ingen J, Supply P, van der Zanden AG.** 2010. Microevolution of *Mycobacterium tuberculosis* in a tuberculosis patient. *J Clin Microbiol* **48:**3813–3816.

47. **Shamputa IC, Jugheli L, Sadradze N, Willery E, Portaels F, Supply P, Rigouts L.** 2006. Mixed infection and clonal representativeness of a single sputum sample in tuberculosis patients from a penitentiary hospital in Georgia. *Respir Res* **7:**99.

48. **Navarro Y, Herranz M, Pérez-Lago L, Martínez Lirola M, Ruiz-Serrano MJ, Bouza E, García de Viedma D, INDAL-TB.** 2011. Systematic survey of clonal complexity in tuberculosis at a population level and detailed characterization of the isolates involved. *J Clin Microbiol* **49:**4131–4137.

49. **Warren RM, Victor TC, Streicher EM, Richardson M, Beyers N, Gey van Pittius NC, van Helden PD.** 2004. Patients with active tuberculosis often have different strains in the same sputum specimen. *Am J Respir Crit Care Med* **169:**610–614.

50. **Andrade MK, Machado SM, Leite ML, Saad MH.** 2009. Phenotypic and genotypic variant of MDR-*Mycobacterium tuberculosis* multiple isolates in the same tuberculosis episode, Rio de Janeiro, Brazil. *Braz J Med Biol Res* **42:**433–437.

51. **Pérez-Lago L, Herranz M, Lirola MM, Bouza E, García de Viedma D, INDAL-TB Group.** 2011. Characterization of microevolution events in *Mycobacterium tuberculosis* strains involved

in recent transmission clusters. *J Clin Microbiol* **49:**3771–3776.

52. **Ijaz K, Yang Z, Matthews HS, Bates JH, Cave MD.** 2002. *Mycobacterium tuberculosis* transmission between cluster members with similar fingerprint patterns. *Emerg Infect Dis* **8:**1257–1259.

53. **Cave MD, Yang ZH, Stefanova R, Fomukong N, Ijaz K, Bates J, Eisenach KD.** 2005. Epidemiologic import of tuberculosis cases whose isolates have similar but not identical IS*6110* restriction fragment length polymorphism patterns. *J Clin Microbiol* **43:**1228–1233.

54. **Martín A, Herranz M, Ruiz Serrano MJ, Bouza E, García de Viedma D.** 2010. The clonal composition of *Mycobacterium tuberculosis* in clinical specimens could be modified by culture. *Tuberculosis (Edinb)* **90:**201–207.

55. **García de Viedma D, Alonso Rodriguez N, Andrés S, Ruiz Serrano MJ, Bouza E.** 2005. Characterization of clonal complexity in tuberculosis by mycobacterial interspersed repetitive unit-variable-number tandem repeat typing. *J Clin Microbiol* **43:**5660–5664.

56. **Pérez-Lago L, Lirola MM, Navarro Y, Herranz M, Ruiz-Serrano MJ, Bouza E, García-de-Viedma D.** 2015. Co-infection with drug-susceptible and reactivated latent multidrug-resistant *Mycobacterium tuberculosis*. *Emerg Infect Dis* **21:**2098–2100.

57. **van Deutekom H, Hoijng SP, de Haas PE, Langendam MW, Horsman A, van Soolingen D, Coutinho RA.** 2004. Clustered tuberculosis cases: do they represent recent transmission and can they be detected earlier? *Am J Respir Crit Care Med* **169:**806–810.

58. **Weis SE, Pogoda JM, Yang Z, Cave MD, Wallace C, Kelley M, Barnes PF.** 2002. Transmission dynamics of tuberculosis in Tarrant county, Texas. *Am J Respir Crit Care Med* **166:**36–42.

59. **Moonan PK, Bayona M, Quitugua TN, Oppong J, Dunbar D, Jost KC Jr, Burgess G, Singh KP, Weis SE.** 2004. Using GIS technology to identify areas of tuberculosis transmission and incidence. *Int J Health Geogr* **3:**23.

60. **Hanekom M, van der Spuy GD, Gey van Pittius NC, McEvoy CR, Hoek KG, Ndabambi SL, Jordaan AM, Victor TC, van Helden PD, Warren RM.** 2008. Discordance between mycobacterial interspersed repetitive-unit-variable-number tandem-repeat typing and IS*6110* restriction fragment length polymorphism genotyping for analysis of *Mycobacterium tuberculosis* Beijing strains in a setting of high incidence of tuberculosis. *J Clin Microbiol* **46:**3338–3345.

61. **Allix-Béguec C, Wahl C, Hanekom M, Nikolayevskyy V, Drobniewski F, Maeda S, Campos-Herrero I, Mokrousov I, Niemann S, Kontsevaya I, Rastogi N, Samper S, Sng LH, Warren RM, Supply P.** 2014. Proposal of a consensus set of hypervariable mycobacterial interspersed repetitive-unit-variable-number tandem-repeat loci for subtyping of *Mycobacterium tuberculosis* Beijing isolates. *J Clin Microbiol* **52:**164–172.

62. **Gardy JL, Johnston JC, Ho Sui SJ, Cook VJ, Shah L, Brodkin E, Rempel S, Moore R, Zhao Y, Holt R, Varhol R, Birol I, Lem M, Sharma MK, Elwood K, Jones SJ, Brinkman FS, Brunham RC, Tang P.** 2011. Whole-genome sequencing and social-network analysis of a tuberculosis outbreak. *N Engl J Med* **364:**730–739.

63. **Walker TM, Ip CL, Harrell RH, Evans JT, Kapatai G, Dedicoat MJ, Eyre DW, Wilson DJ, Hawkey PM, Crook DW, Parkhill J, Harris D, Walker AS, Bowden R, Monk P, Smith EG, Peto TE.** 2013. Whole-genome sequencing to delineate *Mycobacterium tuberculosis* outbreaks: a retrospective observational study. *Lancet Infect Dis* **13:**137–146.

64. **Roetzer A, Diel R, Kohl TA, Rückert C, Nübel U, Blom J, Wirth T, Jaenicke S, Schuback S, Rüsch-Gerdes S, Supply P, Kalinowski J, Niemann S.** 2013. Whole genome sequencing versus traditional genotyping for investigation of a *Mycobacterium tuberculosis* outbreak: a longitudinal molecular epidemiological study. *PLoS Med* **10:**e1001387.

65. **Bryant JM, Schürch AC, van Deutekom H, Harris SR, de Beer JL, de Jager V, Kremer K, van Hijum SA, Siezen RJ, Borgdorff M, Bentley SD, Parkhill J, van Soolingen D.** 2013. Inferring patient to patient transmission of *Mycobacterium tuberculosis* from whole genome sequencing data. *BMC Infect Dis* **13:**110.

66. **Luo T, Yang C, Peng Y, Lu L, Sun G, Wu J, Jin X, Hong J, Li F, Mei J, DeRiemer K, Gao Q.** 2014. Whole-genome sequencing to detect recent transmission of *Mycobacterium tuberculosis* in settings with a high burden of tuberculosis. *Tuberculosis (Edinb)* **94:**434–440.

67. **Pérez-Lago L, Comas I, Navarro Y, González-Candelas F, Herranz M, Bouza E, García-de-Viedma D.** 2014. Whole genome sequencing analysis of intrapatient microevolution in *Mycobacterium tuberculosis*: potential impact on the inference of tuberculosis transmission. *J Infect Dis* **209:**98–108.

68. **Pérez-Lago L, Martínez Lirola M, Herranz M, Comas I, Bouza E, García-de-Viedma D.** 2015. Fast and low-cost decentralized surveillance of transmission of tuberculosis based on strain-specific PCRs tailored from whole genome sequencing data: a pilot study. *Clin Microbiol Infect* **21:**249.e1–249.e9.

69. **Plikaytis BB, Marden JL, Crawford JT, Woodley CL, Butler WR, Shinnick TM.** 1994. Multiplex PCR assay specific for the multidrug-resistant strain W of *Mycobacterium tuberculosis*. *J Clin Microbiol* **32:**1542–1546.

70. **Mokrousov I, Vyazovaya A, Zhuravlev V, Otten T, Millet J, Jiao WW, Shen AD, Rastogi N, Vishnevsky B, Narvskaya O.** 2014. Real-time PCR assay for rapid detection of epidemiologically and clinically significant *Mycobacterium tuberculosis* Beijing genotype isolates. *J Clin Microbiol* **52:** 1691–1693.

71. **Pérez-Lago L, Herranz M, Comas I, Ruiz-Serrano MJ, López Roa P, Bouza E, García-de-Viedma D.** 2016. Ultrafast assessment of the presence of a high-risk *Mycobacterium tuberculosis* strain in a population. *J Clin Microbiol* **54:** 779–781.

72. **Stucki D, Ballif M, Bodmer T, Coscolla M, Maurer AM, Droz S, Butz C, Borrell S, Längle C, Feldmann J, Furrer H, Mordasini C, Helbling P, Rieder HL, Egger M, Gagneux S, Fenner L.** 2015. Tracking a tuberculosis outbreak over 21 years: strain-specific single-nucleotide polymorphism typing combined with targeted whole-genome sequencing. *J Infect Dis* **211:**1306–1316.

73. **Votintseva AA, Pankhurst LJ, Anson LW, Morgan MR, Gascoyne-Binzi D, Walker TM, Quan TP, Wyllie DH, Del Ojo Elias C, Wilcox M, Walker AS, Peto TE, Crook DW.** 2015. Mycobacterial DNA extraction for whole-genome sequencing from early positive liquid (MGIT) cultures. *J Clin Microbiol* **53:**1137–1143.

74. **Briese T, Kapoor A, Mishra N, Jain K, Kumar A, Jabado OJ, Lipkin WI.** 2015. Virome capture sequencing enables sensitive viral diagnosis and comprehensive virome analysis. *mBio* **6:**e01491-e15.

75. **Forero-Castro M, Robledo C, Benito R, Abáigar M, África Martín A, Arefi M, Fuster JL, de Las Heras N, Rodríguez JN, Quintero J, Riesco S, Hermosín L, de la Fuente I, Recio I, Ribera J, Labrador J, Alonso JM, Olivier C, Sierra M, Megido M, Corchete-Sánchez LA, Ciudad Pizarro J, García JL, Ribera JM, Hernández-Rivas JM.** 2016. Genome-wide DNA copy number analysis of acute lymphoblastic leukemia identifies new genetic markers associated with clinical outcome. *PLoS One* **11:**e0148972.

76. **Singh P, Benjak A, Schuenemann VJ, Herbig A, Avanzi C, Busso P, Nieselt K, Krause J,** Vera-Cabrera L, Cole ST. 2015. Insight into the evolution and origin of leprosy bacilli from the genome sequence of *Mycobacterium lepromatosis*. *Proc Natl Acad Sci U S A* **112:**4459–4464.

77. **Mendum TA, Schuenemann VJ, Roffey S, Taylor GM, Wu H, Singh P, Tucker K, Hinds J, Cole ST, Kierzek AM, Nieselt K, Krause J, Stewart GR.** 2014. *Mycobacterium leprae* genomes from a British medieval leprosy hospital: towards understanding an ancient epidemic. *BMC Genomics* **15:**270.

78. **Brown AC, Bryant JM, Einer-Jensen K, Holdstock J, Houniet DT, Chan JZ, Depledge DP, Nikolayevskyy V, Broda A, Stone MJ, Christiansen MT, Williams R, McAndrew MB, Tutill H, Brown J, Melzer M, Rosmarin C, McHugh TD, Shorten RJ, Drobniewski F, Speight G, Breuer J.** 2015. Rapid whole-genome sequencing of *Mycobacterium tuberculosis* isolates directly from clinical samples. *J Clin Microbiol* **53:**2230–2237.

79. **Jolley KA, Maiden MC.** 2010. BIGSdb: scalable analysis of bacterial genome variation at the population level. *BMC Bioinformatics* **11:**595.

80. **Mellmann A, Harmsen D, Cummings CA, Zentz EB, Leopold SR, Rico A, Prior K, Szczepanowski R, Ji Y, Zhang W, McLaughlin SF, Henkhaus JK, Leopold B, Bielaszewska M, Prager R, Brzoska PM, Moore RL, Guenther S, Rothberg JM, Karch H.** 2011. Prospective genomic characterization of the German enterohemorrhagic *Escherichia coli* O104:H4 outbreak by rapid next generation sequencing technology. *PLoS One* **6:** e22751.

81. **Vogel U, Szczepanowski R, Claus H, Jünemann S, Prior K, Harmsen D.** 2012. Ion torrent personal genome machine sequencing for genomic typing of *Neisseria meningitidis* for rapid determination of multiple layers of typing information. *J Clin Microbiol* **50:**1889–1894.

82. **Kohl TA, Diel R, Harmsen D, Rothgänger J, Walter KM, Merker M, Weniger T, Niemann S.** 2014. Whole-genome-based *Mycobacterium tuberculosis* surveillance: a standardized, portable, and expandable approach. *J Clin Microbiol* **52:** 2479–2486.

83. **Jagielski T, van Ingen J, Rastogi N, Dziadek J, Mazur PK, Bielecki J.** 2014. Current methods in the molecular typing of *Mycobacterium tuberculosis* and other mycobacteria. *BioMed Res Int* **2014:**645802.

Breaking Transmission with Vaccines: The Case of Tuberculosis

14

JESUS GONZALO-ASENSIO,[1,2] NACHO AGUILO,[1,2]
DESSISLAVA MARINOVA,[1,2] and CARLOS MARTIN[1,2,3]

INTRODUCTION

Tuberculosis (TB) is the biggest killer of humanity. TB has killed more human beings than any other infectious disease in history, with an estimated loss of over a billion lives in the past 200 years (1). Despite effective treatment, in the WHO 2016 there were an estimated 10.4 million new TB cases and 1.8 million deaths attributed to the disease worldwide, surpassing those caused by AIDS (2). Still more worrying is the rising transmission of multidrug-resistant TB (MDR-TB), caused by mycobacteria that are resistant to treatment with at least two of the most powerful first-line anti-TB drugs, isoniazid and rifampin (2). Nearly half a million new MDR-TB cases are estimated every year, which together with increasing globalization makes TB an alarming global health problem (2). Loss of compliance with the current treatments for TB raises the frightening idea of a return to the pre-antibiotic era, when 50% of TB patients died in the absence of an effective treatment. Dissemination of multi- and extremely drug-resistant *Mycobacterium tuberculosis* strains has adverse implications for TB control in the 21st century.

[1]Department of Microbiology, Preventive Medicine, and Public Health, University of Zaragoza, Zaragoza, Spain; [2]CIBER Enfermedades Respiratorias, Instituto de Salud Carlos III, Madrid, Spain; [3]Servicio de Microbiología, Hospital Miguel Servet, ISS Aragón, Zaragoza, Spain.
Microbial Transmission in Biological Processes
Edited by Fernando Baquero, Emilio Bouza, J.A. Gutiérrez-Fuentes, and Teresa M. Coque
© 2018 American Society for Microbiology, Washington, DC
doi:10.1128/microbiolspec.MTBP-0001-2016

M. tuberculosis complex (MTBC) comprises a group of closely related TB-causing subspecies or ecotypes adapted to different animal hosts, including humans. According to their phylogenetic distances, the MTBC members can be classified into eight major lineages, which include the human-adapted lineages of *M. tuberculosis* and the animal-adapted ecotypes including *M. bovis*, *M. caprae*, and *M. pinnipedii*, among others (3, 4). *M. tuberculosis* and humans seem to have coevolved well before the human migrations out of Africa (5). Transmission from animals to humans has been documented throughout the history of human beings, and there is evidence that human infection caused by members of the MTBC in pre-Columbian mummies could be due to zoonotic transfer of MTBC strains by seals and sea lions between A.D. 700 and 1000 (6). This finding reconciles the presence of TB-causing bacteria in the New World prior to human colonization (6).

At the beginning of the 20th century, before the introduction of pasteurization, *M. bovis* was an important cause of TB in humans and was efficiently transmitted by ingestion of raw milk (Fig. 1). In our day, *M. bovis* is rarely found causing TB outbreaks in humans. However, some particular *M. bovis* strains have adapted to the human host with the ability to transmit between immune-compromised individuals, as discussed later in this chapter. Even in countries with a very high incidence of livestock TB caused by *M. bovis* and high incidence rates of extrapulmonary TB in humans, human infection with *M. bovis* is excluded, as different lineages of *M. tuberculosis* are considered responsible for extrapulmonary TB (7).

Nowadays, *M. tuberculosis* spread in humans is due to airborne person-to-person transmission, posing an enormous public health problem (Fig. 2). Since humans are the only known reservoir for *M. tuberculosis*, to stop the global TB epidemic, transmission must be stopped to prevent new infections and new cases (8). The traditional way to fight TB transmission is active detection of TB cases, with patients then separated safely

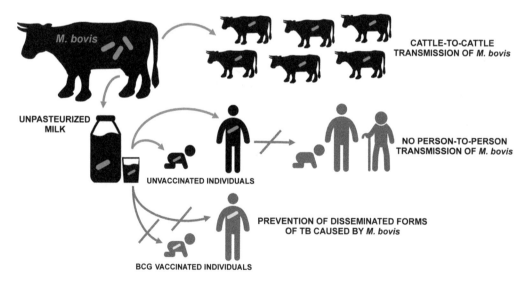

FIGURE 1 *M. bovis* transmission. Infected cattle transmit *M. bovis* bacteria (orange bacilli) to the neighboring herd members and also during milking. Before milk pasteurization was introduced, *M. bovis* was an important cause of cattle-to-human transmission of TB. Now *M. bovis* rarely causes TB outbreaks in humans, and transmission of *M. bovis* strains between humans is infrequent. Vaccination with BCG (schematized as blue bacilli), starting in the 1920s, was efficient to prevent disseminated forms of TB caused by *M. bovis*.

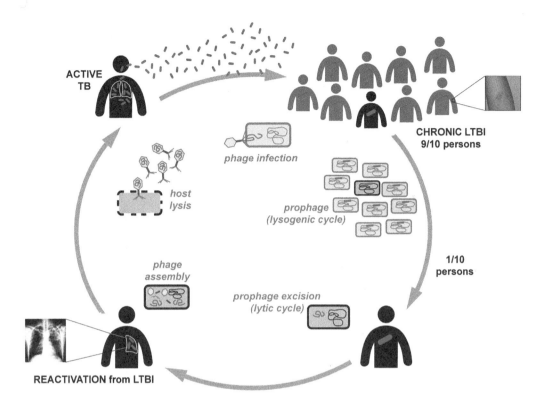

FIGURE 2 *M. tuberculosis* transmission. Humans are the only known reservoir of *M. tuberculosis* (red bacilli). The *M. tuberculosis* infectious cycle starts with the transmission of bacilli by the respiratory route from a patient with active pulmonary disease, who aerosolizes *M. tuberculosis*, placing contacts at risk of infection. Epidemiological data indicate that 9 of every 10 infected individuals are chronically infected in the form of LTBI (gray human shapes); therefore, LTBI constitutes a potential reservoir for transmission. People with LTBI are at risk for TB reactivation at some later time, and 1 of every 10 infected persons will develop clinical disease (black human shapes). The essential question on the natural history of TB is when *M. tuberculosis* decides to either infect and live with its host in the form of LTBI or to cause active pulmonary disease, which without treatment kills the host, searching the transmission to new hosts. The inner circle shows the lambda phage infectious cycles and their similarities to *M. tuberculosis* infection and disease. The lysogenic cycle of lambda phage resembles to LTBI, and the lytic cycle of lambda phage is similar to active TB disease caused by *M. tuberculosis*.

and treated effectively. Prompt initiation of effective antibiotic treatment to rapidly render TB patients noninfectious is crucial for this task. Since TB mainly affects developing and underdeveloped countries, active case-finding is not often implemented in these regions of the world, resulting in long delays in diagnosis and treatment (9). In this context, new TB vaccines with the potential to protect against pulmonary forms of the disease could play an essential role in preventing TB transmission (Fig. 3).

TB INFECTION OR TB DISEASE: THE *M. TUBERCULOSIS* DECISION TO LIVE WITH OR TO KILL ITS HOST

In humans, the *M. tuberculosis* infectious cycle starts with the transmission of the tubercle bacilli by the respiratory route from a patient with active pulmonary disease, placing their contacts at risk of infection (10). Efficient transmission of TB is dependent on the generation of a lesion in the lung, which results in a bacterium-laden cough (Fig. 2).

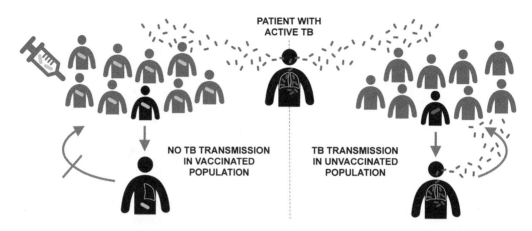

FIGURE 3 Ending TB transmission with vaccines. A patient with active TB disseminates *M. tuberculosis* (red bacilli) to neighboring individuals. One of every 10 persons is susceptible to TB (black human shapes) and therefore will develop clinical disease in the absence of vaccination. A vaccine able to protect against respiratory forms of TB (blue bacilli) will interrupt the TB transmission cycle, contributing enormously to TB control.

When a patient with pulmonary TB coughs, sneezes, or even speaks, the aerosolized *M. tuberculosis* can be inhaled by neighboring individuals; bacteria reach the alveoli, where resident macrophages phagocytose them. *M. tuberculosis* has adapted to an intracellular lifestyle; the fate of most bacteria in the phagosome is often death, but *M. tuberculosis* has developed adaptations to survive and even to escape from the macrophage phagosome. *M. tuberculosis* is able to manipulate both the innate and acquired immune responses of the host. This manipulation results in an effective CD4$^+$ T-cell response that limits bacterial dissemination but can also promote the development of a progressive and destructive lesion in the lungs (11).

The development of lesions in pulmonary disease, the most common form of TB, is the result of the conflict between the invader, *M. tuberculosis*, and the host. TB is the paradigm for diseases caused by an intracellular pathogen. The pathogen is able to multiply within macrophages and monocytes, and the host immune system is thought to control the infection by cell-mediated immunity (CMI) carried out by effector-activated macrophages orchestrated by T-cell-derived lymphokines. The CMI generated in TB is so potent that on average 90% of immunocompetent humans infected with *M. tuberculosis* are able to contain the infection as latent TB infection (LTBI) (Fig. 2) and avoid progression to clinical disease during their lifetimes (12). It is estimated that >2 billion humans have LTBI, and most of them remain infected although asymptomatic. People with latent TB are at risk of disease reactivation at some later time due to a weakened immune system (e.g., as a result of malnutrition, stress, diabetes, or HIV infection), making LTBI individuals potential reservoirs of transmission (Fig. 2). The risk of progression to active TB is higher in the several years following initial infection. The extent to which LTBI reduces the risk of progression to active TB following reexposure and reinfection has been recently reviewed by Andrews et al. (13), who concluded that individuals with LTBI had a 79% lower risk of progressive TB after reinfection than uninfected individuals. Taken together, pulmonary cases of TB represent the tip of the iceberg when compared with the one-third of the world population latently infected with TB.

In a minority of cases (5 to 10% of infected individuals), the caseum of the TB lesion softens and infection with *M. tuberculosis* progresses into TB disease. The intracellular bacilli avoid killing by macrophages by arresting phagosome-lysosome fusion. *M. tuberculosis* is also able to escape from the phagosome to the cytosol, where it continues multiplying, eventually leading to lysis of the infected cell. These extracellular bacilli are then taken up by other macrophages and by blood monocytes that are attracted to the infectious focus and then develop into immature macrophages. The latter cells readily ingest bacilli but are incapable of killing virulent *M. tuberculosis* organisms or inhibiting their growth. This results in the accumulation of an extracellular bacillary population growing in the lung cavity. This actively dividing population, consisting of millions of microorganisms, is responsible for TB transmission. The tuberculous lung cavity with its high bacillary content is discharged into the bronchi and subsequently to other parts of the lung and to the outside environment, allowing human-to-human transmission. Before the antibiotic era, 50% of patients with cavitary lung TB died within 2 years (12). Efficient coevolution of *M. tuberculosis* with its human host has led to a fine-tuned balance between latency, a persistent phase of the infection responsible for a massive reservoir from which active TB cases may emerge, and the infamous ability of the bacterium to cause severe lung pathology that is a prerequisite for aerosol spread (14).

M. tuberculosis has the ability to promote dynamic responses to the host environment in order to guarantee its survival, replication, and transmission. Determinants of *M. tuberculosis* virulence include biologically active secreted proteins such as ESAT-6 (early secretory antigenic target-6), which mediates damage to the mycobacterial phagosomal membrane, which appears to enable the bacteria to replicate in the cytosol, allowing cell-to-cell spread of virulent *M. tuberculosis* (15, 16). Active lipids interact with the host to contribute to the long-term success of the bacteria by modulating intracellular bacterial trafficking, host cell death pathways, and granuloma formation (17).

Some risk factors leading to progression to active disease in LTBI individuals are related to malnutrition and immunodeficiency of the host. Coinfection with other pathogens such as HIV unbalances the CMI of the host and profoundly alters the immune response to *M. tuberculosis* (18). Treatment for diseases such as rheumatoid arthritis and Crohn's disease with TNF antagonists have been found to markedly increase the frequency of TB reactivation. Further, there is increasing evidence highlighting the importance of vitamin D as a potent modulator of human immune responses, with important implications for the control of TB infection (18). When does *M. tuberculosis* take the decision to remain as LTBI or to progress to disease, allowing TB transmission? And how is this decision taken? Both are essential unresolved questions about the natural history of TB, and their answers will greatly help to discover methods to allow control of respiratory transmission of *M. tuberculosis*.

Members of the MTBC are a highly clonal population, which is particularly well reflected by the evolutionary hyperconservation of human T-cell epitopes. Most bacterial pathogens rely on antigenic drift to favor immune escape. However, the hyperconservation of T-cell epitopes in *M. tuberculosis* implies a better recognition of the pathogen by the human immune system, allowing it to subsequently decide whether to cause disease or remain latent (19). Probably this could reflect the need for *M. tuberculosis* to develop pulmonary forms of the disease where bacteria are able to grow extracellularly, allowing transmission to new hosts.

It is tempting to think that *M. tuberculosis* is acting with its human host in the same way that bacteriophages act with their bacterial hosts (Fig. 2). Lambda phage integrates its genome in the *Escherichia coli* chromosome during the lysogenic cycle, ensuring transmission of the prophage every time when bacteria divide. This lysogenic phase reminds us of the LTBI with *M. tuberculosis* dialogue with the host confering advantages as an strong CMI against other infections. When the phage senses that its bacterial host is in danger as a result of starvation or DNA damage, e.g., by UV light among others, lambda decides to start the lytic cycle, producing multiple copies of its genome and the synthesis of its own proteins, causing the destruction of the bacterial host and transmitting to other bacteria. This lytic phase is similar to the active phase of TB disease, where mycobacteria multiply extracellularly, allowing the transmission to a new host (Fig. 2). Similar to lambda phage that senses a damaging environment of its host, *M. tuberculosis* produces active disease when the immune status of the host is impaired, as in the case of an HIV infection when CMI declines, diminishing the CD4 T-cell count. Today, more than 6 decades after the initial discovery of the lambda phage, we have come to decipher its molecular life cycle with *E. coli*. Hopefully, in the very near future, new technologies and smart researchers will allow us to decipher the intimate relationship of *M. tuberculosis* with the human host and to identify the warning stimuli that awaken latent *M. tuberculosis* to complete its transmission cycle.

TRANSMISSION OF MTBC LINEAGES AND ADAPTATION TO THE HOST LIFESTYLE

Comparative genome analyses have identified a series of regions of difference (RDs), also named large sequence polymorphisms (LSPs), which due to their irreversible nature and intralineage conservation have allowed proposal of broad and accurate evolutionary schemes of the *M. tuberculosis* complex that are still valid (3, 20, 21). These studies suggest a strong indication for a clonal population structure of the MTBC, without evidence of ongoing horizontal gene transfer (3). This has made possible the development of molecular methods to characterize circulating strains, such as gold standard restriction fragment length polymorphism (RFLP) analysis (22, 23), spoligotyping (24), mycobacterial interspersed repetitive-unit-variable-number

tandem-repeat analysis (25), and/or multilocus sequencing approaches (26). These molecular epidemiology techniques are valuable tools to study TB transmission patterns suspected from traditional epidemiological investigation, allowing characterization of highly transmissible *M. tuberculosis* strains. The emergence of whole-genome sequencing more recently as an affordable tool for studying genomic content and inferring genetic relationships offers an extraordinarily detailed view on the evolution of *M. tuberculosis* lineages and outbreak clones, with unprecedented possibilities for verification, interpretation, and refinement of hypotheses on the distant and recent evolution of the tubercle bacilli (14).

Comparative genomics has resulted in congruent groupings of MTBC comprising eight major lineages, which include the human-adapted ecotypes *M. tuberculosis* (L1 to L4 and L7), *M. africanum* (L5 and L6), and *M. canettii*, and the animal-adapted ecotypes grouped into L8 (4). According to RD distribution and whole-genome data, the animal-adapted lineages of the MTBC seem to have evolved from RD9-deleted *M. africanum*-like ancestor strains that may well have been adapted to humans. As regards the presence of L2, L3, and L4 lineages, these TbD1-deleted lineages might correspond to "modern" *M. tuberculosis* strains that were introduced into Africa by more recent human contact and colonialism (14).

Epidemiological data suggest that the different phylogenetic lineages of MTBC might have adapted to different human populations. Over all, the phylogenetically "modern" MTBC lineages are more successful in terms of their geographical spread compared with the "ancient" lineages. Interestingly, the global success of modern MTBC correlates with a hypoinflammatory phenotype in macrophages, possibly reflecting higher virulence, and a shorter latency in humans. Finally, various human genetic variants have been associated with different MTBC lineages, suggesting an interaction between human genetic diversity and MTBC variation (8). *M. tuberculosis* organisms belonging to lineages 2, 3, and 4 are more closely related and well extended in urban populations. Contacts exposed to modern MTBC are more likely to develop active TB in a shorter time compared with individuals exposed to ancient MTBC, who develop TB later (27). Additionally, it has been recently found that genetically diverse strains of MTBC vary widely in induction of an early inflammatory response during infection of human macrophages, with a significantly lower response to evolutionarily modern lineages as compared with ancient lineages (19, 28). It would seem that virulence of the strains may be related to populations living in either rural areas, where transmission needs to be slow to ensure dissemination to the next generation, or crowded cities, where population densities are high enough to allow fast transmission of the disease between neighboring individuals.

Host-pathogen coevolution is characterized by reciprocal adaptive changes in interacting species. Host immune pressure and associated pathogen immune evasion are key features of this process, often referred to as an evolutionary arms race. Studies in human pathogenic viruses, bacteria, and protozoa have revealed that genes encoding antigens tend to be highly variable as a consequence of diversifying selection to evade host immunity. However, since all MTBC strains have highly conserved human T-cell epitopes, the ultimate transmission mechanisms rely on the host immune response that contributes to tissue destruction and formation of cavities in the lung (8).

MDR-TB OUTBREAKS: THE RARE CASE OF A PARTICULAR *M. BOVIS* MDR-XDR STRAIN TRANSMITTED BETWEEN HUMANS

Since no plasmids or horizontal gene transfer for antibiotic resistance genes have been detected, *M. tuberculosis* acquires antibiotic resistance by selection of specific mutations in target genes (3). Transmission of MDR-TB (resistant at least to isoniazid and rifampin) strains depends on the fitness cost of the mutations conferring the drug resistance phenotype. In laboratory-derived mutants of *M. tuberculosis*, rifampin resistance could be associated with a competitive fitness cost, and this cost is likely determined by the specific resistance mutation and strain genetic background. In the case of epidemic MDR *M. tuberculosis* clinical isolates, no fitness-impairing mutations have been found (29). Isoniazid-resistant isolates have been used to demonstrate that strain genetic diversity influences the transmission dynamics of drug-resistant bacteria (30). Association between specific drug resistance mutations and the main *M. tuberculosis* lineages allows us to predict that strain fitness is an important determinant of MDR *M. tuberculosis* transmission and demonstrates the important effects of strain diversity. The impact of resistance mutations on the transmission of isoniazid-resistant *M. tuberculosis* is very important; for example, strains with a KatG S315T or *inhA* promoter mutation were more likely to spread than strains with other mutations that have lost their fitness.

In the 1990s, an MDR-TB outbreak was extended from >200 New York City patients and to at least four additional U.S. cities, and transmitted to Europe. The MDR *M. tuberculosis* clonal strain, named "W strain," belongs to lineage 2 (Beijing family). Isolates were typed by IS*6110*-based RFLP, and gene mutations associated with resistance to rifampin and isoniazid were studied. The MDR phenotype in these organisms arose by sequential acquisition of resistance-conferring mutations in several genes, most likely as a consequence of antibiotic selection of randomly occurring mutants in concert with inadequately treated infections (31). The MDR-TB epidemic was the confluence of several factors, including the AIDS epidemic as result of HIV infection, before an effective antiretroviral treatment was available; immigration from countries where TB is endemic; poverty; homelessness; and lack of TB control programs.

In Europe, a high rate of TB reinfection during a nosocomial outbreak of MDR-TB caused by *M. bovis* was detected in the 1990s among AIDS patients (32). The *M. bovis* strain was typed by IS*6110*-based RFLP and named "strain B," and after studying the resistance phenotype of the strain, it was classified as extensively drug-resistant TB (XDR-TB), which is an MDR-TB further resistant to any fluoroquinolone and to at least one of three injectable second-line drugs (i.e., amikacin, kanamycin, or capreomycin) (33). Strain B caused >100 deaths of AIDS patients in different regions throughout Spain (33). Since *M. bovis* exhibits a lower transmissibility among humans than *M. tuberculosis sensu stricto* (Fig. 1), it seems very likely that the higher human-to-human transmission rate of strain B was a consequence of additional fitness gained by this particular isolate. Molecular epidemiology techniques identified the insertion of an IS*6110* mobile element upstream of *phoPR*, leading to overexpression of this operon, which codes for the two-component system PhoPR, which is essential for the virulence of *M. tuberculosis* (34). This finding suggested that PhoPR-associated phenotypes likely favored aerosol transmission of *M. bovis* strain B between humans (35). The discovery of the essential role of the *phoP* gene in this outbreak of MDR-TB was the founding principle for the construction of the attenuated vaccine MTBVAC, now being evaluated in the clinic, as discussed in detail below.

ANIMAL MODELS TO STUDY TB TRANSMISSION

In view of the great difficulty of monitoring TB transmission among humans, future research efforts might be well advised to focus on animal models of transmission (36). The relationship between TB transmission dynamics and the evolution of *M. tuberculosis* has been an important question in TB research for many years. This has not been studied in TB because of the lack of an experimental TB transmission model in a well-controlled system.

One important line of research in TB is the relationship between transmissibility and bacterial genotype. A transmission mouse model has been established to study the hypothesis that increased virulence of the strains was linked to increased transmission (37). By using a BALB/c mouse model of progressive pulmonary TB, authors examined the course of infection in terms of strain virulence (mouse survival, lung bacillary load, and histopathology) and immune response cytokine expression produced by different *M. tuberculosis* strains selected from clinical/epidemiological studies. Animals that were exposed to the more virulent strain developed the hallmark of progressive disease (pneumonic patches) after 2 months of cohousing, whereas the low- or intermediate-virulence strains only induced small granulomas and chronic inflammatory infiltrates. A correlation between virulence, immunopathology, and transmissibility of selected strains of *M. tuberculosis* was found. The research was able to correlate virulent and transmissible phenotypes and markers of community transmission such as tuberculin reactivity among contacts, rapid progression to disease, and cluster status. Nevertheless, as mice lack the cough reflex, this animal model is not considered to mirror the TB transmission mechanisms occurring in humans.

In the case of guinea pigs, due to their high susceptibility to TB, their use as sentinels in hospitals to study direct transmission from human TB patients has been explored (38).

Quantitative studies of disease in animals that develop cavitary, transmissible TB may be key in determining whether the host or the pathogen plays the role in TB transmission. In this regard, an interesting model in cattle has been established to study transmission of bovine TB in a natural transmission setting to examine the efficacy of *M. bovis* BCG for protection against bovine TB in calves under field conditions. The study demonstrated a BCG protective efficacy between 56 and 68% (39).

Goats are highly social and relatively easy-to-handle animals and have been proposed as a reliable ruminant model for research, representing an easier approach than use of larger ruminants (40). Goats are very sensitive to TB infection, exhibiting disease-causing lesions in the lungs similar to humans (41) when infected with different members of the MTBC, including *M. bovis* and *M. caprae* (42). Recent studies have demonstrated an effective and quick rate of TB transmission in this animal model by cohousing TB-infected and -noninfected goats (43). Today, goats represent a very promising ruminant model for the assessment of vaccine efficacy against TB transmission (L. Domingez, personal communication).

BCG: THE ONLY VACCINE IN USE TO PREVENT DISSEMINATED BUT NOT RESPIRATORY FORMS OF TB

BCG is a live attenuated vaccine derived from *M. bovis*, isolated for the first time in 1902 by Edmond Nocard from the milk of a cow suffering from tuberculous mastitis. BCG is almost 100 years old and is currently the only available vaccine for the prevention of human forms of TB. BCG is effective for the disseminated forms of TB and is included as part of the routine immunization schedule in developing countries. Since 1974, BCG vaccination at birth has been included in the World Health Organization Expanded Programme on Immunization, resulting in more than 3 billion cumulative vaccinations worldwide. Today, BCG is the most widely administered vaccine in humans, being one of the vaccines with minimal recorded adverse events.

Since BCG protects against the more severe forms of TB (meningitis and miliary TB) in children, thousands of lives are saved every year (44). The coverage of BCG is nearly 90% all around the world, and >100 million doses are administered every year (44, 45). However, BCG is very variable in protecting against pulmonary TB, responsible for TB transmission. Consequently, BCG is not recommended for use in the United States or other high-income countries considered to have a low burden of TB.

Multiple explanations have been put forward to explain the variable efficacy of the BCG vaccine. It is very likely that BCG is not able to establish effective central memory T cells. Accordingly, BCG protects infants and adolescents for 10 to 15 years, but protection is gradually lost in adults. This may have extraordinary implications for developing new TB vaccines aiming to enhance central memory immunity (46).

As previously described, the experimentally verified human T-cell epitopes of *M. tuberculosis* are the most conserved elements of its genome (19). The genome sequences of different BCG strains were compared to determine T-cell epitope conservation (47). It was found that among the 1,530 human T-cell epitopes, 23% of them are absent in the BCG vaccines. The majority of the absent epitopes in BCG are contained in three proteins: ESAT-6, CFP-10 (10-kDa culture filtrate protein), and PPE68 (cell envelope protein from PPE family that contributes to M. tuberculosis maintenance of infection) all of them encoded in the RD1 region absent in BCG (47). If these epitopes are necessary to complete the pulmonary cycle of *M. tuberculosis*, we could hypothesize that vaccine candidates containing epitopes absent in BCG could confer immunity to protect against pulmonary TB.

THE SEARCH FOR A NEW TB VACCINE TO END TRANSMISSION

In the last 15 years, many vaccine candidates have entered clinical trials. Most are protein-adjuvant formulations and recombinant viral-vectored constructs designed to increase the protection from pulmonary TB in individuals previously vaccinated with BCG (prime-boost strategy) (18). Two live attenuated whole-cell vaccines are in clinical trials for prime vaccination, one based on recombinant BCG and the other based on attenuated *M. tuberculosis* of human origin (18).

Live, rationally attenuated MTBVAC is a derivative of an *M. tuberculosis* isolate belonging to lineage 4 (Euro-American), one of the most widespread lineages of *M. tuberculosis* today. MTBVAC contains antigens present in *M. tuberculosis* strains commonly transmitted between humans by the aerosol route, including those antigens deleted in the RD1 region of *M. bovis* BCG (ESAT-6, CFP-10, and PPE68). MTBVAC contains two independent stable deletion mutations in the virulence genes *phoP* and *fadD26*. These deletions were generated in the absence of antibiotic resistance markers, fulfilling the Geneva consensus requirements for progressing live mycobacterial vaccines to clinical trials (48). PhoP is a transcription factor that controls expression of 2% of the *M. tuberculosis* genome, including production of immunomodulatory cell wall lipids and ESAT-6 secretion (4). Deletion of *fadD26* leads to complete abrogation of synthesis of the virulence surface lipids phthiocerol dimycocerosates. Extensive preclinical studies with the prototype vaccine S02 in mice, guinea pigs, and nonhuman primates (49–51) and final vaccine candidate MTBVAC in mice and guinea pigs have demonstrated attenuation and safety of MTBVAC comparable to BCG, with superior immunogenicity and efficacy against *M. tuberculosis* (48, 52). A first-in-human MTBVAC clinical trial was recently completed successfully in healthy adults in Lausanne, Switzerland (NCT02013245) (53). In this trial, when MTBVAC was given at the same dose as BCG (5×10^5 CFU), there were more responders in the MTBVAC group than in the BCG group, with a greater frequency of polyfunctional CD4$^+$ central memory T cells. However, this study has the limitation, as a phase 1 first-in-human trial, that the secondary objective (immunogenicity) was not powered for statistical analysis. Nevertheless, MTBVAC is the first live attenuated *M. tuberculosis* vaccine to enter clinical trials and to date has shown a comparable safety profile to BCG. A notable finding in the first trial was a transitory ESAT-6- and CFP-10-specific T-cell responses that at the end of the study was negative, suggesting that gamma interferon release assays could be utilized as study endpoints in future efficacy trials to test efficacy against *M. tuberculosis* infection (53). The immunogenicity data show that MTBVAC is at least as immunogenic as BCG, a result congruent with the maintenance of the whole epitope repertoire from an *M. tuberculosis* strain. Altogether, these data supported the advanced clinical development in high-burden countries where TB is endemic. A dose-escalation safety and immunogenicity study to compare MTBVAC to BCG in newborns with a safety arm in adults is currently ongoing in South Africa (NCT02729571). A review on MTBVAC, from discovery to clinical trials in tuberculosis-endemic countries, has been recently published (54).

Due to the lack of a correlation of protection for TB, future efficacy studies with MTBVAC in countries with a high incidence of TB could demonstrate the effectiveness of this vaccine in preventing pulmonary forms of TB. Efficacy studies in new TB transmission animal models, such as the recently developed model in goats (55), are extremely important to demonstrate proof of concept of pulmonary protection to help accelerate clinical development of new TB vaccines toward efficacy trials in humans. Specific response in human to TB vaccinees candidates as potential biomarker of protection could accelerate the clinical trials efficacy evaluation (56).

CONCLUDING REMARKS

Additional threats to TB control include the spread of MDR-TB, the appearance of XDR-TB, and the destructive impact of TB/HIV coinfection. Today, the main strategy to stop TB transmission is via active case-finding and by prompt establishment of an effective treatment as soon as TB is diagnosed. New vaccines against *M. tuberculosis* are essential for preventing infection, disease, and transmission. The development of a new vaccine able to protect against pulmonary forms of TB is essential to overcome this terrible disease, with the final objective to eradicate TB from the planet.

ACKNOWLEDGMENTS

We acknowledge EC HORIZON2020 TBVAC 2020 (contract no. 643381) and the Spanish Ministry of Economy and Competitiveness [BIO2014-5258P].

CONFLICT OF INTEREST

C.M., J.G.-A., and N.A. are coinventors of a patent on a live attenuated TB vaccine held by the University of Zaragoza. There is not any commercial or other association that might pose a conflict of interest.

CITATION

Gonzalo-Asensio J, Aguilo N, Marinova D, Martin C. 2017. Breaking transmission with vaccines: the case of tuberculosis. Microbiol Spectrum 5(4):MTBP-0001-2016.

REFERENCES

1. **Paulson T.** 2013. Epidemiology: a mortal foe. *Nature* **502:**S2–S3.
2. **World Health Organization.** 2015. *World Health Organization Global Tuberculosis Report 2015.* World Health Organization, Geneva, Switzerland.
3. **Brosch R, Gordon SV, Marmiesse M, Brodin P, Buchrieser C, Eiglmeier K, Garnier T, Gutierrez C, Hewinson G, Kremer K, Parsons LM, Pym AS, Samper S, van Soolingen D, Cole ST.** 2002. A new evolutionary scenario for the *Mycobacterium tuberculosis* complex. *Proc Natl Acad Sci U S A* **99:**3684–3689.
4. **Broset E, Martín C, Gonzalo-Asensio J.** 2015. Evolutionary landscape of the *Mycobacterium tuberculosis* complex from the viewpoint of PhoPR: implications for virulence regulation and application to vaccine development. *mBio* **6:**e01289-e15.
5. **Comas I, Coscolla M, Luo T, Borrell S, Holt KE, Kato-Maeda M, Parkhill J, Malla B, Berg S, Thwaites G, Yeboah-Manu D, Bothamley G, Mei J, Wei L, Bentley S, Harris SR, Niemann S, Diel R, Aseffa A, Gao Q, Young D, Gagneux S.** 2013. Out-of-Africa migration and Neolithic coexpansion of *Mycobacterium tuberculosis* with modern humans. *Nat Genet* **45:**1176–1182.
6. **Bos KI, Harkins KM, Herbig A, Coscolla M, Weber N, Comas I, Forrest SA, Bryant JM, Harris SR, Schuenemann VJ, Campbell TJ, Majander K, Wilbur AK, Guichon RA, Wolfe Steadman DL, Cook DC, Niemann S, Behr MA, Zumarraga M, Bastida R, Huson D, Nieselt K, Young D, Parkhill J, Buikstra JE, Gagneux S, Stone AC, Krause J.** 2014. Pre-Columbian mycobacterial genomes reveal seals as a source of New World human tuberculosis. *Nature* **514:**494–497.
7. **Berg S, Schelling E, Hailu E, Firdessa R, Gumi B, Erenso G, Gadisa E, Mengistu A, Habtamu M, Hussein J, Kiros T, Bekele S, Mekonnen W, Derese Y, Zinsstag J, Ameni G, Gagneux S, Robertson BD, Tschopp R, Hewinson G, Yamuah L, Gordon SV, Aseffa A.** 2015. Investigation of the high rates of extrapulmonary tuberculosis in Ethiopia reveals no single driving factor and minimal evidence for zoonotic transmission of *Mycobacterium bovis* infection. *BMC Infect Dis* **15:**112.
8. **Gagneux S.** 2012. Host-pathogen coevolution in human tuberculosis. *Philos Trans R Soc Lond B Biol Sci* **367:**850–859.
9. **Yates TA, Khan PY, Knight GM, Taylor JG, McHugh TD, Lipman M, White RG, Cohen T, Cobelens FG, Wood R, Moore DAJ, Abubakar I.** 2016. The transmission of *Mycobacterium tuberculosis* in high burden settings. *Lancet Infect Dis* **16:**227–238.
10. **Ernst JD.** 2012. The immunological life cycle of tuberculosis. *Nat Rev Immunol* **12:**581–591.
11. **Orme IM, Robinson RT, Cooper AM.** 2015. The balance between protective and pathogenic immune responses in the TB-infected lung. *Nat Immunol* **16:**57–63.
12. **Grosset J.** 2003. *Mycobacterium tuberculosis* in the extracellular compartment: an underestimated adversary. *Antimicrob Agents Chemother* **47:**833–836.
13. **Andrews JR, Noubary F, Walensky RP, Cerda R, Losina E, Horsburgh CR.** 2012. Risk of progression to active tuberculosis following reinfection with *Mycobacterium tuberculosis. Clin Infect Dis* **54:**784–791.
14. **Boritsch EC, Supply P, Honoré N, Seemann T, Stinear TP, Brosch R, Brosch R.** 2014. A glimpse

into the past and predictions for the future: the molecular evolution of the tuberculosis agent. *Mol Microbiol* **93**:835–852.

15. **Aguiló N, Marinova D, Martín C, Pardo J.** 2013. ESX-1-induced apoptosis during mycobacterial infection: to be or not to be, that is the question. *Front Cell Infect Microbiol* **3**:88.

16. **Aguilo JI, Alonso H, Uranga S, Marinova D, Arbués A, de Martino A, Anel A, Monzon M, Badiola J, Pardo J, Brosch R, Martin C.** 2013. ESX-1-induced apoptosis is involved in cell-to-cell spread of *Mycobacterium tuberculosis*. *Cell Microbiol* **15**:1994–2005.

17. **Neyrolles O, Guilhot C.** 2011. Recent advances in deciphering the contribution of *Mycobacterium tuberculosis* lipids to pathogenesis. *Tuberculosis (Edinb)* **91**:187–195.

18. **Marinova D, Gonzalo-Asensio J, Aguilo N, Martin C.** 2013. Recent developments in tuberculosis vaccines. *Expert Rev Vaccines* **12**:1431–1448.

19. **Comas I, Chakravartti J, Small PM, Galagan J, Niemann S, Kremer K, Ernst JD, Gagneux S.** 2010. Human T cell epitopes of *Mycobacterium tuberculosis* are evolutionarily hyperconserved. *Nat Genet* **42**:498–503.

20. **Mostowy S, Inwald J, Gordon S, Martin C, Warren R, Kremer K, Cousins D, Behr MA.** 2005. Revisiting the evolution of *Mycobacterium bovis*. *J Bacteriol* **187**:6386–6395.

21. **Gagneux S, Small PM.** 2007. Global phylogeography of *Mycobacterium tuberculosis* and implications for tuberculosis product development. *Lancet Infect Dis* **7**:328–337.

22. **Otal I, Martín C, Vincent-Lévy-Frebault V, Thierry D, Gicquel B.** 1991. Restriction fragment length polymorphism analysis using IS6110 as an epidemiological marker in tuberculosis. *J Clin Microbiol* **29**:1252–1254.

23. **van Embden JD, Cave MD, Crawford JT, Dale JW, Eisenach KD, Gicquel B, Hermans P, Martin C, McAdam R, Shinnick TM, Small PM.** 1993. Strain identification of *Mycobacterium tuberculosis* by DNA fingerprinting: recommendations for a standardized methodology. *J Clin Microbiol* **31**:406–409.

24. **Kamerbeek J, Schouls L, Kolk A, van Agterveld M, van Soolingen D, Kuijper S, Bunschoten A, Molhuizen H, Shaw R, Goyal M, van Embden J.** 1997. Simultaneous detection and strain differentiation of *Mycobacterium tuberculosis* for diagnosis and epidemiology. *J Clin Microbiol* **35**:907–914.

25. **Supply P, Lesjean S, Savine E, Kremer K, van Soolingen D, Locht C.** 2001. Automated high-throughput genotyping for study of global epidemiology of *Mycobacterium tuberculosis* based on mycobacterial interspersed repetitive units. *J Clin Microbiol* **39**:3563–3571.

26. **Baker L, Brown T, Maiden MC, Drobniewski F.** 2004. Silent nucleotide polymorphisms and a phylogeny for *Mycobacterium tuberculosis*. *Emerg Infect Dis* **10**:1568–1577.

27. **Comas I, Gagneux S.** 2011. A role for systems epidemiology in tuberculosis research. *Trends Microbiol* **19**:492–500.

28. **Portevin D, Gagneux S, Comas I, Young D.** 2011. Human macrophage responses to clinical isolates from the *Mycobacterium tuberculosis* complex discriminate between ancient and modern lineages. *PLoS Pathog* **7**:e1001307.

29. **Gagneux S, Long CD, Small PM, Van T, Schoolnik GK, Bohannan BJM.** 2006. The competitive cost of antibiotic resistance in *Mycobacterium tuberculosis*. *Science* **312**:1944–1946.

30. **Gagneux S, Burgos MV, DeRiemer K, Encisco A, Muñoz S, Hopewell PC, Small PM, Pym AS.** 2006. Impact of bacterial genetics on the transmission of isoniazid-resistant *Mycobacterium tuberculosis*. *PLoS Pathog* **2**:e61.

31. **Bifani PJ, Plikaytis BB, Kapur V, Stockbauer K, Pan X, Lutfey ML, Moghazeh SL, Eisner W, Daniel TM, Kaplan MH, Crawford JT, Musser JM, Kreiswirth BN.** 1996. Origin and interstate spread of a New York City multidrug-resistant *Mycobacterium tuberculosis* clone family. *JAMA* **275**:452–457.

32. **Rivero A, Márquez M, Santos J, Pinedo A, Sánchez MA, Esteve A, Samper S, Martín C.** 2001. High rate of tuberculosis reinfection during a nosocomial outbreak of multidrug-resistant tuberculosis caused by *Mycobacterium bovis* strain B. *Clin Infect Dis* **32**:159–161.

33. **Samper S, Martín C.** 2007. Spread of extensively drug-resistant tuberculosis. *Emerg Infect Dis* **13**:647–648.

34. **Pérez E, Samper S, Bordas Y, Guilhot C, Gicquel B, Martín C.** 2001. An essential role for *phoP* in *Mycobacterium tuberculosis* virulence. *Mol Microbiol* **41**:179–187.

35. **Gonzalo-Asensio J, Malaga W, Pawlik A, Astarie-Dequeker C, Passemar C, Moreau F, Laval F, Daffé M, Martin C, Brosch R, Guilhot C.** 2014. Evolutionary history of tuberculosis shaped by conserved mutations in the PhoPR virulence regulator. *Proc Natl Acad Sci U S A* **111**:11491–11496.

36. **Bishai W.** 2001. Tuberculosis transmission—rogue pathogen or rogue patient? *Am J Respir Crit Care Med* **164**:1104–1105.

37. **Marquina-Castillo B, García-García L, Ponce-de-León A, Jimenez-Corona M-E, Bobadilla-Del Valle M, Cano-Arellano B, Canizales-Quintero S, Martinez-Gamboa A, Kato-Maeda M, Robertson B, Young D, Small P, Schoolnik G, Sifuentes-Osornio J, Hernández-Pando R.**

2009. Virulence, immunopathology and transmissibility of selected strains of *Mycobacterium tuberculosis* in a murine model. *Immunology* **128**: 123–133.

38. Escombe AR, Oeser C, Gilman RH, Navincopa M, Ticona E, Martínez C, Caviedes L, Sheen P, Gonzalez A, Noakes C, Moore DAJ, Friedland JS, Evans CA. 2007. The detection of airborne transmission of tuberculosis from HIV-infected patients, using an in vivo air sampling model. *Clin Infect Dis* **44**:1349–1357.

39. Ameni G, Vordermeier M, Aseffa A, Young DB, Hewinson RG. 2010. Field evaluation of the efficacy of *Mycobacterium bovis* bacillus Calmette-Guerin against bovine tuberculosis in neonatal calves in Ethiopia. *Clin Vaccine Immunol* **17**: 1533–1538.

40. Larsen GD. 2015. A reliable ruminate for research. *Lab Anim (NY)* **44**:337.

41. Sanchez J, Tomás L, Ortega N, Buendía AJ, del Rio L, Salinas J, Bezos J, Caro MR, Navarro JA. 2011. Microscopical and immunological features of tuberculoid granulomata and cavitary pulmonary tuberculosis in naturally infected goats. *J Comp Pathol* **145**:107–117.

42. Bezos J, Casal C, Díez-Delgado I, Romero B, Liandris E, Álvarez J, Sevilla IA, Juan L, Domínguez L, Gortázar C. 2015. Goats challenged with different members of the *Mycobacterium tuberculosis* complex display different clinical pictures. *Vet Immunol Immunopathol* **167**:185–189.

43. Bezos J, Casal C, Puentes E, Díez-Guerrier A, Romero B, Aguiló N, de Juan L, Martín C, Domínguez L. 2015. Evaluation of the immunogenicity and diagnostic interference caused by *M. tuberculosis* SO2 vaccination against tuberculosis in goats. *Res Vet Sci* **103**:73–79.

44. Young D, Dye C. 2006. The development and impact of tuberculosis vaccines. *Cell* **124**:683–687.

45. World Health Organization. 2011. The Immunological Basis for Immunization Series. *Module 5: Tuberculosis.* World Health Organization, Geneva, Switzerland.

46. Orme IM. 2010. The Achilles heel of BCG. *Tuberculosis (Edinb)* **90**:329–332.

47. Copin R, Coscollá M, Efstathiadis E, Gagneux S, Ernst JD. 2014. Impact of in vitro evolution on antigenic diversity of *Mycobacterium bovis* bacillus Calmette-Guerin (BCG). *Vaccine* **32**:5998–6004.

48. Arbués A, Aguilo JI, Gonzalo-Asensio J, Marinova D, Uranga S, Puentes E, Fernandez C, Parra A, Cardona P-J, Vilaplana C, Ausina V, Williams A, Clark S, Malaga W, Guilhot C, Gicquel B, Martin C. 2013. Construction, characterization and preclinical evaluation of MTBVAC, the first live-attenuated *M. tuberculosis*-based

vaccine to enter clinical trials. *Vaccine* **31**:4867–4873.

49. Martin C, Williams A, Hernandez-Pando R, Cardona PJ, Gormley E, Bordat Y, Soto CY, Clark SO, Hatch GJ, Aguilar D, Ausina V, Gicquel B. 2006. The live *Mycobacterium tuberculosis phoP* mutant strain is more attenuated than BCG and confers protective immunity against tuberculosis in mice and guinea pigs. *Vaccine* **24**:3408–3419.

50. Verreck FAW, Vervenne RAW, Kondova I, van Kralingen KW, Remarque EJ, Braskamp G, van der Werff NM, Kersbergen A, Ottenhoff THM, Heidt PJ, Gilbert SC, Gicquel B, Hill AVS, Martin C, McShane H, Thomas AW. 2009. MVA.85A boosting of BCG and an attenuated, *phoP* deficient *M. tuberculosis* vaccine both show protective efficacy against tuberculosis in rhesus macaques. *PLoS One* **4**: e5264.

51. Nambiar JK, Pinto R, Aguilo JI, Takatsu K, Martin C, Britton WJ, Triccas JA. 2012. Protective immunity afforded by attenuated, PhoP-deficient *Mycobacterium tuberculosis* is associated with sustained generation of $CD4^+$ T-cell memory. *Eur J Immunol* **42**:385–392.

52. Aguilo N, Uranga S, Marinova D, Monzon M, Badiola J, Martin C. 2016. MTBVAC vaccine is safe, immunogenic and confers protective efficacy against *Mycobacterium tuberculosis* in newborn mice. *Tuberculosis (Edinb)* **96**:71–74.

53. Spertini F, Audran R, Chakour R, Karoui O, Steiner-Monard V, Thierry A-C, Mayor CE, Rettby N, Jaton K, Vallotton L, Lazor-Blanchet C, Doce J, Puentes E, Marinova D, Aguilo N, Martin C. 2015. Safety of human immunisation with a live-attenuated *Mycobacterium tuberculosis* vaccine: a randomised, double-blind, controlled phase I trial. *Lancet Respir Med* **3**:953–962.

54. Marinova D, Gonzalo-Asensio J, Aguilo N, Martin C. 2017. MTBVAC from discovery to clinical trials in tuberculosis-endemic countries. *Expert Review of Vaccines* **16**(6):565–576.

55. Bezos J, Casal C, Álvarez J, Roy A, Romero B, Rodríguez-Bertos A, Bárcena C, Díez A, Juste R, Gortázar C, Puentes E, Aguiló N, Martín C, de Juan L, Domínguez L. 2017. Evaluation of the Mycobacterium tuberculosis SO2 vaccine using a natural tuberculosis infection model in goats. *Vet J* **223**:60–67. Epub 2017 May 3.

56. Aguilo N, Gonzalo-Asensio J, Alvarez-Arguedas S, Marinova D, Gomez AB, Uranga S, Spallek R, Singh M, Audran R, Spertini F, Martin C. 2017. Reactogenicity to major tuberculosis antigen absent in BCG is linked to improved protection against Mycobacterium tuberculosis. *Nat Commun* **8**:16085.

Transmission, Human Population, and Pathogenicity: the Ebola Case in Point

15

RAFAEL DELGADO[1] and FERNANDO SIMÓN[2]

EBOLA VIRUS AND THE HISTORY OF THE *FILOVIRIDAE* FAMILY

Ebolaviruses are the causative agents responsible for several outbreaks of hemorrhagic fever. *Ebolavirus* is a genus within the family *Filoviridae*. The genus *Ebolavirus* contains five species: *Zaire ebolavirus* (EBOV), *Sudan ebolavirus* (SUDV), *Reston ebolavirus* (RESTV), *Täi Forest ebolavirus* (TAFV), and *Bundibugyo ebolavirus* (BDBV) (1, 2). Ebolaviruses were identified for the first time during two major outbreaks of hemorrhagic fever disease, which took place almost at the same time in Yambuku, Democratic Republic of the Congo (DRC, previously Zaire), and Nzara, Sudan, in 1976 (3, 4), and were demonstrated to be caused respectively by the agents now known as EBOV and SUDV. More than 500 cases were reported in those outbreaks, with a striking mortality rate of 88% in Zaire and of 53% in Sudan. The origin of the name Ebola corresponds to a river in nearby Yambuku, DRC, the first location known to be affected by EBOV (5). Within the *Filoviridae* there is also the genus *Marburgvirus*, with its unique species, *Marburg marburgvirus* (MARV), which shares many epidemiological and pathogenic aspects with EBOV. MARV was actually the first filovirus discovered, in 1967 during an outbreak in Germany and Belgrade, Serbia, that resulted in the infection of several

[1]Department of Microbiology and Instituto de Investigación i+12, Hospital Universitario 12 de Octubre, Madrid, Spain; [2]Center for Health Alerts and Emergencies Coordination, Ministry of Health and CIBERESP, Madrid, Spain.
Microbial Transmission in Biological Processes
Edited by Fernando Baquero, Emilio Bouza, J.A. Gutiérrez-Fuentes, and Teresa M. Coque
© 2018 American Society for Microbiology, Washington, DC
doi:10.1128/microbiolspec.MTBP-0003-2016

laboratory technicians who were manipulating tissues from African monkeys (6). At that time, structures with thread-like morphology were visualized by electron microscopy in organs of infected individuals, and the term filovirus was coined (7) to describe these agents. All ebolaviruses except RESTV have been described in Africa and are highly pathogenic for humans: EBOV and SUDV in 1976, TAFV in 1994, and BDBV in 2007. RESTV comes from Asia (Philippines), and for unknown reasons it is unique in not causing disease in humans, an observation based on a number of documented zoonotic infections, since RESTV can asymptomatically infect swine and eventually be transmitted to humans (8, 9). Intriguingly, despite being nonpathogenic for humans and swine, RESTV is capable of being highly lethal in nonhuman primates (NHPs) (9–15). Recently a third genus of filovirus, *Cuevavirus*, has been described infecting cave bats in northern Spain. The single agent within *Cuevavirus*, named Lloviu virus, has not been replicated in culture although it has been fully characterized by sequencing analysis. Its pathogenic potential for humans is unknown (16, 17).

Since the first outbreaks of EBOV in 1976, little more than two dozen outbreaks have been confirmed in remote areas of Central Africa (Congo, Gabon, Sudan, and Uganda), affecting a relatively small number of individuals (tens to a few hundred). In these cases, the control of the outbreaks by basic public health measures such as rapid identification and isolation of infected individuals, tracing of suspected cases, and proper disposal of corpses has been relatively straightforward since the outbreaks have occurred in poorly served rural areas with reduced mobility of people.

The recent outbreak of EBOV disease (EVD) is unprecedented in many aspects. It has mainly affected Guinea (Conakry), Sierra Leone, and Liberia in West Africa, a distant location from the usual area in Central Africa that had experienced most of the previous Ebola outbreaks. It has acquired a much larger scale, with close to 30,000 cases and more than 11,000 officially reported deaths, according to the World Health Organization (WHO), and according with its magnitude it has produced an international crisis of security (18, 19).

EBOLA VIRUS: THE INFECTIOUS AGENT IN THE 2013–2016 OUTBREAK

As for many emergent viral diseases, EVD is a clear example of a zoonotic infection; however, our knowledge of the ecology of EBOV is only partial, and specifically, information about a crucial aspect of the Ebola cycle, such as the characterization of the viral reservoir in the wild, is quite limited (20). Certain varieties of fruit bats in Africa have been identified as the natural reservoir of the virus; however, these observations are based just on the detection of specific RNA sequences, and EBOV remains to be isolated from wild animals apart from humans (21). If bats are the reservoir of the virus, EBOV in bats could infect other mammals, such as antelopes and monkeys, that could infect humans due to bushmeat hunting and consumption, although direct contact with bats or bat fluids have been implicated in some cases, including the recent outbreak (22). There is also evidence that EBOV can be actively circulating in the wild among NHPs, and some field studies have estimated that EVD could have been an important factor in the recent dramatic reduction of great apes in Africa (23, 24).

EBOV was detected as the causal agent of the recent outbreak in West Africa in March 2014, and a few weeks later the complete sequence of the virus was made available (25). Sequencing analysis showed a close homology with varieties of *Zaire ebolavirus*, the *Ebolavirus* species associated with the highest mortality. The varieties within *Zaire ebolavirus* include, among others, the Mayinga strain from the original 1976 outbreak and the Kikwit strain from an outbreak in 1995 in this location also in the DRC. The new variant from

West Africa has been named Makona (EBOV/ Mak) and exhibits a 3% genetic divergence as compared with the variants of *Zaire ebolavirus* previously reported in Central Africa (25–27). EBOV/Mak is thought to represent a previously undetected variant in parallel evolution with a common ancestor that is circulating through an unknown reservoir in this area, which is several thousand miles from Central Africa, where all the previous outbreaks have been reported (28). The only geographical close antecedent is a single case of infection in 1994 of a scientist infected in Ivory Coast, who was involved in necropsy fieldwork with primates in the Täi Forest. Subsequent studies demonstrated a new species of *Ebolavirus*, TAFV (29). The biological relevance of the genetic divergence of EBOV/ Mak from the classical strains has been a matter of intense debate. Although the unprecedented scale of the outbreak could suggest a different behavior of the virus, no differences have been demonstrated in transmission, infectivity or pathogenesis as compared with previous outbreaks (30, 31). Nevertheless, there are differences between the EBOV/ Mak variant and classical EBOV in terms of cross-immune recognition whose biological relevance remains to be established (32). Preliminary information on vaccines designed with the EBOV/Kikwit variant has shown protection against the new variant in NHPs and humans (33, 34).

EVD

Symptoms of EVD are quite nonspecific, especially in the first stages of the illness, when it can be confused with other common endemic infections such as malaria, dengue, or typhoid. After a few days of incubation (typically 5 to 10 days, maximum incubation period 21 days), EVD begins with fever with important general involvement. As disease progresses, there appears digestive discomfort with abdominal pain, vomiting, and diarrhea that can be very intense, leading to severe dehydration, ionic disorder, and commonly death. In advanced cases, hemorrhages appear as bloody diarrhea and epistaxis. Without supportive treatment to restore fluids and ions and to maintain general condition, mortality reaches over 70%. EVD is mostly, if not always, clearly and rapidly symptomatic, and transmission does not appear to occur during the incubation period. EBOV does not establish latency, so patients were not thought to be infectious once recovered from the acute episode; however, there were observations in previous outbreaks of the persistence of the virus in semen for long periods of time, including an event of sexual transmission in the original Marburg outbreak of 1967 (6). Persistence of EBOV in certain organs has been confirmed in the present outbreaks due to the large population involved, the use of advanced technology, and the unique opportunity to have had EVD patients in modern health facilities in Europe and the United States for the first time. In Africa it has been proved that EBOV RNA is detectable by reverse transcriptase PCR in semen of 100% of convalescent men by 2 to 3 months after the onset of EVD, in 65% by months 4 to 6, and in up to 26% by months 7 to 9 (35). It has also been demonstrated that this can represent viable viral forms in some instances in which there has been documented sexual transmission from male to female 6 months after the index patient recovered from acute infection (36). With such a large population of convalescent patients in the recent outbreak, sexual transmission appears to have played some role in the cluster of cases that have occurred once the circulation of the virus was considered officially over. Likewise, EBOV persistence has been well documented in organs apart from gonads, such as the eye and central nervous system, through the study of episodes of reactivation producing uveitis (37) and meningitis (38), respectively, in patients treated in the United States and Europe.

What makes this infection so lethal? EBOV combines two elements that make it particularly lethal to humans: (i) the ability of the virus to replicate at a very high rate from the beginning of the infection; and (ii) the involvement of critical subsets of immune cells, such as dendritic cells and other varieties of antigen-presenting cells. In the first steps of the infective process, the virus infects primarily dendritic cells and macrophages, which are responsible for detecting pathogens, and starts to interfere with the development of an efficient immune response (39, 40). Additionally, proteins of EBOV such as VP24 and VP35 antagonize the production of interferon (41, 42), which is one of the most important antiviral responses, and the envelope glycoprotein of EBOV known as GP has substantial toxicity for some tissues and especially to the vascular endothelium, which could cause coagulation disorders and bleeding (43).

EBOLA TRANSMISSION

Since the first Ebola epidemic of 1976 in the DRC, EBOV virus behaved as a wave front-like epidemic in a northwestern-southeastern direction, originating from a single epicenter (44). This wave-like epidemic behavior could be explained by environmental factors. Field surveys indicate that mortality excess among primates due to Ebola virus often appears at the end of the dry season (45), a period when food resources are scarce. Clustering of different species of fruit-eating animals such as bats, NHPs, and small terrestrial mammals around a limited number of fruit trees and fallen or partially eaten fruits or spats, during the dry season, would increase the probability of contact between infected and susceptible individuals of both reservoir and secondary host species, and promote virus transmission and disease spread (46). EVD epizooties would increase the opportunity of exposure to Ebola virus in humans living in rural and forest areas and having close contact with bats or secondary host species such as other primates.

Once an index case appears in a human population, contact with secretions and fluids from EVD cases, while either caring for afflicted patients or preparing bodies for funeral, was identified since the first outbreaks as the main transmission mode for the virus (47, 48).

Dynamics of the disease and EVD outbreaks in affected human populations will depend on the number of index cases introduced in that population and, most importantly, on the transmission capacity of the virus.

One of the most useful parameters to measure the transmission capacity of a pathogen is the average number of secondary cases generated by a primary case in a susceptible population, also called basic reproductive number (R_0) (49). R_0 depends on specific factors associated with the pathogen and human host susceptibility to infection and cycle of the pathogen (i.e., the period of time a case is infectious), but it also depends on the intensity and characteristics of social contact patterns and the prevalence of infection-prone behaviors in the affected group; therefore, R_0 for a specific pathogen may vary in different populations (50). Pathogen-associated factors favoring transmission are difficult to modify with human interventions; however, human host susceptibility and cycle of the pathogen, and social contact and risk behaviors could be modified with either medical (i.e., vaccine, prophylaxis, or early treatment) or public health (i.e., isolation, quarantine, or social distancing) countermeasures, resulting in a changing average number of secondary cases generated by a primary case during an outbreak, called effective reproductive number (R_e).

When R_0 associated with a pathogen is high, the epidemic growth will be fast and will affect most of the population in a short period of time. When R_0 is low, outbreak development will be slow, allowing for the implementation of effective transmission control measures and thus a reduction of R_e and of the expected final epidemic size. When R_0 for a pathogen is ≤1, there is no epidemic. An intervention is considered successful if it reduces R_e to <1 (49). There were no effective medical countermeasures for Ebola transmission control during the outbreak in West Africa in 2014–15, and therefore, reductions in R_e were to be achieved by implementing public health interventions.

A study of the dynamics of 1995 Ebola-Zaire virus outbreak in the DRC and the 2000 Ebola-Sudan virus outbreak in Uganda estimated an R_0 of 1.83 and 1.34, respectively, in the absence of control measures. The implementation of transmission control interventions reduced these figures, R_e, to 0.51 in the DRC and 0.66 in Uganda. This study showed, as expected, that the final epidemic size grows exponentially fast, with a 2-week delay in implementing public health control measures resulting in an approximately doubled outbreak size (51). This study found that the infectious period of the cases proposed by Breman et al. of 3.5 to 10.7 days (52) fits well with the evolution of the two studied outbreaks.

Similar R_0s for the 2013–2016 Ebola-Zaire virus epidemic in West Africa were estimated by the WHO Ebola response team: 1.71 (95% confidence interval [CI], 1.44 to 2.01) for Guinea, 1.83 (95% CI, 1.72 to 1.94) for Liberia, and 2.02 (95% CI, 1.79 to 2.26) for Sierra Leone during the initial period of exponential growth. By the end of August, after almost 9 months of outbreak but before widespread and effective implementation of public health control measures, R_e estimations were not very different except for Sierra Leona: 1.81 (95% CI, 1.60 to 2.03) for Guinea, 1.51 (95% CI, 1.41 to 1.60) for Liberia, and 1.38 (95% CI, 1.27 to 1.51) for Sierra Leone. The time for doubling the size of the epidemic in the absence of new control measures was estimated at 15.7 days (95% CI, 12.9 to 20.3) for Guinea, 23.6 days (95% CI, 20.2 to 28.2) for Liberia, and 30.2 days (95% CI, 23.6 to 42.3) for Sierra Leone (53). Another study found a compatible R_0 for the whole area during the same period, 1.44 (95% CI, 0.75 to 1.92) (54). The differences between R_0 and R_e in Sierra Leona observed by the WHO Ebola response

team could be explained by a super-spreader event at the beginning of the outbreak in this country, where up to 365 EVD cases were linked to a single funeral (55). This super-spreader event implied that a vast number of cases were introduced in a very short period of time in Sierra Leone's population, producing a more explosive growth of the outbreak compared with Guinea and Liberia.

Based on R_e estimates we can calculate the percentage of the population at risk that should be protected in order to control the outbreak by applying the formula $R_e - 1/R_e$ (49); in other words, the proportion of potential secondary cases that should be prevented to reduce R_e to ≤1: 45% (95% CI, 38 to 51%) in Guinea, 34% (95% CI, 29 to 38%) in Liberia, and 28% (95% CI, 21 to 34%) in Sierra Leone.

A few weeks after the United Nations Special Summit on Ebola, held in New York on September 25, 2014, and an exponential increase in international investment for implementing effective control measures in West Africa, R_e decreased to around or below 1, Ebola virus transmission was under control in all three affected countries, and the epidemic entered into a decline phase (56).

THE 2013–2016 EBOLA OUTBREAK IN WEST AFRICA

The first EVD outbreak in West Africa was identified and communicated at an international level on March 22, 2014. However, epidemiological investigations traced back the origin of the outbreak to December 2013 (55). A 2-year-old child living in Meliandou, a village in the Nzerekoré region in the southeast of Guinea and close to the border with Liberia and Sierra Leona, felt ill with high fever, black feces, and vomiting on December 26, 2013, and is considered the first case of the biggest Ebola outbreak ever known. The child died 2 days after onset of symptoms.

A few days later, in January 2014, the mother and the sister of the child died presenting similar symptoms and his grandmother was hospitalized in the nearby village of Gueckedou, where she died on January 14. The investigation team could identify five close contacts of this family who died within the following weeks, two in Sierra Leona, one in Conakry, and two traditional midwives who died also at the hospital of Gueckedou.

It was only in March 2014 when health authorities in Guinea suspected Ebola virus (a new disease in this part of Africa) as a possible cause of the "mysterious" disease of Meliandou. The first laboratory results from Pasteur Institute, available on March 22, confirmed Ebola virus infection in seven patients.

The porous border with Liberia and Sierra Leona, easy access to the capital cities of the three countries (Conakry, Monrovia, and Freetown), and family relationships between residents on both sides of the borders favored the rapid international spread of the virus. Unsafe traditional burial practices magnified the outbreak, putting already very fragile health systems under an unbearable pressure.

Nigeria identified on July 22 an imported case of EVD in a Liberian citizen who traveled by plane to Lagos on July 20. This patient, who was sick while traveling, was the first diagnosed in a country not sharing any border with Guinea, where the epidemic originated. He died on July 25 and was the origin of a 20-case outbreak in Nigeria, most of them among health care personnel who attended him. No travel contact of the case became ill, but it was the first sign of the risk of international spread of Ebola virus and the need for effective outbreak containment.

A few days later, on August 2 and 7, three humanitarian health workers, two from the United States and one from Spain, working in Liberia were evacuated to their countries after confirmed diagnoses of EVD.

On August 8, 2014, with 1,779 confirmed, probable, and suspected cases already notified in four countries, including 961 deaths, the general director of the WHO declared the EVD outbreak in West Africa a Public Health Emer-

gency of International Concern (PHEIC). A coordinated international response was considered essential to stop and reverse the largest-ever Ebola outbreak and its international spread. However, it was after the United Nations Special Summit on Ebola, held in New York on September 25, 2014, when there was an exponential increase in international investment in implementing effective control measures in West Africa. A few weeks later, Ebola virus transmission was under control in all three affected countries and the epidemic entered a decline phase (56). In the last week of January 2015, <100 cases were notified, for the first time since June 2014, and the focus shifted from slowing transmission to ending the epidemic. However, to achieve this objective would take a year longer.

Liberia, the country most affected, was first to be declared free of Ebola transmission, on May 9, 2015, 42 days after the death of the last diagnosed case. Unfortunately, two flare-ups were detected: the first on June 29 (declared free of Ebola again on September 3) and the second on November 19. Sierra Leona was declared free of Ebola transmission on November 7, but a flare-up was notified on January 14, 2016. Transmission control measures implemented in Guinea seemed to be less effective, probably due to people's mistrust of public health services, fear of communicating Ebola-related deaths in the community because of restrictions in traditional funerals, and because the outbreak in Guinea spread into rural areas, more difficult to reach by the public health teams (55). Guinea was the last country to be declared free of Ebola, on December 29, but again, as already seen in Liberia and Sierra Leona, two new cases were reported on March 16. A total of thirteen cases were reported in this new flare-up, ten in Guinea and three in Liberia infected from cases in the neighboring country.

Although the general director of the WHO declared the end of the PHEIC on March 29, 2016, Ebola transmission was declared over on June 1 in Guinea and on June

9 in Liberia. Almost two and a half years after it began, the Ebola virus outbreak of West Africa ended.

THE WEST AFRICA EBOLA OUTBREAK AMONG HEALTH CARE PROFESSIONALS

A special mention and acknowledgement is due to health care professionals who participated in the response to and control of the Ebola outbreak.

Health centers, hospitals, and health workers who failed to efficiently apply infection control measures acted as amplifying epidemic hubs for community transmission in previous Ebola outbreaks (57). This effect was observed to a lesser degree in West Africa.

The limited availability of health services and resources in Guinea, Liberia, and Sierra Leona and the extensive use of traditional medicine, self-treatment, and traditional healers could justify the reduced role of hospitals as outbreak amplifiers. This difference with previous outbreaks was more obvious in Guinea, where the capital city was less affected.

Despite the reduced role of health services in Ebola virus transmission, owing to the limited knowledge of the disease, the lack of appropriate triage procedures, insufficient equipment, and inadequate infection control practices during the first year of the epidemic, health care workers were at high risk of exposure to infection both at the health service level and in the community, leading to a high incidence of disease among health professionals (Table 1) (58).

TABLE 1 Cases and deaths among health care professionals, Ebola outbreak in West Africa, 2014–2016

Country	Cases	Deaths
Guinea	196	100
Liberia	378	192
Sierra Leona	307	221
Total	881	513

Source: World Health Organization. Ebola Situation Report, October 21, 2015.

Because of the high number of cases and deaths among health care workers, the population associated health services with high risk of infection. Hospitals were closed, both because of the high death toll among the personnel and because of absenteeism and the population's refusal to attend to those kept open. This situation led to an increase in maternal and infant mortality as well as a disruption of most public health programs, including national immunization programs (59). The reconstruction of the health systems was to be a major task in the postepidemic period.

Furthermore, among the 35 EVD cases identified out of the three countries with extensive transmission, 18 were in health care professionals (11 in Nigeria, 3 in Mali, 3 in the United States, and 1 in Spain). Three of them, the Spanish case and the two of the U.S. cases, infected in October 2014, were the first registered Ebola virus transmissions outside of Africa, except for a few laboratory accidents that occurred during manipulation of the virus for research projects.

EBOLA CASES IN EUROPE AND THE UNITED STATES

Out of the 28,610 registered cases of EVD, 31 were treated in Europe or the United States. Four of these cases were contracted in Africa but the onset of symptoms and diagnosis were in the country of treatment; 24 cases were diagnosed in Africa and then air-evacuated; and for the first time, 3 infections were contracted outside of Africa in the course of treating EVD cases (one in Spain and two in the United States). Most of them, 26 cases, were health care professionals who were infected while treating patients with EVD (55). Five of the European-U.S. cases died, as reported by Uyeki et al. in a study of 27 cases (60), and no other death was reported among this group of cases after their report. The lethality among EVD cases treated outside of Africa was therefore 16.1%, much lower than the

35 to 74% reported in Guinea, Liberia, and Sierra Leona (53, 56, 61–63). Although mortality due to EVD in Europe and United States was still high, close monitoring and aggressive supportive care, including intravenous fluid hydration, correction of electrolyte abnormalities, nutritional support, and critical care management for respiratory and renal failure, can improve survival among patients with EVD (60).

The 28 primary cases (evacuated cases and cases infected in Africa but with onset of symptoms in Europe or the United States) generated 3 secondary cases (all of them among health care professionals), 1 secondary case for every 10.3 primary cases ($R_e \sim 0.11$), despite treating cases with very high median EBOV RNA levels on admission, 2.7×10^7 copies/ml (60), which made them highly infectious. This very low transmission capacity, compared with Africa, was probably due to the application of strict infection control measures and the availability of high-quality personal protection equipment and isolation units.

Treating EVD patients in high-level medical units for the first time helped to improve understanding of the pathogenesis, the evolution of the disease, and the impact of aggressive ICU and supportive and experimental therapies, but also to better understand virus transmission in medical settings and from highly infectious patients. The identification of immunoprivileged sites, such as semen, cerebrospinal fluid, and vitreous humor, where live virus may persist for long periods of time is key for the control of transmission to health care workers, but also to understand the last phase of the outbreak and the observed flare-ups in all three affected African countries.

TRANSMISSION IN THE ERA OF NEXT-GENERATION SEQUENCING

The occurrence of an EVD epidemic involving tens of thousands of individuals and lasting more than 3 years is unique since it is probably the first time in history that such a long-term human-to-human transmission took place. The wide availability of next-generation sequencing (NGS) techniques has even allowed carrying of sequencing instruments in mobile facilities deployed in the field (64–66). This has facilitated the carrying out of evolutionary analysis, almost in real time, in the West Africa Ebola outbreak and the obtaining of valuable information on the complexity of transmission in what has been called "transmission analysis" (31). Application of NGS technology has allowed estimation of the evolutionary rate of virus replication in human hosts—8.2×10^{-4} to 9.6×10^{-4} substitutions/site/year (67)—and description of viral evolution during prolonged human-to-human transmission, pointing out changes in the sequence of EBOV/Mak that are suggestive of adaptation to a new host or escape mutants to humoral or cellular response (31, 66, 68). Also, it has been demonstrated by NGS that infectious doses of EBOV/Mak are large enough for intrahost variants to be transmitted between hosts (31). These evolutionary changes are also important since they might compromise the targets for molecular diagnostic tools or therapeutics with monoclonal antibodies (69, 70). Over all, transmission analysis helps to explain how the virus may have spread between the neighboring countries and has confirmed that the outbreak was initiated in Guinea in late 2013 and was the result of a single introduction of the virus in the human population (25, 66). This information also clarifies the movement of EBOV/Mak within the region and confirms that it moved from Guinea into Sierra Leone most likely in April or early May 2014, and then into Liberia in May or mid-June 2014 (66), also most probably by a single introduction event (70).

These data provide an unprecedented window into the evolution and dynamics of an active viral hemorrhagic fever outbreak and have the enormous value of being used in conjunction with epidemiological information to evaluate the effectiveness of control measures and the impact of public health programs (31, 68).

TREATMENT AND VACCINES FOR EVD

Before this outbreak there were limited data on the clinical utility of therapeutic strategies against EBOV. Due to the unpredictable occurrence of EVD outbreaks, research was limited to *in vitro* testing and experimental animal models consisting of rodents and NHPs. Based on this information, a number of agents were shown to have remarkable efficacy in treating experimentally infected rodents and/or macaques. The most promising compounds consisted of a combination of three monoclonal antibodies (ZMapp) directed against the envelope glycoprotein (GP) of EBOV (71), liposomal-formulated interfering RNA (TKM-130803) (72), and inhibitors of RNA polymerase: favipiravir (T-705) (73) and the new nucleoside analog GS-5734 (74). Despite the impressive results of some of these compounds in treating animals experimentally infected with EBOV, the results obtained in the few clinical trials that have been performed during this outbreak have not demonstrated significant impact on survival (75, 76), including the infusion of plasma from convalescent patients to acute infected individuals (77). Nevertheless, these clinical trials performed in West Africa in Ebola treatment units (ETUs) have been mostly uncontrolled and have involved a relatively small number of patients, too few to exclude a potential clinical impact of the medications. During this outbreak and for the first time, a number of EBOV-infected patients have been treated outside of Africa in modern facilities in Europe and the United States. The mortality in these groups of patients, 5 out of 27 (18.5%), is remarkably lower that that observed in ETUs in Africa (60). Although some of these patients received different experimental compounds as part of their treatment, it is thought that basic supportive therapy and specifically intensive rehydration and electrolyte balance have been the most beneficial factor. This intensive supportive therapy implies close monitoring and restoration of fluid and electrolytes through intravenous

lines, a practice that is mostly out of reach in the treatment facilities currently used in Africa (78).

It is clear that for the control of an outbreak of these characteristics an effective vaccine would have been extraordinarily helpful. As has been the case for drug treatments, several vaccine strategies for EBOV have been undergoing preclinical studies for the last 2 decades. Two main vaccines have proved efficacious in preventing EBOV infection in the NHP model. Both vaccines express GP as the single EBOV component and are virally vectored in chimpanzee adenovirus 3 (ChAD3) (79) and vesicular stomatitis virus (rVSV) (80), respectively. This EVD outbreak has encouraged the completion of the clinical development process of these vaccines in humans, and basically the phase 1 to 3/4 period that typically can last for 5 to 7 years has been compressed to 18 months (81, 82). Despite this fast-tracking of Ebola vaccines by the industry, regulatory agencies, and clinical groups, deployment of the vaccine trials in West Africa after completion of the phase 1 studies started in March 2015, at a time when the epidemics were vanishing in many areas. These circumstances made it very difficult to demonstrate the potential utility of the vaccines, so limited, but very important results are available from the clinical trial using the vaccine based on rVSV performed in Guinea from April to July 2015 (34). In this clinical trial a ring design was adopted to test the efficacy of the EBOV-rVSV vaccine. The design consisted in vaccinating all the close contacts of individuals with a new, confirmed diagnosis of EVD. A total of 90 clusters (rings) with a total population of 7,651 people were included. Clusters were randomized to be vaccinated immediately or after a delay of 21 days. No cases of infection by EBOV were observed in the immediate vaccination arm, whereas 16 cases were reported in the delayed vaccination arm, for an efficacy rate of 100% (95% CI, 74.7 to 100.0%; $P = 0.0036$) (34). This is the first time that a vaccine against EBOV proved to be effective in humans and, despite the relatively small population tested and the limitation of the design, opens a promising perspective to perform clinical trials in developing countries under devastating conditions and to eventually control this type of highly lethal infection.

CITATION

Delgado R, Simón F. 2017. Transmission, human population, and pathogenicity: the Ebola Case in point. Microbiol Spectrum 6(2):MTBP-0003-2016.

REFERENCES

1. **Kuhn JH, Bào Y, Bavari S, Becker S, Bradfute S, Brauburger K, Rodney Brister J, Bukreyev AA, Caì Y, Chandran K, Davey RA, Dolnik O, Dye JM, Enterlein S, Gonzalez JP, Formenty P, Freiberg AN, Hensley LE, Hoenen T, Honko AN, Ignatyev GM, Jahrling PB, Johnson KM, Klenk HD, Kobinger G, Lackemeyer MG, Leroy EM, Lever MS, Mühlberger E, Netesov SV, Olinger GG, Palacios G, Patterson JL, Paweska JT, Pitt L, Radoshitzky SR, Ryabchikova EI, Saphire EO, Shestopalov AM, Smither SJ, Sullivan NJ, Swanepoel R, Takada A, Towner JS, van der Groen G, Volchkov VE, Volchkova VA, Wahl-Jensen V, Warren TK, Warfield KL, Weidmann M, Nichol ST.** 2014. Virus nomenclature below the species level: a standardized nomenclature for filovirus strains and variants rescued from cDNA. *Arch Virol* **159:** 1229–1237.

2. **Kuhn JH, Becker S, Ebihara H, Geisbert TW, Johnson KM, Kawaoka Y, Lipkin WI, Negredo AI, Netesov SV, Nichol ST, Palacios G, Peters CJ, Tenorio A, Volchkov VE, Jahrling PB.** 2010. Proposal for a revised taxonomy of the family *Filoviridae*: classification, names of taxa and viruses, and virus abbreviations. *Arch Virol* **155:**2083–2103.

3. **Johnson KM, Lange JV, Webb PA, Murphy FA.** 1977. Isolation and partial characterisation of a new virus causing acute haemorrhagic fever in Zaire. *Lancet* **1:**569–571.

4. **Bowen ET, Lloyd G, Harris WJ, Platt GS, Baskerville A, Vella EE.** 1977. Viral haemorrhagic fever in southern Sudan and northern Zaire. Preliminary studies on the aetiological agent. *Lancet* **1:**571–573.

5. **Ahmad Z, Din NU, Ahmad A, Imran S, Pervez S, Ahmed R, Kayani N.** 2015. Rhabdomyosarcoma—

6. **Martini GA.** 1973. Marburg virus disease. *Postgrad Med J* **49:**542–546.

7. **Slenczka W, Klenk HD.** 2007. Forty years of Marburg virus. *J Infect Dis* **196**(Suppl 2):S131–S135.

8. **Barrette RW, Metwally SA, Rowland JM, Xu L, Zaki SR, Nichol ST, Rollin PE, Towner JS, Shieh WJ, Batten B, Sealy TK, Carrillo C, Moran KE, Bracht AJ, Mayr GA, Sirios-Cruz M, Catbagan DP, Lautner EA, Ksiazek TG, White WR, McIntosh MT.** 2009. Discovery of swine as a host for the Reston ebolavirus. *Science* **325:**204–206.

9. **Miranda ME, Ksiazek TG, Retuya TJ, Khan AS, Sanchez A, Fulhorst CF, Rollin PE, Calaor AB, Manalo DL, Roces MC, Dayrit MM, Peters CJ.** 1999. Epidemiology of Ebola (subtype Reston) virus in the Philippines, 1996. *J Infect Dis* **179**(Suppl 1):S115–S119.

10. **Feldmann H, Geisbert TW, Jahrling PB, Klenk HD, Netesov SV, Peters CJ, Sanchez A, Swanepoel R, Volchkov V.** 2005. *Family Filoviridae.* Elsevier/Academic Press, San Diego, CA.

11. **Feldmann H, Klenk HD, Sanchez A.** 1993. Molecular biology and evolution of filoviruses. *Arch Virol Suppl* **7:**81–100.

12. **Peters CJ, Sanchez A, Rollin PE, Ksiazek TG, Murphy GA.** 1996. *Filoviridae: Marburg and Ebola Viruses*, **vol 1.** Lippincott-Raven Press, Philadelphia, PA.

13. **Pringle CR.** 1998. Virus taxonomy—San Diego 1998. *Arch Virol* **143:**1449–1459.

14. **Bukreyev AA, Chandran K, Dolnik O, Dye JM, Ebihara H, Leroy EM, Mühlberger E, Netesov SV, Patterson JL, Paweska JT, Saphire EO, Smither SJ, Takada A, Towner JS, Volchkov VE, Warren TK, Kuhn JH.** 2014. Discussions and decisions of the 2012–2014 International Committee on Taxonomy of Viruses (ICTV) Filoviridae Study Group, January 2012–June 2013. *Arch Virol* **159:**821–830.

15. **Rollin PE, Williams RJ, Bressler DS, Pearson S, Cottingham M, Pucak G, Sanchez A, Trappier SG, Peters RL, Greer PW, Zaki S, Demarcus T, Hendricks K, Kelley M, Simpson D, Geisbert TW, Jahrling PB, Peters CJ, Ksiazek TG.** 1999. Ebola (subtype Reston) virus among quarantined nonhuman primates recently imported from the Philippines to the United States. *J Infect Dis* **179** (Suppl 1):S108–S114.

16. **Maruyama J, Miyamoto H, Kajihara M, Ogawa H, Maeda K, Sakoda Y, Yoshida R, Takada A.** 2013. Characterization of the envelope glycopro-

tein of a novel filovirus, Lloviu virus. *J Virol* **88:** 99–109.

17. Negredo A, Palacios G, Vázquez-Morón S, González F, Dopazo H, Molero F, Juste J, Quetglas J, Savji N, de la Cruz Martínez M, Herrera JE, Pizarro M, Hutchison SK, Echevarría JE, Lipkin WI, Tenorio A. 2011. Discovery of an ebolavirus-like filovirus in Europe. *PLoS Pathog* **7:**e1002304.

18. Bogoch II, Creatore MI, Cetron MS, Brownstein JS, Pesik N, Miniota J, Tam T, Hu W, Nicolucci A, Ahmed S, Yoon JW, Berry I, Hay S, Anema A, Tatem AJ, MacFadden D, German M, Khan K. 2014. Assessment of the potential for international dissemination of Ebola virus via commercial air travel during the 2014 west African outbreak. *Lancet* **385:**29–35.

19. Briand S, Bertherat E, Cox P, Formenty P, Kieny MP, Myhre JK, Roth C, Shindo N, Dye C. 2014. The international Ebola emergency. *N Engl J Med* **371:**1180–1183.

20. Groseth A, Feldmann H, Strong JE. 2007. The ecology of Ebola virus. *Trends Microbiol* **15:** 408–416.

21. Leroy EM, Kumulungui B, Pourrut X, Rouquet P, Hassanin A, Yaba P, Délicat A, Paweska JT, Gonzalez JP, Swanepoel R. 2005. Fruit bats as reservoirs of Ebola virus. *Nature* **438:**575–576.

22. Marí Saéz A, Weiss S, Nowak K, Lapeyre V, Zimmermann F, Düx A, Kühl HS, Kaba M, Regnaut S, Merkel K, Sachse A, Thiesen U, Villányi L, Boesch C, Dabrowski PW, Radonić A, Nitsche A, Leendertz SA, Petterson S, Becker S, Krähling V, Couacy-Hymann E, Akoua-Koffi C, Weber N, Schaade L, Fahr J, Borchert M, Gogarten JF, Calvignac-Spencer S, Leendertz FH. 2014. Investigating the zoonotic origin of the West African Ebola epidemic. *EMBO Mol Med* **7:** 17–23.

23. Leroy EM, Rouquet P, Formenty P, Souquière S, Kilbourne A, Froment JM, Bermejo M, Smit S, Karesh W, Swanepoel R, Zaki SR, Rollin PE. 2004. Multiple Ebola virus transmission events and rapid decline of central African wildlife. *Science* **303:**387–390.

24. Walsh PD, Abernethy KA, Bermejo M, Beyers R, De Wachter P, Akou ME, Huijbregts B, Mambounga DI, Toham AK, Kilbourn AM, Lahm SA, Latour S, Maisels F, Mbina C, Mihindou Y, Obiang SN, Effa EN, Starkey MP, Telfer P, Thibault M, Tutin CE, White LJ, Wilkie DS. 2003. Catastrophic ape decline in western equatorial Africa. *Nature* **422:**611–614.

25. Baize S, Pannetier D, Oestereich L, Rieger T, Koivogui L, Magassouba N, Soropogui B, Sow MS, Keïta S, De Clerck H, Tiffany A, Dominguez

G, Loua M, Traoré A, Kolié M, Malano ER, Heleze E, Bocquin A, Mély S, Raoul H, Caro V, Cadar D, Gabriel M, Pahlmann M, Tappe D, Schmidt-Chanasit J, Impouma B, Diallo AK, Formenty P, Van Herp M, Günther S. 2014. Emergence of Zaire Ebola virus disease in Guinea. *N Engl J Med* **371:**1418–1425.

26. Kuhn JH, Andersen KG, Baize S, Bào Y, Bavari S, Berthet N, Blinkova O, Brister JR, Clawson AN, Fair J, Gabriel M, Garry RF, Gire SK, Goba A, Gonzalez JP, Günther S, Happi CT, Jahrling PB, Kapetshi J, Kobinger G, Kugelman JR, Leroy EM, Maganga GD, Mbala PK, Moses LM, Muyembe-Tamfum JJ, N'Faly M, Nichol ST, Omilabu SA, Palacios G, Park DJ, Paweska JT, Radoshitzky SR, Rossi CA, Sabeti PC, Schieffelin JS, Schoepp RJ, Sealfon R, Swanepoel R, Towner JS, Wada J, Wauquier N, Yozwiak NL, Formenty P. 2014. Nomenclature- and database-compatible names for the two Ebola virus variants that emerged in Guinea and the Democratic Republic of the Congo in 2014. *Viruses* **6:**4760–4799.

27. Hoenen T, Groseth A, Feldmann F, Marzi A, Ebihara H, Kobinger G, Günther S, Feldmann H. 2014. Complete genome sequences of three Ebola virus isolates from the 2014 outbreak in West Africa. *Genome Announc* **2:**e01331-14.

28. de La Vega MA, Stein D, Kobinger GP. 2015. Ebolavirus evolution: past and present. *PLoS Pathog* **11:**e1005221.

29. Le Guenno B, Formenty P, Wyers M, Gounon P, Walker F, Boesch C. 1995. Isolation and partial characterisation of a new strain of Ebola virus. *Lancet* **345:**1271–1274.

30. Marzi A, Feldmann F, Hanley PW, Scott DP, Günther S, Feldmann H. 2015. Delayed disease progression in cynomolgus macaques infected with Ebola virus Makona strain. *Emerg Infect Dis* **21:**1777–1783.

31. Park DJ, Dudas G, Wohl S, Goba A, Whitmer SL, Andersen KG, Sealfon RS, Ladner JT, Kugelman JR, Matranga CB, Winnicki SM, Qu J, Gire SK, Gladden-Young A, Jalloh S, Nosamiefan D, Yozwiak NL, Moses LM, Jiang PP, Lin AE, Schaffner SF, Bird B, Towner J, Mamoh M, Gbakie M, Kanneh L, Kargbo D, Massally JL, Kamara FK, Konuwa E, Sellu J, Jalloh AA, Mustapha I, Foday M, Yillah M, Erickson BR, Sealy T, Blau D, Paddock C, Brault A, Amman B, Basile J, Bearden S, Belser J, Bergeron E, Campbell S, Chakrabarti A, Dodd K, Flint M, Gibbons A, Goodman C, Klena J, McMullan L, Morgan L, Russell B, Salzer J, Sanchez A, Wang D, Jungreis I, Tomkins-Tinch C, Kislyuk A, Lin MF, Chapman S, MacInnis B, Matthews A, Bochicchio J, Hensley LE, Kuhn

JH, Nusbaum C, Schieffelin JS, Birren BW, Forget M, Nichol ST, Palacios GF, Ndiaye D, Happi C, Gevao SM, Vandi MA, Kargbo B, Holmes EC, Bedford T, Gnirke A, Ströher U, Rambaut A, Garry RF, Sabeti PC. 2015. Ebola virus epidemiology, transmission, and evolution during seven months in Sierra Leone. *Cell* **161**: 1516–1526.

32. Luczkowiak J, Arribas JR, Gómez S, Jiménez-Yuste V, de la Calle F, Viejo A, Delgado R. 2016. Specific neutralizing response in plasma from convalescent patients of Ebola Virus Disease against the West Africa Makona variant of Ebola virus. *Virus Res* **213**:224–229.

33. Marzi A, Robertson SJ, Haddock E, Feldmann F, Hanley PW, Scott DP, Strong JE, Kobinger G, Best SM, Feldmann H. 2015. EBOLA VACCINE. VSV-EBOV rapidly protects macaques against infection with the 2014/15 Ebola virus outbreak strain. *Science* **349**:739–742.

34. Henao-Restrepo AM, Longini IM, Egger M, Dean NE, Edmunds WJ, Camacho A, Carroll MW, Doumbia M, Draguez B, Duraffour S, Enwere G, Grais R, Gunther S, Hossmann S, Kondé MK, Kone S, Kuisma E, Levine MM, Mandal S, Norheim G, Riveros X, Soumah A, Trelle S, Vicari AS, Watson CH, Kéïta S, Kieny MP, Røttingen J-A. 2015. Efficacy and effectiveness of an rVSV-vectored vaccine expressing Ebola surface glycoprotein: interim results from the Guinea ring vaccination cluster-randomised trial. *Lancet* **386**:857–866.

35. Deen GF, Knust B, Broutet N, Sesay FR, Formenty P, Ross C, Thorson AE, Massaquoi TA, Marrinan JE, Ervin E, Jambai A, McDonald SL, Bernstein K, Wurie AH, Dumbuya MS, Abad N, Idriss B, Wi T, Bennett SD, Davies T, Ebrahim FK, Meites E, Naidoo D, Smith S, Banerjee A, Erickson BR, Brault A, Durski KN, Winter J, Sealy T, Nichol ST, Lamunu M, Ströher U, Morgan O, Sahr F. 2015. Ebola RNA persistence in semen of Ebola virus disease survivors—preliminary report. *N Engl J Med.*

36. Mate SE, Kugelman JR, Nyenswah TG, Ladner JT, Wiley MR, Cordier-Lassalle T, Christie A, Schroth GP, Gross SM, Davies-Wayne GJ, Shinde SA, Murugan R, Sieh SB, Badio M, Fakoli L, Taweh F, de Wit E, van Doremalen N, Munster VJ, Pettitt J, Prieto K, Humrighouse BW, Ströher U, DiClaro JW, Hensley LE, Schoepp RJ, Safronetz D, Fair J, Kuhn JH, Blackley DJ, Laney AS, Williams DE, Lo T, Gasasira A, Nichol ST, Formenty P, Kateh FN, De Cock KM, Bolay F, Sanchez-Lockhart M, Palacios G. 2015. Molecular evidence of sexual transmission of Ebola virus. *N Engl J Med* **373**: 2448–2454.

37. Varkey JB, Shantha JG, Crozier I, Kraft CS, Lyon GM, Mehta AK, Kumar G, Smith JR, Kainulainen MH, Whitmer S, Ströher U, Uyeki TM, Ribner BS, Yeh S. 2015. Persistence of Ebola virus in ocular fluid during convalescence. *N Engl J Med* **372**:2423–2427.

38. Jacobs M, Rodger A, Bell DJ, Bhagani S, Cropley I, Filipe A, Gifford RJ, Hopkins S, Hughes J, Jabeen F, Johannessen I, Karageorgopoulos D, Lackenby A, Lester R, Liu RS, MacConnachie A, Mahungu T, Martin D, Marshall N, Mepham S, Orton R, Palmarini M, Patel M, Perry C, Peters SE, Porter D, Ritchie D, Ritchie ND, Seaton RA, Sreenu VB, Templeton K, Warren S, Wilkie GS, Zambon M, Gopal R, Thomson EC. 2016. Late Ebola virus relapse causing meningoencephalitis: a case report. *Lancet* **388**:498–503.

39. Alvarez CP, Lasala F, Carrillo J, Muñiz O, Corbí AL, Delgado R. 2002. C-type lectins DC-SIGN and L-SIGN mediate cellular entry by Ebola virus in cis and in trans. *J Virol* **76**:6841–6844.

40. Dominguez-Soto A, Aragoneses-Fenoll L, Martin-Gayo E, Martinez-Prats L, Colmenares M, Naranjo-Gomez M, Borras FE, Munoz P, Zubiaur M, Toribio ML, Delgado R, Corbi AL. 2007. The DC-SIGN-related lectin LSECtin mediates antigen capture and pathogen binding by human myeloid cells. *Blood* **109**:5337–5345.

41. Edwards MR, Liu G, Mire CE, Sureshchandra S, Luthra P, Yen B, Shabman RS, Leung DW, Messaoudi I, Geisbert TW, Amarasinghe GK, Basler CF. 2016. Differential regulation of interferon responses by Ebola and Marburg virus VP35 proteins. *Cell Rep* **14**:1632–1640.

42. Xu W, Edwards MR, Borek DM, Feagins AR, Mittal A, Alinger JB, Berry KN, Yen B, Hamilton J, Brett TJ, Pappu RV, Leung DW, Basler CF, Amarasinghe GK. 2014. Ebola virus VP24 targets a unique NLS binding site on karyopherin alpha 5 to selectively compete with nuclear import of phosphorylated STAT1. *Cell Host Microbe* **16**:187–200.

43. Yang ZY, Duckers HJ, Sullivan NJ, Sanchez A, Nabel EG, Nabel GJ. 2000. Identification of the Ebola virus glycoprotein as the main viral determinant of vascular cell cytotoxicity and injury. *Nat Med* **6**:886–889.

44. Walsh PD, Biek R, Real LA. 2005. Wave-like spread of Ebola Zaire. *PLoS Biol* **3**:e371.

45. Pinzon JE, Wilson JM, Tucker CJ, Arthur R, Jahrling PB, Formenty P. 2004. Trigger events: enviroclimatic coupling of Ebola hemorrhagic fever outbreaks. *Am J Trop Med Hyg* **71**:664–674.

46. Gonzalez JP, Pourrut X, Leroy E. 2007. Ebolavirus and other filoviruses. *Curr Top Microbiol Immunol* **315**:363–387.

47. **Anonymous.** 1978. Ebola haemorrhagic fever in Sudan, 1976. Report of a WHO/International Study Team. *Bull World Health Organ* **56**:247–270.

48. **Anonymous.** 1978. Ebola haemorrhagic fever in Zaire, 1976. *Bull World Health Organ* **56**:271–293.

49. **Anderson RM, May RM.** 1991. *Infectious Diseases of Humans.* Oxford University Press, Oxford, United Kingdom.

50. **Edmunds WJ, Gay NJ, Kretzschmar M, Pebody RG, Wachmann H, ESEN Project. European Sero-epidemiology Network.** 2000. The prevaccination epidemiology of measles, mumps and rubella in Europe: implications for modelling studies. *Epidemiol Infect* **125**:635–650.

51. **Chowell G, Hengartner NW, Castillo-Chavez C, Fenimore PW, Hyman JM.** 2004. The basic reproductive number of Ebola and the effects of public health measures: the cases of Congo and Uganda. *J Theor Biol* **229**:119–126.

52. **Breman JG, Heymann DL, Lloyd G, McCormick JB, Miatudila M, Murphy FA, Muyembé-Tamfun JJ, Piot P, Ruppol JF, Sureau P, van der Groen G, Johnson KM.** 2016. Discovery and description of Ebola Zaire virus in 1976 and relevance to the West African epidemic during 2013–2016. *J Infect Dis* **214**(suppl 3):S93–S101.

53. **Team WHOER, WHO Ebola Response Team.** 2014. Ebola virus disease in West Africa—the first 9 months of the epidemic and forward projections. *N Engl J Med* **371**:1481–1495.

54. **Barbarossa MV, Dénes A, Kiss G, Nakata Y, Röst G, Vizi Z.** 2015. Transmission dynamics and final epidemic size of Ebola virus disease outbreaks with varying interventions. *PLoS One* **10**:e0131398.

55. **World Health Organization.** Sierra Leone: a traditional healer and a funeral. http://www.who.int/csr/disease/ebola/ebola-6-months/sierra-leone/en/. Accessed July 20, 2016.

56. **Agua-Agum J, Ariyarajah A, Aylward B, Blake IM, Brennan R, Cori A, Donnelly CA, Dorigatti I, Dye C, Eckmanns T, Ferguson NM, Formenty P, Fraser C, Garcia E, Garske T, Hinsley W, Holmes D, Hugonnet S, Iyengar S, Jombart T, Krishnan R, Meijers S, Mills HL, Mohamed Y, Nedjati-Gilani G, Newton E, Nouvellet P, Pelletier L, Perkins D, Riley S, Sagrado M, Schnitzler J, Schumacher D, Shah A, Van Kerkhove MD, Varsaneux O, Wijekoon Kannangarage N, WHO Ebola Response Team.** 2015. West African Ebola epidemic after one year—slowing but not yet under control. *N Engl J Med* **372**:584–587.

57. **Peters CJ, LeDuc JW.** 1999. An introduction to Ebola: the virus and the disease. *J Infect Dis* **179** (Suppl 1):ix–xvi.

58. **Grinnell M, Dixon MG, Patton M, Fitter D, Bilivogui P, Johnson C, Dotson E, Diallo B, Rodier G, Raghunathan P.** 2015. Ebola virus disease in health care workers—Guinea, 2014. *MMWR Morb Mortal Wkly Rep* **64**:1083–1087.

59. **Evans DK, Goldstein M, Popova A.** 2015. Health-care worker mortality and the legacy of the Ebola epidemic. *Lancet Glob Health* **3**:e439–e440.

60. **Uyeki TM, Mehta AK, Davey RT, Jr, Liddell AM, Wolf T, Vetter P, Schmiedel S, Grünewald T, Jacobs M, Arribas JR, Evans L, Hewlett AL, Brantsaeter AB, Ippolito G, Rapp C, Hoepelman AI, Gutman J, Working Group of the U.S.-European Clinical Network on Clinical Management of Ebola Virus Disease Patients in the U.S. and Europe.** 2016. Clinical management of Ebola virus disease in the United States and Europe. *N Engl J Med* **374**:636–646.

61. **Schieffelin JS, Shaffer JG, Goba A, Gbakie M, Gire SK, Colubri A, Sealfon RS, Kanneh L, Moigboi A, Momoh M, Fullah M, Moses LM, Brown BL, Andersen KG, Winnicki S, Schaffner SF, Park DJ, Yozwiak NL, Jiang PP, Kargbo D, Jalloh S, Fonnie M, Sinnah V, French I, Kovoma A, Kamara FK, Tucker V, Konuwa E, Sellu J, Mustapha I, Foday M, Yillah M, Kanneh F, Saffa S, Massally JL, Boisen ML, Branco LM, Vandi MA, Grant DS, Happi C, Gevao SM, Fletcher TE, Fowler RA, Bausch DG, Sabeti PC, Khan SH, Garry RF, KGH Lassa Fever Program, Viral Hemorrhagic Fever Consortium, WHO Clinical Response Team.** 2014. Clinical illness and outcomes in patients with Ebola in Sierra Leone. *N Engl J Med* **371**:2092–2100.

62. **Bah EI, Lamah MC, Fletcher T, Jacob ST, Brett-Major DM, Sall AA, Shindo N, Fischer WA II, Lamontagne F, Saliou SM, Bausch DG, Moumié B, Jagatic T, Sprecher A, Lawler JV, Mayet T, Jacquerioz FA, Méndez Baggi MF, Vallenas C, Clement C, Mardel S, Faye O, Faye O, Soropogui B, Magassouba N, Koivogui L, Pinto R, Fowler RA.** 2015. Clinical presentation of patients with Ebola virus disease in Conakry, Guinea. *N Engl J Med* **372**:40–47.

63. **Qin E, Bi J, Zhao M, Wang Y, Guo T, Yan T, Li Z, Sun J, Zhang J, Chen S, Wu Y, Li J, Zhong Y.** 2015. Clinical features of patients with Ebola virus disease in Sierra Leone. *Clin Infect Dis* **61**:491–495.

64. **Quick J, Loman NJ, Duraffour S, Simpson JT, Severi E, Cowley L, Bore JA, Koundouno R, Dudas G, Mikhail A, Ouédraogo N, Afrough B, Bah A, Baum JH, Becker-Ziaja B, Boettcher JP, Cabeza-Cabrerizo M, Camino-Sánchez Á, Carter LL, Doerrbecker J, Enkirch T, García-Dorival I, Hetzelt N, Hinzmann J, Holm T,**

Kafetzopoulou LE, Koropogui M, Kosgey A, Kuisma E, Logue CH, Mazzarelli A, Meisel S, Mertens M, Michel J, Ngabo D, Nitzsche K, Pallasch E, Patrono LV, Portmann J, Repits JG, Rickett NY, Sachse A, Singethan K, Vitoriano I, Yemanaberhan RL, Zekeng EG, Racine T, Bello A, Sall AA, Faye O, Faye O, Magassouba N, Williams CV, Amburgey V, Winona L, Davis E, Gerlach J, Washington F, Monteil V, Jourdain M, Bererd M, Camara A, Somlare H, Camara A, Gerard M, Bado G, Baillet B, Delaune D, Nebie KY, Diarra A, Savane Y, Pallawo RB, Gutierrez GJ, Milhano N, Roger I, Williams CJ, Yattara F, Lewandowski K, Taylor J, Rachwal P, Turner DJ, Pollakis G, Hiscox JA, Matthews DA, O'Shea MK, Johnston AM, Wilson D, Hutley E, Smit E, Di Caro A, Wölfel R, Stoecker K, Fleischmann E, Gabriel M, Weller SA, Koivogui L, Diallo B, Keïta S, Rambaut A, Formenty P, Günther S, Carroll MW. 2016. Real-time, portable genome sequencing for Ebola surveillance. *Nature* **530:**228–232.

65. Hoenen T, Groseth A, Rosenke K, Fischer RJ, Hoenen A, Judson SD, Martellaro C, Falzarano D, Marzi A, Squires RB, Wollenberg KR, de Wit E, Prescott J, Safronetz D, van Doremalen N, Bushmaker T, Feldmann F, McNally K, Bolay FK, Fields B, Sealy T, Rayfield M, Nichol ST, Zoon KC, Massaquoi M, Munster VJ, Feldmann H. 2016. Nanopore sequencing as a rapidly deployable Ebola outbreak tool. *Emerg Infect Dis* **22:** 331–334.

66. Carroll MW, Matthews DA, Hiscox JA, Elmore MJ, Pollakis G, Rambaut A, Hewson R, García-Dorival I, Bore JA, Koundouno R, Abdellati S, Afrough B, Aiyepada J, Akhilomen P, Asogun D, Atkinson B, Badusche M, Bah A, Bate S, Baumann J, Becker D, Becker-Ziaja B, Bocquin A, Borremans B, Bosworth A, Boettcher JP, Cannas A, Carletti F, Castilletti C, Clark S, Colavita F, Diederich S, Donatus A, Duraffour S, Ehichioya D, Ellerbrok H, Fernandez-Garcia MD, Fizet A, Fleischmann E, Gryseels S, Hermelink A, Hinzmann J, Hopf-Guevara U, Ighodalo Y, Jameson L, Kelterbaum A, Kis Z, Kloth S, Kohl C, Korva M, Kraus A, Kuisma E, Kurth A, Liedigk B, Logue CH, Lüdtke A, Maes P, McCowen J, Mély S, Mertens M, Meschi S, Meyer B, Michel J, Molkenthin P, Muñoz-Fontela C, Muth D, Newman EN, Ngabo D, Oestereich L, Okosun J, Olokor T, Omiunu R, Omomoh E, Pallasch E, Pályi B, Portmann J, Pottage T, Pratt C, Priesnitz S, Quartu S, Rappe J, Repits J, Richter M, Rudolf M, Sachse A, Schmidt KM, Schudt G, Strecker T, Thom R, Thomas S, Tobin E, Tolley H, Trautner J, Vermoesen T, Vitoriano I, Wagner M, Wolff S,

Yue C, Capobianchi MR, Kretschmer B, Hall Y, Kenny JG, Rickett NY, Dudas G, Coltart CE, Kerber R, Steer D, Wright C, Senyah F, Keita S, Drury P, Diallo B, de Clerck H, Van Herp M, Sprecher A, Traore A, Diakite M, Konde MK, Koivogui L, Magassouba N, Avšič-Županc T, Nitsche A, Strasser M, Ippolito G, Becker S, Stoecker K, Gabriel M, Raoul H, Di Caro A, Wölfel R, Formenty P, Günther S. 2015. Temporal and spatial analysis of the 2014–2015 Ebola virus outbreak in West Africa. *Nature* **524:** 97–101.

67. Hoenen T, Safronetz D, Groseth A, Wollenberg KR, Koita OA, Diarra B, Fall IS, Haidara FC, Diallo F, Sanogo M, Sarro YS, Kone A, Togo AC, Traore A, Kodio M, Dosseh A, Rosenke K, de Wit E, Feldmann F, Ebihara H, Munster VJ, Zoon KC, Feldmann H, Sow S. 2015. Virology. Mutation rate and genotype variation of Ebola virus from Mali case sequences. *Science* **348:**117–119.

68. Gire SK, Goba A, Andersen KG, Sealfon RS, Park DJ, Kanneh L, Jalloh S, Momoh M, Fullah M, Dudas G, Wohl S, Moses LM, Yozwiak NL, Winnicki S, Matranga CB, Malboeuf CM, Qu J, Gladden AD, Schaffner SF, Yang X, Jiang PP, Nekoui M, Colubri A, Coomber MR, Fonnie M, Moigboi A, Gbakie M, Kamara FK, Tucker V, Konuwa E, Saffa S, Sellu J, Jalloh AA, Kovoma A, Koninga J, Mustapha I, Kargbo K, Foday M, Yillah M, Kanneh F, Robert W, Massally JL, Chapman SB, Bochicchio J, Murphy C, Nusbaum C, Young S, Birren BW, Grant DS, Scheiffelin JS, Lander ES, Happi C, Gevao SM, Gnirke A, Rambaut A, Garry RF, Khan SH, Sabeti PC. 2014. Genomic surveillance elucidates Ebola virus origin and transmission during the 2014 outbreak. *Science* **345:**1369–1372.

69. Kugelman JR, Kugelman-Tonos J, Ladner JT, Pettit J, Keeton CM, Nagle ER, Garcia KY, Froude JW, Kuehne AI, Kuhn JH, Bavari S, Zeitlin L, Dye JM, Olinger GG, Sanchez-Lockhart M, Palacios GF. 2015. Emergence of Ebola virus escape variants in infected nonhuman primates treated with the MB-003 antibody cocktail. *Cell Rep* **12:**2111–2120.

70. Kugelman JR, Wiley MR, Mate S, Ladner JT, Beitzel B, Fakoli L, Taweh F, Prieto K, Diclaro JW, Minogue T, Schoepp RJ, Schaecher KE, Pettitt J, Bateman S, Fair J, Kuhn JH, Hensley L, Park DJ, Sabeti PC, Sanchez-Lockhart M, Bolay FK, Palacios G, US Army Medical Research Institute of Infectious Diseases, National Institutes of Health, Integrated Research Facility–Frederick Ebola Response Team 2014-2015. 2015. Monitoring of Ebola virus Makona evolution through establishment

of advanced genomic capability in Liberia. *Emerg Infect Dis* **21**:1135–1143.

71. Qiu X, Wong G, Audet J, Bello A, Fernando L, Alimonti JB, Fausther-Bovendo H, Wei H, Aviles J, Hiatt E, Johnson A, Morton J, Swope K, Bohorov O, Bohorova N, Goodman C, Kim D, Pauly MH, Velasco J, Pettitt J, Olinger GG, Whaley K, Xu B, Strong JE, Zeitlin L, Kobinger GP. 2014. Reversion of advanced Ebola virus disease in nonhuman primates with ZMapp. *Nature* **514**:47–53.

72. Geisbert TW, Lee ACH, Robbins M, Geisbert JB, Honko AN, Sood V, Johnson JC, de Jong S, Tavakoli I, Judge A, Hensley LE, Maclachlan I. 2010. Postexposure protection of non-human primates against a lethal Ebola virus challenge with RNA interference: a proof-of-concept study. *Lancet* **375**:1896–1905.

73. Oestereich L, Lüdtke A, Wurr S, Rieger T, Muñoz-Fontela C, Günther S. 2014. Successful treatment of advanced Ebola virus infection with T-705 (favipiravir) in a small animal model. *Antiviral Res* **105**:17–21.

74. Warren TK, Jordan R, Lo MK, Ray AS, Mackman RL, Soloveva V, Siegel D, Perron M, Bannister R, Hui HC, Larson N, Strickley R, Wells J, Stuthman KS, Van Tongeren SA, Garza NL, Donnelly G, Shurtleff AC, Retterer CJ, Gharaibeh D, Zamani R, Kenny T, Eaton BP, Grimes E, Welch LS, Gomba L, Wilhelmsen CL, Nichols DK, Nuss JE, Nagle ER, Kugelman JR, Palacios G, Doerffler E, Neville S, Carra E, Clarke MO, Zhang L, Lew W, Ross B, Wang Q, Chun K, Wolfe L, Babusis D, Park Y, Stray KM, Trancheva I, Feng JY, Barauskas O, Xu Y, Wong P, Braun MR, Flint M, McMullan LK, Chen SS, Fearns R, Swaminathan S, Mayers DL, Spiropoulou CF, Lee WA, Nichol ST, Cihlar T, Bavari S. 2016. Therapeutic efficacy of the small molecule GS-5734 against Ebola virus in rhesus monkeys. *Nature* **531**:381–385.

75. Sissoko D, Laouenan C, Folkesson E, M'Lebing AB, Beavogui AH, Baize S, Camara AM, Maes P, Shepherd S, Danel C, Carazo S, Conde MN, Gala JL, Colin G, Savini H, Bore JA, Le Marcis F, Koundouno FR, Petitjean F, Lamah MC, Diederich S, Tounkara A, Poelart G, Berbain E, Dindart JM, Duraffour S, Lefevre A, Leno T, Peyrouset O, Irenge L, Bangoura N, Palich R, Hinzmann J, Kraus A, Barry TS, Berette S, Bongono A, Camara MS, Chanfreau Munoz V, Doumbouya L, Souley Harouna, Kighoma PM, Koundouno FR, Réné Lolamou, Loua CM, Massala V, Moumouni K, Provost C, Samake N, Sekou C, Soumah A, Arnould I, Komano MS, Gustin L, Berutto C, Camara D, Camara FS, Colpaert J, Delamou L, Jansson L, Kourouma E, Loua M, Malme K, Manfrin E, Maomou A, Milinouno A, Ombelet S, Sidiboun AY, Verreckt I, Yombouno P, Bocquin A, Carbonnelle C, Carmoi T, Frange P, Mely S, Nguyen VK, Pannetier D, Taburet AM, Treluyer JM, Kolie J, Moh R, Gonzalez MC, Kuisma E, Liedigk B, Ngabo D, Rudolf M, Thom R, Kerber R, Gabriel M, Di Caro A, Wölfel R, Badir J, Bentahir M, Deccache Y, Dumont C, Durant JF, El Bakkouri K, Gasasira Uwamahoro M, Smits B, Toufik N, Van Cauwenberghe S, Ezzedine K, D'Ortenzio E, Pizarro L, Etienne A, Guedj J, Fizet A, Barte de Sainte Fare E, Murgue B, Tran-Minh T, Rapp C, Piguet P, Poncin M, Draguez B, Allaford Duverger T, Barbe S, Baret G, Defourny I, Carroll M, Raoul H, Augier A, Eholie SP, Yazdanpanah Y, Levy-Marchal C, Antierrens A, Van Herp M, Günther S, de Lamballerie X, Keïta S, Mentre F, Anglaret X, Malvy D, JIKI Study Group. 2016. Experimental treatment with favipiravir for Ebola virus disease (the JIKI trial): a historically controlled, single-arm proof-of-concept trial in Guinea. *PLoS Med* **13**:e1001967.

76. Dunning J, Sahr F, Rojek A, Gannon F, Carson G, Idriss B, Massaquoi T, Gandi R, Joseph S, Osman HK, Brooks TJ, Simpson AJ, Goodfellow I, Thorne L, Arias A, Merson L, Castle L, Howell-Jones R, Pardinaz-Solis R, Hope-Gill B, Ferri M, Grove J, Kowalski M, Stepniewska K, Lang T, Whitehead J, Olliaro P, Samai M, Horby PW, RAPIDE-TKM trial team. 2016. Experimental treatment of Ebola virus disease with TKM-130803: a single-arm phase 2 clinical trial. *PLoS Med* **13**:e1001997.

77. van Griensven J, Edwards T, de Lamballerie X, Semple MG, Gallian P, Baize S, Horby PW, Raoul H, Magassouba N, Antierens A, Lomas C, Faye O, Sall AA, Fransen K, Buyze J, Ravinetto R, Tiberghien P, Claeys Y, De Crop M, Lynen L, Bah EI, Smith PG, Delamou A, De Weggheleire A, Haba N, Ebola-Tx Consortium. 2016. Evaluation of convalescent plasma for Ebola virus disease in Guinea. *N Engl J Med* **374**:33–42.

78. Lamontagne F, Clément C, Fletcher T, Jacob ST, Fischer WA II, Fowler RA. 2014. Doing today's work superbly well—treating Ebola with current tools. *N Engl J Med* **371**:1565–1566.

79. Stanley DA, Honko AN, Asiedu C, Trefry JC, Lau-Kilby AW, Johnson JC, Hensley L, Ammendola V, Abbate A, Grazioli F, Foulds KE, Cheng C, Wang L, Donaldson MM, Colloca S, Folgori A, Roederer M, Nabel GJ, Mascola J, Nicosia A, Cortese R, Koup RA, Sullivan NJ. 2014. Chimpanzee adenovirus vaccine generates acute and durable protective

immunity against ebolavirus challenge. *Nat Med* **20**:1126–1129.

80. Marzi A, Feldmann H, Geisbert TW, Falzarano D. 2011. Vesicular stomatitis virus-based vaccines for prophylaxis and treatment of filovirus infections. *J Bioterror Biodef* **S1**:2157-2526-S1-004.

81. Ledgerwood JE, DeZure AD, Stanley DA, Novik L, Enama ME, Berkowitz NM, Hu Z, Joshi G, Ploquin A, Sitar S, Gordon IJ, Plummer SA, Holman LA, Hendel CS, Yamshchikov G, Roman F, Nicosia A, Colloca S, Cortese R, Bailer RT, Schwartz RM, Roederer M, Mascola JR, Koup RA, Sullivan NJ, Graham BS. 2017. Chimpanzee Adenovirus Vector Ebola Vaccine. *N Engl J Med* **376**(10):928–938.

82. Agnandji ST, Huttner A, Zinser ME, Njuguna P, Dahlke C, Fernandes JF, Yerly S, Dayer JA, Kraehling V, Kasonta R, Adegnika AA, Altfeld M, Auderset F, Bache EB, Biedenkopf N, Borregaard S, Brosnahan JS, Burrow R, Combescure C, Desmeules J, Eickmann M, Fehling SK, Finckh A, Goncalves AR, Grobusch MP, Hooper J, Jambrecina A, Kabwende AL, Kaya G, Kimani D, Lell B, Lemaître B, Lohse AW, Massinga-Loembe M, Matthey A, Mordmüller B, Nolting A, Ogwang C, Ramharter M, Schmidt-Chanasit J, Schmiedel S, Silvera P, Stahl FR, Staines HM, Strecker T, Stubbe HC, Tsofa B, Zaki S, Fast P, Moorthy V, Kaiser L, Krishna S, Becker S, Kieny MP, Bejon P, Kremsner PG, Addo MM, Siegrist CA. 2016. Phase 1 trials of rVSV Ebola vaccine in Africa and Europe. *N Engl J Med* **374**: 1647–1660.

EXPERIMENTAL AND THEORETICAL MODES OF TRANSMISSION

Quantifying Transmission

16

MARK WOOLHOUSE[1]

INTRODUCTION

Transmissibility is the defining attribute of infectious diseases, and it has profound consequences for their epidemiology. In contrast to noncommunicable diseases, the risk of an individual contracting an infectious disease increases with the number of infected and infectious individuals present in the population. This is positive feedback, and it makes the epidemiology of infectious diseases considerably more complex and often hard to understand intuitively. For example, reducing the per capita transmission rate is expected to decrease the size of an epidemic, but it is difficult to estimate by how much; because of the positive feedback, there is not a proportional (or linear) relationship between epidemic size and transmission rate. Less obvious still is the expectation that decreasing transmission rate may increase rather than decrease the duration of an outbreak (1).

A quantitative understanding of transmission is therefore central to infectious disease epidemiology and to evidence-based decisions on prevention and control strategies. Nonetheless, measuring transmission either retrospectively (estimating how many transmission events have occurred) or prospectively (estimating transmission risk) is often a formidable technical challenge.

[1]Centre for Immunity, Infection and Evolution, University of Edinburgh, Edinburgh, United Kingdom.
Microbial Transmission in Biological Processes
Edited by Fernando Baquero, Emilio Bouza, J.A. Gutiérrez-Fuentes, and Teresa M. Coque
© 2018 American Society for Microbiology, Washington, DC
doi:10.1128/microbiolspec.MTBP-0005-2016

In this chapter, I review some of the various approaches used to quantify transmissibility at both the individual and population levels.

TRANSMISSION EVENTS

Retrospective investigation of transmission events is a well-established activity that contributes to standard public health procedures such as epidemiological tracing, outbreak investigation, and forensic epidemiology (2). These are usually empirical exercises based on knowledge of transmission routes, contact histories (i.e., transmission opportunities), epidemiological risk factors, and the so-called natural history of infection, which indicates the possible relative timings of key events such as exposure, the onset of infectiousness, and the onset of clinical signs (Fig. 1). These techniques are widely used for a range of infectious diseases such as measles (3) and foot-and-mouth disease (FMD) (4). Epidemiological data may be supplemented by pathogen typing data, preferably as detailed as possible to maximize the ability to discriminate between dissimilar strains in two or more hosts, thus ruling out a transmission event. The outputs of epidemiological tracing studies typically take the form of a (sometimes subjective) assessment of the likelihood that individual X infected individual Y.

Much greater levels of confidence may be achieved where pathogen sequence data are available. The analysis of sequence data to establish transmission pathways—"who infected whom"—is known as forensic phylogenetics. Forensic phylogenetics takes advantage of the high nucleotide substitution rates in fast-evolving RNA viruses (of the order of 1×10^{-3} to 5×10^{-3} per site per year), making it possible to use sequences isolated from different individuals at different times in order to estimate time-resolved phylogenetic trees. Forensic phylogenetics has been used, for example, in suspected cases of HIV/AIDS transmission and can confirm or rule out transmission events with a high level of certainty (5).

INDIVIDUAL TRANSMISSIBILITY

Empirical studies of individual transmissibility can be considered under two subheadings: (i) infectiousness, i.e., the potential of an infected individual to infect others given the opportunity to do so; and (ii) opportunities to transmit, as determined by some measure of the behavior or other attributes of the infected individual relevant to a pathogen's route of transmission.

Infectiousness may be most straightforwardly measured by quantifying pathogens exiting from the host body in feces (e.g., *Escherichia coli* bacteria counts in stool samples) or urine (e.g., egg counts for *Schistosoma haematobium*), as aerosols (e.g., influenza virus particles in droplets), or as the successful infection of vectors (e.g., tsetse vectors of trypanosomes). More indirect measures are also used (e.g., density of malaria gametocytes in host blood). Simple assays of viremia or bacteremia in the blood are the most widely used as measures of infectiousness, but these are less satisfactory if transmission is not via the blood (e.g., influenza virus).

The gold standard determination of infectiousness is experimental exposure of sus-

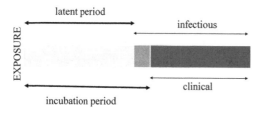

FIGURE 1 Time line of exposure, infectiousness, and clinical signs. Following exposure to infection, there is a period when the host is infected but not yet infectious—the latent period (yellow)—and a period when the host is infected but not yet showing clinical signs—the incubation period (yellow and orange). In this example, there is a (brief) period when the host is infectious but asymptomatic (orange), as occurs for infections such as influenza or FMD.

ceptible hosts to infected hosts, though this is far less frequently attempted, especially for natural hosts (e.g., humans, cattle, and pigs) as opposed to model systems. Importantly, such studies have the ability to distinguish between pathogen detection and sufficient levels of pathogen excretion to infect other hosts. For example, an experimental study of FMD virus (FMDV) transmission between cattle (6) suggested that the period for which infected cattle could infect in-contact cattle was substantially less than the period for which virus could be detected (often at very low levels) in the blood, and that cattle were typically infectious for only a short period before clinical signs appeared (Fig. 2). This has important implications for what are termed reactive control measures, i.e., imple-

menting preventive measures once clinical disease is detected, since if clinical cases are detected and removed early enough, then transmission rates can be greatly reduced (6).

Estimating an individual's opportunities to transmit infection requires information on behaviors associated with a risk of transmission. A straightforward example is commercial sex workers and the transmission of sexually transmitted infections. Identification of sex workers and their sexual contacts enables the provision of health interventions that would benefit the individuals concerned and also be beneficial in public health terms by reducing the risk of onward transmission.

More generally, contact tracing is a standard public health tool that can be used not only retrospectively (as described above) but also prospectively to identify at-risk individuals who have been exposed to an infected individual and might require preventive interventions (e.g., quarantine or vaccination) or therapy. Contact tracing is widely used during infectious disease outbreaks, such as the 2014–2015 ebolavirus epidemic in West Africa (7). This kind of approach is useful for pathogens transmitted by direct contact or close proximity of individuals (e.g., HIV or influenza) but usually not for those transmitted indirectly, such as via the fecal-oral route (e.g., cholera) or by vectors (e.g., malaria or Zika virus).

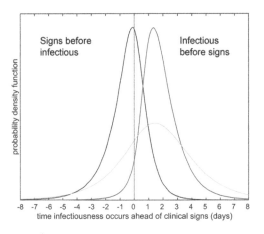

FIGURE 2 Infectiousness of FMDV in experimental infections of cattle. Distribution of the incubation period minus the latent period, predicted using a Bayesian analysis, where a negative value indicates when clinical signs appear before an animal is infectious. The plot shows that when infectiousness is measured directly by the exposure of in-contact susceptible cattle, the analysis indicates that only a small fraction of infectiousness is found to occur before the appearance of clinical signs (black line). In contrast, if infectiousness is measured indirectly using virus isolation from blood (red) or nasal fluid (green), the bulk of infectiousness is estimated to occur well before clinical signs appear. Data from reference 6; figure kindly supplied by Simon Gubbins.

Factors affecting individual transmissibility (infectiousness and transmission opportunities) can, in principle, be investigated and their effects quantified using standard epidemiological risk analyses. However, in marked contrast to the vast number of empirical studies of risk factors for becoming infected (susceptibility and exposure), few studies of transmissibility of this kind have been published. There are some obvious reasons for this lack of attention. First, it is often much harder to establish that an individual has transmitted infection than that it has acquired infection. Second, the sample size available is not the total population but the infected population (each of whom may or may not have transmitted infection onwards), typically a much smaller number with a corresponding loss of statistical power to identify risk factors. Examples of quantitative analysis of the risk of onward transmission include farms infected with FMD (8) and *E. coli* O157 on cattle farms (9).

POPULATION-LEVEL TRANSMISSIBILITY

Contact tracing can, in principle, be scaled up from the individual to the population level if the distribution of the key risk factors across the population is known. An example is the reconstruction of transmission "trees" for the spread of FMD between livestock farms in the United Kingdom in 2001 based on the dates on which FMD was detected and the distances between farms, given that inter-farm distance was known to be a major risk factor (10). Applied in real time, with the incorporation of information on additional risk factors where available, such methods enable estimation of the case reproduction number (the average number of cases generated per case) and therefore projections of epidemic trajectory (11). In general, population-level contact tracing is likely to be less accurate than individual-level contact tracing since many of the detailed risk factors, e.g., movement of people from one household to another or sexual contacts, are not knowable for the entire population. Even so, demographic and geographic variables may represent useful proxies for individual risk behaviors and thus be used to generate good approximations of transmission patterns at the population level.

In recent years, the availability of pathogen genome sequences coupled with advances in bioinformatics analysis have led to the increasing use of phylogeographic approaches to understanding transmission patterns at the population level. As an early example, phylogenetic analyses of FMDV genome sequence data from a subset of affected farms from the 2001 U.K. epidemic largely supported the results of contact tracing studies, but did suggest some revisions to those assessments (12). More recently, ebolavirus genome sequences from West Africa in 2014-15 were analyzed to obtain estimates of the case reproduction rate, infectious period, and sampling fraction, and provided important supporting data for projections of epidemic trajectory based on case reports (13).

A potentially powerful application of phylogeographic methods is to quantify the frequency with which a pathogen moves between populations, representing different locations, e.g., cities, or different host species. Given that only a fraction, often a very small fraction, of cases provide sequence data, these methods do not provide estimates of absolute rates of transmission but can show whether transmission has occurred and, in principle, indicate the relative importance of different routes. Examples include the transmission of the SAT2 topotype of FMDV between different ungulate species in Africa (14) and the transmission of the CC398 clade of methicillin-resistant *Staphylococcus aureus* between humans and livestock (15).

These two studies covered time spans of several decades; using sequence data to resolve epidemiological questions is challenging due to the short time scales, and therefore few nucleotide substitutions, involved. However, phylogeographic techniques have been used during epidemics, for example, to investigate the geographic origins and spread of H1N1 influenza A in 2009 (16). Similarly, this approach has been used to determine the source of outbreaks. For example, Middle East respiratory syndrome outbreaks tend to occur as genetically distant lineages persisting for only a few months each, suggesting multiple introductions from an animal reservoir with limited human-to-human transmission (17). In contrast, both the 2009 H1N1 influenza pandemic and 2014 West Africa ebolavirus disease epidemic consisted of single rapidly expanding lineages, suggesting single introductions followed by sustained human-to-human transmission.

A key parameter in interpreting sequence data is the time to most recent common ancestor (TMRCA) of the cases. From sequences obtained during an outbreak, however sparsely sampled, a TMRCA much longer ago than the first reported case suggests an unobserved epidemic, e.g., in a reservoir population, and multiple origins for the current outbreak. For outbreaks that spread entirely within the host population, the TMRCA of the sequenced cases will be closer to the date of the first infection (whether sampled or not) and provides an estimate of when the pathogen was introduced into that population.

MODELING

Mathematical models have been used in infectious disease epidemiology for more than 100 years (18). A key parameter in such models is the per capita transmission rate, often designated as β. β is a composite parameter, encompassing infectiousness, opportunities to transmit the infection, and susceptibility. It is also a component of the basic reproduction number, R_0, the average number of infections generated by a single infection introduced into a large population of previously uneHxposed hosts. The threshold $R_0 > 1$ is a condition for a large outbreak or epidemic to be possible.

Rapid and accurate estimation of β and R_0 are therefore extremely important for predicting the trajectory of an infectious disease outbreak. Neither parameter is likely to be known precisely in advance of an outbreak since they vary with the characteristics of the pathogen (e.g., strain differences) and the host population (demography, contact patterns, and risk behavior). Comparative assessments may be possible; e.g., for pathogens transmitted by direct contact, such as measles or influenza A, transmission rates may be higher in higher-density host populations. However, even for these kinds of pathogens the common assumption that β scales linearly with host density—so-called density-dependent transmission—may be overly simplistic, for example, in spatially structured populations (19). Often, quantitative estimates for a specific pathogen in a specific host population are only possible once an outbreak is occurring.

The standard approach to obtaining quantitative estimates of β and R_0 is to fit an appropriate epidemiological model to time series data on epidemic progression, usually based on clinical cases but sometimes on diagnosis of infection or of exposure (e.g., by serology). This exercise requires additional information on the generation time, i.e., the average interval between the time of infection of a host and onward transmission of infection by that host. It also requires accurate data, which may be problematic. For example, data collection was poor during the early stages of the West African ebolavirus epidemic, and the majority of H1N1 cases were subclinical and unreported during the 2009 pandemic. Model assumptions may also be critical, especially whether or not the host population can be regarded as homogeneous from the perspective of pathogen transmission (see next section).

Recently, methods have been developed for estimating population transmission rates using pathogen genome sequence data. These methods are based on estimates of changes in the effective population size of the pathogen over time. They were used for both the 2009 influenza A pandemic and the 2014–2015 ebolavirus epidemic (17) and were helpful in supporting or challenging estimates made using epidemiological data. In order to inform public health responses during an infectious disease outbreak, pathogen sequences need to be obtained and made available for analysis in real time. This has recently become technically feasible, and is likely to become a more widely used epidemiological tool for outbreak management (17). In the future, the most accurate estimates of transmission parameters, requiring the minimum of data, are likely to come from the integrated analysis of combinations of epidemiological and pathogen sequence data (20).

HETEROGENEITIES

Individual variation in infectiousness, contact behavior, and susceptibility can have consequences for infectious disease epidemiology at the population level (21, 22). These include potentially substantial effects on the likelihood that an outbreak will take off, the initial rate of growth, and the scale and duration of the outbreak. Such variation may also favor targeted intervention strategies that not only protect those most at risk of infection but also prevent the onward transmission of infection from those most likely to do so.

Heterogeneities in infectiousness may involve a phenomenon termed "super-shedding," meaning that a small proportion of individuals are substantially more infectious than the median (23). Super-shedding has been reported for a number of different infections, including severe acute respiratory syndrome coronavirus, bovine tuberculosis, paratuberculosis, norovirus, and influenza (24). Super-shedding is particularly well characterized for *E. coli* O157 in cattle. *E. coli* O157 is fecally transmitted, and bacterial counts in feces demonstrate marked heterogeneities (Fig. 3A). The mechanism underlying super-shedding is known (23): super-shedding infections involve bacterial colonization at the rectal-anal junction—these infections are more productive and more persistent than transient infections of the gut lumen. Model-based studies have suggested that super-shedders are associated with much higher herd prevalences, and in the absence of super-shedding R_0 for *E. coli* O157 in cattle is <1 (25).

Heterogeneities in contact behavior may promote "super-spreading," meaning that a small proportion of individuals have substan-

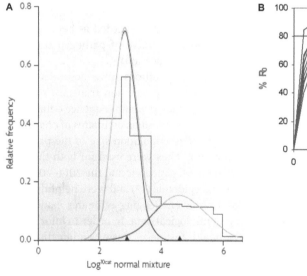
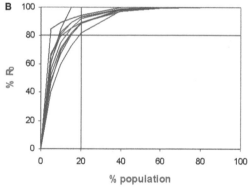

FIGURE 3 Transmission heterogeneities. **(A)** Heterogeneous infectiousness. Frequency distribution of bacterial counts for *E. coli* O157 in cattle fecal samples (horizontal axis, log scale). Raw data (histogram) are compared with a fitted mixture distribution log normal model that identified two distributions (red lines) and their sum (green). Arrowheads indicate the mean for each distribution. Reproduced with permission from reference 23. **(B)** Heterogeneous contact rates. The graph shows the cumulative, fractional contribution to the value of R_0 of individuals arranged in order (highest to lowest along the horizontal axis) of their observed contact rates. For a range of infectious diseases (multiple examples covering HIV/AIDS, malaria, schistosomiasis, and leishmaniasis), 20% of the population contribute 80% of the basic reproduction number, R_0, as estimated given observed heterogeneities in contact behavior (sexual contacts, vector biting rates, water contact, as appropriate). Data from reference 21.

tially more opportunities to infect other hosts than the median (23). Super-spreading is a property of individual hosts, whereas super-shedding is a property of individual infections, as determined by the host-pathogen interaction. Super-spreading has been widely reported for many different kinds of infection, particularly those transmitted sexually or by vectors (21), but may be less apparent for those transmitted by direct contact (22). For infectious diseases in the former category, e.g., HIV/AIDS, malaria, and schistosomiasis, a useful rule of thumb is that 20% of individuals are responsible for at least 80% of R_0, the so-called 20–80 rule (Fig. 3B).

Heterogeneities in host susceptibility to infection are commonly studied and are commonly found; note that here we are concerned only with heterogeneity in susceptibility to infection, not disease, since it is this that influences the population-level transmission rate. Heterogeneities in susceptibility may be due to multiple causes including host genetics, physiology, and immune status (19), but I do not review these in depth here.

Heterogeneities in infectiousness, contact behavior, and susceptibility clearly all have the potential to influence the ways in which a pathogen spreads through a host population. Often these heterogeneities are ignored in estimating transmission parameters; however, in some circumstances, estimation of R_0 requires knowledge of not only the mean but also the variance of the transmission rate (21). This situation arises when there is a correlation between the propensity of a host to infect and the propensity of a host to be infected. Often there will not be an a priori reason to suspect that a highly susceptible individual will also be highly infectious if infected (a super-shedder), although this is certainly conceivable, for example, with immune-compromised patients. However, for contact behavior there may be circumstances when a correlation is expected between behavior that increases onward transmission and behavior that increases exposure to infection. This is the case, for example, with sexually transmitted or vector-borne infec-

tions, although it is not necessarily so, for example, with fecal-oral transmission.

In circumstances in which the variance in transmission rate is high and there is a strong positive correlation between propensity to infect and propensity to be infected, transmission heterogeneities can have a very substantial impact on the absolute value of R_0 (21). A corollary is that the variance in transmission rates contributes more to the absolute value of R_0 than does the mean. Moreover, in addition to the second-order effects captured by the variance, there may be higher-order effects on R_0 captured only by the full matrix of rates of (direct or indirect) transmission between subsets of the population (26, 27).

One study of these effects concerned the potential for infectious disease transmission between cattle farms as a result of the movement of cattle between farms (28). Here, β was broken down into the number of farms per unit time from which cattle are moved onto a given farm, designated β_1, and the number of farms per unit time to which cattle are moved from a given farm, designated β_2 (so $\beta = \beta_1\beta_2$). R_0 is given by the expression

$$R_0 \propto \frac{1}{N}\sum \beta_1\beta_2 = \beta_1\beta_2 + \sigma(\beta_1)\sigma(\beta_2)r_{\beta_1\beta_2}$$

where $\sigma(\bullet)$ represents the standard deviation, r is the linear correlation coefficient, N is the number of farms, and the right-hand term represents the average of the cross-products over all farms. For cattle farms in the United Kingdom, β_1 and β_2 had high standard deviations but were not correlated, so there was little impact on the absolute value of R_0, although because of high variance in the value of the product $\beta_1\beta_2$ across farms, the population still followed the 20–80 rule (28).

In general, quantifying these effects requires estimation of the distribution of the components of transmission across individuals in the population and knowledge of the extent that transmission rates from and to subpopulations or individuals are correlated. This information is, in principle, relatively straightforward to collect where contact behaviors are observable, e.g., movements between locations, sexual contacts, or vector biting rates. There has also been progress in methodologies to observe patterns of proximity between individuals that are relevant to transmission by direct contact such as influenza (29). Another approach is to fit models explicitly incorporating transmission heterogeneities to outbreak data (22).

CONCLUDING REMARKS

Four aspects of infectious disease transmission have been reviewed here: tracing transmission events, phylogenetics, mathematical modeling, and heterogeneities in transmission rates. Each of these is an important topic in its own right, but I anticipate that the most significant future developments in quantifying transmissibility will involve integrating these components. This will require both the integration of data—case data, demographic and behavioral data, and pathogen sequence data—and methods for integrated data analysis. Some progress has already been made. There has been recent work on ways of analyzing sequence data using a framework based explicitly on epidemiological models (30). Estimates of the transmission chain from temporal sequence data can be improved by incorporating additional information on the date of onset of individual cases, duration of latent and infectious periods, and overall prevalence (31), and there has also been work on integrating sequence analysis with contact tracing (20). Although we still have some way to go before a truly integrated analysis of multiple data types is available as an epidemiological tool, this does look to be an achievable goal, and one which would be a powerful aid to understanding and controlling infectious disease outbreaks of all kinds.

Citation

Woolhouse M. 2017. Quantifying transmission. Microbiol Spectrum 5(4):MTBP-0005-2016.

REFERENCES

1. **Woolhouse M.** 2011. How to make predictions about future infectious disease risks. *Philos Trans R Soc Lond B Biol Sci* **366:**2045–2054.
2. **Dworkin MS.** 2011. *Cases in Field Epidemiology: A Global Perspective.* Jones & Bartlett, Sudbury, MA.
3. **Chen RT, Goldbaum GM, Wassilak SG, Markowitz LE, Orenstein WA.** 1989. An explosive point-source measles outbreak in a highly vaccinated population. Modes of transmission and risk factors for disease. *Am J Epidemiol* **129:** 173–182.
4. **Gibbens JC, Sharpe CE, Wilesmith JW, Mansley LM, Michalopoulou E, Ryan JB, Hudson M.** 2001. Descriptive epidemiology of the 2001 foot-and-mouth disease epidemic in Great Britain: the first five months. *Vet Rec* **149:**729–743.
5. **Hué S, Brown AE, Ragonnet-Cronin M, Lycett SJ, Dunn DT, Fearnhill E, Dolling DI, Pozniak A, Pillay D, Delpech VC, Leigh Brown AJ, UK Collaboration on HIV Drug Resistance and the Collaborative HIV, Anti-HIV Drug Resistance Network (CHAIN).** 2014. Phylogenetic analyses reveal HIV-1 infections between men misclassified as heterosexual transmissions. *AIDS* **28:**1967–1975.
6. **Charleston B, Bankowski BM, Gubbins S, Chase-Topping ME, Schley D, Howey R, Barnett PV, Gibson D, Juleff ND, Woolhouse ME.** 2011. Relationship between clinical signs and transmission of an infectious disease and the implications for control. *Science* **332:**726–729.
7. **Greiner AL, Angelo KM, McCollum AM, Mirkovic K, Arthur R, Angulo FJ.** 2015. Addressing contact tracing challenges-critical to halting Ebola virus disease transmission. *Int J Infect Dis* **41:**53–55.
8. **Bessell PR, Shaw DJ, Savill NJ, Woolhouse ME.** 2010. Estimating risk factors for farm-level transmission of disease: foot and mouth disease during the 2001 epidemic in Great Britain. *Epidemics* **2:**109–115.
9. **Chase-Topping ME, McKendrick IJ, Pearce MC, MacDonald P, Matthews L, Halliday J, Allison L, Fenlon D, Low JC, Gunn G, Woolhouse ME.** 2007. Risk factors for the presence of high-level shedders of *Escherichia coli* O157 on Scottish farms. *J Clin Microbiol* **45:**1594–1603.
10. **Haydon DT, Chase-Topping M, Shaw DJ, Matthews L, Friar JK, Wilesmith J, Woolhouse ME.** 2003. The construction and analysis of epidemic trees with reference to the 2001 UK foot-and-mouth outbreak. *Proc Biol Sci* **270:**121–127.
11. **Woolhouse M, Chase-Topping M, Haydon D, Friar J, Matthews L, Hughes G, Shaw D,**

Wilesmith J, Donaldson A, Cornell S, Keeling M, Grenfell B. 2001. Epidemiology. Foot-and-mouth disease under control in the UK. *Nature* **411:**258–259.

12. Cottam EM, Haydon DT, Paton DJ, Gloster J, Wilesmith JW, Ferris NP, Hutchings GH, King DP. 2006. Molecular epidemiology of the foot-and-mouth disease virus outbreak in the United Kingdom in 2001. *J Virol* **80:**11274–11282.

13. Stadler T, Kühnert D, Rasmussen DA, du Plessis L. 2014. Insights into the early epidemic spread of Ebola in Sierra Leone provided by viral sequence data. *PLoS Curr* **6:**ecurrents.outbreaks.02bc6d927 ecee7bbd33532ec8ba6a25f.

14. Hall MD, Knowles NJ, Wadsworth J, Rambaut A, Woolhouse ME. 2013. Reconstructing geographical movements and host species transitions of foot-and-mouth disease virus serotype SAT 2. *mBio* **4:**e00591-e13.

15. Ward MJ, Gibbons CL, McAdam PR, van Bunnik BA, Girvan EK, Edwards GF, Fitzgerald JR, Woolhouse ME. 2014. Time-scaled evolutionary analysis of the transmission and antibiotic resistance dynamics of *Staphylococcus aureus* CC398. *Appl Environ Microbiol* **80:**7275–7282.

16. Lycett S, McLeish NJ, Robertson C, Carman W, Baillie G, McMenamin J, Rambaut A, Simmonds P, Woolhouse M, Leigh Brown AJ. 2012. Origin and fate of A/H1N1 influenza in Scotland during 2009. *J Gen Virol* **93:**1253–1260.

17. Woolhouse ME, Rambaut A, Kellam P. 2015. Lessons from Ebola: improving infectious disease surveillance to inform outbreak management. *Sci Transl Med* **7:**307rv5.

18. Anderson RM, May RM. 1991. *Infectious Diseases of Humans: Dynamics and Control.* Oxford University Press, New York, NY.

19. Keeling MJ, Rohani P. 2008. *Modeling Infectious Diseases in Humans and Animals.* Princeton University Press, Princeton, NJ.

20. Cottam EM, Thébaud G, Wadsworth J, Gloster J, Mansley L, Paton DJ, King DP, Haydon DT. 2008. Integrating genetic and epidemiological data to determine transmission pathways of foot-and-mouth disease virus. *Proc Biol Sci* **275:**887–895.

21. Woolhouse ME, Dye C, Etard JF, Smith T, Charlwood JD, Garnett GP, Hagan P, Hii JL, Ndhlovu PD, Quinnell RJ, Watts CH,

Chandiwana SK, Anderson RM. 1997. Heterogeneities in the transmission of infectious agents: implications for the design of control programs. *Proc Natl Acad Sci U S A* **94:**338–342.

22. Lloyd-Smith JO, Schreiber SJ, Kopp PE, Getz WM. 2005. Superspreading and the effect of individual variation on disease emergence. *Nature* **438:**355–359.

23. Chase-Topping M, Gally D, Low C, Matthews L, Woolhouse M. 2008. Super-shedding and the link between human infection and livestock carriage of *Escherichia coli* O157. *Nat Rev Microbiol* **6:**904–912.

24. Canini L, Woolhouse MEJ, Maines TR, Carrat F. 2016. Heterogeneous shedding of influenza by human subjects and its implications for epidemiology and control. *Sci Rep* **6:**38749.

25. Matthews L, Low JC, Gally DL, Pearce MC, Mellor DJ, Heesterbeek JAP, Chase-Topping M, Naylor SW, Shaw DJ, Reid SWJ, Gunn GJ, Woolhouse ME. 2006. Heterogeneous shedding of *Escherichia coli* O157 in cattle and its implications for control. *Proc Natl Acad Sci U S A* **103:** 547–552.

26. Woolhouse ME, Watts CH, Chandiwana SK. 1991. Heterogeneities in transmission rates and the epidemiology of schistosome infection. *Proc Biol Sci* **245:**109–114.

27. Gates MC, Woolhouse ME. 2015. Controlling infectious disease through the targeted manipulation of contact network structure. *Epidemics* **12:**11–19.

28. Woolhouse ME, Shaw DJ, Matthews L, Liu WC, Mellor DJ, Thomas MR. 2005. Epidemiological implications of the contact network structure for cattle farms and the 20-80 rule. *Biol Lett* **1:**350–352.

29. Read JM, Edmunds WJ, Riley S, Lessler J, Cummings DA. 2012. Close encounters of the infectious kind: methods to measure social mixing behaviour. *Epidemiol Infect* **140:**2117–2130.

30. Hall M, Woolhouse M, Rambaut A. 2015. Epidemic reconstruction in a phylogenetics framework: transmission trees as partitions of nodes. *PLoS Comput Biol* **11:**e1004613.

31. Volz EM, Kosakovsky Pond SL, Ward MJ, Leigh Brown AJ, Frost SD. 2009. Phylodynamics of infectious disease epidemics. *Genetics* **183:**1421–1430.

Experimental Epidemiology of Antibiotic Resistance: Looking for an Appropriate Animal Model System

17

PABLO LLOP,[1] AMPARO LATORRE,[1,2,3*] and ANDRÉS MOYA[1,2,3*]

TRANSMISSION OF ANTIBIOTIC RESISTANCE: THE PROBLEM

The problem of antibiotic resistance in hospital bacteria and the human community has been recognized by various organizations (1–3) as one of the greatest challenges to public health, which calls into question the maintenance and progress of modern medicine (4, 5). This alarm is based on the inability to treat and prevent infections caused by microorganisms that are resistant to all therapeutic alternatives available. In recent years, there have been some unexpected circumstances that have acted synergistically and have worsened the problem, namely, (i) a general failure to discover new antimicrobials; (ii) the exponential development of antibiotic resistance in overcrowded countries with serious health deficits and the global spread of multiresistant bacteria; (iii) the invasion by resistant bacteria of ecosystems (surface water and sewage, soil, animals, and food) and, particularly, the invasion of human intestinal microbiota; and (iv) a pollution environment with high concentrations of antibiotics, metals, and biocides that favor the selection of multiresistant bacteria and their persistence. An estimated 25,000 people die each year in Europe and the United States from antibiotic resistance (5).

[1]Foundation for the Promotion of Sanitary and Biomedical Research in the Valencian Region (FISABIO), València, Spain; [2]Integrative Systems Biology Institute, Universitat de València, València, Spain; [3]Network Research Center for Epidemiology and Public Health (CIBERESP), Madrid, Spain.

Microbial Transmission in Biological Processes
Edited by Fernando Baquero, Emilio Bouza, J.A. Gutiérrez-Fuentes, and Teresa M. Coque
© 2018 American Society for Microbiology, Washington, DC
doi:10.1128/microbiolspec.MTBP-0007-2016

The antibiotic resistance problem has been addressed during the last quarter of a century under the highly orthodox approach of "thinking" based on (i) the need to develop new antibiotics, (ii) reduced consumption of antimicrobials, and (iii) the control and preventive isolation of patients carrying resistant bacteria in hospitals. These strategies were effective in very early stages of the invasion by resistant bacteria and even in developed countries with high standards of public health. Unfortunately, the focus of the pharmaceutical companies on other areas of therapeutic research and the planetary globalization of resistance with the invasion of populations and ecosystems has radically changed the landscape for actions based on the above premises (6). In parallel with this conceptual stagnation, advances in molecular genetics and the biology of bacterial populations that have revealed the explosive evolution of resistance (it has been compared to a chain reaction where the same resistance gene in India emerging as the β-lactamase NDM-1 appears a few months later in the rest of the world) allow us to speculate that the spread is due to the interaction of transmission chain events that occur at different levels of the biological hierarchy (7).

It is no longer the classical transmission of bacteria from one space to another, but swarms of clonal complexes, the gene exchange of communities and even fragments of microbiota or complete microbiota (8–10), which requires attention. Antibiotic resistance genes (ABRs) can be located in transposons, integrons, and plasmids that are integrated in a bacterial cell, either in the chromosome or in replicons that form part of a community of bacteria that belong to a particular host that lives in a particular environment. In other words, ABRs can be successively located at different subcellular, cellular, and supracellular nested levels of the full ecosystem. All the previously mentioned ABR carriers are units of selection that can be simultaneously and independently chosen at the different environmental levels. Understanding ABR evolution is complex, since it is not just the result of antibiotic-driven selection of mutant resistant bacterial clones but, more properly, the consequence of a variety of trans-hierarchical interactions between all biological vehicles involved in the dissemination of the genetic information encompassing ABRs. Such multilevel complexity is difficult to address as a whole. Within each of these levels there are "epidemic" resistance genes and gene vectors (plasmids, transposons, or integrons) that accelerate global spread. However, is it possible to predict the dissemination of resistance?

THE ROLE OF MICROBIOTA IN ANTIBIOTIC RESISTANCE

The gut microbiome is a complex community of microorganisms that live in the digestive tracts of humans and other animals. It is essential to maintain homeostasis and the health of the host, since it is responsible for vitamin synthesis, energy supply, immune cell maturation, and defense against infectious pathogens, among other properties (11). In humans, there are large numbers of microorganisms (up to 10^{12} CFU/g material). Although the composition of this microbiota determines the health status of the organism, it is not a stable organization, undergoing a series of changes during human development. In contrast, an unbalanced microbiota (dysbiosis) is associated with many gastrointestinal as well as nongastrointestinal diseases (1, 4, 12). Anaerobic bacteria in particular, and more specifically those of the *Bacteroides* genus, are the most common bacterial species in the human microbiota, according to metagenomic studies (13). Intestinal bacteria, on the other hand, not only exchange resistance genes between them but can interact with bacteria passing through the colon, causing the acquisition and transmission of ABRs (14).

The increase in the number of ABRs is attributed to different causes including the composition of human gut microbiota, the selective pressure generated by the massive use of antibiotics, and social changes that have increased the transmission of resistant organisms (15, 16). Other factors include the age of individuals (17, 18) and social interchange (19). We should also add the fact that farm-raised animals are often treated with antibiotics in large quantities to improve their quality and prevent infection. Thus, pathogenic-resistant organisms propagated in livestock are a source of introduction to the food supply and could be widely disseminated in food products (20). The problem occurs when all these factors and treatments cause the emergence of resistant bacteria and the increase of their propagation (16).

EXPERIMENTAL EPIDEMIOLOGY: THE CONCEPT

It is not easy to measure the transmission of ABRs in human populations. However, we can mimic the process by using appropriate experimental models in which to test interventions and, ultimately, encourage public health recommendations. Experimental epidemiology began nearly a century ago, but its development has been very slow and it is currently an area of knowledge that remains poorly treated (21–25), particularly in its evolutionary and predictive aspects. Nevertheless, over the last few years new studies using several model systems with different levels of microbial complexity have been assayed and have revealed how host genes affect the microbiome and how the microbiome regulates host genetic programs (26). Model organisms are the best way to perform, under controlled conditions, different host-microbiome interactions and relationship experiments that are not affordable in human studies. In many cases, the genetic and genomic studies of hosts and microbes have proven essential in identifying key factors that enable symbiosis. Model systems are also revealing roles for the microbiome in host physiology ranging from mate selection (27) to skeletal biology (28) and lipid metabolism (29), to cite a few. With the increasing number of microbiome studies completed and underway, experimental systems using model organisms are proving to be essential tools to interrogate and validate the associations identified between the human microbiome and disease.

The gut microbiotas of many animals are reservoirs of ABRs, and it is a matter of how to choose an appropriate experimental system to observe and measure the processes that determine the spread of resistance genes in populations, considering different units of selection by the antibiotic. In this sense, arranged hierarchically we can study (i) resistance genes, (ii) elements of horizontal transfer carriers of these genes (integrons, transposons, and/or plasmids), and (iii) bacterial lineages and bacterial communities with horizontal transfer exchange. Our chosen model system was the German cockroach *Blatella germanica*, which has been suggested as a useful animal system in previous work (30, 31).

WHY CHOOSE *B. GERMANICA* AS AN EXPERIMENTAL MODEL SYSTEM?

B. germanica is a cosmopolitan species of cockroach (32). Cockroaches are omnivorous insects that harbor a rich and complex gut microbiota, similar in some characteristics to human gut microbiota (33, 34), and may contain bacteria with many ABRs that can be a reservoir to be transferred to humans (32). They are found mostly in buildings and homes, sheltered in small, damp places such as bathrooms or kitchens, since the best conditions for them are high humidity (60%) and warm temperatures (between 26 and 28°C) (35). In addition, this and other cockroach species have been detected in areas like hospital rooms and in intensive care areas, sometimes acting as pathogenic vectors (34, 36). They are responsible for generating allergic reactions due to their feces, and their behavior is regulated by pheromones (35). It has been found that many of the bacteria present in the human digestive tract are also present in that of cockroaches, where they coexist with many pathogens and opportunists that can cause disease in humans (37). Therefore, B. germanica is considered a natural reservoir of human pathogens, and its characterization may be helpful for biomedical research, given that many isolates identified from its external body and internal gut show antibiotic multiresistance (32, 38).

Cockroaches are insects that maintain two types of symbiotic systems. One is the intracellular symbiont Blattabacterium cuenoti, a Gram-negative bacterium belonging to the phylum Bacteroidetes, located in bacteriocytes (special host cells) in the fat body; and the other group, the gut microbiota proper, is formed mostly by ectosymbionts located in particular areas of the intestinal tract (39). The endosymbiont is key in recycling nitrogen and contains urease, an enzyme absent in mammals and many other animals that is capable of degrading urea (40). On the other hand, the gut microbiota of cockroaches also plays an important role in host metabolism because it helps to process the complex diet of an omnivorous insect like B. germanica (39, 41). It is still unknown how cockroaches obtain their microbiota in each generation, but the presumption is that it is via trophallaxis (mouth-to-mouth or anus-to-mouth feeding), coprophagy (consumption of feces), or body/ootheca licking or from the environment. A relevant result obtained by our group is that the endosymbiont Blattabacterium was the only bacterium found in the ootheca, which clearly indicates that there is no vertical transmission and thus there must be horizontal acquisition of the intestinal microbiota in each generation by any of the previous proposed mechanisms (39, 41).

The ontogenetic development of the microbial community also remains unknown. The gut contents of nymphs are similar but are different from that of adult cockroaches. Bacteroidetes (60%), Firmicutes (30%), and Proteobacteria (10%) were the phyla most commonly found in all the stages except in embryos and in nymphal stage 1 (n1), where Blattabacterium was the only (embryo) or the most present (n1) bacterium (39).

Some of the interesting characteristics of B. germanica in proposing it as an experimental animal model are its relatively short life cycle and the ease with which it is maintained in the laboratory. Although variable, the B. germanica life cycle from eggs lasts ~100 days. The nymphs go through six stages before becoming adults, which occurs in ~36 days, with a life expectancy of adults of 9 to 10 months. The population under study belong to an original population maintained in the lab for 30 years and kindly provided by Xavier Belles from the Institut de Biologia Evolutiva (Barcelona, Spain) in 2013, being reared since then in the chambers of the Institut Cavanilles (València, Spain) in lunch boxes with aeration at 26°C, 70% humidity, and a photoperiod of 12-h light/12-h darkness. The normal diet in lab-reared animals is dog food (Teklad 2021C; Harlan UK Ltd, Bicester), which provides the animal with a complete set of nutrients.

The digestive tract of the insect is divided into three parts: foregut, midgut, and hindgut. There are few or no microbiota at all in either the foregut or the midgut. Thus, the hindgut concentrates the vast majority of bacterial species that constitute the intestinal bacterial microbiota of this insect (33, 34, 39). Another important part of the insect is the fat body, which contains three types of cells: adipocytes, uricocytes, and bacteriocytes, the special eukaryotic cells harboring Blattabacterium, which, as already stated, plays an essential role in the metabolism of cockroaches, allowing them to recycle the excess of nitrogen stored in the uricocytes and used as a nitrogen source (40). This means that the cockroach is capable of generating a reservoir and of recycling nitrogen by means of a new metabolic pathway in collaboration with the endosymbiont (40, 42). In this way, the insect-endosymbiont relationship can convert an excretory product into a valuable metabolic reserve (43). The relationship between both partners (B. germanica and Blattabacterium) is mutualistic, meaning that both host and symbionts need each other to survive. Thus, any experimental setting with *B. germanica* needs to keep *Blattabacterium* alive, or somehow be able to play its role.

Before starting with the experimental epidemiology itself, two major types of questions should be addressed. The first is related to the composition, function, and transmission of gut microbiota in *B. germanica*, and more precisely the role played in host physiology and how symbionts, particularly the gut microbiota, are transmitted and/or acquired throughout generations, and how different diets affect gut microbiota and host fitness. The second type of questions are related to the presence of ABRs in natural and lab-reared populations and how the fitness of *B. germanica* is affected when it is treated with different antibiotics.

Large differences in bacterial community composition have been observed among individuals of the same cockroach species that are associated with the accumulation of different microbial products that influence the health status of the host (34). Similar variations among individuals in bacterial communities from the same habitat have also been reported for mammals, including humans (44) and pigs (45), and are believed to have appeared from the random acquisition of microorganisms in diet and the environment (45). Apart from these two factors, host phylogeny is also considered as an important issue that affects the composition and abundance of the gut communities of mammals (46). The impact of host phylogeny on the composition of gut microbiota has also been demonstrated in cockroaches. Thus, cockroaches share a high presence of *Proteobacteria* and *Fusobacteria* with their sister group wood-feeding termites. In addition, the gut microbiota of these animals has many elements in common with the gut communities of more distantly related animals, such as cow rumen and the intestinal tracts of mice and humans (33). This suggests the existence of common environmental factors that determine the composition of resident microbiota in the intestinal habitat. In

humans, bacterial populations in the gut have an impact on host physiological functions through their metabolic activity, because they are performing essential metabolic functions and produce small bioactive molecules that interact with the host (47–49). Similarly, in insects, several works have demonstrated the diverse roles played by gut microbiota in host physiology leading, in extreme cases where some groups are absent, to host mortality (50–53). In the case of our model, *B. germanica*, preliminary work has shown changes in bacterial abundance and composition across insect development (37), although no further information regarding the associated metabolic roles of the involved bacteria is yet available (work in progress).

As already stated, *Blattabacterium* is located in the bacteriocytes, specialized cells 20 μm in diameter, which originated phylogenetically from intestinal epithelium cells infected by a free-living ancestor via food intake (54). Bacteriocytes, in turn, are internalized in the abdominal fat body of cockroaches (55). They are also localized in the follicular epithelium of the ovarioles, the structures that group ovaries. Transmission is vertical, i.e., maternal by transovarial infection (54). The transfer begins with the invasion of ovarioles by bacteriocytes that are attached to the oocytes. *Blattabacterium* is then released from the bacteriocyte and migrates through its own tunic and follicular epithelium into the space between the latter and the oocyte (56). Then the bacteria are "endocytosed" by the pseudopodia of the egg membrane, and are internalized. Finally, they migrate to the center of the egg (57).

The dependency of microbiota on diet is a matter that has been widely observed, and in cockroaches the subject has been studied first by observing morphological and developmental aspects (58), and later by studying the effect of synthetic diets and how they affect the insect and the microbiota (34, 59, 60). In previous studies in our group on the dynamics of microbiota across time, the bacterial load was determined by quantitative PCR (qPCR) and the bacterial composition of gut microbiota was established by pyrosequencing the 16S rRNA gene gene in the egg, five nymphal stages, and adult (38). It was observed that bacterial load increased by 2 orders of magnitude from n1 to n2, coinciding with the incorporation of the majority of bacterial taxa. As in humans, there is an ecological succession from nymphs to adults, and important changes in the bacterial composition between the adult and the nymphs have been found. The effect of diet on the composition and evolution of gut microbiota in this animal model has also been studied in previous work (39, 41). To assess the effect of protein content in the females of *B. germanica*, three types of diet—high protein content (50%), no protein content (0%), and control diet or dog food (24% protein content)—at two different adult stages (8 and 13 days) were used. It was found that the variations in the bacterial community were due mainly to changes in the protein content of the diet and also the time analyzed (39). Clustering analyses proved that samples tended to be grouped by diet, indicating that protein content is a very important element in modulating the structure of the gut microbial ecosystem in cockroaches. In the same work, the gut microbiota of wild adult cockroaches was analyzed. Remarkably, the highest diversity was found in the wild animals, and the composition was more similar to that of the cockroaches fed with no protein content and for 13 days, indicating the low protein content that cockroaches must cope with in natural conditions.

EFFECT OF ANTIBIOTIC ON SYMBIOTIC SYSTEMS: MICROBIOTA AND FITNESS CHANGES DUE TO ANTIBIOTIC TREATMENT IN *B. GERMANICA*

As stated above, before starting experimental epidemiology with *B. germanica*, it is necessary (i) to have knowledge about the effect of antibiotics in *B. germanica* symbionts (either endosymbionts or gut microbiota) and in the

fitness of the host and (ii) to explore the presence of ABRs in the microbiota of wild *B. germanica* by metagenome analyses.

Regarding the first point, several preliminary experiments were carried out. In the first series, two antibiotics with two different intensities of antibiotic exposure were employed: chlortetracycline (1 and 10 mg/ml) and rifampin (2 and 20 mg/ml). Several parameters were then measured: (i) fitness (weight of the individuals at established time points, time of development, and fecundity measured as number of females with ootheca at established time points) and (ii) qualitative PCR and qPCR determination assays, with primers targeting the gene *ureC* specific to *Blattabacterium*, as a measure of the amount of genomes and, thus, of endosymbionts. For the qPCR assay, genomic DNA samples prepared from previously dissected fat bodies were measured and unified to a concentration of 5 ng/µl, and 3 µl of each sample mixed with 17 µl of a PCR mixture using SYBR green in an AriaMx real-time PCR system (Agilent Technologies, Santa Clara, CA). The sequences of the primers were UC1F, 5'-GTCCAGCAACTGGAACTAT AGCCA-3', and UC1R, 5'-GTCCAGCAACTG GAACTATAGCCA-3', giving an amplification fragment of 166 nucleotides.

With antibiotic treatments there was observed, in general, a statistically significant decrease in the three fitness parameters measured: weight, developmental time, and fecundity. Significant differences in weight after 25 days of treatment were obtained for both antibiotics and treatments (see Fig. 1 to see the general observation of a decrease in size and weight). The developmental time, measured as the proportion of individuals that reached the adult stage, showed no significant differences between chlortetracycline and the control at low exposures. However, significant differences were observed at high doses. It should be noted that this result is in agreement with recent findings of the bactericidal effect of chlortetracycline on bacteria harboring low numbers of ribosomes, as in the case

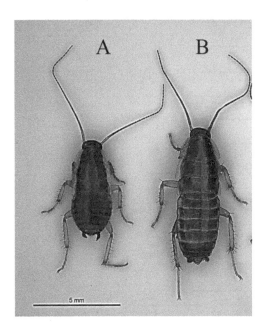

FIGURE 1 Loss of weight and size in *B. germanica* due to antibiotic treatment after 25 days. (A) Insect treated with chlortetracycline 1 mg/ml. (B) Insect not treated with antibiotics.

of *Blattabacterium* (61). Under treatment with rifampicin both concentrations clearly affected development, which was more noticeable at the highest concentration. The appearance of oothecas (i.e., fecundity) was also clearly affected as a result of antibiotic treatments. Both treatments with the two exposures differed from the corresponding control. After the treatments, fewer females had oothecas, and they were smaller and took longer to appear.

Quantitative analyses were carried out using the same gene as the target and real-time qPCR with SYBR green, using four control samples and four individuals treated, each with three replicates. The results of the abundance of endosymbionts in parental chlortetracycline-treated samples revealed a decrease in the amount of the *ureC* gene compared to the control cockroaches. The ones treated with rifampicin showed no differences in the amount, with no decrease in the endosymbionts. The qPCR in the progeny

(F1) of *B. germanica* treated with chlortetracycline revealed a marked reduction in the amount of DNA compared to control cockroaches, by nearly 6 orders of magnitude (Fig. 2). In addition, the appearance of individuals in this F1 was different, with a lighter color and smaller size compared to the control. The average weight per individual was also lower compared to the control. Rifampicin-treated samples could not be analyzed due to the death of all the samples of the progeny with both antibiotic doses, which shows the strong effect of this antibiotic in the insect.

In a second series of experiments, additional trials were carried out with rifampicin with a dose 10 times below the lowest dose previously employed, using a population that was fed dog food until the adults appeared. This population was divided in two; the control was fed dog food, and rifampicin (0.2 mg/ml) was added to the water supply of the other group. The gut and fat body of three individuals at different time points (10, 20, and 30 days) were analyzed to monitor two parameters: (i) the amount of *Blattabacterium* by qPCR, using the *ureC* gene as target DNA; and (ii) the changes in the bacterial composition by 16S rRNA gene sequencing. Once the new individuals appeared, the antibiotic-treated population was subdivided into another two groups; one continued with the antibiotic supply and the other returned to its dog food diet for 10 days. The qPCR analyses did not show any significant differences in the quantification of the endosymbiont of the antibiotic-treated individuals versus dog food diet recipients in the original two populations. However, the two populations derived from the antibiotic-treated one showed a reduction in the *Blattabacterium* population of 5 log units in all of the samples, compared to the amounts of the original antibiotic-treated and dog food-receiving populations.

Changes in the microbiota composition from these antibiotic treatments were analyzed using the Illumina (San Diego, CA)

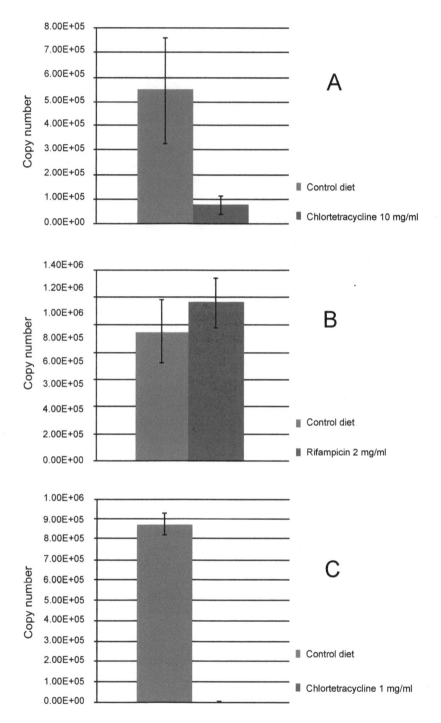

FIGURE 2 Copy number of gene *ureC* of *Blattabacterium* genome in *B. germanica* treated with chlortetracycline 10 mg/ml (A) and rifampicin 2 mg/ml (B). There is a strong reduction in the number of endosymbionts with chlortetracycline, whereas with rifampin at low dose no effect is observed. (C) Copy number of gene *ureC* of *Blattabacterium* genome in F1 progeny of *B. germanica* treated with chlortetracycline 1 mg/ml.

MiSeq platform to amplify and sequence the 16S rRNA gene (amplicons). These regions are frequently used for phylogenetic classifications in microbial populations (62). The analysis of the sequences was accomplished by using the MiSeq system in the Illumina analysis cloud environment BaseSpace (www.basespace.illumina.com). The taxonomic information for the 16S rDNA sequences was obtained by comparison against the Ribosomal Database Project-II (RDP). For species identification, the taxonomic assignment was also performed with RDP and a bootstrap threshold of 60%. Additional Web-based matching against type strain sequences was conducted with RDP SeqMatch (http://rdp.cme.msu.edu/seqmatch/seqmatch_intro.jsp). Abundances were Hellinger transformed and a principal component analysis based on the covariance matrix of transformed abundances was performed. Subsequently, the QIIME application was used for analysis (63). The FastQC application was used as a quality control for the sequences (https://www.bioinformatics.babraham.ac.uk/projects/fastqc/). With the 16S Metagenomics application, the taxonomic classification was determined. This application performs a taxonomic classification using the Greengenes Database (64).

The results obtained in the original two populations showed that the microbiota was greatly affected in the antibiotic-treated samples compared to the control ones. In the new population formed with the newborns of the antibiotic-treated populations, but with no antibiotic in the diet, the microbiota recovered almost to the same composition of the samples that were fed the control diet. That is to say, the microbiota recovered simply by suspending the treatment of rifampicin, while if the treatment continued, it produced a drastic reduction in the composition of the microbiota. In this case, the treatment with rifampicin had a rapid effect on the microbiota composition in one generation, while the endosymbiont population (qPCR experiments) seemed to be affected in the next generation, despite the suppression of the

treatment. The morphological features of the population (size, weight, and developmental time of insects) were affected by the antibiotic, with a delay in all these parameters (unpublished data).

In terms of the second goal (to explore the presence of ABRs in the microbiota of wild *B. germanica* by metagenome analyses), metagenomics analyses of three wild animals were also performed to determine their bacterial composition and abundances (Fig. 3) and also to identify ABRs and their possible taxon origin (Table 1). In these analyses, we applied a bioinformatics pipeline from raw DNA sequencing data that included demultiplexing and quality filtering, OTU picking, taxonomic assignment, phylogenetic reconstruction, diversity analyses, and visualizations. The search for resistance genes in the predicted open reading frames was performed by a blastp analysis against the Antibiotic Resistance Genes Database (http://ardb.cbcb.umd.edu/), through local alignments for the location of gene sequences belonging to resistant genes.

The results of all these experiments were of great interest, helping us to observe what could be expected in the experimental model with the different antibiotics and the dose to be employed.

HUMANIZING THE BACTERIAL MICROBIOTA OF *B. GERMANICA*

A fundamental question that we had in mind was the following: Is it possible to humanize the bacterial microbiota of cockroaches? By that, we mean to introduce human bacterial species harboring ABRs into the gut microbiota of *B. germanica*. In a first approach, the idea was to use bacteria naturally occurring in cockroaches, so the system would be as natural as possible. A search for antibiotic-resistant bacterial isolates was carried out and these were analyzed to look for the presence of plasmids that could be responsible for resistance. Finally, a system to analyze the population of the endosymbiont was also

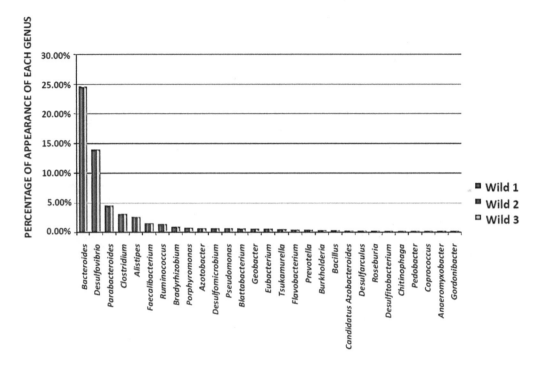

FIGURE 3 **Percentage of genus abundance (>1.5%) from three wild *B. germanica* females.**

required, to evaluate the effect of different antibiotics on *Blattabacterium* survival. In summary, for this specific project we had to look for natural cultured antibiotic-resistant bacterial strains in natural and lab-reared populations, and locate which of the resistance genes observed were in plasmids. The results obtained allowed the identification of bacterial species also present in humans and harboring antibiotic resistance; thus, this idea of "humanizing" the gut microbiota was no longer necessary because we can use bacteria present in both systems.

Previous work on the analysis of cultivable microbiota in the hindgut of different species of cockroaches used several culture media and conditions (rich and specific media, incubation temperature of 37°C). All previous research was addressed to find human-pathogenic bacteria and measure the risk of this insect as a vector for the spread of disease (65, 66). In our case, screening of the gut microbiota using culturing methods was performed as previ-

ously described (65, 67). Some bacterial strains showing ABRs in wild and in lab-reared animals were obtained, with some isolates presenting multiresistance (Table 2). The idea was to increase the chance of finding target antibiotic-resistant organisms of clinical interest by means of isolation in general media with different antibiotics, to look for the presence of plasmids that were resistant to one or several antibiotics, and finally to tag the plasmid with green fluorescent protein (GFP) to monitor its possible transfer between insects harboring it. After checking several media, the best results were obtained using brain heart infusion (Pronadisa, Madrid, Spain), a general medium rich in nutrients and suitable for the growth and development of various bacterial groups including many types of pathogens (68). Two more media, specifically for enterococci (*Enterococcus* agar; Difco, Le Pont de Claix, France) and enterobacteria (MacConkey agar; bioMérieux, Marcy l'Etoile, France), were also employed to increase the

TABLE 1 Antibiotic resistance genes found in the metagenomic analyses performed on three wild *B. germanica* females

Resistance gene	Description	Resistance profile
acra, acrb	Resistance-nodulation-cell division transporter system. Multidrug resistance efflux pump	Aminoglycoside, glycylcycline, β-lactam, macrolide, acriflavine
adeb	Resistance-nodulation-cell division transporter system. Multidrug resistance efflux pump	Chloramphenicol, aminoglycoside
amrb	Resistance-nodulation-cell division transporter system. Multidrug resistance efflux pump	Aminoglycoside, macrolide, acriflavine
aph33ib, aph6id	Aminoglycoside O-phosphotransferase	Streptomycin
arna	Bifunctional enzyme that catalyzes the oxidative decarboxylation of UDP-glucuronic acid (UDP-GlcUA) to UDP-4-keto-arabinose (UDP-Ara4O)	Polymyxin
baca	Undecaprenyl pyrophosphate phosphatase	Bacitracin
bcra	ABC transporter system, bacitracin efflux pump	Bacitracin
bl1_ampc, bl1_sm, bl1_mox	Class C β-lactamase	Cephalosporin
bl2b_tem	Class A β-lactamase	Cephalosporin, penicillin
bl2b_tem1	Class A β-lactamase	Cephalosporin ii, penicillin, Cephalosporin i
cata2, mdtl	Group A chloramphenicol acetyltransferase	Chloramphenicol
ceob	Resistance-nodulation-cell division transporter system	Chloramphenicol
ermf	rRNA adenine N-6-methyltransferase	Streptogramin B, lincosamide, macrolide
fosx	Glutathione transferase, metalloglutathione transferase	Fosfomycin
ksga	Dimethylates two adjacent adenosines in the 16S rRNA in the 30S particle	Kasugamycin
lsa	ABC efflux family that is resistant to macrolides-lincosamides-streptogramin B	Streptogramin B, lincosamide, macrolide
macb	Resistance-nodulation-cell division transporter system. Multidrug resistance efflux pump	Macrolide
mdtf	Resistance-nodulation-cell division transporter system. Multidrug resistance efflux pump	Doxorubicin, erythromycin
mdth, mdtg	Major facilitator superfamily transporter. Multidrug resistance efflux pump	Deoxycholate, fosfomycin
mdtk	Major facilitator superfamily transporter. Multidrug resistance efflux pump	Enoxacin, norfloxacin
mexi, mexw, mexd, oprj	Resistance-nodulation-cell division transporter system. Multidrug resistance efflux pump	Glycylcycline, fluoroquinolone, erythromycin, roxithromycin
mexy	Resistance-nodulation-cell division transporter system. Multidrug resistance efflux pump	Aminoglycoside, glycylcycline
pbp1b, pbp2	Penicillin-insensitive transglycosylase N-terminal domain	Penicillin
qnrb	Pentapeptide repeat family	Fluoroquinolone
rosa, rosb	Efflux pump/potassium antiporter system. RosA: major facilitator superfamily transporter; RosB: potassium antiporter	Fosmidomycin
smeb, smed, smee	Resistance-nodulation-cell division transporter system. Multidrug resistance efflux pump	Fluoroquinolone
sul2	Sulfonamide-resistant dihydropteroate synthase	Sulfonamide
tet32, tetm	Ribosomal protection protein	Tetracycline
tet37	Flavoproteins. Only one such protein found in oral metagenome	Tetracycline
tolc	Resistance-nodulation-cell division transporter system. Multidrug resistance efflux pump	Aminoglycoside, glycylcycline, β-lactam, macrolide, acriflavin
vand, vanrd	VanD-type vancomycin resistance operon genes	Vancomycin, teicoplanin
vanra, vansa, vanrc	VanA-type vancomycin resistance operon genes	Vancomycin, teicoplanin
vatb	Virginiamycin A acetyltransferase	Streptogramin A

TABLE 2 Species identified and the antibiotics to which they show resistance after isolation of colonies belonging to the gut microbiota of 12 wild and 5 lab-reared *B. germanica* individuals

	Antibiotics and concentrations used					
Isolate	Kanamycin (50 µg/ml)	Vancomycin (10 µg/ml)	Ampicillin (100 µg/ml)	Gentamicin (20 µg/ml)	Gram reaction	Identification (16S rRNA gene)
Wild1	S	R	R	S	−	*Klebsiella oxytoca*
Wild2	S	R	R	S	−	*Klebsiella oxytoca*
Wild3	R	R	R	R	−	*Pseudomonas nitroreducens*
Wild4	S	R	R	S	−	*Pseudomonas nitroreducens*
Wild5	S	R	R	S	−	*Klebsiella oxytoca*
Wild6	S	S	S	S	+	*Enterococcus pallens*
Wild7	S	R	R	S	−	*Pseudomonas nitroreducens*
Wild8	S	R	R	S	−	*Klebsiella oxytoca*
Wild9	R	R	S	R	+	*Enterococcus malodoratus*
Wild10	R	R	R	R	+	*Enterococcus avium*
Wild11	R	R	S	R	+	*Enterococcus avium/Enterococcus gilvus*
Wild12	R	R	S	R	+	*Enterococcus malodoratus*
Lab1	R	R	R	R	−	*Stenotrophomonas pavanii*
Lab2	R	R	R	S	+	*Enterococcus durans*
Lab3	R	R	R	R	+	*Staphylococcus hominis*
Lab4	S	S	R	S	−	*Klebsiella oxytoca*
Lab5	R	R	R	R	+	*Enterococcus canis*

R: antibiotic resistant; S: antibiotic sensible

chance of finding antibiotic-resistant bacteria. The incubation temperature was chosen to be as similar as possible to cockroaches' natural conditions (28°C) instead of the conditions found inside the human body (37°C). The colonies isolated were analyzed for antibiotic resistance with four antibiotics at the standard concentrations of use in microbiology (gentamicin, 20 µg/ml; kanamycin, 50 µg/ml; vancomycin, 10 µg/ml; and ampicillin, 100 µg/ml) and identified by sequencing the 16S rRNA gene (using Sanger platform) and blastn searches using the 16S rRNA sequences database. Bacterial isolates resistant to all the antibiotics assayed were found after analyzing a few individuals (Table 2). From several isolates showing resistance to more than one antibiotic, plasmid extractions were performed and analyzed by gel electrophoresis. Different plasmids were found, ranging in size from 1 to >50 kb (Fig. 4), but the restriction analyses performed did not show similarities to plasmids previously analyzed from the same species (69–71). Consequently, due to the difficulties found in using the plasmids observed because of the lack of sequence information,

we used previously analyzed plasmids pRE25 (72) and pIP501 (73) showing resistance to different antibiotics. pRE25 is a conjugative and mobilizing multiresistance plasmid of 50 kb

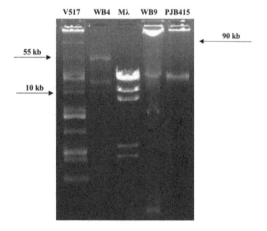

FIGURE 4 Plasmid profiles of some of the isolates from the hindgut. V517 and PJB415, marker plasmids; Mλ, marker λ HindIII; V517, *Escherichia coli* strain with plasmids used as markers; WB4, *Pseudomonas nitroreducens*; WB9, *K. oxytoca*; PJB415, plasmid marker 90 kb.

from *Enterococcus faecalis* strain RE25 (74). Plasmid pRE25 encodes resistance to 12 antimicrobials belonging to five structural classes. These include aminoglycosides, lincosamides, macrolides, chloramphenicol, and streptothricin. These genes are closely related to the ABRs already detected in human pathogens, including kanamycin, neomycin, streptomycin, erythromycin, roxithromycin, tylosin, and chloramphenicol, among others. Similar resistance determinants have been found in Gram-positive and Gram-negative bacteria, bacteria isolated from animal environments and other sources, which reveals the widespread dissemination of antibiotic resistance traits among Gram-positive and Gram-negative bacteria. This important genetic exchange may lead to a dramatic limitation of the potential of antibiotics to combat human infection (75). Accordingly, pRE25 may contribute to the further spread of antibiotic-resistant microorganisms via food in the human community.

Plasmid pIP501 (30 kbp) is a broad-host-range, conjugative plasmid originally isolated from a clinical strain of *Streptococcus agalactiae* in 1975 (76). When compared to relevant sequences of pRE25, an overall nucleotide identity of 98% was observed. pRE25 can be transferred by conjugation to *E. faecalis*, *Listeria innocua*, and *Lactococcus lactis* by means of a transfer region that is similar to that of pIP501, and in addition, a 30.5-kb segment is almost identical to this plasmid. At the time being the protocol for measuring antibiotic resistance transfer is based on the use of these plasmids, hosted by *Klebsiella oxytoca* and *Enterococcus avium*, isolated from the *Blatella* gut.

Two *gfp* genes, one placed in the broad-range-host vector pSEVA237M harboring a promoterless monomeric superfolder *gfp* gene (77), and another GFP with the strong constitutive promoter J23104 cloned in the pUC57-Amp plasmid (78), were employed. The following step was to introduce these *gfp* genes into the plasmids pRE25 and pIP501 and, once the emission of green fluorescence had been confirmed, transform these labeled plasmids into natural bacterial isolates that

did not show resistance to the antibiotic under study (*K. oxytoca* and *Enterococcus pallens*; Table 2). These bacteria were provided to a population of cockroaches with a water supply that had been modified with the same antibiotic to introduce selective pressure to increase the resistant bacteria harboring the markers, mimicking a hospital population. Another population fed without antibiotic, as a normal population, was mixed with the antibiotic-treated cockroaches.

EXPERIMENTAL EPIDEMIOLOGY DESIGN: A PROPOSAL TO MEASURE THE ANTIBIOTIC RESISTANCE TRANSMISSION RATE

The two populations grew in two different hospital and community environments (Fig. 5), with the possibility of migrating from one population to another being simulated, which means the study was metapopulational. The first consisted of individuals previously colonized by bacteria resistant to one antibiotic, whereas the second consisted of individuals with possible natural resistance. The hospital environment was supplied with water containing antibiotic. Each blue box corresponds to a roach with its particular microbiota. The green boxes are bacteria that, in turn, can harbor different plasmids (red and dark-blue boxes). The arrows mean trans-hierarchical horizontal transfer events of bacteria and plasmids, represented by the discontinuous boxes. Then migration was allowed to facilitate the transmission of resistant bacteria to the untreated population.

The methodology proposed intends to establish a reproducible model of the transmission of antibiotic resistance using an animal model system to understand the dynamics of ABRs in human populations. This type of complex scenario, where bacteria-resistant populations and their genetic platforms containing ABRs move because they are selected, and evolve because of their promiscuous migration, establishes the precondition to visu-

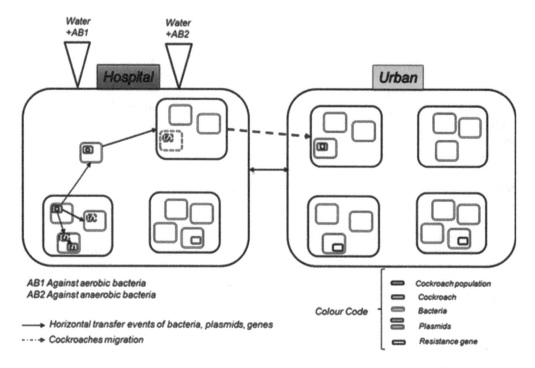

FIGURE 5 Experimental model of transmission of information about antibiotic resistance using an experimental model system with the aim of simulating the evolution of antibiotic (AB) resistance genes in human communities mimicking hospital and urban environments.

alize ABRs not only as a biological function but also as the processing of an information flow.

According to the current situation in this field of research, we aim to combine new developments in molecular microbiology, metagenomics, bacterial population biology and metapopulation, evolutionary biology, and computational biology and systems. The project has been divided into five levels.

1. *Theory:* the issue of trans-hierarchical relations between evolutionary objects. If a resistance gene is in a specific gene vector in a bacterial population and this is housed in a microbiota of a particular host and if genes, vectors, populations, and guests are independently subjected to selective processes, could we predict the spread of resistance, given the dynamics of these biological objects and selection conditions?

2. *Computational:* we aim to test the hypothesis that transmission processes can be defined computationally when resistance genes and genetic vectors can be formalized (see below). If this is confirmed, a computer model can be made based on the processes under study to formulate new hypotheses to return the focus of computing to biology through new experiments. In addition to the description and resolution of this problem for the first time, modeling techniques based on membrane computing can be applied.

3. *Experimental:* a model system for experimental epidemiology with *B. germanica* populations in order to measure where they will represent both hierarchical levels of study, the population conditions and selection, to help test the model.

4. *Clinical:* the model of *B. germanica* also constitutes a model of evolution of anti-

biotic resistance in hospitals and in the community and will be compared with epidemiological field experiences in these areas.

5. *Intervention:* the targets will be detected for interventions to prevent the spread of resistant organisms.

COMPUTER MODELING OF THE TRANSMISSION OF ABRS

In parallel with the experimental epidemiology on ABRs, we developed a computer model (31) that captures the transmission of genetic information across different levels of the biological hierarchy, from metapopulations of a given species (ecology) to the genetic units of bacteria harboring ABRs in the corresponding animal microbiotas (79). The model and the associated software, entitled ARES (Antibiotic Resistance Evolution Simulator), aims to simulate and measure the antibiotic resistance transmission rate under different population scenarios and exposure regimes to antibiotics. ARES simulates P-system model scenarios with five types of nested computing membranes to emulate the following nested compartments: (i) a peripheral ecosystem, (ii) different local environments, (iii) a reservoir of supplies, (iv) an animal host, and (v) host-associated microbiota. The computational objects emulating molecular entities, such as plasmids, ABRs, antimicrobials, and/or other substances, can be properly introduced in the ARES framework and may interact and evolve together with the membranes, based on a set of pre-established rules and specifications. ARES has been implemented as an online server and offers additional tools for storage and model editing and downstream analysis (31). ARES can be accessed at http://gydb.org/ares. The experimental epidemiology design with *B. germanica* offers empirical values for the transmission rates of ABRs on the above-mentioned hierarchical levels, which will also be simulated by ARES under a similar design

(i.e., two populations of animals, with a given migration rate of animals, different exposure to antibiotics, etc.). Accordingly, this will validate ARES as a tool to apply it to other regimes. In fact, ARES offers the chance to model predictive multilevel scenarios of antibiotic resistance evolution that can be interrogated, edited, and resimulated if necessary, with different parameters, until a correct model description of the process in the real world is convincingly approached.

CONCLUSIONS AND FUTURE WORK

This chapter presents a research program to experimentally (with the cockroach *B. germanica*) and computationally (by means of P-system membrane computing) evaluate the transferability of ABRs across different biological elements (microbiota, clones, and plasmids) and establish a model of experimental epidemiology of antibiotic resistance. Prolonged use of antibiotics or the intake of processed food increases the proportion of resistant bacteria (79), implying that the study of the emergence, persistence, and transfer mode of antibiotic resistance between hosts is necessary for the design of new antibiotics, health measures, vaccination campaigns, and epidemiological risk prediction (8–10, 80). *B. germanica* is a model to investigate the evolution of resistance because it has a very rich intestinal microbiota with human-like complexity (40), capable of incorporating antibiotic-resistant bacteria. It can be grown in the laboratory and has a short generation time (4 months), enabling both the size and nature of the bacterial inoculum, as well as the dose of the various antibiotics, to be manipulated.

The outcomes of this project will be important to estimate the critical parameters that feed ARES, a membrane computational model to investigate the transmission of antibiotic resistance across hierarchical levels. The results obtained by the simulator will, in turn, serve to refine the experiments. *B. germanica* also constitutes a model of evolution of antibiotic resistance in hospitals and in the community and will be compared with epidemiological field experiences in these areas.

ACKNOWLEDGMENTS

This work was supported by grants to A.M. and A.L. from the Spanish Ministry of Economy and Competitiveness, co-financed by ERDF funds (projects SAF2012-31187, SAF2013-49788-EXP, SAF2015-65878-R, and BFU2015-64322-C2-1-R), Carlos III Institute of Health (projects PIE14/00045 and AC15/00022), and Valencian Regional Government (project PrometeoII/2014/065). Plasmids pRE25 and pIP501 were kindly provided by T. Coque and F. Baquero (University Hospital Ramón y Cajal, Madrid, Spain).

CITATION

Llop P, Latorre A, Moya A. 2017. Experimental epidemiology of antibiotic resistance: looking for an appropriate animal model system. Microbiol Spectrum 6(1):MTBP-0007-2016.

REFERENCES

1. **Centers for Disease Control and Prevention.** 2017. Antibiotic resistance threats in the United States. 2013. http://www.cdc.gov/drugresistance/threat-report-2013/. Accessed February 20th, 2017.
2. **Foreign and Commonwealth Office.** 2013. G8 Science Ministers Statement. https://www.gov.uk/government/news/g8-science-ministers-statement. Accessed February 20th, 2017.
3. **World Health Organization.** 2016. Antimicrobial resistance. Fact sheet No. 194. http://www.who.int/mediacentre/factsheets/fs194/en/. Accessed February 20th, 2017.
4. **Carlet J, Jarlier V, Harbarth S, Voss A, Goossens H, Pittet D, Participants of the 3rd World Healthcare-Associated Infections Forum.** 2012. Ready for a world without antibiotics? The Pensières Antibiotic Resistance Call to Action. *Antimicrob Resist Infect Control* 1:11.
5. **Laxminarayan R, Duse A, Wattal C, Zaidi AKM, Wertheim HFL, Sumpradit N, Vlieghe E, Hara GL, Gould IM, Goossens H, Greko C, So AD, Bigdeli M, Tomson G, Woodhouse W, Ombaka E, Peralta AQ, Qamar FN, Mir F, Kariuki S, Bhutta ZA, Coates A, Bergstrom R, Wright GD, Brown ED, Cars O.** 2013. Antibiotic resistance—the need for global solutions. *Lancet Infect Dis* 13:1057–1098.
6. **Jarlier V, Carlet J, McGowan J, Goossens H, Voss A, Harbarth S, Pittet D, Participants of the 3rd World Healthcare-Associated Infections Forum.** 2012. Priority actions to fight antibiotic resistance: results of an international meeting. *Antimicrob Resist Infect Control* 1:17.
7. **Rolain JM, Parola P, Cornaglia G.** 2010. New Delhi metallo-beta-lactamase (NDM-1): towards a new pandemia? *Clin Microbiol Infect* 16:1699–1701.
8. **Baquero F.** 2004. From pieces to patterns: evolutionary engineering in bacterial pathogens. *Nat Rev Microbiol* 2:510–518.
9. **Baquero F, Coque TM, de la Cruz F.** 2011. Ecology and evolution as targets: the need for novel eco-evo drugs and strategies to fight antibiotic resistance. *Antimicrob Agents Chemother* 55:3649–3660.
10. **Baquero F, Tedim AP, Coque TM.** 2013. Antibiotic resistance shaping multi-level population biology of bacteria. *Front Microbiol* 4:15.
11. **Sekirov I, Russell SL, Antunes LC, Finlay BB.** 2010. Gut microbiota in health and disease. *Physiol Rev* 90:859–904.
12. **Dethlefsen L, McFall-Ngai M, Relman DA.** 2007. An ecological and evolutionary perspective on human-microbe mutualism and disease. *Nature* 449:811–818.
13. **Arumugam M, Raes J, Pelletier E, Le Paslier D, Yamada T, Mende DR, Fernandes GR, Tap J, Bruls T, Batto JM, Bertalan M, Borruel N, Casellas F, Fernandez L, Gautier L, Hansen T, Hattori M, Hayashi T, Kleerebezem M, Kurokawa K, Leclerc M, Levenez F, Manichanh C, Nielsen HB, Nielsen T, Pons N, Poulain J, Qin J, Sicheritz-Ponten T, Tims S, Torrents D, Ugarte E, Zoetendal EG, Wang J, Guarner F, Pedersen O, de Vos WM, Brunak S, Doré J; MetaHIT Consortium, Antolín M, Artiguenave F, Blottiere HM, Almeida M, Brechot C, Cara C, Chervaux C, Cultrone A, Delorme C, Denariaz G, Dervyn R, Foerstner KU, Friss C, van de Guchte M, Guedon E, Haimet F, Huber W, van Hylckama-Vlieg J, Jamet A, Juste C, Kaci G, Knol J, Lakhdari O, Layec S, Le Roux K, Maguin E, Mérieux A, Melo Minardi R, M'rini C, Muller J, Oozeer R, Parkhill J, Renault P, Rescigno M, Sanchez N, Sunagawa S, Torrejon A, Turner K, Vandemeulebrouck G, Varela E, Winogradsky Y, Zeller G, Weissenbach J, Ehrlich SD, Bork P.** 2011. Enterotypes of the human gut microbiome. *Nature* 473:174–180.

14. **Salyers AA, Gupta A, Wang Y.** 2004. Human intestinal bacteria as reservoirs for antibiotic resistance genes. *Trends Microbiol* 12:412–416.

15. **Francino MP.** 2014. Early development of the gut microbiota and immune health. *Pathogens* 3:769–790.

16. **Francino MP.** 2016. Antibiotics and the human gut microbiome: dysbioses and accumulation of resistances. *Front Microbiol* 6:1543.

17. **Moore AM, Ahmadi S, Patel S, Gibson MK, Wang B, Ndao MI, Deych E, Shannon W, Tarr PI, Warner BB, Dantas G.** 2015. Gut resistome development in healthy twin pairs in the first year of life. *Microbiome* 3:27.

18. **Lu N, Hu Y, Zhu L, Yang X, Yin Y, Lei F, Zhu Y, Du Q, Wang X, Meng Z, Zhu B.** 2014. DNA microarray analysis reveals that antibiotic resistance-gene diversity in human gut microbiota is age related. *Sci Rep* 4:4302.

19. **von Wintersdorff CJ, Penders J, Stobberingh EE, Oude Lashof AM, Hoebe CJ, Savelkoul PH, Wolffs PF.** 2014. High rates of antimicrobial drug resistance gene acquisition after international travel, The Netherlands. *Emerg Infect Dis* 20:649–657.

20. **Hu Y, Yang X, Lu N, Zhu B.** 2014. The abundance of antibiotic resistance genes in human guts has correlation to the consumption of antibiotics in animal. *Gut Microbes* 5:245–249.

21. **Ebert D, Lipsitch M, Mangin KL.** 2000. The effect of parasites on host population density and extinction: experimental epidemiology with *Daphnia* and six microparasites. *Am Nat* 156:459–477.

22. **Flexner S.** 1922. Experimental epidemiology. *J Exp Med* 36:9–14.

23. **Greenwood M, Hill AB, Topley WWC, Wilson J.** 1936. *Experimental Epidemiology.* Medical Research Council Special Report No. 209. Medical Research Council, London, United Kingdom.

24. **May RM, Anderson RM.** 1979. Population biology of infectious diseases: part II. *Nature* 280:455–461.

25. **Webster LT.** 1932. Experimental epidemiology. *Medicine* 11:321–344.

26. **Kostic AD, Howitt MR, Garrett WS.** 2013. Exploring host-microbiota interactions in animal models and humans. *Genes Dev* 27:701–718.

27. **Sharon G, Segal D, Ringo JM, Hefetz A, Zilber-Rosenberg I, Rosenberg E.** 2010. Commensal bacteria play a role in mating preference of *Drosophila melanogaster. Proc Natl Acad Sci U S A* 107:20051–20056.

28. **Cho I, Yamanishi S, Cox L, Methé BA, Zavadil J, Li K, Gao Z, Mahana D, Raju K, Teitler I, Li H, Alekseyenko AV, Blaser MJ.** 2012. Antibiotics in early life alter the murine colonic microbiome and adiposity. *Nature* 488:621–626.

29. **Semova I, Carten JD, Stombaugh J, Mackey LC, Knight R, Farber SA, Rawls JF.** 2012. Microbiota regulate intestinal absorption and metabolism of fatty acids in the zebrafish. *Cell Host Microbe* 12:277–288.

30. **Baquero F.** 2015. Causes and interventions: need of a multiparametric analysis of microbial ecobiology. *Environ Microbiol Rep* 7:13–14.

31. **Campos M, Llorens C, Sempere JM, Futami R, Rodriguez I, Carrasco P, Capilla R, Latorre A, Coque TM, Moya A, Baquero F.** 2015. A membrane computing simulator of trans-hierarchical antibiotic resistance evolution dynamics in nested ecological compartments (ARES). *Biol Direct* 10:41.

32. **Akinjogunla OJ, Odeyemi AT, Udoinyang EP.** 2012. Cockroaches (*Periplaneta americana* and *Blattella germanica*): reservoirs of multi drug resistant (MDR) bacteria in Uyo, Akwa Ibom State. *Sci J Biol Sci* 1:19–30.

33. **Schauer C, Thompson CL, Brune A.** 2012. The bacterial community in the gut of the Cockroach *Shelfordella lateralis* reflects the close evolutionary relatedness of cockroaches and termites. *Appl Environ Microbiol* 78:2758–2767.

34. **Engel P, Moran NA.** 2013. The gut microbiota of insects—diversity in structure and function. *FEMS Microbiol Rev* 37:699–735.

35. **Siegfried BD, Scott SC.** 1996. Insecticide resistance mechanisms in the German cockroach, *Blatella germanica. Am Chem Soc* 96:218–229.

36. **Dubus JC, Guerra MT, Bodiou AC.** 2001. Cockroach allergy and asthma. *Allergy* 56:351–352.

37. **Menasria T, Moussa F, El-Hamza S, Tine S, Megri R, Chenchouni H.** 2014. Bacterial load of German cockroach (*Blattella germanica*) found in hospital environment. *Pathog Glob Health* 108:141–147.

38. **Pai HH, Chen WC, Peng CF.** 2005. Isolation of bacteria with antibiotic resistance from household cockroaches (*Periplaneta americana* and *Blattella germanica*). *Acta Trop* 93:259–265.

39. **Carrasco P, Pérez-Cobas AE, van de Pol C, Baixeras J, Moya A, Latorre A.** 2014. Succession of the gut microbiota in the cockroach *Blattella germanica. Int Microbiol* 17:99–109.

40. **López-Sánchez MJ, Neef A, Peretó J, Patiño-Navarrete R, Pignatelli M, Latorre A, Moya A.** 2009. Evolutionary convergence and nitrogen metabolism in *Blattabacterium* strain Bge, primary endosymbiont of the cockroach *Blattella germanica. PLoS Genet* 5:e1000721.

41. **Pérez-Cobas AE, Maiques E, Angelova A, Carrasco P, Moya A, Latorre A.** 2015. Diet shapes the gut microbiota of the omnivorous cockroach

Blattella germanica. FEMS Microbiol Ecol **91:** fiv022.

42. **Patiño-Navarrete R, Moya A, Latorre A, Peretó J.** 2013. Comparative genomics of *Blattabacterium cuenoti*: the frozen legacy of an ancient endosymbiont genome. *Genome Biol Evol* **5:**351–361.

43. **Sabree ZL, Kambhampati S, Moran NA.** 2009. Nitrogen recycling and nutritional provisioning by *Blattabacterium*, the cockroach endosymbiont. *Proc Natl Acad Sci U S A* **106:**19521–19526.

44. **Blekhman R, Goodrich JK, Huang K, Sun Q, Bukowski R, Bell JT, Spector TD, Keinan A, Ley RE, Gevers D, Clark AG.** 2015. Host genetic variation impacts microbiome composition across human body sites. *Genome Biol* **16:**191.

45. **Thompson CL, Wang B, Holmes AJ.** 2008. The immediate environment during postnatal development has long-term impact on gut community structure in pigs. *ISME J* **2:**739–748.

46. **Hoy YE, Bik EM, Lawley TD, Holmes SP, Monack DM, Theriot JA, Relman DA.** 2015. Variation in taxonomic composition of the fecal microbiota in an inbred mouse strain across individuals and time. *PLoS One* **10:**e0142825.

47. **Ley RE, Hamady M, Lozupone C, Turnbaugh PJ, Ramey RR, Bircher JS, Schlegel ML, Tucker TA, Schrenzel MD, Knight R, Gordon JI.** 2008. Evolution of mammals and their gut microbes. *Science* **320:**1647–1651.

48. **Pluznick JL.** 2014. Gut microbes and host physiology: what happens when you host billions of guests? *Front Endocrinol (Lausanne)* **5:**91.

49. **Krishnan S, Alden N, Lee K.** 2015. Pathways and functions of gut microbiota metabolism impacting host physiology. *Curr Opin Biotechnol* **36:**137–145.

50. **Yano JM, Yu K, Donaldson GP, Shastri GG, Ann P, Ma L, Nagler CR, Ismagilov RF, Mazmanian SK, Hsiao EY.** 2015. Indigenous bacteria from the gut microbiota regulate host serotonin biosynthesis. *Cell* **161:**264–276.

51. **Gross EM, Brune A, Walenciak O.** 2008. Gut pH, redox conditions and oxygen levels in an aquatic caterpillar: potential effects on the fate of ingested tannins. *J Insect Physiol* **54:**462–471.

52. **Ryu JH, Kim SH, Lee HY, Bai JY, Nam YD, Bae JW, Lee DG, Shin SC, Ha EM, Lee WJ.** 2008. Innate immune homeostasis by the homeobox gene caudal and commensal-gut mutualism in *Drosophila. Science* **319:**777–782.

53. **Ke J, Sun JZ, Nguyen HD, Singh D, Lee KC, Beyenal H, Chen SL.** 2010. *In-situ* oxygen profiling and lignin modification in guts of wood-feeding termites. *Insect Sci* **17:**277–290.

54. **Brooks MA, Richards AG.** 1955. Intracellular symbiosis in cockroaches. I. Production of aposymbiotic cockroaches. *Biol Bull* **109:**22–39.

55. **Sacchi L, Nalepa CA, Bigliardi E, Lenz M, Bandi C, Corona S, Grigolo A, Lambiase S, Laudani U.** 1998. Some aspects of intracellular symbiosis during embryo development of *Mastotermes darwiniensis* (Isoptera: Mastotermitidae). *Parassitologia* **40:**309–316.

56. **Sacchi L, Grigolo A.** 1989. Endocytobiosis in *Blattella germanica* L. (BLATTODEA): recent acquisitions. *Endocytobiosis Cell Res* **6:**121–147.

57. **Sacchi L, Corona S, Grigolo A, Laudani U, Selmi MG, Bigliardi E.** 1996. The fate of the endocytobionts of *Blattella germanica* (Blattaria: Blattellidae) and *Periplaneta americana* (Blattaria: Blattidae) during embryo development. *Ital J Zool (Modena)* **63:**1–11.

58. **Aguilera L, Marquetti MC, Fuentes O, Navarro A.** 1998. Efecto de 2 dietas sobre aspectos biológicos de *Blattella germanica* (Dictyoptera: Blattellidae) en condiciones de laboratorio. *Rev Cubana Med Trop* **50:**143–149.

59. **Colman DR, Toolson EC, Takacs-Vesbach CD.** 2012. Do diet and taxonomy influence insect gut bacterial communities? *Mol Ecol* **21:**5124–5137.

60. **Yun JH, Roh SW, Whon TW, Jung MJ, Kim MS, Park DS, Yoon C, Nam YD, Kim YJ, Choi JH, Kim JY, Shin NR, Kim SH, Lee WJ, Bae JW.** 2014. Insect gut bacterial diversity determined by environmental habitat, diet, developmental stage, and phylogeny of host. *Appl Environ Microbiol* **80:**5254–5264.

61. **Levin BR, McCall IC, Perrot V, Weiss H, Ovesepian A, Baquero F.** 2017. A numbers game: ribosome densities, bacterial growth, and antibiotic-mediated stasis and death. *mBio* **8:**e02253-16.

62. **Fadrosh DW, Ma B, Gajer P, Sengamalay N, Ott S, Brotman RM, Ravel J.** 2014. An improved dual-indexing approach for multiplexed 16S rRNA gene sequencing on the Illumina MiSeq platform. *Microbiome* **2:**6.

63. **Caporaso JG, Kuczynski J, Stombaugh J, Bittinger K, Bushman FD, Costello EK, Fierer N, Peña AG, Goodrich JK, Gordon JI, Huttley GA, Kelley ST, Knights D, Koenig JE, Ley RE, Lozupone CA, McDonald D, Muegge BD, Pirrung M, Reeder J, Sevinsky JR, Turnbaugh PJ, Walters WA, Widmann J, Yatsunenko T, Zaneveld J, Knight R.** 2010. QIIME allows analysis of high-throughput community sequencing data. *Nat Methods* **7:**335–336.

64. **DeSantis TZ, Hugenholtz P, Larsen N, Rojas M, Brodie EL, Keller K, Huber T, Dalevi D, Hu P, Andersen GL.** 2006. Greengenes, a chimera-checked 16S rRNA gene database and workbench compatible with ARB. *Appl Environ Microbiol* **72:**5069–5072.

65. **Hammad KM, Mahdy HM.** 2012. Antibiotic resistant-bacteria associated with the cockroach, *Periplaneta americana* collected from different habitat in Egypt. *N Y Sci J* **5:**198–206.

66. **Haghi FM, Nikookar H, Hajati H, Harati MR, Shafaroudi MM, Yazdani-Charati J, Ahanjan M.** 2014. Evaluation of bacterial infection and antibiotic susceptibility of the bacteria isolated from cockroaches in educational hospitals of Mazandaran University of medical sciences. *Bull Environ Pharmacol Life Sci* **3:**25–28.

67. **Wannigama DL, Dwivedi R, Zahraei-Ramazani A.** 2013. Prevalence and antibiotic resistance of gram-negative pathogenic bacteria species isolated from *Periplaneta americana* and *Blattella germanica* in Varanasi, India. *J Arthropod Borne Dis* **8:**10–20.

68. **Atlas RM.** 2010. *Handbook of Microbiological Media*, 4th ed. ASM Press, Washington, DC, and CRC Press, Boca Raton, FL.

69. **Wu SW, Dornbusch K, Kronvall G, Norgren M.** 1999. Characterization and nucleotide sequence of a *Klebsiella oxytoca* cryptic plasmid encoding a CMY-type β-lactamase: confirmation that the plasmid-mediated cephamycinase originated from the *Citrobacter freundii* AmpC β-lactamase. *Antimicrob Agents Chemother* **43:**1350–1357.

70. **Huang TW, Wang JT, Lauderdale TL, Liao TL, Lai JF, Tan MC, Lin AC, Chen YT, Tsai SF, Chang SC.** 2013. Complete sequences of two plasmids in a *bla*$_{NDM-1}$-positive *Klebsiella oxytoca* isolate from Taiwan. *Antimicrob Agents Chemother* **57:**4072–4076.

71. **Akingbade A, Balogun SA, Ojo DA, Afolabi RO, Motayo BO, Okerentugba PO, Okonko IO.** 2012. Plasmid profile analysis of multidrug resistant *Pseudomonas aeruginosa* isolated from wound infections in South West, Nigeria. *World Appl Sci J* **20:**766–775.

72. **Schwarz FV, Perreten V, Teuber M.** 2001. Sequence of the 50-kb conjugative multiresistance plasmid pRE25 from *Enterococcus faecalis* RE25. *Plasmid* **46:**170–187.

73. **Thompson JK, Collins MA.** 2003. Completed sequence of plasmid pIP501 and origin of spontaneous deletion derivatives. *Plasmid* **50:**28–35.

74. **Perreten V, Teuber M.** 1995. Antibiotic resistant bacteria in fermented dairy products. A new challenge for raw milk cheeses? *In* Proceedings of the Symposium on Residues of Antimicrobial Drugs and other Inhibitors in Milk, 28-31 August 1995, Kiel, Germany. International Dairy Federation, Brussels, Belgium.

75. **Tauch A, Krieft S, Kalinowski J, Pühler A.** 2000. The 51,409-bp R-plasmid pTP10 from the multi-resistant clinical isolate *Corynebacterium striatum* M82B is composed of DNA segments initially identified in soil bacteria and in plant, animal, and human pathogens. *Mol Gen Genet* **263:**1–11.

76. **Horodniceanu T, Bouanchaud DH, Bieth G, Chabbert YA.** 1976. R plasmids in *Streptococcus agalactiae* (group B). *Antimicrob Agents Chemother* **10:**795–801.

77. **Silva-Rocha R, Martínez-García E, Calles B, Chavarría M, Arce-Rodríguez A, de Las Heras A, Páez-Espino AD, Durante-Rodríguez G, Kim J, Nikel PI, Platero R, de Lorenzo V.** 2013. The Standard European Vector Architecture (SEVA): a coherent platform for the analysis and deployment of complex prokaryotic phenotypes. *Nucleic Acids Res* **41**(D1)**:**D666–D675.

78. **Vilanova C, Tanner K, Dorado-Morales P, Villaescusa P, Chugani D, Frías A, Segredo E, Molero X, Fritschi M, Morales L, Ramón D, Peña C, Peretó J, Porcar M.** 2015. Standards not that standard. *J Biol Eng* **9:**17.

79. **Marshall BM, Levy SB.** 2011. Food animals and antimicrobials: impacts on human health. *Clin Microbiol Rev* **24:**718–733.

80. **Martínez JL, Baquero F, Andersson DI.** 2007. Predicting antibiotic resistance. *Nat Rev Microbiol* **5:**958–965.

Transmission in the Origins of Bacterial Diversity, From Ecotypes to Phyla

18

FREDERICK M. COHAN[1]

IN SEARCH OF THE ORIGINS OF MICROBIAL DIVERSITY

In recent decades, microbiologists have discovered an astounding disparity of prokaryotic life. Our field has identified the most anciently divergent prokaryotic lineages, and we have found them to be utterly different in every aspect of their being: their cell architecture, biochemistry, physiology, genome content, and how they make a living. Our understanding of the prokaryotes' phylogenetic diversity began in large part with Carl Woese's tree of all life, based on the universal 16S rRNA gene (1). His universal tree yielded the surprising result that the not-yet-named archaea and bacteria, already known to be extremely different in cell structure, represented the deepest divisions of life. Subsequent surveys of 16S diversity, using cultivation-free methods, led to discovery of vast numbers of uncultivated prokaryotic taxa, at all levels from species to phyla, in even the most familiar of habitats (2). While cultivation has yielded discovery of ∼30 bacterial phyla, cultivation-free methods focusing on 16S have expanded the number of bacterial phyla to nearly 100 (3). Moreover, we can extrapolate that among rare, presently uncultivable organisms, we will eventually discover ∼1,300 phyla (4)! Most recently, single-cell genomic approaches have yielded much greater resolution for prokaryotic phylogeny and

[1]Department of Biology, Wesleyan University, Middletown, CT.
Microbial Transmission in Biological Processes
Edited by Fernando Baquero, Emilio Bouza, J.A. Gutiérrez-Fuentes, and Teresa M. Coque
© 2018 American Society for Microbiology, Washington, DC
doi:10.1128/microbiolspec.MTBP-0014-2016

have revealed a totally unexpected super-phylum at the base of the bacteria tree. This group is predominated by phyla with limited metabolic capabilities and a shared stubbornness against cultivation (5). These are all exciting forays into estimating the vastness and organization of prokaryotic diversity, but these purely phylogenetic approaches fail to portray the profound distinctness among the most anciently divergent prokaryotes.

What makes the discovery of all these phyla so interesting is their great disparity in cell architectures, physiologies, genomes, and ecologies (6). In some cases, it is clear how ancient architectural differences have generated disparate ways of making a living. For example, the multilayered peptidoglycans of the *Firmicutes'* cell walls give these organisms constitutive resistance to the osmotic stresses of drought and rewetting found in desert soils (7). Also, the photosynthetic capabilities of the various phototrophic phyla do not emerge from their enzymes alone; their photosynthetic functions depend on complex architectural membrane structures (8). Cells of the *Planctomycetes* phylum (as well as the *Caulobacterales* of the *Alphaproteobacteria*) sport stalk and holdfast structures that raise the cell above the still water at the surface of the seabed, and so provide access to a greater flow of water and nutrients (9–11). It will be interesting to discover how architecture has led to distinct ways of making a living in other phyla.

The unique capabilities of phyla are based on long-standing, highly conserved differences that are not transferred across taxa (although some transfers were involved early on in the origins of complex traits [12]). That is, the familiar horizontal transfers of simple traits like antibiotic resistance and virulence, which plague public health (13, 14), do not apply to phylum-defining qualities such as the *Firmicutes'* Gram-positive cell wall. The nontransferable nature of phylum-defining traits suggests that these are complex adaptations based on many genes and proteins (15, 16). Indeed, all *Cyanobacteria* share hundreds

of genes that are unique to that phylum (and the derivative eukaryotic chloroplasts) (17), and similar results hold for other phyla (18). It will be fascinating to find out what novel physiologies those 1,300 or so undiscovered phyla might be capable of. Genomics will yield some of the secrets (19), as will studies of habitat differences among phyla (18, 20), but eventual cultivation of these organisms will tell us so much more (21). Fortunately, new high-throughput culture methods promise to make isolates available for many taxa that resist cultivation (22).

Whence did this profound disparity emerge? We cannot yet identify the history of architectural and physiological changes leading to each phylum, but there is one kind of historical moment shared in the emergence of all anciently divergent groups. That is, all lineages, no matter how distant they are now, began their divergence as one population splitting to become two lineages that could coexist indefinitely (23). By addressing the origin of species, population biology can help explain the origins of the deepest divisions of life. My goal here is to explore how one population may split into two lineages that can coexist indefinitely.

As we shall see, this splitting of lineages involves a "transmission" of part of the old lineage into a new ecological niche: the new niche may in some cases be a novel microhabitat with different resources; in other cases, the new microhabitat may hold different physical and chemical conditions; in pathogens and other endosymbionts, the niches may be different hosts or different host tissues; in still other cases, the niches may not be in different places at all but instead represent different sets of resources in the same microhabitat. Whether ecological divergence between lineages brings about their persistence in the same or different habitats, we will refer to the outcome of persistence as "coexistence." How do these splits happen, and what is necessary for newly divergent lineages to ride the long haul of time to eventually become profoundly different creatures?

THE DYNAMIC PROPERTIES OF SPECIES

Let us begin with what speciologists have described as the quintessential attributes of species (24, 25). First, species are understood to be ecologically distinct, since ecological distinctness is required for the groups to coexist into the future. Then there is the property of cohesion within but not between species. That is, lineages within a species are constrained in their divergence, while lineages from different species are not. In the case of the bacteria, we'll see that cohesion within species involves a force called "periodic selection," which purges the diversity genome-wide within but not between species-like populations (26). The flip side of cohesion is that upon speciation, two lineages lose their cohesion and can for the first time diverge indefinitely (although we will give a caveat to the meaning of *indefinite* divergence). After they have become different species, two lineages can no longer fuse back into one, and so species lineages are irreversibly separate (25). Finally, at some point in their divergence, species become recognizable as sequence clusters for most genes in the genome as they accumulate neutral sequence divergence (27).

The species-like property of irreversible separateness, whereby species can coexist indefinitely, is necessary for two lineages to eventually diverge to the point of becoming two genera, or two families, or even two phyla. However, this property is clearly not sufficient—only the rarest pair of newly divergent species will become two phyla! So, in what sense can we say that two new species have the potential to diverge "indefinitely"?

Two species should at least be ecologically different enough that one will not globally outcompete the other to extinction (28), noting that very small ecological differences can in principle lead to indefinitely long coexistence (29, 30). However, new species are not immune to the vicissitudes of nature that may extinguish them, and so pairs of new species are unlikely to persist indefinitely, regardless of how much they diverge from one another. For example, two new species may fail to coexist into the indefinite future if they have diversified within a single individual host but fail to be transmitted before the host dies. We may think of this as "shortsighted" speciation, analogous to the shortsighted evolution discussed by Levin and Bull, when a pathogen evolves high virulence within a host but fails to be transmitted (31). Here I will attempt to identify the properties of newly divergent species that give them a chance of coexisting into the remote future.

How can bacteriologists study the origins of species? Studies of animal and plant speciation have long focused on the origins of sexual isolation, owing to the influence of Ernst Mayr's ideas on speciation through much of the 20th century (32). That is, the quintessential element of species' origins was thought to be the evolution of inability to interbreed and exchange genes. In this view, unless the propensity to interbreed is reduced drastically between two groups, the groups are prevented from diverging, a process known as "Mayr's brake" on diversification (33). In recent decades, however, zoologists and botanists have accumulated evidence that very little sexual isolation is needed for indefinite divergence, sometimes just the physical distance between two adjacent types of microhabitat (34–36).

In the case of bacteria, a growing literature of experimental evolution experiments indicates the potential for ecological diversification within a single vessel and without any sexual isolation. In some cases, there is some spatial separation of populations (scum on the surface versus the water column) (37, 38), but in other cases, there is no spatial separation whatsoever, and newly evolved populations differ ecologically only in the soluble resources they utilize (39, 40).

Nevertheless, several recent studies have claimed that sexual isolation is a necessary precondition for ecological divergence among bacterial populations (41–43). Their evidence was finding that closely related, ecologically distinct clades had reduced capacity for exchanging genes with one another, while lineages within each clade showed little or no sexual isolation. They concluded that the higher rates of recombination within the clades prevented ecological diversification. However, these studies did not actually attempt to determine whether the more rapidly recombining close relatives within the clades may have diversified ecologically, without the benefit of sexual isolation (44). My colleagues and I recently investigated, in hot spring *Synechococcus*, the possibility of ecological diversification among extremely close relatives that were not sexually isolated, and we found that the highest rates of recombination within clades did not prevent their ecological diversification (44). Where it has been investigated in bacteria, an absence of sexual isolation has not precluded ecological diversification among closest relatives (45). We may conclude that sexual isolation is not a prerequisite for ecological diversification in bacteria, and that sexual isolation is more likely to be the effect than the cause of ecological divergence.

More such studies will be desirable, given the hegemony of Mayrian ideas in speciology, but for theoretical reasons we should not expect to find an important role for sexual isolation in bacterial diversification. That is, recurrent genetic exchange is unlikely to prevent ecological divergence among bacterial populations (46, 47). J. B. S. Haldane showed long ago that when a niche-specifying allele is beneficial for one population but is harmful for another, natural selection can limit the niche-specifying allele to negligible frequency in any population where it is harmful (48). Haldane's model predicts the frequency of a harmful, foreign allele to be c_b/s, where c_b is the rate of recombination between populations and s is the intensity of selection against the foreign allele; because the rate of recombination between bacterial populations is extremely low ($\sim 10^{-6}$ or less per gene per generation) (47), adaptive divergence between bacterial populations will not be stifled by recombination between them.

I will therefore not focus here on the origins of sexual divergence in bacteria. Instead, I will show that we can more usefully focus on the origins of *ecological* divergences that allow bacterial populations to coexist (46, 49, 50).

THE FOCAL SPECIES OF BACTERIAL SPECIOLOGY

Speciologists have traditionally studied the origins of species by focusing on the species taxa recognized by systematists and characterizing their divergence. If species taxa are newly divergent enough, the differences among new species may be reasonably attributed to the process of species splitting, and not to divergence that happened after the lineages had split (51). This is not a bad approximation for animal and plant species, but it is not so useful for bacterial speciology. A recognized bacterial taxon is typically already extremely diverse in physiology, genome content, and ecology, and contains multiple lineages that each hold the species-like properties we have discussed (52–56).

The problem is that while the classification scheme of bacterial systematics has focused on finding species that are significantly different from one another in DNA sequence identity, genome content, and physiology (57), the classification is not aimed to ensure that each individual species is homogeneous in any characteristic (52, 54, 55, 58). To pick on a particularly notable example, we would not learn much about speciation by studying the divergence between the closely related *Escherichia coli* and *Escherichia fergusonii* species taxa, as lineages within *E. coli* are already hugely diversified. Some populations of *E. coli* are specialized as pathogens and others as commensals; within one host species, some lineages of *E. coli* may be specialized to colonize the large intestine and others the urinary tract (59, 60); populations may be specialized to different hosts (61) or even to living outside of any host (62, 63). These environments reflect vast differences in temperature, pH, and extracellular secretions and matrices; moreover, the ecological and physiological adaptations to these environments are based on huge genomic differences (60, 64). Most other named species also contain a high diversity of ecologically, physiologically, and genomically distinct populations (45, 65–75). In addition, genome sequencing is suggesting substantial ecological differences among closely related isolates within a given species taxon (43, 76, 77). Studying the divergence between the species taxa recognized by bacterial taxonomy is clearly not the way to study speciation; we need to zoom in within species taxa to find the origins of the most newly divergent lineages with species-like properties.

My colleagues and I have studied the dynamics of bacterial speciation by focusing on the origins of "ecotypes" (78–80). We define ecotypes as the most newly divergent, ecologically distinct bacterial populations that can coexist indefinitely as a result of their ecological differences. (As noted earlier, by indefinite coexistence we mean only that newly diverged ecotypes will not outcompete one another to extinction.) Ecotypes are defined such that lineages within an ecotype are largely homogeneous; to the extent that there are ecological differences within an ecotype, they are defined to be too small to allow indefinite coexistence (81) (Fig. 1). We will consider ecotypes to be the most newly divergent bacterial species, and we will refer to the origins of ecotypes as speciation, following recent usage by microbial ecologists (43, 45, 55, 78).

I will first discuss progress toward identifying the most newly divergent ecotypes. I will then explain how these efforts have allowed us to characterize the genetic basis of ecotype divergence, to find the ecological dimensions along which ecotypes have diverged, to identify the species-like characteristics held by bacterial ecotypes, and to estimate the tempo of bacterial speciation. In particular, I will address how the lifestyle of a

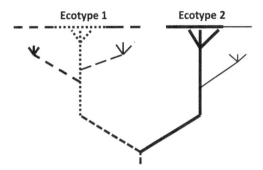

FIGURE 1 Ecological divergence between ecotypes and ecological homogeneity within ecotypes. The ecological divergence between ecotypes is sufficient for them to coexist into the indefinite future. Ecotypes are defined so that any ecological differences among lineages within ecotypes are not sufficient to allow them to coexist indefinitely. We may thus refer to ecologically distinct lineages within ecotypes as "ephemeral ecotypes." The different styles of dashed lines within ecotype 1 refer to different ephemeral ecotypes; note that only one of these lineages persists to the present. The different weights of solid lines represent different ephemeral ecotypes within ecotype 2 (52). Used with permission from Elsevier.

bacterial group and the genetic basis of speciation can affect the dynamic attributes of speciation and the likelihood of long-term coexistence. I will focus on pathogens wherever possible.

TO IDENTIFY THE MOST NEWLY DIVERGENT ECOTYPES

Bacterial systematists have approached species demarcation under the premise that each species should contain a standard and large level of sequence diversity, for example, a level of ~1% divergence in the 16S rRNA molecule (82). As we have seen, the universal molecular criteria for demarcating species have led to species taxa like *E. coli* that are notably diverse in their physiology and ecology. In contrast, several algorithms use sequence data from the taxon of focus to identify the appropriate level of sequence diversity for distinguishing groups likely to have the dynamic properties of species. These include Ecotype Simulation (83), BAPS (84), GMYC (85), AdaptML (45), Minimum Entropy Decomposition (MED) (86), and Accessory Gene Network Analysis (77). For example, Ecotype Simulation identifies sequence clusters that are consistent with ecotypes, assuming that new ecotypes form and cohesive forces purge diversity within ecotypes at rates that the algorithm infers from the sequence data (79).

The algorithm AdaptML requires the habitat of isolation as input data, while Ecotype Simulation, MED, BAPS, and GMYC are blind to ecology and demarcate ecotypes based solely on patterns of sequence clustering. Ecology-blind and ecology-informed approaches both have their advantages (87). The ecology-informed AdaptML is useful when the investigators have hypothesized one or more environmental parameters they believe to be important in ecotype divergence. For example, Dana Hunt and colleagues believed that newly divergent ecotypes in marine *Vibrio* would differ in the size of small particles they inhabit, and they were right (45)! The ecology-informed algorithms not only discover the putative ecotypes, but they also confirm their ecological distinctness by testing for significant differences in habitat preferences. In contrast, the ecology-blind algorithms can identify ecotypes even when the researcher is ignorant of the environmental differences that might be important in ecotype divergence. Moreover, ecology-blind methods can discover ecotypes even when they do not differ in their preferred habitats (83).

So, how successful are these algorithms in finding the most closely related ecotypes? We must require two properties of the "putative ecotypes" that are hypothesized and demarcated by the algorithms. One requirement is that the putative ecotypes must be ecologically distinct from one another; the second requirement is that each putative ecotype must be ecologically homogeneous. By and large, when these algorithms have predicted putative ecotypes, these groups have been

confirmed to be ecologically distinct based on their habitat differences (45, 58, 79, 80). For example, putative ecotypes of soil *Bacillus* hypothesized by Ecotype Simulation have been shown to differ in preferences for solar exposure, soil texture, rhizospheres, elevation, and geochemical stressors (78, 79); putative ecotypes of *Synechococcus* from hot spring mats have differed in their temperature and depth associations (58, 80); putative ecotypes of *Legionella* have differed in the amoebae they can infect (that is, they differ in their host ranges) (88); and putative ecotypes within *Vibrio splendidus* differed in the sizes of particles they were attached to and in their seasons of abundance (45). In addition, many ecologists have noted that very closely related sequence clusters (demarcated by intuition rather than by algorithm) were different in their habitat associations (62, 72, 89–91). Over all, putative ecotypes identified as closely related sequence clusters in a great diversity of phyla (*Actinobacteria, Cyanobacteria, Firmicutes, Proteobacteria,* and *Spirochaetes*) have shown ecological distinctness through habitat preferences.

Microbial ecologists have also confirmed the ecological distinctness of putative ecotypes by finding the physiological and genomic differences that underlie their habitat associations. For example, putative ecotypes of *Bacillus subtilis* and *Bacillus simplex* that are associated with more direct solar exposure have been shown to have membranes yielding greater thermal tolerances (78, 92). Putative ecotypes of *Synechococcus* farther from the source of the hot spring (and living in cooler water) were found to be less tolerant of extremely high temperatures (93), and they had genes enabling utilization of ions that are relatively more abundant downstream (94, 95).

Do the putative ecotypes meet the second requirement for ecotypes, that they must be ecologically homogeneous? We should note that attempts to identify putative ecotypes have so far drawn from low-resolution phylogenies, based on only one to three genes. If speciation is occurring rapidly, one to three genes might not provide enough resolution to find the most recently divergent ecotypes as sequence clusters, and so each putative ecotype could actually be an amalgam of many newly divergent ecotypes. When we explore the rates of speciation for various bacterial phyla, we shall see that the ecological homogeneity within putative ecotypes varies across lifestyles. The hypothesized putative ecotypes are in some cases the most newly divergent ecological species; in other cases, they are not, but they at least represent an early phase of ecological diversification.

We'll next consider the genetic and ecological basis of early diversification in bacteria.

THE GENETIC BASIS OF EARLY DIVERSIFICATION

Bacteria can evolve to change their ecology through various kinds of genetic changes: mutations in genes they already have, replacement of one allele by another at a genetic locus through homologous recombination, and acquisition of suites of novel genes either by horizontal genetic transfer (HGT) of chromosomal genes or through infection by a plasmid or a phage (47, 96, 97). As we shall see, the genetic basis of divergence may have implications for the long-term coexistence of ecologically distinct lineages.

Like the animals and plants, bacteria can diversify ecologically through changes in the genes they already have. The capacity for mutation-driven diversification has been demonstrated many times in laboratory evolution experiments, where a single bacterial clone diversifies by mutation into multiple coexisting ecotypes (37, 98–100). In addition, mutations have been shown to be responsible for bacterial diversification in nature, primarily in pathogens. Mutations have resulted in diversification of populations specializing in different mammalian host species in *Borrelia* (91, 101); mutations have also resulted in diversification of populations specializing in different tissues and microhabitats within

hosts by *E. coli* (102), *Pseudomonas aeruginosa* (103, 104), and *Bartonella bacilliformis* (105, 106). Also, mutations in *Salmonella enterica* have resulted in a "top-down" diversification, in which populations are differentiated by their defenses against amoebic predators (107). Mutation alone can even generate biochemical novelty (e.g., utilization of a new carbohydrate), especially when the gene involved has been duplicated (108).

While bacteria and the higher organisms share mutation as a driver of diversification, bacteria are distinguished by the huge role that HGT plays in their diversification. This is in part because transfer can occur across vast phylogenetic distances in the prokaryotes (109) but also because transfer is usually limited to a small stretch of DNA (47), ranging from several thousand bases in genetic transformation (110) to several hundred thousand in conjugation (111, 112). The short lengths transferred provide that a recipient can acquire a small adaptive set of genes from a donor without also acquiring a huge number of genes ("genetic baggage") that would be maladaptive for the recipient (110).

A horizontal transfer event can profoundly alter the ecology of a recipient bacterium in a single step and may constitute an instantaneous speciation event. That is, acquisition of DNA by horizontal transfer may cause the recipient lineage to differ markedly from the preexisting lineage in the resources it can utilize or the conditions it can tolerate (113, 114), such that the two lineages can coexist indefinitely.

We should note that horizontal transfer of an adaptation does not necessarily make the donor and recipient lineages more similar ecologically. Instead, a transferred adaptation can allow the recipient to build on its unique, preexisting adaptations to either invade a new niche or improve its performance in its current niche (87). For example, *E. coli* and *Burkholderia cepacia* share a niche-transcending adaptation that does not make these lineages more similar ecologically. The shared class 5 fimbriae allow each lineage to better attack the epithelial cells of its respective niche, whether in the small intestine for *E. coli* or in the lung for *B. cepacia* (in cystic fibrosis [CF] patients) (115), but these lineages nevertheless still attack different tissues (28, 87). Likewise, when ecologically disparate human pathogens acquire the same antibiotic resistance factors by HGT (116), their ecological niches are not converging beyond their response to natural selection by antibiotics.

We have noted that once two populations have diverged ecologically, sexual isolation is not required for maintaining their ecological divergence (47). However, sexual isolation can impact the *creation* of ecological divergence by limiting the opportunities for HGT. This is because bacteria are much more likely to acquire genes through HGT from close relatives, both because lower sequence divergence will foster homology-facilitated illegitimate recombination (117) and because closer relatives are more likely to share habitats (109).

What might be the scope of transferable adaptations that can bring about speciation? Transfer of adaptations is limited by the short length of DNA segments that can be transferred by the various mechanisms of recombination. An ecology-changing horizontal transfer can be as small as a single gene, even a small set of nucleotides within a gene. This is the case for homologous recombination of penicillin resistance alleles that have been transferred from one *Neisseria* species to another and from one strain of *Streptococcus pneumoniae* to another (118).

Also, an adaptation *coded by several genes* may be transferred in one event, provided that the genes lie contiguously on a small segment of chromosome. For example, the *lac* operon, which has been studied so famously in *E. coli* (119), was acquired by an *Escherichia* ancestor by HGT, as evidenced by the operon's unusual codon usage (120). The operon has all the components needed for uptake and metabolism of lactose, as well as regulation of the whole transcription unit.

Jeffrey Lawrence's "selfish operon" theory explains that many metabolic capabilities have transferred between lineages owing to the operon organization of the genes involved (121). The selfish operon model predicts that natural selection will favor the contiguous arrangement of a functionally related set of genes as an operon, enabling the gene set to be successfully transferred as a single, functional element across taxa; that is, natural selection acts on the operon itself rather than on the organism (121–123). Operons may thus make possible a wholesale transfer of metabolic capabilities even in the context of very short recombined segments. Beyond carbohydrate utilization functions, transferable units include the sets of genes coding for synthesis of siderophores (113), synthesis of outer membrane structures (124, 125), heavy-metal resistance (126), and antibiotic resistance (127). Many such transfers have created new populations that are ecologically distinct from their parental populations.

Microbiologists have become accustomed to evolution of adaptations through HGT, to the extent that HGT is seen as a deus ex machina that can solve any ecological challenge. For example, when a pathogen needs a new outer surface structure to evade the immune system, it can just grab it from another species through HGT (128). HGT makes possible the saltational evolution toward "hopeful monsters" that was hypothesized long ago by Richard Goldschmidt for animal evolution (129).

But there are limits to the complexity of adaptations that can be transferred: the genes coding the adaptation must fit on a transferable piece of DNA and the adaptation must be compatible with the physiology and architecture of the recipient (47). For example, the extremely resilient cell wall of the *Firmicutes* is a remarkable structure that grants constitutive resistance to osmotic stress. Surely, other organisms would do well with the osmotic resistance of the *Firmicutes'* cell wall, but this structure has never been transferred across phyla. We can imagine that the complexity of the *Firmicutes'* cell wall architecture cannot be coded on a small piece of

DNA, nor would it be compatible with the existing architecture of some other phylum. Likewise, the stalked structure of the *Planctomycetes* phylum is highly adaptive in raising a cell above the still water at the surface of the seabed, and we can imagine that a stalk structure would provide greater nutrients to any other bacteria residing in that habitat. However, this structure has not been transferred either, likely for being too complex to travel across phyla. While HGT is a marvelous device for acquiring simple adaptations, there are clearly limits to what can be transferred (18).

Bacteria can also change their ecology by acquiring a plasmid that comes fully adapted to change the ecological niche of its host. For example, a *Rhizobium* cell may be adapted to infect and provide nitrogen fixation for a given legume species by virtue of its "symbiosis" plasmid. A *Rhizobium* lineage may change its host adaptation by gaining a symbiosis plasmid for one plant host and losing the plasmid for another, or it may adapt to life in free soil by losing all its symbiosis plasmids (47, 130). Also, within *E. coli* there are several pathogenic populations whose virulence capabilities are determined by plasmids (e.g., enteroinvasive, enterotoxigenic, and enteroaggregative *E. coli*), and one virulence type is determined by a phage (enterohemorrhagic *E. coli*). These extrachromosomal elements can all move readily from one lineage to another, thereby converting an *E. coli* lineage to a new ecology (131, 132). Likewise, lineages within *Bacillus cereus sensu lato* can move from the niche of a gut pathogen of mammals (*B. cereus*) to that of causing systemic infection in mammals (*Bacillus anthracis*) to that of an insect pathogen (*Bacillus thuringiensis*) by acquiring and losing different plasmids. These dynamics each present a paradoxical case where the various niches may persist into the remote future, yet those bacteria inhabiting those niches may never diverge as independent and irreversibly separate lineages. Their divergence is prevented by any given bacterial lineage being thrust from one ecotype into another and then back again through recurrent transfer of plasmids (81).

There is one circumstance where plasmid determination of niches can help precipitate irreversible divergence among bacterial lineages. This is the case when closely related bacterial lineages diversify, perhaps gradually, to specialize on the services of different plasmids. This appears to be happening within agricultural lineages of *Rhizobium leguminosarum*, where there are five sequence clusters that can each be infected by various symbiosis plasmids that adapt the bacteria to either vetch or clover (133). While these clusters have no known physiological features that would explain their coexistence, they appear to differ in their propensities to be infected by the various symbiosis plasmids (52). Differences in association between plasmid adaptations and bacterial sequence clusters cause the clusters to differ dramatically in the plants they infect. It is not clear why the sequence clusters differ in their frequencies of infection by different plasmids, but this could represent an early stage of irreversible ecological diversification of the *Rhizobium* sequence clusters.

A later stage of permanent diversification of bacteria through specialization on different plasmids was observed among *R. leguminosarum* lineages, in this case sampled from nonagricultural species of clover (134). Here, three chromosomally defined sequence clusters were each infected by a different plasmid lineage, and so the *Rhizobium* lineages largely infected different species of clover. This study concluded that plasmids can promote indefinite coexistence of different bacterial lineages. Likely the specialization on different plasmids was fostered by a slow rate of transfer of plasmids, yielding a long residence time of plasmids in any given bacterial lineage; this would give a particular bacterial chromosomal lineage an opportunity to adapt to its plasmid before the plasmid leaves for another lineage.

To what extent can HGT of *chromosome-based* genes lead to reversible ecological divergence? One possibility is that the transfer of an operon could first create a new population that is ecologically distinct from its parental population; then, if the new population should lose the operon, the divergence between the new and old populations would be reversed. However, there is little evidence that ecological divergence can be reversed in this way, and indeed two factors appear to prevent ecological reversals through acquisition and then loss of chromosome-based genes.

One limiting factor is that the rates of acquisition and loss of chromosome-based functions are not likely to be as high as for plasmid-based genes, except possibly in the case of homologous recombination of niche-determining alleles. For example, penicillin-binding protein alleles can be recurrently gained and lost through homologous recombination among close relatives of *Neisseria*, thus converting lineages from one ecologically defined population to another (135).

Another factor limiting the reversibility of ecological divergence is that horizontally acquired genes can create secondary selection to improve the adaptations they provide. In contrast to plasmids circulating continuously through a given bacterial clade, the adaptations provided by a novel suite of genes from a distant taxon often are not fully adapted to a given recipient. As a result, many horizontally acquired genes engender a round of ameliorative evolution that improves the adaptation's compatibility with its new genetic background (47, 136, 137). Modes of ameliorative evolution include changes in genes whose products interact with the new adaptation (138–140) and in some cases changes in the transferred genes themselves (137). Moreover, the incompatibilities brought by a transferred adaptation can yield a cascade of evolutionary changes (141).

We can expect that the ameliorative evolution following a horizontal transfer complicates the possibility of reversible evolution. Whereas a *Rhizobium* lineage can return to its previous ecological niche by simply losing its symbiosis plasmid, a lineage that has changed its ecology by acquiring a transfer from a distant relative cannot so easily return to its previous niche. The ameliorative changes that have occurred in the rest of the genome might not be easily reversible (142).

In summary, we can hypothesize that the most easily reversible ecological divergences will involve acquisitions and losses of plasmids that circulate through a given taxon, as seen in *R. leguminosarum* (133), *E. coli* (131), and *B. cereus* (143). Perhaps next easiest is acquisition of an adaptation through homologous recombination, as in the case of antibiotic resistance in *Neisseria* (135), although even a single gene can create ameliorative evolution (139, 142). Less reversible will be evolution brought about by a horizontal transfer from a distant relative, given the abundant opportunities for ameliorative evolution to follow the transfer (136). Finally, we may hypothesize that the least reversible evolutionary transitions will be those effected by a series of mutations, since there will be many events that each must be reversed.

THE ECOLOGICAL DIMENSIONS OF EARLY DIVERSIFICATION

What are the ecological changes that have allowed one population to diverge into two ecologically distinct and coexisting lineages? There are two fundamental ways that populations may distinguish themselves ecologically. First, populations may diverge in their habitat preferences, and may coexist because they are each the superior competitor in different habitats. This is the classic meaning of "ecotype" from the botanical literature, where, for example, closely related populations within a plant species taxon may each be the superior competitor at different elevations (144). Alternatively, populations may coexist in the same microhabitat because they prefer different resources within that habitat. In the animal world, this is commonly seen among closely related species that specialize on different food resources from the same habitat (145). As we shall see, most of the bacterial ecotypes characterized thus far have diverged by habitat type, probably because these differences are easier to document.

We need to take into account that an adaptation yielding an ecological change is not by itself sufficient for ecological diversification. If a new genotype is to found a new population that can coexist indefinitely with the old population, the genetic change must come with a trade-off in fitness. If instead an adaptive mutation were to convey a new resource at no cost in utilizing the old resource, the adaptation would simply be an improvement in the old population. The new mutation would sweep through the old population, and in the end we would have one improved population, not two different populations (47) (Fig. 2).

One possibility is that a trade-off comes intrinsically with the ability to use some new resource. For example, suppose we begin with a cyanobacterial population that is adapted to low levels of light. A new mutant that utilizes high levels of light can coexist as a separate population with the low-light population if the mutation comes at a cost to utilizing low light (30, 80). An intrinsic trade-off can yield coexistence of a new population with the old, even when the populations are living in the same microhabitat (sympatric speciation) or when the populations live in different microhabitats that are in easy dispersal range of the populations (parapatric speciation) (47, 146).

However, trade-offs that yield coexistence need not be intrinsic to the new adaptations. An alternative is possible when nascent ecotypes are geographically isolated (allopatric speciation). In this case, a population may adapt to some new microhabitat with no intrinsic losses in its ability to compete in the old microhabitat; nevertheless, adaptations that are specific to the old microhabitat may be costly to keep in the new habitat and may disappear (147). Even without intrinsic trade-offs, each population eventually evolves to be superior in its own microhabitat and inferior in the other's (148).

We may divide the ecological dimensions of speciation into changes in tolerances to physical and chemical conditions versus changes in resources consumed. Of course, changes in the conditions tolerated will ultimately result in consumption of resources from microhabitats that differ in their conditions (149).

Physical and Chemical Conditions

In the *Cyanobacteria*, hot spring *Synechococcus* and marine *Prochlorococcus* have both been studied for early diversification in temperature tolerances. For hot spring *Synechococcus*, temperature has proved a difficult dimension on which to diversify, at least more difficult than diversification by resources. We found two temperature ecotones, one at 61 to 62°C and another at 64 to 65°C, over which evolutionary transitions have been rare (80). That is, comparatively large clades are found nearly entirely on one side of a temperature ecotone or the other, but within each clade, there are many ecotypes that have recently diverged in resource adaptations (e.g., by light and oxygen levels) (150).

However, studies on *Prochlorococcus* show a contrasting pattern. Here the most newly divergent clades within *P. marinus* differ in their temperature adaptations, but only the most anciently divergent clades differ in the light levels they are adapted to (151). What is easiest and what is hardest varies with taxa, even among *Cyanobacteria*!

Diversification in temperature adaptations between newly divergent ecotypes has occurred also in heterotrophic *Bacillus*. Following the "Evolution Canyon" paradigm (152), organisms were sampled from soil of the north- and south-facing slopes of an east-west desert canyon. The principle of Evolution Canyon is that, at least for very shallow soil samples, the south-facing slope has much more intense solar exposure and higher day-

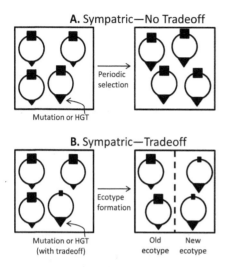

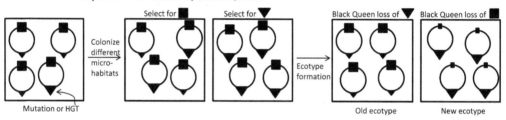

FIGURE 2 The consequences of fitness trade-offs in ecological diversification. Improvement of an ecological function by mutation or HGT (indicated by the enlarged triangle) can lead to a periodic selection event (A) or an ecotype formation event (B or C). Each individual is represented by a circle, and each individual's degree of adaptation to two resources (or conditions) is indicated by the sizes of the square and triangle, respectively. In panel A, adaptation to the triangle resource or condition is increased in one individual (indicated by increased triangle size), and the resultant strain is now able to outcompete the membership of its ecotype by virtue of its more generalist ecology. In panel B, the increase in adaptation to the triangle resource intrinsically decreases the adaptation to the square resource. Thus, increase in one ecological capability comes at the expense of a preexisting capability. In this case, acquisition of the new function leads to a new ecotype, which can coexist with the preexisting ecotype. This has been seen repeatedly in experimental populations of E. coli that primarily used glucose for carbon; a mutation to utilize secreted acetate created a new ecotype because the acetate-utilizing bacteria were less able to utilize glucose (39, 47). An alternative possibility is shown in panel C, where there is no intrinsic trade-off to the new adaptation yet a new ecotype can form. Here the new genotype invades a new habitat where the new adaptation is selected for. If the "square" adaptation is not utilized in one habitat and the "triangle" adaptation is not utilized in the other, under the Black Queen hypothesis, the unnecessary adaptations may be lost (147). This will make each ecotype the superior competitor in its own microhabitat. Adapted with permission from reference 47.

time temperatures (153), indeed even different plant species (78). This approach led to the discovery that very closely related putative ecotypes of *Bacillus* differed significantly in their associations with solar exposure (78, 79, 92). Moreover, those putative ecotypes associated with greater solar exposure were found to be better adapted to higher temperatures through greater abundance of lipids conferring reduced membrane flexibility (78, 92).

Adaptations to chemical conditions appear to evolve very quickly in *Bacillus*. Along a geochemical gradient with toxic levels of various metals and metalloids, there was an astounding diversity of tolerance even among extremely close relatives within a single putative ecotype (154). This was an indication that the putative ecotypes demarcated in *Bacillus* by one or several genes do not provide the resolution to identify the most newly divergent ecotypes.

Resource Differences among Newly Divergent Free-Living Organisms

Beyond light levels, another resource dimension of diversification for newly divergent lineages of *Cyanobacteria* is the set of mineral nutrients they consume. In hot spring *Synechococcus*, upstream and downstream populations differ, beyond temperature, in their nutrient utilization capabilities. Phosphate, the easiest phosphorus ion to utilize, is depleted by the upstream populations, leaving the more difficult ions for the downstream populations (94). In addition, the downstream clades showed a genomic capacity for storage of nitrogen, a nutrient largely depleted by the upstream populations (94). Similarly, closely related clades of *Prochlorococcus* differ in their abilities to take up inorganic minerals (155).

Generalist heterotrophs are likely to change their resource base frequently (156). All that is needed is HGT of a functional set of genes conferring metabolism of a new resource. We have seen that operons make possible a wholesale transfer of metabolic capabilities even in the context of very small recombination events (120). For example, *Bacillus* is a generalist heterotroph with a history of rapid change in metabolic capabilities: subspecies taxa within *B. subtilis* are different in utilization of scores of carbohydrates (81).

Instead of diverging in the sets of resources they can metabolize, generalist heterotrophs may also diverge *quantitatively* in the extent to which they utilize the same set of resources. For example, within a single putative ecotype of *B. subtilis*, a genome comparison found only quantitative ecological divergence—all the lineages studied shared the same set of resources but differed in the ability to utilize some of these resources. For example, while all the lineages were able to use maltose, one lineage had additional genes for metabolizing this resource and was superior to other lineages when maltose was the only carbon source (81).

With generalist heterotrophs, ecological divergence can take place within the same microhabitat. What is needed is specialization to different soluble compounds within one habitat. This has been observed repeatedly in experimental microcosms, most often when one ecotype cross-feeds from the exudate of another ecotype within the same vessel (39, 40) but also when the medium contains a rich diversity of organic compounds (38, 157). There are probably many instances of sympatric diversification among closely related heterotrophic ecotypes in nature, but much more attention has been paid to diversification by microhabitat type (43, 158).

More-specialized heterotrophs appear less likely to change resources frequently than generalists (156). Some phylogenetic groups specialize on a particular single-carbon (C1) molecule, and many ecotypes and even taxonomic species in these groups share the same organic resources. For example, different taxonomic species of *Methylobacter* appear to be limited to consuming methane as an organic carbon source. Nevertheless, speciation is possible in other resource dimensions, as closely related clades within *Methylobacter* are adapted to different depths (and oxygen levels) in a crater lake (159). In some C1 heterotrophs, speciation is possible by changing specialization from one C1 molecule to another (160).

Resource Differences among Pathogens

Pathogens may diversify by specializing on different host species. For example, in the *Mycobacterium tuberculosis* complex, which is responsible for tuberculosis, sequence clusters correspond to different clades of hosts (humans, artiodactyls, pinnipeds) (161). Also, within the species *Anaplasma phagocytophilum*, the pathogen responsible for tick-borne fever, sequence clusters are associated with different mammalian hosts (70). Within *Borrelia burgdorferisensu stricto*, the North American Lyme disease spirochete, some sequence clusters are associated with different rodent species (101, 162), although it is not yet clear whether the adaptations to specific hosts are genome-wide adaptations or are due primarily to a single outer-surface protein (163). In some cases, host specificity is determined by plasmids, and the bacteria can adapt from one host species to another with acquisition of plasmids, as seen in legume-infecting *Rhizobium* ecotypes (133) or mammal-versus insect-infecting ecotypes in *B. cereus sensu lato* (143).

Phylogenetic approaches can address the rate that a pathogen group moves from one host species to another. For example, consider the case of aphids and the obligately endosymbiotic *Buchnera* lineages that infect them. The aphids and their bacteria have congruent phylogenies, in that a splitting of aphid lineages corresponds to a splitting of their *Buchnera* endosymbionts, implying that nearly all *Buchnera* diversification has emerged as cospeciation with aphids (164). A *Buchnera* lineage rarely ventures into a new host lineage except by passive vertical transmission. This pattern of passive transmission and cospeciation occurs also in some viruses, with hantaviruses rarely transmitting to a new lineage; in contrast, the arenaviruses frequently change host lineages (165).

Can we predict the host species most likely to share pathogens? Humans are a good place to start, as obviously there is a lot of interest in discovering the animal species that are most likely to share their contagions with us. Relatedness is a predictor of the probability of a pathogen spillover, as the primates have given us ~10% of our novel pathogens in the last 3 decades (166). However, the much more distantly related ungulates, rodents, and bats

have introduced us to many more diseases in recent decades. There is clearly a role of shared environment (ecological opportunity) here, as rodents infect us through cohabiting our housing and cities with us (167), and our caring for domestic ungulates has introduced us to novel diseases from ancient times to the present (168, 169). Bats have introduced (and reintroduced) us to several diseases in recent decades through sharing their environment with our domestic animals: Middle East respiratory syndrome through camels (170), Nipah through pigs (171), and Hendra through horses (172). Bats have also introduced severe acute respiratory syndrome to us through infecting civets in a bushmeat market (173). In addition, bats have directly and recurrently transmitted Ebola to us (174).

Daniel Streicker has recently investigated the parameters that determine the likelihood of a pathogen moving to another host species and then becoming established there (175). Focusing on lineages of rabies virus that infect different species of bats, he found that the most important determinants were sharing the same geographic range and the relatedness of the bat hosts. Less important was a shared ecology among the bat species, for example, having the same roosting behavior.

The Streicker study suggests that there may be many more host shifts than we appreciate, given the tendency of microbial systematics to lump ecologically distinct lineages into a single taxon. When we see a particular microbe taxon, e.g., rabies virus, infecting a huge diversity of bat species, the established taxonomy does not make clear whether we have a generalist virus that can infect dozens of host species or whether there are many specialist viruses that each primarily infect one host lineage. Streicker's work shows the latter, and implores us to fine-tune our systematics to accommodate rapid diversification of pathogens (52).

Pathogens may also diversify by the host tissues they infect. For example, *Yersinia pseudotuberculosis* is a gut pathogen transmitted by the fecal-oral route, but it has the capacity to be lethal when it (rarely) invades the lungs or blood (176). The plague bacterium, *Yersinia pestis*, which is derived from *Y. pseudotuberculosis*, inherited its ancestor's capacity for systemic infection, but it evolved to reside *primarily* in the hosts' blood through transmission by fleas (177). Similarly, ecotypes within *Streptococcus pyogenes* are differentiated to infect the throat, causing strep throat, versus the skin, causing impetigo (178).

Pathogens with a free-living phase have many more opportunities for ecological diversification than obligate pathogens. Living outside of hosts allows diversification of ecotypes by specialization to different environmental carbon sources, for example, as seen in some members of the *Enterobacteriaceae* such as *E. coli* (179) or in some *Firmicutes* such as *Listeria* (180).

MODELS OF SPECIATION: SLOWLY SPECIATING, LONG-LIVED TAXA

As we have discussed, the properties attributed to species include (i) ecological distinctness and irreversible separateness of different species, (ii) cohesion within species but not across species, and (iii) distinguishability of species as sequence clusters. Earlier ecotype models assumed that all of these species-like properties would follow once two populations diverged to be ecologically distinct (26). However, it now appears that these properties follow ecological divergence only under certain circumstances (28, 43, 124, 156).

We begin with the stable ecotype model of speciation, where all the species-like properties hold. Here, each ecotype is assumed to be long-lived, and speciation is infrequent (Fig. 3). The long-term coexistence of ecotypes may be fostered by a *qualitative* ecological divergence, where each ecotype can use at least some resource that is not used by its close relatives (81). Such ecotypes are most likely to persist into the long haul of time because the ecotypes' unique resources provide a haven protecting them from

extinction by competition from one another (52). Nonsharing of resources may be facilitated by HGT, whereby novel resources or capabilities can become available to a recipient ecotype (96), but changes in expression of existing genes can also lead to utilization of novel resources (181). Whether ecotypes will coexist into the indefinite future will depend also on whether their unshared resources will persist into the future.

Newly divergent ecotypes are unlikely to fuse to become a single ecotype once again (28). While fusion may be possible for closely related animal and plant species, owing to their higher rates of recombination (182), the low rates of recombination in bacteria (183) make population fusion unlikely. We have discussed how natural selection against niche-specifying alleles from other populations will hold those alleles to negligible frequencies and thereby prevent species fusion (47, 48). So the only way fusion can occur is if the preferred niches of two ecotypes disappear and there emerges a new niche to which hybrids are adapted. Studies on *Campylobacter* by Sam Sheppard and colleagues have demonstrated the emergence of a new agricultural niche for hybrids between *C. coli* and *C. jejuni*. However, this is not a fusion because the two original species remain adapted to and persist in their respective niches (184).

We might hypothesize that ecotype fusion is most likely among free-living ecotypes that have adapted to infinitesimally different regions of a continuous environmental gradient. However, even a continuous gradient will result in a discontinuity of ecotypes that are adapted to discretely different points on the gradient, as modeled for continuous light variation in a photosynthetic mat (30). If niche-specifying genes from one such ecotype were transferred into another ecotype adapted to a discretely different point on the gradient, it is likely that selection against the maladaptive, foreign genes would prevail and prevent fusion (47). In bacteria, the impetus for irreversible diversification, Fernando Baquero's *ex unibus plurum*, appears much

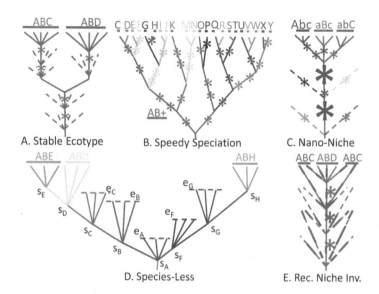

FIGURE 3 Models of bacterial speciation. Ecotypes are represented by different colors, periodic selection events are indicated by asterisks, and extinct lineages are represented by dashed lines. The letters at the top represent the resources that each group of organisms can utilize. In cases where ecotypes utilize the same set of resources but in different proportions, the predominant resource of each ecotype is noted by a capital letter. (A) The stable ecotype model. In the stable ecotype model, each ecotype endures many periodic selection events during its long lifetime. The stable ecotype model generally yields a one-to-one correspondence between ecotypes and sequence clusters because ecotypes are formed at a low rate. The ecotypes are able to coexist indefinitely because each has a resource not shared with the others. (B) The speedy speciation model. This model is much like the stable ecotype model, except that speciation occurs so rapidly that most newly divergent ecotypes cannot be detected as sequence clusters in multilocus analyses. (C) The nano-niche model of bacterial speciation. In the figure, there are three nano-niche ecotypes that use the same set of resources but in different proportions (noted by Abc, aBc, and abC). Each nano-niche ecotype can coexist with the other two because they have partitioned their resources, at least quantitatively. However, because the ecotypes share all their resources, each is vulnerable to a possible speciation-quashing mutation that may arise in the other ecotypes. (D) The species-less model. Here the diversity within an ecotype is limited not by periodic selection but instead by the short time from the ecotype's invention as a single mutant until its extinction. The origination and extinction of each ecotype i is indicated by s_i and e_i, respectively. In the absence of periodic selection, each extant ecotype that has given rise to another ecotype is a paraphyletic group, and each recent ecotype that has not yet given rise to another ecotype is monophyletic (81). (E) Recurrent niche invasion model. Here a lineage may move, frequently and recurrently, from one ecotype to another, usually by acquisition and loss of niche-determining plasmids. Red lines indicate the times in which a lineage is in the plasmid-containing ecotype; blue lines indicate the times when the lineage is in the plasmid-absent ecotype. Periodic selection events within one ecotype extinguish only the lineages of the same ecotype. For example, in the most ancient periodic selection event shown, which is in the plasmid-absent (blue) ecotype, only the lineages missing the plasmid at the time of periodic selection are extinguished, while the plasmid-containing lineages (red) persist. Ecotypes determined by a plasmid are not likely to be discoverable as sequence clusters. Reproduced from reference (81).

greater than the opposite impetus for reunification, *ex pluribus unum* (185).

The longevity of ecotypes in the stable ecotype model fosters two species-like properties. First, over the long lifetime of an ecotype, ample opportunity is provided for the ecotype to acquire a unique set of neutral mutations in each gene in the genome. Thus, each ecotype will eventually become distinguishable as a sequence cluster. Second, there may be opportunity for many incidences of cohesion during the long life of an ecotype.

What provides cohesion for a bacterial ecotype? Owing to the rarity of recombination in bacteria, natural selection favoring each adaptive mutation purges the diversity within an ecotype to near zero across the genome, the process of periodic selection (28). Periodic selection purges the diversity within but not between ecotypes, and may occur many times during the long lifetime of an ecotype (Fig. 4).

We may test whether the stable ecotype model applies by first using an algorithm to hypothesize ecotypes from sequence diversity, e.g., with Ecotype Simulation. We may then test whether the putative ecotypes are ecologically distinct and finally whether the putative ecotypes are each ecologically homogeneous. If the putative ecotypes are predicted to each contain up to 0.5 to 2.0% average nucleotide divergence (a divergence great enough to detect ecotypes with the reso-

lution of a single gene of 1,000 bp or more), finding ecological homogeneity would indicate a slow rate of speciation (156). This would mean that in the time the average gene has accumulated 0.5% neutral divergence or more, no speciation events have occurred.

So, what bacteria abide by the stable ecotype model? Our surveys of diversity in the photoautotrophic *Synechococcus* of Yellowstone hot springs indicate slow speciation and long-lived species in this group. Each putative ecotype contains ~0.5% sequence diversity genome-wide and appears to be ecologically homogeneous (80, 95). One piece of evidence for ecological homogeneity was that each putative ecotype consisted of several sequence types that maintained the same relative frequencies across a great range of environments. These environments included different hot springs and different depths and

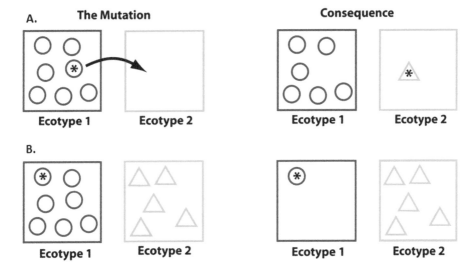

FIGURE 4 The dynamics of ecotype formation and periodic selection within an ecotype. Circles represent different genotypes, and asterisks represent adaptive mutations. (A) Ecotype formation event. A mutation or a recombination event allows the cell to occupy a new ecological niche, founding a new ecotype. A new ecotype can be formed only if the founding organism has undergone a fitness trade-off, whereby it cannot compete successfully with the parental ecotype in the old. (B) Periodic selection event. A periodic selection mutation improves the fitness of an individual such that the mutant and its descendants outcompete all other cells within the ecotype; these mutations do not affect the diversity within other ecotypes because ecological differences between ecotypes prevent direct competition. Periodic selection leads to the distinctness of ecotypes by purging the divergence within but not between ecotypes. Reproduced with permission from reference 193.

temperatures within the same hot spring, as well as experimental manipulations of temperature and light. Note that if the different sequence types within a putative ecotype had been specialized to different environments, we would have expected the frequencies of the constituent sequences to vary across environments. Another piece of evidence emerged from comparing multiple genome sequences. Within a given putative ecotype, there was no indication of different histories of positive selection (95), which would have suggested ecological diversity (186). So, in the time it took 0.5% sequence diversity to accumulate, apparently no speciation events had occurred. While it is possible that lineages within a putative ecotype had diverged to accommodate fine differences in conditions (29), there is no evidence that they have done so.

On the other hand, the generalist heterotroph *B. subtilis* and its close relatives in Death Valley soils have shown extremely rapid ecological diversification. We surveyed genome sequence diversity within one putative ecotype and found that every lineage studied had a unique history of positive selection, suggesting that each isolate represented a different ecotype (81). This supported Ford Doolittle's hypothesis that bacterial diversification is so rapid that any given cell is unlikely to be ecologically identical to any beyond its immediate offspring (187).

The contrast between *Synechococcus* and *Bacillus* suggests a general hypothesis for predicting rates of speciation and the circumstances under which the stable ecotype model applies. Among free-living bacteria, we may predict that generalist heterotrophs like *Bacillus*, with many options for metabolic diversification, will speciate rapidly (156). Alternatively, photoautotrophs and any other ecological guilds that consume few or no organic resources will have limited options for metabolic diversification and will speciate slowly (156).

This hypothesis was supported by a recent metagenomic survey of diversity over time within an acidic lake in Wisconsin, United States (156, 188). Matthew Bendall and coworkers assembled metagenome sequences into clusters with usually up to 2% sequence divergence within them. One such cluster was shown to lose its diversity in a genome-wide sweep over 8 years, providing direct evidence for a periodic selection event in nature. The authors also found evidence that some genome-wide sweeps had taken place in the community before their study began. Each cluster that was swept genome-wide of its diversity was interpreted as being ecologically homogeneous, such that an adaptive mutant could outcompete all the lineages within the cluster. Because these clusters did not diversify in the time that 2% divergence accumulated, we may conclude that diversification within these clusters occurred at a slow rate consistent with the stable ecotype model.

So, what did those clusters abiding by the stable ecotype model have in common? While they were from several phyla, both photosynthetic and heterotrophic, all but one cluster appeared limited in its carbon sources. These clusters included photoautotrophs of the phylum *Chlorobi* as well as heterotrophs limited to consuming single-carbon molecules from various phyla (156). The one possible exception was a genome-wide sweep within a cluster from the *Rickettsia*, a genus of obligately intracellular pathogens. Nevertheless, two aspects of the *Rickettsia* lifestyle may have contributed to slow diversification: its radically reduced metabolism (189) and the reduced opportunity for an obligately intracellular pathogen to infect new host species. The stable ecotype model may be limited to the ecological guilds of photoautotrophs, C1 heterotrophs, and obligately intracellular pathogens.

The metagenomic study also identified various taxa that had less profound sweeps, where only a small chromosomal region was swept of diversity while the rest of the genome remained heterogeneous (188). Bendall and colleagues argued that a genome-wide sweep was prevented in these clusters by high recombination rates; however, they did not supply evidence for a recombination-based explanation. Likewise, other authors finding single-gene sweeps in other systems have drawn on recombination to explain their results (43, 187, 190, 191). However, periodic selection is predicted to cause a genome-wide sweep *only within an ecotype* (192), and in many of these cases, the single-gene sweep was known to have traversed across ecologically distinct populations (43, 187, 190, 191). Moreover, recombination is too rare in bacteria to prevent genome-wide sweeps within an ecotype (183, 193).

A more likely explanation for the single-gene sweeps found in the metagenome study and elsewhere is offered by the "adapt globally, act locally" model (194) and the negative frequency-dependent selection model (195) (Fig. 5). Following these models, the metagenome clusters showing single-gene sweeps may be interpreted to each contain a heterogeneous amalgam of many ecotypes. Assuming that an adaptive mutation driving periodic selection confers a fitness benefit to each of the ecotypes within a cluster, here is the sequence of events that could lead to a single-region sweep. First, an adaptive mutation appears in one ecotype, and the resulting periodic selection drives a genome-wide sweep within that ecotype; then the small region containing the adaptation transfers into another ecotype and causes a genome-wide sweep within that ecotype; and so on, until the adaptive mutation has swept to fixation in all the constituent ecotypes of the cluster. The result is that the cluster will be swept of diversity in the region containing the adaptive mutation, but the cluster will maintain its genetic heterogeneity elsewhere on the chromosome.

Thus, those clusters from the metagenome survey that showed a single-region chromosomal sweep could be interpreted as containing multiple ecotypes within the cluster's 2% sequence divergence, owing to rapid speciation (156). The taxa showing single-

region sweeps in the metagenome study were largely generalist heterotrophs, like *Bacillus*, and supported the hypothesis that a highly plastic metabolism yields rapid speciation (52).

To sum up, the data for free-living organisms (plus *Rickettsia*) largely support the hypothesis that taxa with little opportunity to diversify tend to speciate slowly and abide by the stable ecotype model, whereas those taxa that can use a vast diversity of organic resources tend to speciate rapidly.

Where do pathogens fit in between the extremes of metabolic plasticity from *Bacillus* to *Synechococcus*? Those pathogens that diversify primarily by changes in host range or host tissue may be most likely to speciate slowly, especially when there are only a small number of hosts or tissues that a particular pathogenic lineage can adapt to. That is, transmission to a new host or tissue may be a rare event. We have seen that in several groups of pathogens (including the *M. tuberculosis* complex of species [161], *A. phagocytophilum* [70], and *B. burgdorferi sensu stricto* [162]), each sequence cluster corresponds to a specialist to a different host species; moreover, each cluster appears to be ecologically homogeneous (52). Likewise, the stable ecotype model may apply to ecotypes that have diverged to infect different tissues of the same host species, for example, the case of *Y. pseudotuberculosis*, focusing on the gut, versus *Y. pestis*, specialized toward systemic infection and transmission by fleas. Each *Yersinia* taxon appears homogeneous in its ecology and so may be considered an ecotype specialized to a different tissue, while each is a generalist with respect to host species.

We may hypothesize that the longevity of newly divergent ecotypes that are specialized to different host species may be short, especially if the host species are closely related. This is because two closely related host species would be likely to be extinguished by the same environmental disturbances (196, 197). On the other hand, ecotypes such as *Y. pseu-*

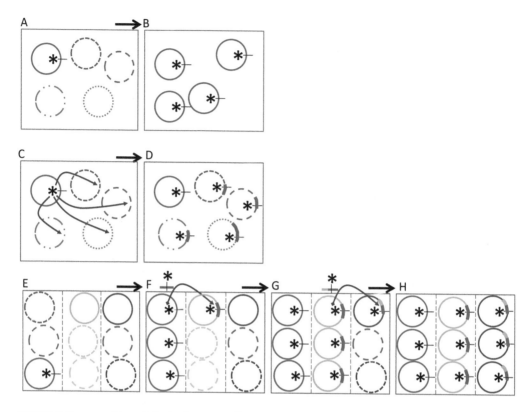

FIGURE 5 Genome-wide and single-chromosomal-region sweeps within a sequence cluster of closely related bacteria. Each row of panels represents a different model of sweep within a metagenome cluster: (A to B) a genome-wide sweep, where the metagenome cluster is populated by only a single ecotype, and where recombination is rare enough to allow a genome-wide sweep within an ecotype (28); (C to D) a narrow sweep (homogenizing only the chromosomal region near the adaptive mutation), where again the metagenome cluster is populated by a single ecotype, but here recombination (indicated by purple arrows) is frequent enough to prevent a genome-wide sweep within an ecotype (model favored by Bendall et al. [188]); and (E to H) a narrow sweep, where the metagenome cluster is populated by many ecotypes (in this case, three), and recombination is rare enough to allow genome-wide sweeps within an ecotype but frequent enough to allow an adaptive mutation to recombine (it need happen only once!) between one ecotype and another (46). In each row, the wide horizontal arrows represent the course of time. In each panel, the rectangle represents one metagenome cluster and each circle represents a single organism. The asterisk represents an adaptive mutation, which allows its carrier to outcompete other organisms in the same ecotype but not organisms from other ecotypes. In panels A to D, the metagenome cluster is ecologically homogeneous, and in panels E to H, the metagenome cluster is ecologically heterogeneous and represents three ecotypes, separated by the vertical dashed lines; the different ecotypes are coded by blue, green, and red. The sequence diversity within an ecotype is represented by different shades of the ecotype color and by different styles of line (dotted, dashed, and solid). In the case of low recombination rates (A to B and E to H), the adaptive mutation causes a genome-wide sweep within the ecotype containing the mutation. In panels E to H, the adaptive mutation is potentially beneficial in different ecotypes and can transfer on a short chromosomal segment to another ecotype, where it precipitates a new genome-wide sweep within its new ecotype. Reproduced with permission from reference (156).

dotuberculosis and *Y. pestis* may be destined to coexist into the far future. Because they are both generalists with respect to host species, they are not likely to become extinguished with the extinction of an individual host species. On the other hand, the two tissue sets to which these ecotypes are specialized are likely to persist into the indefinite future.

Some pathogens may speciate at a quick rate, owing to many more opportunities for ecological diversification. One possibility is that those pathogens with a free-living phase can diversify by the resources and physical and chemical conditions available to them outside of their hosts, as seen among ecotypes within *Burkholderia seminalis* (181). Another possibility for rapid diversification in pathogens is that they can diversify as they escape the immune system, an issue to which we will return.

In sum, at least some bacterial groups abide by the stable ecotype model, where speciation is slow and ecotypes hold all the species-like properties conceived by speciologists. Some of these ecotypes may persist into the indefinite future. On the other hand, it is clear that many bacteria undergo speciation rapidly. As we shall see, there are several models of rapid bacterial speciation, and in each model, ecotypes are missing at least one of the species-like properties.

MODELS OF SPECIATION: RAPIDLY SPECIATING TAXA

The Speedy Speciation Model

Speedy speciation is a model of adaptive radiation, where opportunities for niche diversification are plentiful (Fig. 3). As in the stable ecotype model, ecotypes are cohesive owing to recurrent periodic selection events. In speedy speciation, the rate of speciation is too high to allow the individual ecotypes to be identified as sequence clusters based on one or a few genes—more resolution is needed to distinguish these newly divergent lineages, perhaps even the resolution of the entire genome. Ecotypes abiding by the speedy speciation model may persist into the indefinite future, depending on whether the ecotypes have some unique resources and on whether their resources are likely to persist into the future.

The speedy speciation model appears to apply to some human pathogens, especially in cases where a host individual is usually infected by only a single clone. The infecting clone can then diversify by specializing into all the niches available to it within the host, provided that specialists already adapted to these niches are not likely to follow the original clone into the host. This pattern appears to hold in *P. aeruginosa* following lung infection of a CF patient. From a single inoculating clone, the descendant bacteria evolve into multiple populations with different nutrient requirements, antibiotic resistance, and virulence (198). This within-host diversification is frequently aided by evolution of higher mutation rates (199) and eventually an attenuation of virulence that could foster coexistence among the populations (200, 201). If instead CF patients were infected by multiple *P. aeruginosa* lineages already specialized to the various lung niches, there would not be the opportunity for *in situ* diversification under the speedy speciation model. It is the shortsightedness of the diversification (in not leading to transmission to other CF patients, *sensu* Levin and Bull) (31) that allows this diversification to occur from scratch in many CF patients.

Similarly, adaptive radiation appears to occur when *M. tuberculosis* infects a human host individual. An individual patient is likely to host an *in situ* diversification of ecologically divergent ecotypes (202), often facilitated by evolution of hypermutation (203). While specialized ecotypes of *P. aeruginosa* and *M. tuberculosis* may be transmitted from one host to another, it is unlikely that a suite of ecotypes will be transmitted, making possible *in situ* adaptive radiation from a single inoculating clone. In this model of within-host diversification, persistence of newly diversified ecotypes is unlikely to extend beyond the life of a single host individual.

Another possibility for rapid speciation in pathogens is diversification in their free-living stage between their times in hosts. The free-living stage may have the same opportunity for diversification as free-living generalist heterotrophs. Pathogens with free-living stages include many members of the *Proteobacteria*, including *E. coli* (62) and *B. seminalis* (181), as well as the *Firmicutes*, including members of the genus *Listeria* (180).

The Species-less Model

The species-less model differs profoundly from all other models of bacterial speciation, which assume a force of cohesion within species (Fig. 3). The species-less model assumes both rapid speciation and rapid extinction, with a high turnover of species. These species are lacking in cohesion because they do not exist long enough to experience even a single periodic selection event (28, 204).

In the species-less model, ecotypes evolve not by becoming more efficient in utilizing their current ecological niche but instead by evolving to invade a new ecological niche. We recently provided evidence that, at least in an experimental microcosm, a lineage of *Bacillus* will split to form new ecotypes at about the same rate that existing ecotypes improve their adaptations (38). This suggests that under the right circumstances, the rate of speciation may be fast enough to make periodic selection unlikely. Little is generally known, however, about the rate of extinction of ecotypes in nature.

However, pathogens may provide a case for both rapid formation and extinction of ecotypes. Mutations that provide an escape from the immune system may each found a new ephemeral ecotype (28, 205, 206), so the species-less model may apply to the diversification of epitope diversity. The species-less model may also apply in cases of bacterial succession, particularly when the descendants of a single colonizing individual at a site must adapt to rapidly changing conditions. For example, successions that occur on mine tailings, with pH and oxidation levels changing rapidly, may yield the high turnover of ecotypes that is compatible with the species-less model (207). Like the case we discussed earlier for *in situ* diversification of *P. aeruginosa* and *M. tuberculosis* within one

patient, the *in situ* diversification in a succession is most likely if dispersal to the site brings only a single founding ecotype. Rapid speciation would not occur if dispersal between different mine tailing sites provided all the ecotypes necessary for each successional stage. Provided that each succession engenders a novel diversification of ecotypes, and the products of each succession are not likely to disperse to other similar habitats, the products of diversification will be short-lived. They will not become the stuff on which novel higher taxa are founded.

The Nano-Niche Model

In the nano-niche model, closely related ecotypes are subtly and only *quantitatively* different in their ecology (52). "Nano-niche" ecotypes use the same set of resources and conditions, but they coexist much like closely related animal species by using their shared resources and conditions *in different proportions* (Fig. 3). Not having any unique resources that might constitute a haven from competition from other ecotypes, each ecotype is expected to be ephemeral and vulnerable to extinction from competition with other ecotypes. For a time, the various ephemeral ecotypes may coexist, and each may even have its own private periodic selection events. At some point, however, an extremely competitive adaptive mutant (which we call a speciation-quashing mutation) from one ephemeral ecotype may extinguish not only the other members of its own population but also other closely related ecotypes (193). In the nano-niche model, divergence among very closely related ephemeral ecotypes is limited by these speciation-quashing mutations. We should not expect any nano-niche ecotypes to coexist long enough to form any higher-level taxa.

Genome comparisons have provided evidence for the nano-niche model in *B. subtilis* (81). Five extremely closely related isolates were found ecologically distinct on the basis of different histories of positive selection, but the genome content differences indicated no unique resources for any of the isolates. The isolates appear to have diverged by specializing quantitatively on resources that they all share (e.g., with one strain being a superior competitor on maltose), supporting the nano-niche model. We suspect that the high-throughput genome sequencing that is now available will provide examples of quantitative divergence, if researchers focus on sequencing sets of extremely closely related isolates.

The nano-niche model may also apply to bacterial ecotypes that adapt over a long course of infection within a host individual, for example, within the gut. Among closely related bacteria, the course of evolutionary adaptation to each human body may lead to each human having its own ecotype, each adapted to the peculiarities of the host's physiology, diet, and the other bacteria coinhabiting the gut. However, the individual hosts might not be different enough to support indefinite coexistence of individual-specific ecotypes. Any speciation-quashing mutation, which makes an individual bacterium superior not just in its own host individual but also in other hosts, would put an end to the speciation among the various nano-niche ecotypes adapting to different host individuals.

Recurrent Niche Invasion Model

In the recurrent niche invasion model, plasmids or phages determine the niches of their bacterial hosts (Fig. 3). We have seen that *Rhizobium* lineages may move from one ecological niche to another by simply gaining the symbiosis plasmid adapting the bacteria to one plant host while losing another symbiosis plasmid, and similar dynamics are seen for plasmids providing virulence to lineages of *E. coli* and *B. cereus sensu lato*. In this model, ecological divergence is in principle reversible, provided that the host lineages do not have an opportunity to adapt and specialize to a given plasmid that is infecting

them. When hosts fail to specialize to their plasmids, host lineages will move back and forth between plasmid-defined populations and will not diverge irreversibly. Nevertheless, the niches made available by the plasmids may persist into the indefinite future.

On the other hand, sometimes different host lineages may specialize to their own plasmids. This may occur if the plasmids are not fully compatible with all their potential hosts and if the plasmids reside in a given lineage long enough for evolution toward compatibility to occur. We have seen various stages of permanent accommodation of host lineages to different niche-defining plasmids (52). As seen in the case where *R. leguminosarum* lineages are completely associated with different symbiosis plasmids (134), a host-plasmid system can leave the recurrent niche invasion model's realm of reversible divergence and enter the stable ecotype model's realm of irreversible divergence. Here the plasmids are providing the same dynamics of diversification as any chromosome-based gene that was originally acquired by HGT.

CONCLUDING REMARKS AND FUTURE DIRECTIONS

We began by challenging the field of population biology to explain the origins of profoundly disparate creatures within the bacterial world. Each pair of higher-level taxa began their divergence long ago as one ordinary population that split to become two lineages that would coexist to our time. So, we may think of the rate of origin of a higher-level taxon level as a product—the rate of speciation times the probability that two new species coexist long enough to reach a particular level of divergence. Here I have tried to use population biology to give insights into these two parameters of disparification.

I have focused on speciation as a process where one population splits into two ecologically distinct lineages that can coexist indefinitely as a result of their ecological divergence. I have hypothesized that the rate of speciation varies among taxa, depending on the ecological opportunities available for invading a new niche (156). I have suggested three ecological guilds where speciation may be restricted by a small number of niches available to a given lineage: photoautotrophs, C1 heterotrophs, and obligately intracellular pathogens. Generalist heterotrophs, with many more opportunities for resource-based diversification, appear to have much higher rates of speciation. The longitudinal metagenome survey approach launched by Bendall and colleagues (188) holds great promise for testing these hypotheses and exploring other lifestyles that may promote slow or fast speciation.

I have identified several features of nascent species that may promote their coexistence into the remote future. First, ecological diversification should not be easily reversed by losing the adaptation that creates the new niche. Two factors contributing to irreversibility are a slow rate of gain and loss of niche-defining adaptations and a fitness cost created by the original adaptation, which causes a secondary round of ameliorative evolution. Also, two nascent species are most likely to coexist into the distant future if they each utilize some resources that are unavailable to the other (47). This is likely to occur when HGT adds a new resource to a recipient's repertoire, at a trade-off cost of diminishing access to an established resource. Also, we can predict that long-term coexistence of lineages will depend on long-term coexistence of their resources.

We may add to these hypothesized conditions for long-term coexistence through a systematic approach pioneered by Laurent Philippot and Noah Fierer and their respective colleagues (18, 20). They have aimed to discover whether "ecological coherence" may exist for higher-level taxa. By comparing both genomes and habitats of many taxa, they discovered properties that were shared, for example, by all the members of a particular

phylum but not by other phyla. For example, the *Acidobacteria* are found largely in acidic soils, in contrast to other related phyla, and we now know some of the genomic basis of their acid tolerance. This approach holds promise for identifying the traits that enable long-term coexistence of newly divergent lineages. We can hypothesize that those traits distinguishing the genera or families within a given phylum are responsible for granting the long-term coexistence of the higher-order taxa. Thus, we may predict that when new species diverge in these traits, they may have a greater probability than average of coexisting into the remote future.

In sum, bacterial diversification depends on transmission of bacteria into new habitats and resources, whereby one lineage splits into two that can coexist as a result of their ecological differences. Population biologists and historians of life will be challenged to identify those transmissions that yield lineages capable of coexisting for billions of years.

ACKNOWLEDGMENTS

I am grateful for Teresa Coque, Fernando Baquero, Emilio Bouza, and José Antonio Gutiérrez-Fuentes for their invitation to participate in the symposium on transmission in microbiology. This work was supported by grants from Wesleyan University.

CITATION

Cohan FM. 2017. Transmission in the origins of bacterial diversity, from ecotypes to phyla. Microbiol Spectrum 5(5):MTBP-0014-2016.

REFERENCES

1. **Woese CR.** 1987. Bacterial evolution. *Microbiol Rev* **51:**221–271.
2. **Rappé MS, Giovannoni SJ.** 2003. The uncultured microbial majority. *Annu Rev Microbiol* **57:**369–394.
3. **Schloss PD, Handelsman J.** 2004. Status of the microbial census. *Microbiol Mol Biol Rev* **68:**686–691.

4. **Yarza P, Yilmaz P, Pruesse E, Glöckner FO, Ludwig W, Schleifer KH, Whitman WB, Euzéby J, Amann R, Rosselló-Móra R.** 2014. Uniting the classification of cultured and uncultured bacteria and archaea using 16S rRNA gene sequences. *Nat Rev Microbiol* **12**:635–645.

5. **Hug LA, Baker BJ, Anantharaman K, Brown CT, Probst AJ, Castelle CJ, Butterfield CN, Hernsdorf AW, Amano Y, Ise K, Suzuki Y, Dudek N, Relman DA, Finstad KM, Amundson R, Thomas BC, Banfield JF.** 2016. A new view of the tree of life. *Nat Microbiol* **1**:16048.

6. **Sutcliffe IC.** 2010. A phylum level perspective on bacterial cell envelope architecture. *Trends Microbiol* **18**:464–470.

7. **Schimel J, Balser TC, Wallenstein M.** 2007. Microbial stress-response physiology and its implications for ecosystem function. *Ecology* **88**:1386–1394.

8. **Adams PG, Cadby AJ, Robinson B, Tsukatani Y, Tank M, Wen J, Blankenship RE, Bryant DA, Hunter CN.** 2013. Comparison of the physical characteristics of chlorosomes from three different phyla of green phototrophic bacteria. *Biochim Biophys Acta* **1827**:1235–1244.

9. **Ward NL.** 2010. Phylum XXV. Planctomycetes Garrity and Holt 2001, 137 emend. Ward (this volume), p 879–925. *In* Krieg NR, Staley JT, Brown DR, Hedlund BP, Paster BJ, Ward NL, Ludwig W, Whitman WB (ed), Bergey's Manual of Systematic Bacteriology, 2nd ed, **vol 4**. *The Bacteroidetes, Spirochaetes, Tenericutes (Mollicutes), Acidobacteria, Fibrobacteres, Fusobacteria, Dictyoglomi, Gemmatimonadetes, Lentisphaerae, Verrucomicrobia, Chlamydiae, and Planctomycetes.* Springer, New York, NY.

10. **Klein EA, Schlimpert S, Hughes V, Brun YV, Thanbichler M, Gitai Z.** 2013. Physiological role of stalk lengthening in *Caulobacter crescentus*. *Commun Integr Biol* **6**:e24561.

11. **Wagner JK, Setayeshgar S, Sharon LA, Reilly JP, Brun YV.** 2006. A nutrient uptake role for bacterial cell envelope extensions. *Proc Natl Acad Sci U S A* **103**:11772–11777.

12. **Brochier-Armanet C, Talla E, Gribaldo S.** 2009. The multiple evolutionary histories of dioxygen reductases: implications for the origin and evolution of aerobic respiration. *Mol Biol Evol* **26**:285–297.

13. **Summers AO.** 2006. Genetic linkage and horizontal gene transfer, the roots of the antibiotic multi-resistance problem. *Anim Biotechnol* **17**:125–135.

14. **Ray A, Kinch LN, de Souza Santos M, Grishin NV, Orth K, Salomon D.** 2016. Proteomics analysis reveals previously uncharacterized virulence factors in *Vibrio proteolyticus*. *mBio* **7**:e01077-e16.

15. **Cohan FM.** 2010. Synthetic biology: now that we're creators, what should we create? *Curr Biol* **20**:R675–R677.

16. **Martiny JB, Jones SE, Lennon JT, Martiny AC.** 2015. Microbiomes in light of traits: a phylogenetic perspective. *Science* **350**:aac9323.

17. **Mulkidjanian AY, Koonin EV, Makarova KS, Mekhedov SL, Sorokin A, Wolf YI, Dufresne A, Partensky F, Burd H, Kaznadzey D, Haselkorn R, Galperin MY.** 2006. The cyanobacterial genome core and the origin of photosynthesis. *Proc Natl Acad Sci U S A* **103**:13126–13131.

18. **Philippot L, Andersson SG, Battin TJ, Prosser JI, Schimel JP, Whitman WB, Hallin S.** 2010. The ecological coherence of high bacterial taxonomic ranks. *Nat Rev Microbiol* **8**:523–529.

19. **Antunes LC, Poppleton D, Klingl A, Criscuolo A, Dupuy B, Brochier-Armanet C, Beloin C, Gribaldo S.** 2016. Phylogenomic analysis supports the ancestral presence of LPS-outer membranes in the Firmicutes. *eLife* **5**:e14589.

20. **Fierer N, Bradford MA, Jackson RB.** 2007. Toward an ecological classification of soil bacteria. *Ecology* **88**:1354–1364.

21. **Tindall BJ, Rosselló-Móra R, Busse HJ, Ludwig W, Kämpfer P.** 2010. Notes on the characterization of prokaryote strains for taxonomic purposes. *Int J Syst Evol Microbiol* **60**:249–266.

22. **Lagier JC, Khelaifia S, Alou MT, Ndongo S, Dione N, Hugon P, Caputo A, Cadoret F, Traore SI, Seck EH, Dubourg G, Durand G, Mourembou G, Guilhot E, Togo A, Bellali S, Bachar D, Cassir N, Bittar F, Delerce J, Mailhe M, Ricaboni D, Bilen M, Dangui Nieko NP, Dia Badiane NM, Valles C, Mouelhi D, Diop K, Million M, Musso D, Abrahão J, Azhar EI, Bibi F, Yasir M, Diallo A, Sokhna C, Djossou F, Vitton V, Robert C, Rolain JM, La Scola B, Fournier PE, Levasseur A, Raoult D.** 2016. Culture of previously uncultured members of the human gut microbiota by culturomics. *Nat Microbiol* **1**:16203.

23. **Lerat E, Daubin V, Ochman H, Moran NA.** 2005. Evolutionary origins of genomic repertoires in bacteria. *PLoS Biol* **3**:e130.

24. **de Queiroz K.** 2005. Ernst Mayr and the modern concept of species. *Proc Natl Acad Sci U S A* **102** (Suppl 1):6600–6607.

25. **Cohan FM.** 2017. Species. *In* Osmanaj B, Escalante Santos L (ed), *Reference Module in Life Sciences* HYPERLINK doi.org/10.1016/B978-0-12-809633-8.07184-3. Elsevier.

26. **Cohan FM.** 1994. The effects of rare but promiscuous genetic exchange on evolutionary divergence in prokaryotes. *Am Nat* **143**:965–986.

27. **Mallet J.** 1995. A species definition for the modern synthesis. *Trends Ecol Evol* **10**:294–299.

28. **Cohan FM.** 2011. Are species cohesive?—A view from bacteriology, p 43–65. *In* Walk S, Feng P (ed), *Bacterial Population Genetics: A Tribute to Thomas S Whittam.* American Society for Microbiology Press, Washington, DC.

29. **Negri MC, Lipsitch M, Blázquez J, Levin BR, Baquero F.** 2000. Concentration-dependent selection of small phenotypic differences in TEM β-lactamase-mediated antibiotic resistance. *Antimicrob Agents Chemother* **44:**2485–2491.

30. **Ward DM, Cohan FM.** 2005. Microbial diversity in hot spring cyanobacterial mats: pattern and prediction, p 185–202. *In* Inskeep WP, McDermott T (ed), *Geothermal Biology and Geochemistry in Yellowstone National Park.* Thermal Biology Institute, Bozeman, MT.

31. **Levin BR, Bull JJ.** 1994. Short-sighted evolution and the virulence of pathogenic microorganisms. *Trends Microbiol* **2:**76–81.

32. **Mayr E.** 1963. *Animal Species and Evolution.* Belknap Press of Harvard University Press, Cambridge, MA.

33. **Wilkins JS.** 2009. *Species: A History of the Idea.* University of California, Berkeley, CA.

34. **Cohan FM.** 2013. Species, p 56–511. *In* Maloy S, Hughes K (ed), *Brenner's Encyclopedia of Genetics,* 2nd ed. Elsevier, Amsterdam, The Netherlands.

35. **Mallet J.** 2008. Hybridization, ecological races and the nature of species: empirical evidence for the ease of speciation. *Philos Trans R Soc Lond B Biol Sci* **363:**2971–2986.

36. **Schluter D.** 2009. Evidence for ecological speciation and its alternative. *Science* **323:**737–741.

37. **Rainey PB, Travisano M.** 1998. Adaptive radiation in a heterogeneous environment. *Nature* **394:** 69–72.

38. **Koeppel AF, Wertheim JO, Barone L, Gentile N, Krizanc D, Cohan FM.** 2013. Speedy speciation in a bacterial microcosm: new species can arise as frequently as adaptations within a species. *ISME J* **7:**1080–1091.

39. **Treves DS, Manning S, Adams J.** 1998. Repeated evolution of an acetate-crossfeeding polymorphism in long-term populations of *Escherichia coli. Mol Biol Evol* **15:**789–797.

40. **Blount ZD, Borland CZ, Lenski RE.** 2008. Historical contingency and the evolution of a key innovation in an experimental population of *Escherichia coli. Proc Natl Acad Sci U S A* **105:**7899–7906.

41. **Ellegaard KM, Klasson L, Näslund K, Bourtzis K, Andersson SG.** 2013. Comparative genomics of *Wolbachia* and the bacterial species concept. *PLoS Genet* **9:**e1003381.

42. **Cadillo-Quiroz H, Didelot X, Held NL, Herrera A, Darling A, Reno ML, Krause DJ, Whitaker RJ.** 2012. Patterns of gene flow define species of thermophilic Archaea. *PLoS Biol* **10:**e1001265.

43. **Shapiro BJ, Friedman J, Cordero OX, Preheim SP, Timberlake SC, Szabó G, Polz MF, Alm EJ.** 2012. Population genomics of early events in the ecological differentiation of bacteria. *Science* **336:**48–51.

44. **Melendrez MC, Becraft ED, Wood JM, Olsen MT, Bryant DA, Heidelberg JF, Rusch DB, Cohan FM, Ward DM.** 2016. Recombination does not hinder formation or detection of ecological species of *Synechococcus* inhabiting a hot spring cyanobacterial mat. *Front Microbiol* **6:** 1540.

45. **Hunt DE, David LA, Gevers D, Preheim SP, Alm EJ, Polz MF.** 2008. Resource partitioning and sympatric differentiation among closely related bacterioplankton. *Science* **320:**1081–1085.

46. **Cohan FM.** 2016. Prokaryotic species concepts, p 119–129. *In* Kliman RM (ed), *Encyclopedia of Evolutionary Biology,* **vol X.** Academic Press, Oxford, United Kingdom.

47. **Wiedenbeck J, Cohan FM.** 2011. Origins of bacterial diversity through horizontal genetic transfer and adaptation to new ecological niches. *FEMS Microbiol Rev* **35:**957–976.

48. **Haldane JB.** 1932. *The Causes of Evolution.* Longmans, Green, and Co, London, United Kingdom.

49. **Ward DM, Cohan FM, Bhaya D, Heidelberg JF, Kühl M, Grossman A.** 2008. Genomics, environmental genomics and the issue of microbial species. *Heredity (Edinb)* **100:**207–219.

50. **Konstantinidis KT, Tiedje JM.** 2005. Genomic insights that advance the species definition for prokaryotes. *Proc Natl Acad Sci U S A* **102:**2567–2572.

51. **Coyne JA, Orr HA.** 2004. *Speciation.* Sinauer Associates, Sunderland, MA.

52. **Cohan FM, Kopac SM.** 2017. A theory-based pragmatism for discovering and classifying newly divergent species of bacterial pathogens, p 25–49. *In* Tibayrenc M (ed), *Genetics and Evolution of Infectious Diseases,* 2nd ed. Elsevier, Oxford, United Kingdom.

53. **Cohan FM.** 2016. Bacterial species concepts, p 119–129. *In* Kliman RM (ed), *Encyclopedia of Evolutionary Biology,* **vol 1.** Academic Press, Oxford, United Kingdom.

54. **Staley JT.** 2006. The bacterial species dilemma and the genomic-phylogenetic species concept. *Philos Trans R Soc Lond B Biol Sci* **361:**1899–1909.

55. **Sikorski J.** 2008. Populations under microevolutionary scrutiny: what will we gain? *Arch Microbiol* **189:**1–5.

56. **Ward DM.** 1998. A natural species concept for prokaryotes. *Curr Opin Microbiol* **1:**271–277.

57. **Rosselló-Mora R, Amann R.** 2001. The species concept for prokaryotes. *FEMS Microbiol Rev* **25**:39–67.

58. **Ward DM, Bateson MM, Ferris MJ, Kühl M, Wieland A, Koeppel A, Cohan FM.** 2006. Cyanobacterial ecotypes in the microbial mat community of Mushroom Spring (Yellowstone National Park, Wyoming) as species-like units linking microbial community composition, structure and function. *Philos Trans R Soc Lond B Biol Sci* **361**:1997–2008.

59. **Touchon M, Hoede C, Tenaillon O, Barbe V, Baeriswyl S, Bidet P, Bingen E, Bonacorsi S, Bouchier C, Bouvet O, Calteau A, Chiapello H, Clermont O, Cruveiller S, Danchin A, Diard M, Dossat C, Karoui ME, Frapy E, Garry L, Ghigo JM, Gilles AM, Johnson J, Le Bouguénec C, Lescat M, Mangenot S, Martinez-Jéhanne V, Matic I, Nassif X, Oztas S, Petit MA, Pichon C, Rouy Z, Ruf CS, Schneider D, Tourret J, Vacherie B, Vallenet D, Médigue C, Rocha EP, Denamur E.** 2009. Organised genome dynamics in the *Escherichia coli* species results in highly diverse adaptive paths. *PLoS Genet* **5**:e1000344.

60. **Walk ST, Alm EW, Gordon DM, Ram JL, Toranzos GA, Tiedje JM, Whittam TS.** 2009. Cryptic lineages of the genus *Escherichia*. *Appl Environ Microbiol* **75**:6534–6544.

61. **Gordon DM, Lee J.** 1999. The genetic structure of enteric bacteria from Australian mammals. *Microbiology* **145**:2673–2682.

62. **Walk ST, Alm EW, Calhoun LM, Mladonicky JM, Whittam TS.** 2007. Genetic diversity and population structure of *Escherichia coli* isolated from freshwater beaches. *Environ Microbiol* **9**:2274–2288.

63. **Cohan FM, Kopac SM.** 2011. Microbial genomics: *E. coli* relatives out of doors and out of body. *Curr Biol* **21**:R587–R589.

64. **Welch RA, Burland V, Plunkett G III, Redford P, Roesch P, Rasko D, Buckles EL, Liou SR, Boutin A, Hackett J, Stroud D, Mayhew GF, Rose DJ, Zhou S, Schwartz DC, Perna NT, Mobley HL, Donnenberg MS, Blattner FR.** 2002. Extensive mosaic structure revealed by the complete genome sequence of uropathogenic *Escherichia coli*. *Proc Natl Acad Sci U S A* **99**:17020–17024.

65. **Lefébure T, Stanhope MJ.** 2007. Evolution of the core and pan-genome of *Streptococcus*: positive selection, recombination, and genome composition. *Genome Biol* **8**:R71.

66. **Paul S, Dutta A, Bag SK, Das S, Dutta C.** 2010. Distinct, ecotype-specific genome and proteome signatures in the marine cyanobacteria *Prochlorococcus*. *BMC Genomics* **11**:103.

67. **Vernikos GS, Thomson NR, Parkhill J.** 2007. Genetic flux over time in the *Salmonella* lineage. *Genome Biol* **8**:R100.

68. **Marri PR, Hao W, Golding GB.** 2006. Gene gain and gene loss in *Streptococcus*: is it driven by habitat? *Mol Biol Evol* **23**:2379–2391.

69. **Aboal M, Werner O, García-Fernández ME, Palazón JA, Cristóbal JC, Williams W.** 2016. Should ecomorphs be conserved? The case of *Nostoc flagelliforme*, an endangered extremophile cyanobacteria. *J Nat Conserv* **30**:52–64.

70. **Dugat T, Lagrée AC, Maillard R, Boulouis HJ, Haddad N.** 2015. Opening the black box of *Anaplasma phagocytophilum* diversity: current situation and future perspectives. *Front Cell Infect Microbiol* **5**:61.

71. **Kettler GC, Martiny AC, Huang K, Zucker J, Coleman ML, Rodrigue S, Chen F, Lapidus A, Ferriera S, Johnson J, Steglich C, Church GM, Richardson P, Chisholm SW.** 2007. Patterns and implications of gene gain and loss in the evolution of *Prochlorococcus*. *PLoS Genet* **3**:e231.

72. **Oh PL, Benson AK, Peterson DA, Patil PB, Moriyama EN, Roos S, Walter J.** 2010. Diversification of the gut symbiont *Lactobacillus reuteri* as a result of host-driven evolution. *ISME J* **4**:377–387.

73. **Choudhary DK, Johri BN.** 2011. Ecological significance of microdiversity: coexistence among casing soil bacterial strains through allocation of nutritional resource. *Indian J Microbiol* **51**:8–13.

74. **Jaspers E, Overmann J.** 2004. Ecological significance of microdiversity: identical 16S rRNA gene sequences can be found in bacteria with highly divergent genomes and ecophysiologies. *Appl Environ Microbiol* **70**:4831–4839.

75. **García-Martínez J, Acinas SG, Massana R, Rodríguez-Valera F.** 2002. Prevalence and microdiversity of *Alteromonas macleodii*-like microorganisms in different oceanic regions. *Environ Microbiol* **4**:42–50.

76. **Zimmerman AE, Martiny AC, Allison SD.** 2013. Microdiversity of extracellular enzyme genes among sequenced prokaryotic genomes. *ISME J* **7**:1187–1199.

77. **Lanza VF, Baquero F, de la Cruz F, Coque TM.** 2017. AcCNET (Accessory Genome Constellation Network): comparative genomics software for accessory genome analysis using bipartite networks. *Bioinformatics* **33**:283–285.

78. **Connor N, Sikorski J, Rooney AP, Kopac S, Koeppel AF, Burger A, Cole SG, Perry EB, Krizanc D, Field NC, Slaton M, Cohan FM.** 2010. Ecology of speciation in the genus *Bacillus*. *Appl Environ Microbiol* **76**:1349–1358.

79. **Koeppel A, Perry EB, Sikorski J, Krizanc D, Warner A, Ward DM, Rooney AP, Brambilla E, Connor N, Ratcliff RM, Nevo E, Cohan FM.** 2008. Identifying the fundamental units of bacterial diversity: a paradigm shift to incorporate

ecology into bacterial systematics. *Proc Natl Acad Sci U S A* **105:**2504–2509.

80. **Becraft ED, Wood JM, Rusch DB, Kühl M, Jensen SI, Bryant DA, Roberts DW, Cohan FM, Ward DM.** 2015. The molecular dimension of microbial species: 1. Ecological distinctions among, and homogeneity within, putative ecotypes of *Synechococcus* inhabiting the cyanobacterial mat of Mushroom Spring, Yellowstone National Park. *Front Microbiol* **6:**590.

81. **Kopac S, Wang Z, Wiedenbeck J, Sherry J, Wu M, Cohan FM.** 2014. Genomic heterogeneity and ecological speciation within one subspecies of *Bacillus subtilis. Appl Environ Microbiol* **80:**4842–4853.

82. **Stackebrandt E, Ebers J.** 2006. Taxonomic parameters revisited: tarnished gold standards. *Microbiol Today* **33:**152–155.

83. **Francisco JC, Cohan FM, Krizanc D.** 2014. Accuracy and efficiency of algorithms for the demarcation of bacterial ecotypes from DNA sequence data. *Int J Bioinform Res Appl* **10:**409–425.

84. **Corander J, Marttinen P, Sirén J, Tang J.** 2008. Enhanced Bayesian modelling in BAPS software for learning genetic structures of populations. *BMC Bioinformatics* **9:**539.

85. **Barraclough TG, Hughes M, Ashford-Hodges N, Fujisawa T.** 2009. Inferring evolutionarily significant units of bacterial diversity from broad environmental surveys of single-locus data. *Biol Lett* **5:**425–428.

86. **Eren AM, Morrison HG, Lescault PJ, Reveillaud J, Vineis JH, Sogin ML.** 2015. Minimum entropy decomposition: unsupervised oligotyping for sensitive partitioning of high-throughput marker gene sequences. *ISME J* **9:**968–979.

87. **Cohan FM, Koeppel AF.** 2008. The origins of ecological diversity in prokaryotes. *Curr Biol* **18:**R1024–R1034.

88. **Cohan FM, Koeppel A, Krizanc D.** 2006. Sequence-based discovery of ecological diversity within *Legionella,* p 367–376. *In* Cianciotto NP, Abu Kwaik Y, Edelstein PH, Fields BS, Geary DF, Harrison TG, Joseph C, Ratcliff RM, Stout JE, Swanson MS (ed), Legionella: *State of the Art 30 Years after Its Recognition.* ASM Press, Washington, DC.

89. **Manning SD, Motiwala AS, Springman AC, Qi W, Lacher DW, Ouellette LM, Mladonicky JM, Somsel P, Rudrik JT, Dietrich SE, Zhang W, Swaminathan B, Alland D, Whittam TS.** 2008. Variation in virulence among clades of *Escherichia coli* O157:H7 associated with disease outbreaks. *Proc Natl Acad Sci U S A* **105:**4868–4873.

90. **Smith NH, Gordon SV, de la Rua-Domenech R, Clifton-Hadley RS, Hewinson RG.** 2006. Bottle-

necks and broomsticks: the molecular evolution of *Mycobacterium bovis. Nat Rev Microbiol* **4:**670–681.

91. **Brisson D, Dykhuizen DE.** 2004. *ospC* diversity in *Borrelia burgdorferi*: different hosts are different niches. *Genetics* **168:**713–722.

92. **Sikorski J, Brambilla E, Kroppenstedt RM, Tindall BJ.** 2008. The temperature-adaptive fatty acid content in *Bacillus simplex* strains from 'Evolution Canyon', Israel. *Microbiology* **154:**2416–2426.

93. **Allewalt JP, Bateson MM, Revsbech NP, Slack K, Ward DM.** 2006. Effect of temperature and light on growth of and photosynthesis by *Synechococcus* isolates typical of those predominating in the octopus spring microbial mat community of Yellowstone National Park. *Appl Environ Microbiol* **72:**544–550.

94. **Bhaya D, Grossman AR, Steunou AS, Khuri N, Cohan FM, Hamamura N, Melendrez MC, Bateson MM, Ward DM, Heidelberg JF.** 2007. Population level functional diversity in a microbial community revealed by comparative genomic and metagenomic analyses. *ISME J* **1:**703–713.

95. **Olsen MT, Nowack S, Wood JM, Becraft ED, LaButti K, Lipzen A, Martin J, Schackwitz WS, Rusch DB, Cohan FM, Bryant DA, Ward DM.** 2015. The molecular dimension of microbial species: 3. Comparative genomics of *Synechococcus* strains with different light responses and *in situ* diel transcription patterns of associated putative ecotypes in the Mushroom Spring microbial mat. *Front Microbiol* **6:**604.

96. **Gogarten JP, Townsend JP.** 2005. Horizontal gene transfer, genome innovation and evolution. *Nat Rev Microbiol* **3:**679–687.

97. **Ochman H, Lawrence JG, Groisman EA.** 2000. Lateral gene transfer and the nature of bacterial innovation. *Nature* **405:**299–304.

98. **Bantinaki E, Kassen R, Knight CG, Robinson Z, Spiers AJ, Rainey PB.** 2007. Adaptive divergence in experimental populations of *Pseudomonas fluorescens.* III. Mutational origins of wrinkly spreader diversity. *Genetics* **176:**441–453.

99. **Koeppel AF, Wertheim JO, Barone L, Gentile N, Krizanc D, Cohan FM.** 2013. Speedy speciation in a bacterial microcosm: New species can arise as frequently as adaptations within a species. *ISME J* **7:**1080–1091.

100. **Blount ZD, Barrick JE, Davidson CJ, Lenski RE.** 2012. Genomic analysis of a key innovation in an experimental *Escherichia coli* population. *Nature* **489:**513–518.

101. **Becker NS, Margos G, Blum H, Krebs S, Graf A, Lane RS, Castillo-Ramírez S, Sing A, Fingerle V.** 2016. Recurrent evolution of host and vector

association in bacteria of the *Borrelia burgdorferi* sensu lato species complex. *BMC Genomics* **17:** 734.

102. **Sokurenko EV, Chesnokova V, Dykhuizen DE, Ofek I, Wu XR, Krogfelt KA, Struve C, Schembri MA, Hasty DL.** 1998. Pathogenic adaptation of *Escherichia coli* by natural variation of the FimH adhesin. *Proc Natl Acad Sci U S A* **95:**8922–8926.

103. **D'Argenio DA, Wu M, Hoffman LR, Kulasekara HD, Déziel E, Smith EE, Nguyen H, Ernst RK, Larson Freeman TJ, Spencer DH, Brittnacher M, Hayden HS, Selgrade S, Klausen M, Goodlett DR, Burns JL, Ramsey BW, Miller SI.** 2007. Growth phenotypes of *Pseudomonas aeruginosa lasR* mutants adapted to the airways of cystic fibrosis patients. *Mol Microbiol* **64:**512–533.

104. **Mowat E, Paterson S, Fothergill JL, Wright EA, Ledson MJ, Walshaw MJ, Brockhurst MA, Winstanley C.** 2011. *Pseudomonas aeruginosa* population diversity and turnover in cystic fibrosis chronic infections. *Am J Respir Crit Care Med* **183:**1674–1679.

105. **Chaloner GL, Palmira Ventosilla, Birtles RJ.** 2011. Multi-locus sequence analysis reveals profound genetic diversity among isolates of the human pathogen *Bartonella bacilliformis*. *PLoS Negl Trop Dis* **5:**e1248.

106. **Paul S, Minnick MF, Chattopadhyay S.** 2016. Mutation-driven divergence and convergence indicate adaptive evolution of the intracellular human-restricted pathogen, *Bartonella bacilliformis*. *PLoS Negl Trop Dis* **10:**e0004712.

107. **Wildschutte H, Lawrence JG.** 2007. Differential *Salmonella* survival against communities of intestinal amoebae. *Microbiology* **153:**1781–1789.

108. **Toll-Riera M, San Millan A, Wagner A, MacLean RC.** 2016. The genomic basis of evolutionary innovation in *Pseudomonas aeruginosa*. *PLoS Genet* **12:** e1006005.

109. **Popa O, Dagan T.** 2011. Trends and barriers to lateral gene transfer in prokaryotes. *Curr Opin Microbiol* **14:**615–623.

110. **Zawadzki P, Cohan FM.** 1995. The size and continuity of DNA segments integrated in *Bacillus* transformation. *Genetics* **141:**1231–1243.

111. **Derbyshire KM, Gray TA.** 2014. Distributive conjugal transfer: new insights into horizontal gene transfer and genetic exchange in mycobacteria. *Microbiol Spectr* **2:**MGM2-0022-2013.

112. **Novais C, Tedim AP, Lanza VF, Freitas AR, Silveira E, Escada R, Roberts AP, Al-Haroni M, Baquero F, Peixe L, Coque TM.** 2016. Co-diversification of *Enterococcus faecium* core genomes and PBP5: evidences of *pbp5* horizontal transfer. *Front Microbiol* **7:**1581.

113. **Lassalle F, Campillo T, Vial L, Baude J, Costechareyre D, Chapulliot D, Shams M, Abrouk D, Lavire C, Oger-Desfeux C, Hommais F, Guéguen L, Daubin V, Muller D, Nesme X.** 2011. Genomic species are ecological species as revealed by comparative genomics in *Agrobacterium tumefaciens*. *Genome Biol Evol* **3:**762–781.

114. **Gogarten JP, Townsend JP.** 2005. Horizontal gene transfer, genome innovation, and evolution. *Nat Rev Microbiol* **3:**679–687.

115. **Anantha RP, McVeigh AL, Lee LH, Agnew MK, Cassels FJ, Scott DA, Whittam TS, Savarino SJ.** 2004. Evolutionary and functional relationships of colonization factor antigen I and other class 5 adhesive fimbriae of enterotoxigenic *Escherichia coli*. *Infect Immun* **72:**7190–7201.

116. **Fondi M, Fani R.** 2010. The horizontal flow of the plasmid resistome: clues from inter-generic similarity networks. *Environ Microbiol* **12:**3228–3242.

117. **Amarir-Bouhram J, Goin M, Petit MA.** 2011. Low efficiency of homology-facilitated illegitimate recombination during conjugation in *Escherichia coli*. *PLoS One* **6:**e28876.

118. **Smith JM, Dowson CG, Spratt BG.** 1991. Localized sex in bacteria. *Nature* **349:**29–31.

119. **Jacob F, Monod J.** 1961. Genetic regulatory mechanisms in the synthesis of proteins. *J Mol Biol* **3:**318–356.

120. **Lawrence JG, Ochman H.** 1998. Molecular archaeology of the *Escherichia coli* genome. *Proc Natl Acad Sci U S A* **95:**9413–9417.

121. **Lawrence JG, Roth JR.** 1996. Selfish operons: horizontal transfer may drive the evolution of gene clusters. *Genetics* **143:**1843–1860.

122. **Lawrence JG.** 1997. Selfish operons and speciation by gene transfer. *Trends Microbiol* **5:**355–359.

123. **Lawrence JG.** 1999. Gene transfer, speciation, and the evolution of bacterial genomes. *Curr Opin Microbiol* **2:**519–523.

124. **Kashtan N, Roggensack SE, Rodrigue S, Thompson JW, Biller SJ, Coe A, Ding H, Marttinen P, Malmstrom RR, Stocker R, Follows MJ, Stepanauskas R, Chisholm SW.** 2014. Single-cell genomics reveals hundreds of coexisting subpopulations in wild *Prochlorococcus*. *Science* **344:**416–420.

125. **López-Pérez M, Gonzaga A, Rodriguez-Valera F.** 2013. Genomic diversity of "deep ecotype" *Alteromonas macleodii* isolates: evidence for Pan-Mediterranean clonal frames. *Genome Biol Evol* **5:**1220–1232.

126. **Arsène-Ploetze F, Koechler S, Marchal M, Coppée JY, Chandler M, Bonnefoy V, Brochier-Armanet C, Barakat M, Barbe V, Battaglia-Brunet F, Bruneel O, Bryan CG, Cleiss-Arnold J, Cruveiller S, Erhardt M, Heinrich-Salmeron A,**

Hommais F, Joulian C, Krin E, Lieutaud A, Lièvremont D, Michel C, Muller D, Ortet P, Proux C, Siguier P, Roche D, Rouy Z, Salvignol G, Slyemi D, Talla E, Weiss S, Weissenbach J, Médigue C, Bertin PN. 2010. Structure, function, and evolution of the *Thiomonas* spp. genome. *PLoS Genet* **6:**e1000859.

127. **Barlow M.** 2009. What antimicrobial resistance has taught us about horizontal gene transfer. *Methods Mol Biol* **532:**397–411.

128. **Croucher NJ, Klugman KP.** 2014. The emergence of bacterial "hopeful monsters". *mBio* **5:** e01550-e14.

129. **Goldschmidt R.** 1933. Some aspects of evolution. *Science* **78:**539–547.

130. **Segovia L, Piñero D, Palacios R, Martínez-Romero E.** 1991. Genetic structure of a soil population of nonsymbiotic *Rhizobium leguminosarum*. *Appl Environ Microbiol* **57:**426–433.

131. **Robins-Browne RM, Holt KE, Ingle DJ, Hocking DM, Yang J, Tauschek M.** 2016. Are *Escherichia coli* pathotypes still relevant in the era of whole-genome sequencing? *Front Cell Infect Microbiol* **6:**141.

132. **Lanza VF, de Toro M, Garcillán-Barcia MP, Mora A, Blanco J, Coque TM, de la Cruz F.** 2014. Plasmid flux in *Escherichia coli* ST131 sublineages, analyzed by plasmid constellation network (PLACNET), a new method for plasmid reconstruction from whole genome sequences. *PLoS Genet* **10:**e1004766.

133. **Kumar N, Lad G, Giuntini E, Kaye ME, Udomwong P, Shamsani NJ, Young JP, Bailly X.** 2015. Bacterial genospecies that are not ecologically coherent: population genomics of *Rhizobium leguminosarum*. *Open Biol* **5:**140133.

134. **Wernegreen JJ, Harding EE, Riley MA.** 1997. *Rhizobium* gone native: unexpected plasmid stability of indigenous *Rhizobium leguminosarum*. *Proc Natl Acad Sci U S A* **94:**5483–5488.

135. **Smith JM, Smith NH, O'Rourke M, Spratt BG.** 1993. How clonal are bacteria? *Proc Natl Acad Sci U S A* **90:**4384–4388.

136. **Baltrus DA.** 2013. Exploring the costs of horizontal gene transfer. *Trends Ecol Evol* **28:**489–495.

137. **Hao W, Golding GB.** 2006. The fate of laterally transferred genes: life in the fast lane to adaptation or death. *Genome Res* **16:**636–643.

138. **Andersson DI, Levin BR.** 1999. The biological cost of antibiotic resistance. *Curr Opin Microbiol* **2:**489–493.

139. **Cohan FM, King EC, Zawadzki P.** 1994. Amelioration of the deleterious pleiotropic effects of an adaptive mutation in *Bacillus subtilis*. *Evolution* **48:**81–95.

140. **Maisnier-Patin S, Paulander W, Pennhag A, Andersson DI.** 2007. Compensatory evolution re-veals functional interactions between ribosomal proteins S12, L14 and L19. *J Mol Biol* **366:**207–215.

141. **Dougherty K, Smith BA, Moore AF, Maitland S, Fanger C, Murillo R, Baltrus DA.** 2014. Multiple phenotypic changes associated with large-scale horizontal gene transfer. *PLoS One* **9:**e102170.

142. **Levin BR, Perrot V, Walker N.** 2000. Compensatory mutations, antibiotic resistance and the population genetics of adaptive evolution in bacteria. *Genetics* **154:**985–997.

143. **Liu Y, Lai Q, Göker M, Meier-Kolthoff JP, Wang M, Sun Y, Wang L, Shao Z.** 2015. Genomic insights into the taxonomic status of the *Bacillus cereus* group. *Sci Rep* **5:**14082.

144. **Clausen J, Keck DD, Hiesey WM.** 1947. Heredity of geographically and ecologically isolated races. *Am Nat* **81:**114–133.

145. **Summers RW, Broome A.** 2012. Associations between crossbills and North American conifers in Scotland. *For Ecol Manage* **271:**37–45.

146. **Wilson DS, Yoshimura J.** 1994. On the coexistence of specialists and generalists. *Am Nat* **144:** 692–707.

147. **Morris JJ.** 2015. Black Queen evolution: the role of leakiness in structuring microbial communities. *Trends Genet* **31:**475–482.

148. **Fry JD.** 1996. The evolution of host-specialization: are trade-offs overrated? *Am Nat* **148:**S84–S107.

149. **Cui B, He Q, Zhang K, Chen X.** 2011. Determinants of annual-perennial plant zonation across a salt-fresh marsh interface: a multistage assessment. *Oecologia* **166:**1067–1075.

150. **Becraft ED, Cohan FM, Kühl M, Jensen SI, Ward DM.** 2011. Fine-scale distribution patterns of *Synechococcus* ecological diversity in microbial mats of Mushroom Spring, Yellowstone National Park. *Appl Environ Microbiol* **77:**7689–7697.

151. **Martiny AC, Tai AP, Veneziano D, Primeau F, Chisholm SW.** 2009. Taxonomic resolution, ecotypes and the biogeography of *Prochlorococcus*. *Environ Microbiol* **11:**823–832.

152. **Nevo E.** 2014. Evolution in action: adaptation and incipient sympatric speciation with gene flow across life at "Evolution Canyon", Israel. *Isr J Ecol Evol* **60:**85–98.

153. **Perry EB.** 2007. Sequence-based discovery of ecological diversity in *Bacillus* from natural communities. M.S thesis. Wesleyan University, Middletown, CT.

154. **Kopac SM.** 2014. Ecological dimensions of significance in speciation in *Bacillus subtilis* and *Bacillus licheniformis*. Ph.D. dissertation. Wesleyan University, Middletown, CT.

155. **Feingersch R, Philosof A, Mejuch T, Glaser F, Alalouf O, Shoham Y, Béjà O.** 2012. Potential for

phosphite and phosphonate utilization by *Pro-chlorococcus. ISME J* **6:**827–834.

156. **Cohan FM.** 2016. Bacterial speciation: genetic sweeps in bacterial species. *Curr Biol* **26:**R112–R115.

157. **Puentes-Téllez PE, van Elsas JD.** 2015. Differential stress resistance and metabolic traits underlie coexistence in a sympatrically evolved bacterial population. *Environ Microbiol* **17:**889–900.

158. **Deng J, Brettar I, Luo C, Auchtung J, Konstantinidis KT, Rodrigues JLM, Höfle M, Tiedje JM.** 2014. Stability, genotypic and phenotypic diversity of *Shewanella baltica* in the redox transition zone of the Baltic Sea. *Environ Microbiol* **16:**1854–1866.

159. **Biderre-Petit C, Jézéquel D, Dugat-Bony E, Lopes F, Kuever J, Borrel G, Viollier E, Fonty G, Peyret P.** 2011. Identification of microbial communities involved in the methane cycle of a freshwater meromictic lake. *FEMS Microbiol Ecol* **77:**533–545.

160. **Kalyuzhnaya MG, Lapidus A, Ivanova N, Copeland AC, McHardy AC, Szeto E, Salamov A, Grigoriev IV, Suciu D, Levine SR, Markowitz VM, Rigoutsos I, Tringe SG, Bruce DC, Richardson PM, Lidstrom ME, Chistoserdova L.** 2008. High-resolution metagenomics targets specific functional types in complex microbial communities. *Nat Biotechnol* **26:**1029–1034.

161. **Smith NH, Kremer K, Inwald J, Dale J, Driscoll JR, Gordon SV, van Soolingen D, Hewinson RG, Smith JM.** 2006. Ecotypes of the *Mycobacterium tuberculosis* complex. *J Theor Biol* **239:**220–225.

162. **Mechai S, Margos G, Feil EJ, Barairo N, Lindsay LR, Michel P, Ogden NH.** 2016. Evidence for host-genotype associations of *Borrelia burgdorferi* sensu stricto. *PLoS One* **11:**e0149345.

163. **Vuong HB, Canham CD, Fonseca DM, Brisson D, Morin PJ, Smouse PE, Ostfeld RS.** 2014. Occurrence and transmission efficiencies of *Borrelia burgdorferi ospC* types in avian and mammalian wildlife. *Infect Genet Evol* **27:**594–600.

164. **Clark MA, Moran NA, Baumann P, Wernegreen JJ.** 2000. Cospeciation between bacterial endosymbionts (*Buchnera*) and a recent radiation of aphids (*Uroleucon*) and pitfalls of testing for phylogenetic congruence. *Evolution* **54:**517–525.

165. **Jackson AP, Charleston MA.** 2004. A cophylogenetic perspective of RNA-virus evolution. *Mol Biol Evol* **21:**45–57.

166. **Woolhouse M, Gaunt E.** 2007. Ecological origins of novel human pathogens. *Crit Rev Microbiol* **33:**231–242.

167. **Himsworth CG, Parsons KL, Jardine C, Patrick DM.** 2013. Rats, cities, people, and pathogens: a systematic review and narrative synthesis of literature regarding the ecology of rat-associated zoonoses in urban centers. *Vector Borne Zoonotic Dis* **13:**349–359.

168. **Azhar EI, El-Kafrawy SA, Farraj SA, Hassan AM, Al-Saeed MS, Hashem AM, Madani TA.** 2014. Evidence for camel-to-human transmission of MERS coronavirus. *N Engl J Med* **370:**2499–2505.

169. **Mindell DP.** 2006. The Evolving World: Evolution in Everyday Life. Harvard University Press, Cambridge, MA.

170. **Reusken CB, Raj VS, Koopmans MP, Haagmans BL.** 2016. Cross host transmission in the emergence of MERS coronavirus. *Curr Opin Virol* **16:**55–62.

171. **Lo Presti A, Cella E, Giovanetti M, Lai A, Angeletti S, Zehender G, Ciccozzi M.** 2016. Origin and evolution of Nipah virus. *J Med Virol* **88:**380–388.

172. **Field HE.** 2016. Hendra virus ecology and transmission. *Curr Opin Virol* **16:**120–125.

173. **Han HJ, Wen HL, Zhou CM, Chen FF, Luo LM, Liu JW, Yu XJ.** 2015. Bats as reservoirs of severe emerging infectious diseases. *Virus Res* **205:**1–6.

174. **Marí Saéz A, Weiss S, Nowak K, Lapeyre V, Zimmermann F, Düx A, Kühl HS, Kaba M, Regnaut S, Merkel K, Sachse A, Thiesen U, Villányi L, Boesch C, Dabrowski PW, Radonić A, Nitsche A, Leendertz SA, Petterson S, Becker S, Krähling V, Couacy-Hymann E, Akoua-Koffi C, Weber N, Schaade L, Fahr J, Borchert M, Gogarten JF, Calvignac-Spencer S, Leendertz FH.** 2015. Investigating the zoonotic origin of the West African Ebola epidemic. *EMBO Mol Med* **7:**17–23.

175. **Streicker DG, Turmelle AS, Vonhof MJ, Kuzmin IV, McCracken GF, Rupprecht CE.** 2010. Host phylogeny constrains cross-species emergence and establishment of rabies virus in bats. *Science* **329:**676–679.

176. **Fisher ML, Castillo C, Mecsas J.** 2007. Intranasal inoculation of mice with *Yersinia pseudotuberculosis* causes a lethal lung infection that is dependent on *Yersinia* outer proteins and PhoP. *Infect Immun* **75:**429–442.

177. **Sun YC, Jarrett CO, Bosio CF, Hinnebusch BJ.** 2014. Retracing the evolutionary path that led to flea-borne transmission of *Yersinia pestis. Cell Host Microbe* **15:**578–586.

178. **Bessen DE.** 2009. Population biology of the human restricted pathogen, *Streptococcus pyogenes. Infect Genet Evol* **9:**581–593.

179. **Gonzales-Siles L, Sjöling Å.** 2016. The different ecological niches of enterotoxigenic *Escherichia coli. Environ Microbiol* **18:**741–751.

180. **Linke K, Rückerl I, Brugger K, Karpiskova R, Walland J, Muri-Klinger S, Tichy A, Wagner M, Stessl B.** 2014. Reservoirs of *Listeria* species in three environmental ecosystems. *Appl Environ Microbiol* **80:**5583–5592.

181. **Zhu B, Ibrahim M, Cui Z, Xie G, Jin G, Kube M, Li B, Zhou X.** 2016. Multi-omics analysis of niche specificity provides new insights into ecological adaptation in bacteria. *ISME J* **10:**2072–2075.

182. **Cutter AD, Gray JC.** 2016. Ephemeral ecological speciation and the latitudinal biodiversity gradient. *Evolution* **70:**2171–2185.

183. **Vos M, Didelot X.** 2009. A comparison of homologous recombination rates in bacteria and archaea. *ISME J* **3:**199–208.

184. **Sheppard SK, McCarthy ND, Jolley KA, Maiden MC.** 2011. Introgression in the genus *Campylobacter*: generation and spread of mosaic alleles. *Microbiology* **157:**1066–1074.

185. **Baquero F.** 2011. The 2010 Garrod Lecture: The dimensions of evolution in antibiotic resistance: *ex unibus plurum et ex pluribus unum*. *J Antimicrob Chemother* **66:**1659–1672.

186. **Vos M.** 2011. A species concept for bacteria based on adaptive divergence. *Trends Microbiol* **19:**1–7.

187. **Doolittle WF, Zhaxybayeva O.** 2009. On the origin of prokaryotic species. *Genome Res* **19:**744–756.

188. **Bendall ML, Stevens SL, Chan LK, Malfatti S, Schwientek P, Tremblay J, Schackwitz W, Martin J, Pati A, Bushnell B, Froula J, Kang D, Tringe SG, Bertilsson S, Moran MA, Shade A, Newton RJ, McMahon KD, Malmstrom RR.** 2016. Genome-wide selective sweeps and gene-specific sweeps in natural bacterial populations. *ISME J* **10:**1589–1601.

189. **Fuxelius HH, Darby A, Min CK, Cho NH, Andersson SG.** 2007. The genomic and metabolic diversity of *Rickettsia*. *Res Microbiol* **158:**745–753.

190. **Papke RT, Zhaxybayeva O, Feil EJ, Sommerfeld K, Muise D, Doolittle WF.** 2007. Searching for species in haloarchaea. *Proc Natl Acad Sci U S A* **104:**14092–14097.

191. **Guttman DS, Dykhuizen DE.** 1994. Detecting selective sweeps in naturally occurring *Escherichia coli*. *Genetics* **138:**993–1003.

192. **Kopac SM, Cohan FM.** 2012. Comment on "Population genomics of early events in the ecological differentiation of bacteria". *Science* **336:**48–51. http://comments.sciencemag.org/content/10.1126/science.1218198#comments.

193. **Cohan FM.** 2005. Periodic selection and ecological diversity in bacteria, p 78–93. *In* Nurminsky D (ed), *Selective Sweep*. Landes Bioscience, Georgetown, TX.

194. **Majewski J, Cohan FM.** 1999. Adapt globally, act locally: the effect of selective sweeps on bacterial sequence diversity. *Genetics* **152:**1459–1474.

195. **Takeuchi N, Cordero OX, Koonin EV, Kaneko K.** 2015. Gene-specific selective sweeps in bacteria and archaea caused by negative frequency-dependent selection. *BMC Biol* **13:**20.

196. **Roy K, Hunt G, Jablonski D.** 2009. Phylogenetic conservatism of extinctions in marine bivalves. *Science* **325:**733–737.

197. **Dunn RR, Harris NC, Colwell RK, Koh LP, Sodhi NS.** 2009. The sixth mass coextinction: are most endangered species parasites and mutualists? *Proc Biol Sci* **276:**3037–3045.

198. **Jorth P, Staudinger BJ, Wu X, Hisert KB, Hayden H, Garudathri J, Harding CL, Radey MC, Rezayat A, Bautista G, Berrington WR, Goddard AF, Zheng C, Angermeyer A, Brittnacher MJ, Kitzman J, Shendure J, Fligner CL, Mittler J, Aitken ML, Manoil C, Bruce JE, Yahr TL, Singh PK.** 2015. Regional isolation drives bacterial diversification within cystic fibrosis lungs. *Cell Host Microbe* **18:**307–319.

199. **Oliver A, Cantón R, Campo P, Baquero F, Blázquez J.** 2000. High frequency of hypermutable *Pseudomonas aeruginosa* in cystic fibrosis lung infection. *Science* **288:**1251–1254.

200. **López-Collazo E, Jurado T, de Dios Caballero J, Pérez-Vázquez M, Vindel A, Hernández-Jiménez E, Tamames J, Cubillos-Zapata C, Manrique M, Tobes R, Máiz L, Cantón R, Baquero F, Del Campo R.** 2015. *In vivo* attenuation and genetic evolution of a ST247-SCC*mec*I MRSA clone after 13 years of pathogenic bronchopulmonary colonization in a patient with cystic fibrosis: implications of the innate immune response. *Mucosal Immunol* **8:**362–371.

201. **Hoboth C, Hoffmann R, Eichner A, Henke C, Schmoldt S, Imhof A, Heesemann J, Hogardt M.** 2009. Dynamics of adaptive microevolution of hypermutable *Pseudomonas aeruginosa* during chronic pulmonary infection in patients with cystic fibrosis. *J Infect Dis* **200:**118–130.

202. **Warner DF, Koch A, Mizrahi V.** 2015. Diversity and disease pathogenesis in *Mycobacterium tuberculosis*. *Trends Microbiol* **23:**14–21.

203. **Ebrahimi-Rad M, Bifani P, Martin C, Kremer K, Samper S, Rauzier J, Kreiswirth B, Blazquez J, Jouan M, van Soolingen D, Gicquel B.** 2003. Mutations in putative mutator genes of *Mycobacterium tuberculosis* strains of the W-Beijing family. *Emerg Infect Dis* **9:**838–845.

204. **Cohan FM, Perry EB.** 2007. A systematics for discovering the fundamental units of bacterial diversity. *Curr Biol* **17:**R373–R386.

205. **Achtman M, Wagner M.** 2008. Microbial diversity and the genetic nature of microbial species. *Nat Rev Microbiol* **6:**431–440.

206. **Baldan R, Testa F, Lorè NI, Bragonzi A, Cichero P, Ossi C, Biancardi A, Nizzero P, Moro M, Cirillo DM.** 2012. Factors contributing to epi-demic MRSA clones replacement in a hospital setting. *PLoS One* **7:**e43153.

207. **Remonsellez F, Galleguillos F, Moreno-Paz M, Parro V, Acosta M, Demergasso C.** 2009. Dynamic of active microorganisms inhabiting a bioleaching industrial heap of low-grade copper sulfide ore monitored by real-time PCR and oligonucleotide prokaryotic acidophile microarray. *Microb Biotechnol* **2:**613–624.

Tracking the Rules of Transmission and Introgression with Networks

19

CHLOÉ VIGLIOTTI*,[1] CÉDRIC BICEP*,[1] ERIC BAPTESTE,[1] PHILIPPE LOPEZ,[1] and EDUARDO COREL[1]

INTRODUCTION

It has been proposed that an organism and its microbes form an assemblage called a holobiont (1, 2). The human body and human genome along with gut microbes and their genomes can be seen as a dynamic holobiont system (3–5), i.e., a superorganism amalgamating microbial and human attributes (6). In this multipartite holobiont, the host genome provides the primary genome, while microbial genes constitute the "second human genome," which is in fact a prokaryotic pangenome (3, 7, 8). Whether the holobionts are units of selection is actively debated (9–11), yet other aspects of their biology are less controversial, and holobionts are becoming a major object of study in biology. Among these uncontroversial features lies the observation that, by definition, a holobiont is home to several different modes of genetic transmission. In nuclear transmission, the genetic material is inherited from one individual (in parthenogenesis, for example) or, most of the time, from two individuals, whereas in organelle transmission (of mitochondria, for example), the material is mostly inherited from the mother, in animals (12). Both types of trans-

[1]Sorbonne Université, CNRS, Institut de Biologie Paris Seine (IBPS), Laboratoire Evolution Paris Seine, F-75005 Paris, France.

Microbial Transmission in Biological Processes
Edited by Fernando Baquero, Emilio Bouza, J.A. Gutiérrez-Fuentes, and Teresa M. Coque
© 2018 American Society for Microbiology, Washington, DC
doi:10.1128/microbiolspec.MTBP-0008-2016

mission result directly from the reproduction of the host. This stands in contrast to transmission of the microbiota, that is, the acquisition (or loss) of microbes between host generations. In mammals, at birth, the microbiota is inherited from the mother, but this is not always the case for other animal groups, where it could also be inherited from the environment (12, 13). During the life of the individual, the microbiota may even evolve, depending on different factors, which are currently not well characterized (e.g., host constraints, diet, environment, and transmission between different hosts) (14). The transmission of microbiomes differs in turn from the transmission of microbiotas, since it is no longer (or at least not only) microbes that are exchanged, acquired, or lost, but genes themselves. These genes may be carried by microbes, but also by viruses, plasmids, or other classes of mobile genetic elements (MGEs). For example, transmissions in the gut microbiome are in part due to horizontal gene transfer (HGT) (4, 15, 16) because of the high cell density in microorganisms, and mediated by viruses—especially temperate prophages (17, 18)—integrases, recombinases (19), and conjugative transposons (20). Finally, the transmission of microbes from the environment to the host has not been systematically taken into account (11). As with any transmission, microbial transmission can be transient or permanent (Fig. 1).

These complex transmissions endow the holobiont with characteristics inherited either from a macroorganism, as in nuclear transmission, or from its microbes, as in microbiome transmission, and even from the coexistence of the host and its microbes (21, 22). The host can exert some control on the microbial species in its microbiota (e.g., by genetic regulation) (23), and it can indirectly influence the genetic content of these microbes, its distribution and transmission. For example, a mutation in the gene *MEFV* (which encodes a protein involved in regulation of innate immunity) affects the gut microbiota composition at the taxon level (e.g., proportions of *Enterobacteriaceae*, *Acidaminococcaceae*, *Ruminococcus*, and *Megasphaera* are affected by the human gene mutation) and the gut microbiota diversity (23). Reciprocally, microbes may play a role in the host ability to digest food (e.g., cellulose in acquisition of a plant-based diet), in host protection, and in host development (24). The gut microbiome encodes indispensable metabolisms for human life, contributes to human nutrition, and affects the development of our immune system and protection against pathogens (20, 25). Coevolution, however, can be difficult to distinguish from mere coexistence of a host and its microbes (3, 11, 12, 26).

Studying already established transmissions may allow us to find associations between a host (maybe with specific characteristics) and its microbiota and its microbiome. This paper first introduces sequence similarity networks and illustrates, with an application to human gut microbiomes, how these networks can be integrated into the study of genetic transmission. Next, it introduces bipartite networks and illustrates how they may be theoretically used to enhance analyses of microbes and of gene transmissions in holobionts, with a particular focus on the microbiomes of populations of lizards with different diets. Over all, network analyses enhance the focus on an important process of genetic transmission, i.e., gene externalization between mobile elements and cellular chromosomes.

INTRODUCING SEQUENCE SIMILARITY NETWORKS

Network-based methods are useful to study the evolution of gene family (27), gene transfer, composite genes and genomes, evolutionary transitions, and holobionts (26, 28–31). More specifically, networks can be used to search for rules of association between genes and their microbial, viral, or animal hosts and to identify putative cases of gene introgres-

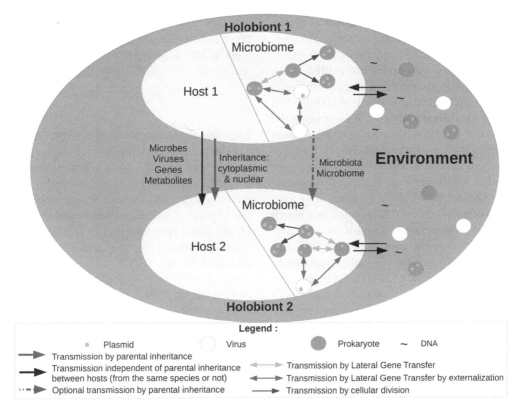

FIGURE 1 Different types of transmission in holobionts. This figure presents different transmissions between holobionts, and between a holobiont and its environment. The holobiont is composed of two parts: the host and its microbial communities (microbiome from gut, skin, oral, etc.). When a host gives birth to another, the parent brings to its offspring mitochondria, cytoplasm, and genes (pink arrows). The transmission is from the parent to the progeny. In some cases, like in mammals, the mother gives microbiota and microbiome to her children (pink dashed arrow). A host from a holobiont may also bring to the microbial community of another holobiont microbes, MGEs (viruses and plasmids), genes, or metabolites (black arrow between holobionts). Otherwise, a holobiont may exchange with the environment MGEs (plasmids and viruses) or microbes (black arrows between holobiont and environment). Then, in a microbial community there are transmissions between the different elements: transmissions between microbes (for example, by reproduction [purple arrows] or lateral gene transfer [green arrows]) or transmission between microbes and MGEs (red arrows). In this case we talk about externalization.

sion. Gene introgression occurs when the genetic material of a particular evolutionary unit propagates into different host structures and is replicated within these host structures (26, 32). By contrast, tree-based methods are more routinely used to describe divergences from a last common ancestor. Stated simply, the tree representation of evolutionary processes does not show the same thing as a network representation. Indeed, the tree representation allows observation of the evolu-tion from one individual to many individuals, while the network representation includes the evolution from several individuals to one individual. These methods do not show the same paths of transmission; therefore it can be argued that network-based methods are more adapted than trees to study the processes where organisms form a collective system of complex genetic transmission, including patterns of vertical inheritance when they exist, since the tree is included in the network (33).

A sequence similarity network is a network representation of sequence similarities, where each node of the network represents a sequence, and two nodes are related by an edge if the sequences have a higher similarity than a predefined threshold of identity and cover (34). Such a network is built using the BLASTP algorithm (in a BLASTP all-against-all run on the set of sequences). In this process, an amino acid sequence is considered similar to another (i.e., the two corresponding nodes are linked by an edge) if at least 80% of each sequence is included in a match (mutual cover criterion) and if the sequence similarity over the covering region (percentage of identity criterion) is higher than a given percentage, e.g., 95% (34, 35). Because of this thresholding scheme, in a sequence similarity network some groups of nodes have no connection, not even an indirect one. Such groups are called connected components (CCs) and can be used to approximate gene families (Fig. 2, i) (27, 36).

Building networks at different thresholds allows one to see differences in transmissions (1, 2). Although the network is filtered for 80% mutual cover, several networks can be produced at different thresholds of percentage of identity: 70, 75, 80, 85, 90, and 95%. If one considers, in a first approximation, that sequences evolve by point mutation (rather than by recombination) and that these mutations accumulate linearly over time, then sequences that have been diverging for a longer time period should contain more mutations than sequences derived from a recent last common ancestor. While such a schematic molecular clock cannot be realistically assumed, since the mutation rates of different gene families can be very different, and so similar percentages of identity can be found for families with very different ages, the use of percentage of identity thresholds can nonetheless serve as a proxy for a relative dating of transmissions (37). Then it provides a lower bound, since this procedure will admittedly underestimate the age of sequences that were affected by recent recombination events leading to gene conversion (since these events changed different, diverged sequences into identical ones).

Application of Sequence Similarity Networks to Human Microbiome Data

Although there is a growing interest in the mobilome of the mammalian and human gastrointestinal tract (17, 38, 39), little is known about the population of MGEs residing in the human gut. In other words, investigations of the "human + gut microbiota" holobiont (3, 15, 40) could turn into studies of a tripartite "mobile elements + gut microbes + human individual" system, taking into account three types of potential partners: gut MGEs, their direct cellular hosts (i.e., the microbial community within which these MGEs circulate), and the human individuals hosting these microbes.

To study this tripartite system, a simple bioinformatics protocol can be used to organize the predicted open reading frames (ORFs) from 31 human gut microbiomes (18 from American and 13 from Japanese individuals) into 21,525 clusters encompassing at least four sequences with significant similarity (Fig. 3). Then genes from the gut microbiota of these humans can be classified into resident families (defining a resident metagenome) and into externalized and highly externalized families (both defining the gut externalized metagenome). This latter terminology indicates that a gene family has undergone horizontal transfer at some point between different types of genomes, i.e., between cells and viruses; between cells and plasmids; or between cells, viruses, and plasmids. This partition allows us to propose a testable hypothesis about genetic transmission: genes externalized on more types of MGEs are shared more broadly both in gut microbial communities and across their human hosts. The methodology underlying the construction and analyses of these networks is detailed below, in order to allow the reader to perform similar studies.

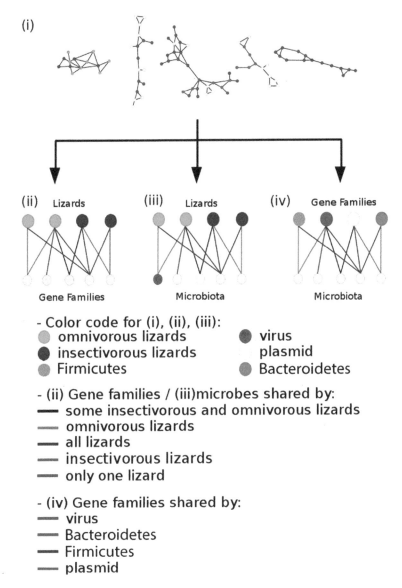

(i)

(ii) Lizards

(iii) Lizards

(iv) Gene Families

Gene Families

Microbiota

Microbiota

- Color code for (i), (ii), (iii):
  - omnivorous lizards
  - insectivorous lizards
  - Firmicutes
  - virus
  - plasmid
  - Bacteroidetes

- (ii) Gene families / (iii)microbes shared by:
  - ▬ some insectivorous and omnivorous lizards
  - ▬ omnivorous lizards
  - ▬ all lizards
  - ▬ insectivorous lizards
  - ▬ only one lizard

- (iv) Gene families shared by:
  - ▬ virus
  - ▬ Bacteroidetes
  - ▬ Firmicutes
  - ▬ plasmid

FIGURE 2 Networks as tools for describing relationships between holobionts and transmission in lizards' gut microbiomes. (i) Sequence similarity network (SSN). The SSN is built by comparing ORFs from all lizards' gut microbiomes, using an all-against-all BLASTP. The SSN contains five CCs, also called gene families. Nodes are ORFs and are colored depending on their taxonomic annotation (see legend). If two nodes are similar at a determined percentage of identity (e.g., 95%), then they are linked by an edge. (ii) Bipartite graph of lizards-gene families. Type I nodes are lizards, colored depending on their diet, and type II nodes are the five gene families described in part i. There is an edge between a type I node and a type II node if in the gene family you can find a sequence that is contained in the lizards' gut microbiomes of the type I node. (iii) Bipartite graph of lizards-microbial classes. Type I nodes are lizards, and type II nodes are microbial classes. If in one lizard's gut microbiome a microbial class is found, then there is a link between the type I node associated and the type II node associated. Type I nodes are colored depending on the diet of the lizard, and type II nodes are colored depending on the microbial class of ORFs. (iv) Bipartite graph of microbial classes-gene families. Type I nodes are microbial classes, and type II nodes are the five gene families described in part i. There is an edge between a type I node and a type II node if at least one ORF of the gene family of the type II node is from the microbial class of the type I node.

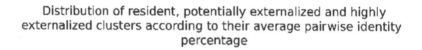

Distribution of resident, potentially externalized and highly externalized clusters according to their average pairwise identity percentage

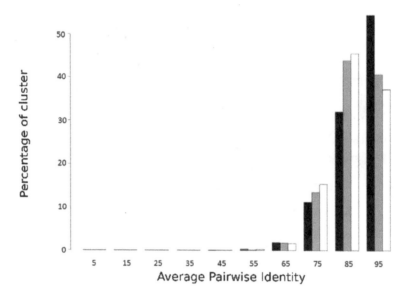

FIGURE 3 Distribution of resident, potentially externalized, and highly externalized clusters according to their average pairwise identity percentage. Functional distributions were plotted for the three classes of clusters; resident clusters are in black, potentially externalized clusters in gray, and potentially highly externalized clusters in white.

Clustering Microbiome Sequences into Groups with Different Degrees of Externalization

Using nucleotide sequences from references 20 and 41 as inputs for MetageneAnnotator (42) (default parameters), 311,265 ORFs were predicted from the gut microbiomes of 13 Japanese individuals and 195,521 ORFs were predicted from the gut microbiomes of 18 U.S. individuals, thus yielding 506,786 similarly predicted ORFs. Unquestionably, assembly problems could create chimeric sequences, which could potentially be misclassified. However, the study below is based on assembled and unassembled reads from two independent data sets, which corroborate one another. These ORFs were compared with 748,688 sequences corresponding to all the proteins from phages, plasmids, and integrons publicly available at the time of the analysis from the NCBI and ACID (annotation of cassette and integron

data) (43), and with all spacers from 52,267 sequences from human gut prokaryotes' clustered regularly interspaced short palindromic repeats (CRISPRs) obtained from reference 44, because spacers in these CRISPRs are expected to correspond to fragments of viruses infecting gut microbes.

All sequences described above were compared by an all-against-all BLASTP with –e set to 1e-20 and other parameters set to default for the nonunique 506,786 predicted ORFs and 748,688 mobile sequences, and the 506,786 predicted ORFs were compared to the 52,267 sequences from human gut prokaryotes' CRISPRs by a BLASTn (parameter –e set to 1e-5, and other parameters set to default) to assign a label to the gut predicted ORFs identical to a spacer. ORFs present in multiple copies were not removed from the data set before performing the analysis. Indeed, some genes might be abundant in the human gut microbiome, such as genes involved in metabolism of carbohydrates, which might be frequently transferred and/or duplicated (45), and this important information was therefore not lost. BLAST outputs were converted to a sequence similarity network using EGN (35). In this network, each protein sequence corresponded to one node, and two nodes were directly connected when their best hit displayed ≥20% identity for a BLAST E value of ≤1e-20. This threshold is sufficiently low to identify divergent homologs, even though it is true that sequences with greater divergence could still be homologs. However, below 20%, BLAST detection is closer to a gray zone and false positives cannot be excluded. These analyses, which took 4 days to be completed, were performed on a computer with two quad-core Intel Xeon E5430 CPUs running at 2.66 GHz.

This inclusive protocol produced 74,615 CCs, defining a first set of clusters of sequences. Each human gut predicted ORF was characterized by a label reflecting its origin: "virus" (for phages or sequences with 100% identity to a spacer), "plasmid," "integron" (altogether corresponding to "MGE"), and "gut predicted ORF." These labels were then used to classify sequence clusters based on their content. Clusters of sequences exclusively encompassing sequences from gut predicted ORFs were considered as a proxy of the "resident gut metagenome," and their gut predicted ORFs were referred to as "resident." We found 13,259 such resident clusters. Clusters of sequences that included sequences both from predicted ORFs and from MGEs were considered as a proxy of the "gut externalized metagenome." These latter clusters were further distinguished into two groups: those with only one type of MGE (only virus, or only plasmid, or only integron), for which gut predicted ORFs were referred to as "potentially externalized," and those with >1 type of MGE, for which gut predicted ORFs were referred to as "potentially highly externalized," because more than one type of vector could intervene in

the transfer of their genes. We found 7,468 potentially externalized clusters and 798 potentially highly externalized clusters.

Sequences with a Higher Degree of Externalization Encode Biased Functions

The sequence similarity network was then simplified by removing nodes corresponding to MGEs, further splitting resident, potentially externalized, and highly externalized clusters into clusters exclusively comprising gut predicted ORFs. We then focused on the 21,525 clusters of resident ORFs and of ORFs from the gut externalized metagenome that comprised ≥4 ORFs (i.e., the minimal number of sequences for significant dN/dS analyses). Each ORF in these 21,525 clusters was individually, taxonomically, and functionally annotated, using RPS-BLAST against the COG database (27, 46) and MG-RAST (47). A majority rule was used to assign a COG category to each cluster (the most frequent COG category associated with ORFs from the cluster determined a general functional assignation for that cluster). This categorization allows one to test whether clusters with resident, potentially externalized, and potentially highly externalized genes were enriched in different functional COG categories (hypergeometric test, P-value threshold of 0.01, adjusted for multiple testing using a Bonferroni correction). The taxonomic diversity was computed based on MG-RAST annotations at different ranks of the taxonomy, from phyla to genera, as the number of different taxa represented in the gut microbiota, using the Vegan package (48). The number of human hosts with sequences in each cluster was quantified for all clusters of sequences.

As a result, we found that resident, potentially externalized, and highly externalized clusters encompass genes encoding significantly distinct functions (hypergeometric test, $P < 0.01$) (Fig. 4). The functional profiling shows that a homology-based separation of genes into resident, potentially externalized, and potentially highly externalized clus-

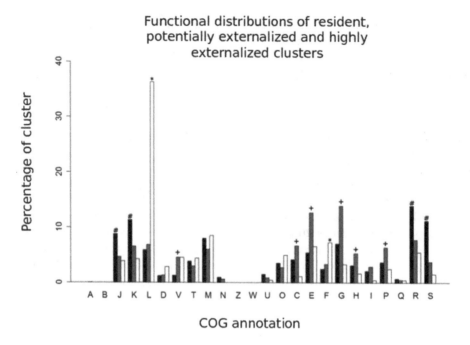

FIGURE 4 Functional distributions of resident, potentially externalized, and highly externalized clusters. Each cluster was assigned a COG annotation. (A) RNA processing and modification; (B) chromatin structure and dynamics; (C) energy production and conversion; (D) cell cycle control and mitosis; (E) amino acid metabolism and transport; (F) nucleotide metabolism and transport; (G) carbohydrate metabolism and transport; (H) coenzyme metabolism; (I) lipid metabolism; (J) translation; (K) transcription; (L) replication and repair; (M) cell wall/membrane/envelope biogenesis; (N) cell motility; (O) posttranslational modification, protein turnover, chaperone functions; (P) inorganic ion transport and metabolism; (Q) secondary structure; (R) general functional prediction only; (S) function unknown; (T) signal transduction; (U) intracellular trafficking and secretion; (V) Defense mechanisms; (W) Extracellular structures; (Z) cytoskeleton. Functional distributions were plotted for the three classes of clusters; resident clusters are in black, potentially externalized clusters in gray, and potentially highly externalized clusters in white. For each class of clusters, significantly enriched functional categories (P < 0.01; hypergeometric test, after adjusting for multiple testing) are identified by # (resident), + (potentially externalized), and * (potentially highly externalized).

ters is compatible with former knowledge of the functions of genes from the mobilome. Genes involved in translation, ribosomal structure and biogenesis, and transcription, as well as genes with poorly predicted functions, were significantly overrepresented in the resident clusters. Accordingly, such informational genes are generally considered less transferred (49–51), while the limited distribution of genes with poorly predicted functions fits well with their lack of functional annotation. Most externalized genes, especially when adaptive, are present in more than one genome, enhancing chances for externalized genes to have been annotated. Con-

sistently, the externalized clusters of the gut microbiome were enriched in genes involved in various metabolic pathways and microbial interactions. More precisely, potentially externalized clusters were significantly enriched in defense mechanisms; energy production and conversion; metabolism; and transport of amino acids, carbohydrates, coenzymes, and inorganic ions. Potentially highly externalized clusters were significantly enriched in genes encoding replication and repair, as well as nucleotide metabolism and transport. These differences are in line with previous knowledge on the gut mobilome. For example, HGT is thought to largely explain CAZyme (carbohydrate active enzyme) convergence across gut bacterial genomes (52), and in our data set, genes diagnosed as potentially externalized that encode enzymes involved in carbohydrate metabolism and transport are indeed overrepresented. Likewise, there is a documented selective pressure in the gut to enrich the microbial community in genes involved in DNA repair since ingested food, secondary bile acids, and nitroso compounds synthetized by gut microbes increase the amount of genotoxic substances in the intestine (20). Such genes are overrepresented in the most externalized clusters. For example, well-known "genetic goods" (53) include ABC-type multidrug transport systems found on contigs associated with TN*1549*-like conjugative transposons (20) and plasmid genes coding community functions, mitigating the toxic effects of bile acids, or promoting adherence to host epithelial cells (15).

MGEs can also be seen as providing a second type of community service for the potentially externalized and highly externalized clusters detected in our analyses. These clusters could contribute to the functional stability of the gut microbiota because the presence of their sequences on MGE genomes generates functional redundancy (3). The risk of losing these functions when a particular bacterial lineage gets eliminated from the competitive gut environment or fails to survive phage attacks (16) is reduced through the externalization of gene copies. This dynamic MGE-mediated genetic redundancy is a key feature of the "mobile elements + gut microbes + human individual" system, as will be shown below.

The Gut Externalized Metagenome Encompasses Genes Benefiting the Gut Microbial Community

Amongst the externalized clusters, genes that can be considered public genetic goods are recovered (53). Since they are externalized, they are likely to benefit a broader range of microbial hosts than strictly vertically inherited genes, and are also likely to favor survival of the gut community. Consistently, genes already reported as beneficial for gut microbes and overrepresented in microbiomes featured within the most abundant of our potentially externalized and highly externalized clusters. For example, the most abundant clusters within the defense mechanism category encoded an ABC-type multidrug transport system, ATPase and permease components (COG1132), and an ABC-type antimicrobial peptide transport system, permease component (COG0577), commonly enriched both in Japanese adult microbiomes (20) and in obese monozygotic twins (41), as well as a cation/multidrug efflux pump (COG0841), which is also enriched in these obese twins. Since host intestinal cells produce various cationic antimicrobial peptides, and many microorganisms also do so to compete with other microbes, the enrichment of antimicrobial peptide transporters and the multidrug efflux pump possibly plays a primary role in stable colonization of gut microbes in the adult intestine by conferring resistance to cationic antimicrobial peptides (20).

Sequences with Different Externalization Degrees Are under Similar Selective Pressure in the Gut

The ratio of nonsynonymous to synonymous mutations (i.e., substitutions in DNA leading to a change in amino acids) in clusters of gut microbial sequences can be computed. Since nonsynonymous mutations can be deleterious, and tend to be eliminated by purifying selection, a dN/dS ratio of <1 indicates that sequences are under this kind of selective pressure. However, dN/dS analyses are ideally performed at an even finer level of granularity than the clusters defined above, i.e., from clusters of sequences presenting even stronger similarities, so that all sequences can be aligned together over most of their length. Thus, we used the BLASTClust program (ftp://ftp.ncbi.nlm.nih.gov; minimum sequence similarity threshold, >70%; bidirectional coverage L, >90%, other parameters by default) to construct stringent clusters of very similar predicted ORFs, which were aligned with MUSCLE (54) (default parameters) when they comprised ≥4 ORFs. Phylogenetic trees were reconstructed from these protein alignments with PhyML (55) (-d aa -m WAG -f e v e). Corresponding nucleotides were aligned, based on these templates, with transAlign (56). Aligned nucleotides and phylogenetic trees were used as input in PAML (57) for estimating one *dN/dS* ratio for each stringent cluster by maximum likelihood. This basic model was fitted by specifying model = 0, NSsites = 0, in the codeml control file.

This protocol allowed us to compare the *dN/dS* distributions for the three classes of clusters. While resident, potentially externalized, and potentially highly externalized clusters showed distinct functional profiles, their molecular sequences were in stark contrast, under comparable selective pressures (Mann-Whitney-Wilcoxon test, *P* > 0.01) (Fig. 5). Most clusters in the gut microbiome were under purifying selection. Thus, just like resident sequences, potentially externalized and highly externalized sequences did not appear to be pseudogenes, nor to represent inactivated prophages that no longer contribute to the active gut externalized metagenome. Instead, sequences from potentially externalized and highly externalized clusters were likely exploited by their microbial hosts. This observation does not mean that, in general, externalized sequences cannot undergo pseudogenization, but that in our study the bioinformatic pipeline effectively discarded pseudogenes. That most such clusters were under purifying selection does not mean that sequences within a cluster would not show genetic divergence. When we estimated genetic variation for each cluster, by computing the mean percentage of identity between all its pairs of connected sequences in the similarity network, we observed that resident clusters comprised significantly more similar sequences than

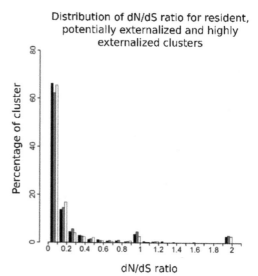

FIGURE 5 Distributions of *dN/dS* ratio for resident, potentially externalized, and highly externalized clusters. Resident, potentially externalized, and highly externalized clusters are colored in black, gray, and white, respectively. The three distributions are not significantly different (Mann-Whitney-Wilcoxon test, *P* < 0.01). *dN/dS* ratios of >2 were pooled to simplify the display.

potentially externalized and highly externalized clusters (Mann-Whitney-Wilcoxon test, *P* < 0.01) (Fig. 3). Thus, sequences from the gut externalized metagenome were in general more divergent than sequences from the resident microbiome but not less affected by purifying selection. This latter observation is consistent with the description of fast-evolving phages in gut microbial communities (58, 59): these phages and their genes are under selection and diverge faster in this environment.

Sequences with Higher Externalization Degree Have Broader Microbial and Human Host Ranges

The distribution of ORFs across inferred microbial host phyla and microbial host genera strongly suggests that partitioning sequences from human gut microbiomes into resident, potentially externalized, and highly externalized clusters effectively captured aspects of the differential mobility of these sequences. Each predicted ORF in a cluster was assigned to its best matching microbial phylum and genus, using RAST annotation server (http://rast.nmpdr.org/, default parameters). Thus, the taxonomic diversity within each cluster could be estimated as the number of distinct microbial host phyla or genera associated with sequences for this cluster. Remarkably, clusters with the highest externalization degree were also the ones with the significantly broadest taxonomic diversity. Clusters of sequences with similarity to more than one type of MGE were more ubiquitous in the gut community (Fig. 6). Some potentially highly externalized clusters were even found in ≥4 phyla, a host range compatible with findings

in reference 60, which, using the most significant BLAST alignment to determine the origin of phage-encoded bacterial genes, found that 97% of these mobile genes were attributed to the four dominant phyla known in the gut (60). These results (Fig. 7) are compatible with the literature. Recent work representing gene-sharing networks of the mobilome (61–63), e.g., what genomes of MGEs share what genes or gene fragments with what other MGE genomes, and even broader gene-sharing networks of both the mobilome and the cellular genomes (64), reported that some genetic material can eventually be shared between different types of MGEs (between viruses and plasmids, between viruses and virophages, etc.). Thus, some sequences from the microbiome are possibly carried around by a greater number

Distribution of the taxonomic diversity for resident, potentially externalized and highly externalized clusters

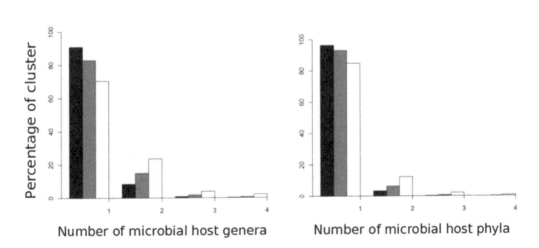

FIGURE 6 Distributions of the taxonomic diversity for resident, potentially externalized, and highly externalized clusters. (Left) Distribution of clusters across microbial host genera; (right) distribution of clusters across microbial host phyla. Clusters are color-coded as above. Potentially externalized clusters have a significantly broader host range than resident clusters, and potentially highly externalized clusters have a significantly broader host range than resident clusters and potentially externalized clusters (Mann-Whitney-Wilcoxon test, $P < 0.01$). Taxonomic diversities of >4 were pooled to simplify the display.

Distribution of resident, potentially
externalized and highly externalized clusters
across human hosts

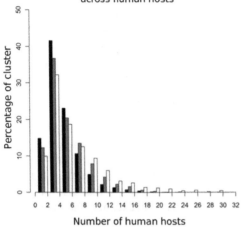

FIGURE 7 Distribution of resident, potentially externalized, and highly externalized clusters across human hosts. Clusters are color-coded as above. Potentially externalized clusters have a significantly broader host range than resident clusters, and potentially highly externalized clusters have a significantly broader host range than resident clusters and potentially externalized clusters (Mann-Whitney-Wilcoxon test, $P < 0.01$).

of types of MGEs (see, for example, reference 15) and are more successful in a broader diversity of genomic contexts than others.

Remarkably, just like for microbial hosts, sequences inferred to be more externalized in the gut community were also the ones with the broader human host range clusters (Mann-Whitney-Wilcoxon test, $P < 0.01$) (Fig. 8). Resident clusters were typically found in a smaller number of individuals than potentially externalized clusters, while potentially highly externalized clusters were found in the largest number of humans (0.8% of these potentially highly externalized clusters were even present in ≥28 out of 31 individuals, and 75% of these clusters from the gut externalized metagenome were shared between ≥4 individuals). Thus, the shared microbiome encoded on the gut externalized metagenome was larger than the shared resident microbiome at the level of human hosts for this data set.

The Gut Externalized Metagenome Is Partly Common to Humans

The sparser distribution of resident genes in comparison to externalized genes across humans may seem counterintuitive. However, it is likely explained by two possibilities. First, the gut microbiome is obviously undersampled, which means that bona fide core genes, present in all prokaryotic lineages and in all human individuals, were missed since they were not sequenced. However, importantly, this undersampling could have equally affected resident and externalized genes. The two broader host distributions for externalized genes than for resident genes is therefore consistent with the notion that gene externalization, producing numerous copies of the same genes in the gut microbial community, introduces genetic redundancy. If so, externalized genes are likely to be more prone to being sequenced than resident genes, and this may explain why they appear to be more broadly distributed. Importantly, all sorts of genes can be externalized: for example, while housekeeping genes are likely to be part of a core microbiome because prokaryotes host these genes in their genomes, it does not mean that housekeeping genes are not being externalized and are exclusively resident. Typically, some *recA* or *gyrB* sequences were classified as highly externalized and present in up to 19 and 22 human hosts, respectively. The second possibility is that externalized genes could be expected to be prominent members of the core microbiome, since not only prokaryotes but also MGEs, i.e., multiple types of genomes, host them and multiply these genes.

This second result is better interpreted in the light of studies focusing on MGEs, which reported contrasting observations about the sharing of the gut mobilome between holobionts. On the one hand, MGE compositions were shown to display high interindividual variation (3). Remarkable interpersonal variations in gut viromes and their encoded functions were described (58), demonstrating that

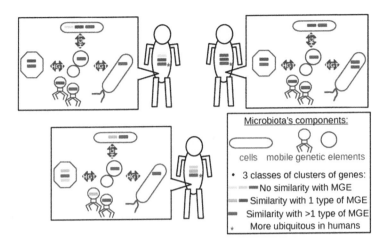

FIGURE 8 A schematic representation of gene sharings within and between three "mobile elements + gut microbes + human individual" holobionts. Combinations of MGEs and of their direct hosts, e.g., the gut microbial cells, as well as of the human body, itself hosting gut microbes, form an integrated, multilevel, multipartite, dynamic biological system, also referred to as a holobiont. For each individual human, the black square represents a close-up of its gut microbiota (with gut microbial cells in brown and MGEs in purple) and of its gut microbiome (the genes contained within these microbial cells and MGEs). Genes are represented by colored rectangles; genes with the same color belong to the same gene family. The process of HGT, mediated by MGEs, is responsible for mobilizing genes between microbial cells. We demonstrated that gene families carried by a larger diversity of MGEs are more widely shared not only between gut microbes but also between individual human hosts, as shown for the red gene family. Thus, HGT is a key process for introducing genetic similarity at multiple consecutive host levels within and between holobionts.

gut viromes were unique to individuals (65) even when individuals have similar bacterial community structures (17, 41). But on the other hand, prophages were also reported to be universal in the human gut, their genes amounting to 5% of the minimal gut metagenome (66), and some convergence of viral populations was described for individuals following the same diet (59). Moreover, the persistence over >2.5 years of a small portion of the global virome within individual guts was also established (58), suggesting the possible existence of at least a very partial shared gut mobilome, should viruses with similar gene content be retained across multiple holobionts. In agreement with this conclusion, some gut plasmids and their ORFs were found in human gut microbiomes over large geographic distances (40). Likewise, Kurokawa et al. indicated that Tn*1549*-like conjugative transposons were enriched in most of

the gut microbiomes present in their study, as well as in two fecal samples from American individuals (20), establishing a connection for this gene family between genetic mobility and its distribution in humans.

Network analyses support and amplify the notion that the gut mobilome can be largely spread across humans. Could such externalized clusters provide benefit beyond the gut microbial community to its human host (4, 15, 33)? HGT from marine bacteria colonizing dietary seaweeds into the genomes of gut bacteria was proposed to have introduced genes required for the use of seaweed glycans, benefiting humans with a typical Japanese diet (45). Likewise, for antibiotic-treated mice, direct evidence that phages contribute functional advantages to their gut microbial hosts (detected by an enrichment in genes related to the synthesis of cell wall constituents, or replication- and repair-related pathways) and possibly to their animal host (diagnosed by an enrichment in genes involved in cofactor and vitamin synthesis; starch, cellulose, lactose, and fructan metabolism; and CAZymes) was also reported (60). Such studies must be considered with caution because samples can be biased, and one cannot exclude the possibility of reagent contamination for the library prep and sequencing kits. While the indications of network analyses do not allow us to make such strong assumptions about the benefits of some externalized genes for the human host, they clearly suggest that the gut externalized metagenome has a broad host distribution across humans. The spread of gut externalized metagenome genes, within and across "mobile elements + gut microbes + human individual" systems, could help to explain why humans host a functional core microbiome (25, 41, 66). It stresses the importance of considering multiple transmission channels to explain animal phenotypes.

INTRODUCING BIPARTITE GRAPHS

Beyond the study of shared gene families with sequence similarity networks (by considering in which genome a given sequence is present), another graph structure, namely bipartite graphs, can also be used to study gene and microbe transmission in holobionts. A bipartite graph is a graph with two types of nodes (type I and II nodes) such that an edge only connects nodes of one type with nodes of the other type. For example, in host-gene family bipartite graphs, type I nodes are host organisms, and type II, gene families. These graphs can be used, for instance, to determine gene families that are shared by individuals (26) and possibly related to characteristics from the host (e.g., male/female or dietary groups) and to find gene families exclusive to each group. One advantage of this type of graph is that, while they are equivalent to a presence-absence heat map on the same data, it is straightforward to

apply some concepts and algorithms of graph theory. It is easy to rapidly identify which groups of genes are shared by which groups of genomes (67) (Fig. 2, ii).

In theory, metagenomic data, such as the microbiomes and microbiotas of lizards with different diets, could be investigated using bipartite graphs, and we will briefly indicate how. This example was chosen because such a data set exists and will soon be made available. In 1969, ecologists introduced 10 insectivorous lizards from the Adriatic island of Pod Kopiste (Croatia) to the neighboring island of Pod Mrcaru. It was later realized that the lizards from the species *Podarcis sicula* on Pod Mrcaru had become omnivorous (80% herbivorous) and even changed in morphology. However, changes in their gut microbiomes and microbiotas and the transmission of microbial genes and of microbes between lizards were not investigated. Bipartite graph analyses would allow us to consider the distributions of pairs of entities as diverse as genes, gene families, microbial taxa, and individual lizards, simply by introducing these objects as either type I or type II nodes, and thus to gain knowledge about the effect of transmission in such holobionts.

Detecting the Transmission of Genes between Hosts

One of the striking features of microbiomes is that their gene content is functionally biased (20). The rules of transmission between hosts' microbiomes could be deciphered by considering host-gene family graphs, where type I nodes are hosts (e.g., lizards) and type II nodes are gene families. As explained above, a gene family can be defined as a CC in a sequence similarity network (at ≥80% mutual cover, ≥30% identity, and E value of ≤1e-5). These thresholds were empirically tested in multiple publications (31, 35, 68, 69). They recovered clusters of homologous sequences that are consistent in terms of COG annotation (27) and Pfam annotations, and therefore their use (in particular that of the ≥80% cover) provides a good proxy to define gene families and to assign a family to each gene. Therefore, a host-gene family bipartite graph can be constructed as follows. An edge is drawn between a type I and a type II node if a member of the gene family represented by the type II node is present in the microbiome of the lizard represented by the type I node. Type I nodes may be further colored by characteristics of the hosts (diet, gender, etc.). Gene families that are exclusively present in lizards displaying one characteristic (insectivorous or omnivorous), or shared by the two groups of lizards, or even the core genome, can then be detected (all the gene families shared by all lizards in the network) (Fig. 2, ii). Importantly, because such an analysis would exploit metagenomic data, the quality of network analysis will depend on the quality of the predicted ORFs. Data sets with higher depth of coverage will in particular produce fewer false negatives in the predicted ORFs, and therefore will introduce fewer artificial nodes and relationships in the networks.

Tracking the Transmission of Microbes between Hosts

Transmission can also take place at the level of the microbes themselves: in this case, the rules of transmission can be investigated by constructing a bipartite graph describing what microbes (type II nodes) are present in what microbiomes (type I nodes).

In this case, type I nodes are still hosts (i.e., lizards), but type II nodes are now the microbial assignation of the genes—either to a given operational taxonomic unit (70) or to a given prokaryotic taxon, i.e., a species, a genus, or a phylum, or to an MGE such as a virus or a plasmid (Fig. 2, iii). An edge links a type II node to a type I node if the microbial assignation has been found in the microbiota of the lizard corresponding to the type I node. These assignations can be achieved by various strategies, such as by analyzing reads (or predicted ORFs) with BLAST against a

reference database containing prokaryotes, viruses, and plasmids (64) or by delineating operational taxonomic units using QIIME (70).

The structure of the bipartite graph can then be exploited by decomposing the network into CCs, i.e., all sets of nodes for which there is always an interconnecting path. CCs in bipartite graphs are informative partitions of the data. They can be studied at different stringency levels, using different thresholds of percentage of identity (with the same molecular clock interpretation as for sequence similarity networks). Bipartite graphs (and CCs themselves) can be further decomposed into twins, i.e., groups of nodes having exactly the same set of neighbors in the graph. Applying these two notions to genome-gene family bipartite graphs simultaneously defines groups of gene families and groups of genomes (referred to as the "support" of the CC or the twin). Computing CCs splits the set of genomes into groups that have no genomic content in common, and defines the corresponding disjointed pools of gene families. By definition, gene families associated with disjoint groups of genomes have not been transmitted between these genomes; or, if these genes have moved across the distinct sets of genomes, they have since been lost. In other words, the definition of CC in the genome-gene family network hints at the existence of barriers of genetic transmission between genomes. Identifying twins splits the set of gene families into groups that are present in exactly the same genomes and thus, on the contrary, characterizes groups of genomes that have an exclusive genomic content in common.

Both operations have been implemented specifically for genomic data (13, 26). A particularly interesting distinction when diverse annotations are additionally available (taxonomic, ecological, dietary, etc.) can be done between CCs and twins having a *homogeneous* or *heterogeneous* support. In the theoretical application to the lizard data set, homogeneous twins might be further subdivided between those whose support contains all lizards of one type and those that contain only a subset of them. Accordingly, the partition in twins could show what microbial phyla are shared by all lizards or, on the contrary, which microbial phyla are specific to lizards with a given diet. This may hint at preferential routes of microbe and gene transmissions between hosts with similar ecologies.

Detecting Gene Transmission in Microbial Communities

One further step in unraveling the processes governing these transmission mechanisms would be the study of the transmissions within microbial communities themselves, that is, of genes between microbes, and how these transmissions are made. In this setting, we are interested in the patterns of inheritance, either vertical or horizontal. The latter corresponds not only to the well-characterized notion of lateral gene transfer (30) but also to the process of gene externalization described above.

To this aim, a sound approach would be to construct a microbiota-gene family bipartite graph, which describes the microbe (in the same broad sense of microbial assignation at a given level as before) that is associated with a particular sequence (bipartite graph 2.iv). As before, the definition of gene families requires us to have built a sequence similarity network (bipartite graph 2.i). Indeed, type I nodes are here defined as microbial classes and type II nodes as gene families, while an edge connects a gene family to a microbial class whenever at least one gene in this family is present in at least one microbe belonging to this microbial class.

Patterns of inheritance may be subsumed under broad classes that characterize the availability of a given gene to be transmitted. Consistently with the study of the human microbiome, three kinds of mobility class can be identified. (i) A gene may be externalized

if the gene family is shared by at least one bacterium and one kind of MGE. (ii) A gene may be highly externalized when it is shared by at least one bacterium and more than one kind of MGE. (iii) A gene may also be resident if the gene family it belongs to is not shared at all by MGEs. With this representation, it is easy to compute how many phyla, genera, or species of bacteria/archaea share a given gene family (Fig. 2, iv).

Moreover, the previous mobility information can be related with functional annotation, since each gene family can be associated with a COG category, derived from ORFs predicted on contigs, using the RPS-BLAST tool (71–73). Thus, the bipartite graph allows us also to find what functions and COG categories are represented in which microbial taxonomic levels (in the specific form under which they are present in the lizards' microbiomes), and in particular their mobility pattern. COG categories (or functions) that are highly externalized, externalized, or resident can therefore be detected, and correlations between gene externalization and gene functions can be calculated. This is particularly important to get a more accurate understanding of the possible biases in the transmissions of genes with different functions in the microbiome.

Extension to Multipartite Graphs

After having constructed and analyzed bipartite graphs, it may be worthwhile to extend even further the methodology to the consideration of multipartite graphs that connect more than two levels of information (Fig. 9). Such a structure may help to unravel more-intricate mechanisms of transmission. In the same illustrative example, a tripartite graph can be built involving the three levels of hosts (lizards), microbiota, and gene families. In principle, this structure allows us to detect patterns that are not accessible to the previously presented bipartite analysis: for instance, some gene families are found to be

Tripartite graphs allow to distinguish gene and microbial transmissions.

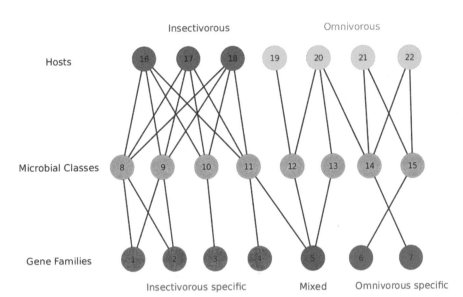

FIGURE 9 Tripartite graphs allow us to distinguish gene and microbial transmissions. In this tripartite graph, type I nodes are the hosts (lizards) and are colored depending on their diet. Middle nodes are microbial classes, and type II nodes are gene families. Type II nodes colored in red are gene families shared by insectivorous lizards only. Type II nodes colored in blue are gene families shared by omnivorous lizards only, and then those colored in purple are shared by insectivorous and omnivorous lizards. The tripartite graph allows division of gene families specific to a diet in two categories: gene families that are shared by microbial classes specific from a diet (group 1: gene families 1 and 2, encircled in red) and gene families that are shared by microbial classes nonspecific from a diet (group 2: gene families 3 and 4, encircled in red). In the first group, gene families are not necessarily involved in the diet of the lizards; they are in insectivorous lizards because all the microbial classes that contain them are specific from insectivorous lizards. In the second group, gene families are more likely involved in the diet because they are present in microbial classes that are not exclusive to insectivory. These two groups correspond to two different ways of transmission: the first group is a microbial transmission, whereas the second group is a gene transmission.

exclusively shared by insectivorous lizards (gene families 1, 2, 3, and 4 in Fig. 9), but some of them are also shared by the same microbes (for example, microbial classes 8 and 9 share gene families 1 and 2), while others are present in different microbes (for example, gene families 3 and 4). In the implied lizard-gene family bipartite graph in Fig. 9, the group of gene families, 1, 2, 3, 4, will be considered as a whole (because these families are equally present in hosts 16, 17, and 18), while in the microbiota-gene family, gene families will be split into three groups: the first group contains gene families 1 and 2

(shared by microbial classes 8 and 9); the second group contains gene family 3; and the third, gene family 4. Only by considering the three levels (Fig. 9) is it possible to find differentially shared gene families. A possible conclusion might be that the first group of genes is shared only because the microbiotas have been transmitted, while the second group of genes (genes present in different microbes yet exclusive to lizards with a specific diet) may indicate that genes coding these functions are present in similarly constrained environments (the insectivorous lizards' gut), irrespective of what microbes carry these genes. Then the transmission of these genes is decoupled from that of the microbes.

CONCLUSION

Holobionts are home to numerous biological transmissions. In this paper, we highlighted the ways of transmission in microbial communities, in particular, the process by which MGEs contribute to the dissemination of genes in an environment, which we have called gene externalization. We propose that gene families present in a higher diversity of MGEs have a broader bacterial and animal host range, and that gene externalization plays a key role in propagating similar material across hosts at two distinct levels of biological organization within this multilevel dynamic system. At the animal level, this gene externalization may therefore contribute to explain the sharing of a core functional microbiome. Under this hypothesis, this core is largely made of externalized genes necessary for microbes to survive in the gut. This claim encourages searching for some structure in the "microbiome + animal" holobiont from a processual perspective (e.g., by characterizing the externalization degree for each shared or not shared gene family), and to reason within the conceptual framework of a "mobile elements + gut microbes + human individual" system.

Accordingly, focusing on the externalized gut metagenome that is shared across humans could encourage future studies taking into account the implication of gut MGEs for human health (4, 18). If gene externalization proves to be a mechanism involved in the constitution of a core microbiome across microbes and humans, for example, variations in introgressive processes and gene mobility are likely to play a role in deviations from the functional core microbiome. Such deviations have already been associated with different physiological states such as leanness or obesity (41), and differences in the abundance of bacteriophages and in pTRACA22, a plasmid

specific to the human gut microbiome, have also already been reported between healthy individuals and those suffering from Crohn's disease and inflammatory bowel disease (3, 4, 74). Highly externalized genes, considering their broad host range within both microbes and humans, especially when involved in antibiotic drug resistance, might prove deleterious to humans (3, 18). These elements of the gut externalized metagenome deserve greater attention in models evaluating antibiotic use (20, 40), because the number of treatment options for many clinical infections makes it critical to understand how the gut externalized metagenome spreads (5).

Moreover, future studies could evaluate whether the number of MGEs carrying externalized genes, and not only the number of types of MGEs on which genes are externalized, contributes to the constitution of the core microbiome. To this end, we have outlined the novel use of bipartite graph structures for the study of genetic transmission in microbial communities. This approach gives a global and synthetic view of the transmissions: what are the externalized gene families and functions, what are the gene families exclusively associated with a particular lifestyle, and what are the microbes exclusively present in a set of microbiomes. Future studies will test the relevance of the network framework in transmission studies.

ACKNOWLEDGMENTS

E.C. and E.B. were funded by the European Research Council (FP7/2007-2013 Grant Agreement 615274) and C.V. by the Labex BCDIV. We thank Paul Dean for kindly proofreading this chapter.

CITATION

Vigliotti C, Bicep C, Bapteste E, Lopez P, Corel E. 2017. Tracking the rules of transmission and introgression with networks. Microbiol Spectrum 6(2):MTBP-0008-2016.

REFERENCES

1. **Bosch TC, McFall-Ngai MJ.** 2011. Metaorganisms as the new frontier. *Zool (Jena)* **114:**185–190.
2. **Bosch TC.** 2012. Understanding complex host-microbe interactions in *Hydra*. *Gut Microbes* **3:**345–351.
3. **Jones BV.** 2010. The human gut mobile metagenome: a metazoan perspective. *Gut Microbes* **1:**415–431.
4. **Lepage P, Leclerc MC, Joossens M, Mondot S, Blottière HM, Raes J, Ehrlich D, Doré J.** 2013. A metagenomic insight into our gut's microbiome. *Gut* **62:**146–158.
5. **Broaders E, Gahan CG, Marchesi JR.** 2013. Mobile genetic elements of the human gastro-intestinal tract: potential for spread of antibiotic resistance genes. *Gut Microbes* **4:**271–280.
6. **Gill SR, Pop M, Deboy RT, Eckburg PB, Turnbaugh PJ, Samuel BS, Gordon JI, Relman DA, Fraser-Liggett CM, Nelson KE.** 2006. Metagenomic analysis of the human distal gut microbiome. *Science* **312:**1355–1359.
7. **Le Chatelier E, Nielsen T, Qin J, Prifti E, Hildebrand F, Falony G, Almeida M, Arumugam M, Batto JM, Kennedy S, Leonard P, Li J, Burgdorf K, Grarup N, Jørgensen T, Brandslund I, Nielsen HB, Juncker AS, Bertalan M, Levenez F, Pons N, Rasmussen S, Sunagawa S, Tap J, Tims S, Zoetendal EG, Brunak S, Clément K, Doré J, Kleerebezem M, Kristiansen K, Renault P, Sicheritz-Ponten T, de Vos WM, Zucker JD, Raes J, Hansen T, MetaHIT consortium, Bork P, Wang J, Ehrlich SD, Pedersen O.** 2013. Richness of human gut microbiome correlates with metabolic markers. *Nature* **500:**541–546.
8. **Relman DA.** 2012. Microbiology: learning about who we are. *Nature* **486:**194–195.
9. **Guerrero R, Margulis L, Berlanga M.** 2013. Symbiogenesis: the holobiont as a unit of evolution. *Int Microbiol* **16:**133–143.
10. **Lloyd EA.** 2016. Holobionts as units of selection: holobionts as interactors, reproducers, and manifestors of adaptation. **1:**1–38.
11. **Moran NA, Sloan DB.** 2015. The hologenome concept: helpful or hollow? *PLoS Biol* **13:**e1002311.
12. **Bordenstein SR, Theis KR.** 2015. Host biology in light of the microbiome: ten principles of holobionts and hologenomes. *PLoS Biol* **13:**e1002226.
13. **Phillips ML.** 2009. Gut reaction: environmental effects on the human microbiota. *Environ Health Perspect* **117:**A198–A205.
14. **Spor A, Koren O, Ley R.** 2011. Unravelling the effects of the environment and host genotype on the gut microbiome. *Nat Rev Microbiol* **9:**279–290.

15. **Ogilvie LA, Firouzmand S, Jones BV.** 2012. Evolutionary, ecological and biotechnological perpectives on plasmids resident in the human gut mobile metagenome. *Bioeng Bugs* **3:**13–31.
16. **Xu J, Mahowald MA, Ley RE, Lozupone CA, Hamady M, Martens EC, Henrissat B, Coutinho PM, Minx P, Latreille P, Cordum H, Van Brunt A, Kim K, Fulton RS, Fulton LA, Clifton SW, Wilson RK, Knight RD, Gordon JI.** 2007. Evolution of symbiotic bacteria in the distal human intestine. *PLoS Biol* **5:**e156.
17. **Duerkop BA, Hooper LV.** 2013. Resident viruses and their interactions with the immune system. *Nat Immunol* **14:**654–659.
18. **Ogilvie LA, Bowler LD, Caplin J, Dedi C, Diston D, Cheek E, Taylor H, Ebdon JE, Jones BV.** 2013. Genome signature-based dissection of human gut metagenomes to extract subliminal viral sequences. *Nat Commun* **4:**2420.
19. **Tasse L, Bercovici J, Pizzut-Serin S, Robe P, Tap J, Klopp C, Cantarel BL, Coutinho PM, Henrissat B, Leclerc M, Doré J, Monsan P, Remaud-Simeon M, Potocki-Veronese G.** 2010. Functional metagenomics to mine the human gut microbiome for dietary fiber catabolic enzymes. *Genome Res* **20:**1605–1612.
20. **Kurokawa K, Itoh T, Kuwahara T, Oshima K, Toh H, Toyoda A, Takami H, Morita H, Sharma VK, Srivastava TP, Taylor TD, Noguchi H, Mori H, Ogura Y, Ehrlich DS, Itoh K, Takagi T, Sakaki Y, Hayashi T, Hattori M.** 2007. Comparative metagenomics revealed commonly enriched gene sets in human gut microbiomes. *DNA Res* **14:**169–181.
21. **Bordenstein SR, O'Hara FP, Werren JH.** 2001. *Wolbachia*-induced incompatibility precedes other hybrid incompatibilities in *Nasonia*. *Nature* **409:**707–710.
22. **Theis KR, Venkataraman A, Dycus JA, Koonter KD, Schmitt-Matzen EN, Wagner AP, Holekamp KE, Schmidt TM.** 2013. Symbiotic bacteria appear to mediate hyena social odors. *Proc Natl Acad Sci U S A* **110:**19832–19837.
23. **Khachatryan ZA, Ktsoyan ZA, Manukyan GP, Kelly D, Ghazaryan KA, Aminov RI.** 2008. Predominant role of host genetics in controlling the composition of gut microbiota. *PLoS One* **3:**e3064.
24. **Selosse MA, Bessis A, Pozo MJ.** 2014. Microbial priming of plant and animal immunity: symbionts as developmental signals. *Trends Microbiol* **22:**607–613.
25. **Lozupone CA, Stombaugh JI, Gordon JI, Jansson JK, Knight R.** 2012. Diversity, stability and resilience of the human gut microbiota. *Nature* **489:**220–230.
26. **Corel E, Lopez P, Méheust R, Bapteste E.** 2016. Network-thinking: graphs to analyze microbial

complexity and evolution. *Trends Microbiol* **24:**224–237.

27. **Tatusov RL, Koonin EV, Lipman DJ.** 1997. A genomic perspective on protein families. *Science* **278:**631–637.

28. **Dagan T, Artzy-Randrup Y, Martin W.** 2008. Modular networks and cumulative impact of lateral transfer in prokaryote genome evolution. *Proc Natl Acad Sci U S A* **105:**10039–10044.

29. **Kloesges T, Popa O, Martin W, Dagan T.** 2011. Networks of gene sharing among 329 proteobacterial genomes reveal differences in lateral gene transfer frequency at different phylogenetic depths. *Mol Biol Evol* **28:**1057–1074.

30. **Skippington E, Ragan MA.** 2011. Lateral genetic transfer and the construction of genetic exchange communities. *FEMS Microbiol Rev* **35:**707–735.

31. **Cheng S, Karkar S, Bapteste E, Yee N, Falkowski P, Bhattacharya D.** 2014. Sequence similarity network reveals the imprints of major diversification events in the evolution of microbial life. *Front Ecol Evol* **2:**72.

32. **Bapteste E, Lopez P, Bouchard F, Baquero F, McInerney JO, Burian RM.** 2012. Evolutionary analyses of non-genealogical bonds produced by introgressive descent. *Proc Natl Acad Sci U S A* **109:**18266–18272.

33. **Zhang S-B, Zhou S-Y, He J-G, Lai J-H.** 2011. Phylogeny inference based on spectral graph clustering. *J Comput Biol* **18:**627–637.

34. **Forster D, Bittner L, Karkar S, Dunthorn M, Romac S, Audic S, Lopez P, Stoeck T, Bapteste E.** 2015. Testing ecological theories with sequence similarity networks: marine ciliates exhibit similar geographic dispersal patterns as multicellular organisms. *BMC Biol* **13:**16.

35. **Halary S, McInerney JO, Lopez P, Bapteste E.** 2013. EGN: a wizard for construction of gene and genome similarity networks. *BMC Evol Biol* **13:**146.

36. **Bittner L, Halary S, Payri C, Cruaud C, de Reviers B, Lopez P, Bapteste E.** 2010. Some considerations for analyzing biodiversity using integrative metagenomics and gene networks. *Biol Direct* **5:**47.

37. **Duchêne S, Holt KE, Weill FX, Le Hello S, Hawkey J, Edwards DJ, Fourment M, Holmes EC.** 2016. Genome-scale rates of evolutionary change in bacteria. *Microb Genom* **2:**e000094.

38. **Breitbart M, Haynes M, Kelley S, Angly F, Edwards RA, Felts B, Mahaffy JM, Mueller J, Nulton J, Rayhawk S, Rodriguez-Brito B, Salamon P, Rohwer F.** 2008. Viral diversity and dynamics in an infant gut. *Res Microbiol* **159:**367–373.

39. **Cadwell K.** 2015. Expanding the role of the virome: commensalism in the gut. *J Virol* **89:**1951–1953.

40. **Jones BV, Sun F, Marchesi JR.** 2010. Comparative metagenomic analysis of plasmid encoded functions in the human gut microbiome. *BMC Genomics* **11:**46.

41. **Turnbaugh PJ, Hamady M, Yatsunenko T, Cantarel BL, Duncan A, Ley RE, Sogin ML, Jones WJ, Roe BA, Affourtit JP, Egholm M, Henrissat B, Heath AC, Knight R, Gordon JI.** 2009. A core gut microbiome in obese and lean twins. *Nature* **457:**480–484.

42. **Noguchi H, Taniguchi T, Itoh T.** 2008. MetaGeneAnnotator: detecting species-specific patterns of ribosomal binding site for precise gene prediction in anonymous prokaryotic and phage genomes. *DNA Res* **15:**387–396.

43. **Joss MJ, Koenig JE, Labbate M, Polz MF, Gillings MR, Stokes HW, Doolittle WF, Boucher Y.** 2009. ACID: annotation of cassette and integron data. *BMC Bioinformatics* **10:**118.

44. **Stern A, Mick E, Tirosh I, Sagy O, Sorek R.** 2012. CRISPR targeting reveals a reservoir of common phages associated with the human gut microbiome. *Genome Res* **22:**1985–1994.

45. **Hehemann JH, Correc G, Barbeyron T, Helbert W, Czjzek M, Michel G.** 2010. Transfer of carbohydrate-active enzymes from marine bacteria to Japanese gut microbiota. *Nature* **464:**908–912.

46. **Galperin MY, Makarova KS, Wolf YI, Koonin EV.** 2015. Expanded microbial genome coverage and improved protein family annotation in the COG database. *Nucleic Acids Res* **43**(D1)**:**D261–D269.

47. **Meyer F, Paarmann D, D'Souza M, Olson R, Glass EM, Kubal M, Paczian T, Rodriguez A, Stevens R, Wilke A, Wilkening J, Edwards RA.** 2008. The metagenomics RAST server—a public resource for the automatic phylogenetic and functional analysis of metagenomes. *BMC Bioinformatics* **9:**386.

48. **Dixon P.** 2003. VEGAN, a package of R functions for community ecology. *J Veg Sci* **14:**927–930.

49. **Cohen O, Gophna U, Pupko T.** 2011. The complexity hypothesis revisited: connectivity rather than function constitutes a barrier to horizontal gene transfer. *Mol Biol Evol* **28:**1481–1489.

50. **Leigh JW, Schliep K, Lopez P, Bapteste E.** 2011. Let them fall where they may: congruence analysis in massive phylogenetically messy data sets. *Mol Biol Evol* **28:**2773–2785.

51. **Jain R, Rivera MC, Lake JA.** 1999. Horizontal gene transfer among genomes: the complexity hypothesis. *Proc Natl Acad Sci U S A* **96:**3801–3806.

52. **Lozupone CA, Hamady M, Cantarel BL, Coutinho PM, Henrissat B, Gordon JI, Knight R.** 2008. The convergence of carbohydrate active

gene repertoires in human gut microbes. *Proc Natl Acad Sci U S A* **105**:15076–15081.

53. **McInerney JO, Pisani D, Bapteste E, O'Connell MJ.** 2011. The public goods hypothesis for the evolution of life on Earth. *Biol Direct* **6**:41.

54. **Edgar RC.** 2004. MUSCLE: multiple sequence alignment with high accuracy and high throughput. *Nucleic Acids Res* **32**:1792–1797.

55. **Guindon S, Delsuc F, Dufayard JF, Gascuel O.** 2009. Estimating maximum likelihood phylogenies with PhyML. *Methods Mol Biol* **537**:113–137.

56. **Bininda-Emonds ORP.** 2005. transAlign: using amino acids to facilitate the multiple alignment of protein-coding DNA sequences. *BMC Bioinformatics* **6**:156.

57. **Yang Z.** 2007. PAML 4: phylogenetic analysis by maximum likelihood. *Mol Biol Evol* **24**:1586–1591.

58. **Minot S, Bryson A, Chehoud C, Wu GD, Lewis JD, Bushman FD.** 2013. Rapid evolution of the human gut virome. *Proc Natl Acad Sci U S A* **110**:12450–12455.

59. **Minot S, Sinha R, Chen J, Li H, Keilbaugh SA, Wu GD, Lewis JD, Bushman FD.** 2011. The human gut virome: inter-individual variation and dynamic response to diet. *Genome Res* **21**:1616–1625.

60. **Modi SR, Lee HH, Spina CS, Collins JJ.** 2013. Antibiotic treatment expands the resistance reservoir and ecological network of the phage metagenome. *Nature* **499**:219–222.

61. **Desnues C, La Scola B, Yutin N, Fournous G, Robert C, Azza S, Jardot P, Monteil S, Campocasso A, Koonin EV, Raoult D.** 2012. Provirophages and transpovirons as the diverse mobilome of giant viruses. *Proc Natl Acad Sci U S A* **109**:18078–18083.

62. **Yutin N, Raoult D, Koonin EV.** 2013. Virophages, polintons, and transpovirons: a complex evolutionary network of diverse selfish genetic elements with different reproduction strategies. *Virol J* **10**:158.

63. **Iranzo J, Krupovic M, Koonin EV.** 2016. The double-stranded DNA virosphere as a modular hierarchical network of gene sharing. *mBio* **7**:e00978-e16.

64. **Halary S, Leigh JW, Cheaib B, Lopez P, Bapteste E.** 2010. Network analyses structure genetic diversity in independent genetic worlds. *Proc Natl Acad Sci U S A* **107**:127–132.

65. **Reyes A, Haynes M, Hanson N, Angly FE, Heath AC, Rohwer F, Gordon JI.** 2010. Viruses in the faecal microbiota of monozygotic twins and their mothers. *Nature* **466**:334–338.

66. **Qin J, Li R, Raes J, Arumugam M, Burgdorf KS, Manichanh C, Nielsen T, Pons N, Levenez F, Yamada T, Mende DR, Li J, Xu J, Li S, Li D, Cao J, Wang B, Liang H, Zheng H, Xie Y, Tap J, Lepage P, Bertalan M, Batto JM, Hansen T, Le Paslier D, Linneberg A, Nielsen HB, Pelletier E, Renault P, Sicheritz-Ponten T, Turner K, Zhu H, Yu C, Li S, Jian M, Zhou Y, Li Y, Zhang X, Li S, Qin N, Yang H, Wang J, Brunak S, Doré J, Guarner F, Kristiansen K, Pedersen O, Parkhill J, Weissenbach J, MetaHIT Consortium, Bork P, Ehrlich SD, Wang J.** 2010. A human gut microbial gene catalogue established by metagenomic sequencing. *Nature* **464**:59–65.

67. **Rivera CG, Vakil R, Bader JS.** 2010. NeMo: Network Module identification in Cytoscape. *BMC Bioinformatics* **11**(Suppl 1):S61.

68. **Haggerty LS, Jachiet PA, Hanage WP, Fitzpatrick DA, Lopez P, O'Connell MJ, Pisani D, Wilkinson M, Bapteste E, McInerney JO.** 2014. A pluralistic account of homology: adapting the models to the data. *Mol Biol Evol* **31**:501–516.

69. **Méheust R, Zelzion E, Bhattacharya D, Lopez P, Bapteste E.** 2016. Protein networks identify novel symbiogenetic genes resulting from plastid endosymbiosis. *Proc Natl Acad Sci U S A* **113**:3579–3584.

70. **Caporaso JG, Kuczynski J, Stombaugh J, Bittinger K, Bushman FD, Costello EK, Fierer N, Peña AG, Goodrich JK, Gordon JI, Huttley GA, Kelley ST, Knights D, Koenig JE, Ley RE, Lozupone CA, McDonald D, Muegge BD, Pirrung M, Reeder J, Sevinsky JR, Turnbaugh PJ, Walters WA, Widmann J, Yatsunenko T, Zaneveld J, Knight R.** 2010. QIIME allows analysis of high-throughput community sequencing data. *Nat Methods* **7**:335–336.

71. **Cock PJA, Chilton JM, Grüning B, Johnson JE, Soranzo N.** 2015. NCBI BLAST+ integrated into Galaxy. *Gigascience* **4**:39.

72. **Camacho C, Coulouris G, Avagyan V, Ma N, Papadopoulos J, Bealer K, Madden TL.** 2009. BLAST+: architecture and applications. *BMC Bioinformatics* **10**:421.

73. **Marchler-Bauer A, Lu S, Anderson JB, Chitsaz F, Derbyshire MK, DeWeese-Scott C, Fong JH, Geer LY, Geer RC, Gonzales NR, Gwadz M, Hurwitz DI, Jackson JD, Ke Z, Lanczycki CJ, Lu F, Marchler GH, Mullokandov M, Omelchenko MV, Robertson CL, Song JS, Thanki N, Yamashita RA, Zhang D, Zhang N, Zheng C, Bryant SH.** 2011. CDD: a Conserved Domain Database for the functional annotation of proteins. *Nucleic Acids Res* **39**(Database):D225–D229.

74. **Riley PA.** 2004. Bacteriophages in autoimmune disease and other inflammatory conditions. *Med Hypotheses* **62**:493–498.

Index